EMG METHODS FOR EVALUATING MUSCLE AND NERVE FUNCTION

Edited by **Mark Schwartz**

EMG Methods for Evaluating Muscle and Nerve Function
Edited by Mark Schwartz

Published by InTech
Janeza Trdine 9, 51000 Rijeka, Croatia

Publishing Process Manager Danijela Duric

Technical Editor Teodora Smiljanic

Cover Designer InTech Design Team

Additional hard copies can be obtained from orders@intechopen.com

EMG Methods for Evaluating Muscle and Nerve Function, Edited by Mark Schwartz
p. cm.
ISBN 978-953-307-793-2

For EU product safety concerns:
IN TECH d.o.o., Prolaz Marije Krucifikse Kozulić 3, 51000 Rijeka, Croatia,
info@intechopen.com or visit our website at intechopen.com.

Meet the editor

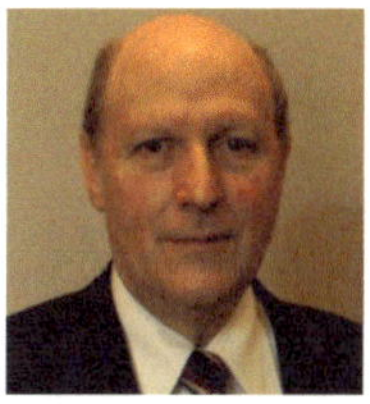

Mark Schwartz has worked in technical education and publishing for over three decades. Starting in the electric utility industry in the 1980s he was responsible for the creation and distribution of videotraining as part of education projects in North America, Africa and Asia. In the 1990s he was in charge of a major software research project in Quebec, Canada in the defense industry involving the creation of simulation software for private industry and universities. For the last 15 years he has worked in the health industry. Currently he is the director of the BFE (Biofeedback Foundation of Europe) Learn from the Best program. In this position he is responsible for over 70 international research and education project teams that create software and courseware on specific topics in neurofeedback, surface electromyography and biofeedback. He also provides consulting services to Thought Technology Ltd. and is on the board of directors of several companies.

Contents

Preface

This is the first of two books on Electromyography (EMG), and it focuses on basic principles of using and analyzing EMG signals. The second book addresses the application of EMG in clinical medicine.

In this first book, there are 6 sections. The first section on principles and methods contains five chapters that cover a wide range of principles and methods, starting with a critical review by Fee discussing proposed improvements for the assessment of muscle interactions using surface EMG. The purpose of this chapter is to propose a mathematical relationship between EMG excitation recorded from muscles in opposition to, or in coordination with each other. The chapter by Nishihara describes the location of electrodes in surface EMG, including the method and sources of variation based on distance from the innervation zone. Kuriki describes the relationship between electromyography and force. This is followed by a chapter by Partanan on EMG in myofascial syndrome. The final chapter, entitled "Clinical implications of muscle- tendon and- force interplay: surface electromyography recordings of *m. vastus lateralis* in renal failure patients undergoing dialysis and of *m. gastrocnemius* in individuals with Achilles tendon damage", was contributed by Dr Harrison.

The second section addresses issues of signal processing and has five chapters, starting with one by Takada. Chapter One is titled "Nonlinear Analysis for Evaluation of Age-Related Muscle Performance by Using Surface Electromyography", which concludes that age-related reductions in muscular function can be detected using an algorithm developed for the nonlinear analysis of surface electromyography signals. The authors examined the *femoral rectus* muscles of the dominant leg, using several measurement parameters, and evaluated changes in these parameters with age. The second chapter in this section is by Phinyomark and covers the usefulness of wavelet transform to reduce noise in the SEMG signal. The third chapter by Sung covers nonlinear analysis of SEMG. The purpose of this chapter is to explore the potential use of nonlinear time series analysis as a tool for the clinical diagnosis of low back pain or neuromuscular dysfunction, especially low back muscle fatigue. Of particular interest is a comparison between methods based on the power spectrum and nonlinear time series analysis of EMG signals. A chapter by Al-Mulla and colleagues then describes the development of a wearable automated muscle fatigue detection system, based on a classification algorithm developed to identify different fatigue states in SEMG signals collected from the *biceps brachii* muscles. In the final chapter in this section, Daikuya and colleagues discuss the importance of the "silent period" of the EMG signal for the evaluation of neuro-muscular function in the field of the sports medicine and rehabilitation. The silent period is the duration of the inhibitory period of muscle contraction detected on surface electromyography, which is due to electrical stimulation at the innervating nerve during tonic muscle contraction.

Section three moves into the area of diagnostics, beginning with a chapter by Turker and colleagues that reviews middle and long latency auditory evoked potentials and their diagnostic application in fibromyalgia and schizophrenia. Recording procedures and appropriate statistical methods for middle latency auditory evoked potentials (MLAEPs) and long latency auditory evoked potentials (LLAEPs) are described. The authors place their findings in the context of the current literature and conclude that "central mechanisms may be important in the evolution of fibromyalgia. CNS dysfunction may be both an etiological factor in the fibromyalgia syndrome and a pathophysiological mechanism explaining the clinical symptoms and signs." In the second chapter of this section, Disselhorst-Klug covers non-invasive diagnosis of neuromuscular disorders by high-spatial-resolution-EMG (HSR-EMG), which is capable of detecting single motor unit activity in a non-invasive way. The chapter provides a clear introduction to the relationship between neuromuscular disorders and changes in the structure of single motor units (MUs) and identifies reasons why conventional SEMG has a limited spatial resolution and is unable to separate the activity of single MUs from simultaneously active adjacent ones. The result is that SEMG is mainly useful for obtaining "global" information about muscle activation, like time or net-intensity of muscle activation within a recording field. The author reviews the evaluation of pathological changes in the HSR-EMG by introducing three sets of parameters that allow a quantitative evaluation of the changes in the pattern typical for each disorder. In the third chapter, Papez and colleagues present "EMG vs. Thermography in severe carpal tunnel syndrome diagnosis of entrapment neuropathy". The authors' conclusions provide a comparison of the use of thermography for CTS with EMG. In the final chapter of the section on diagnostics, Naito writes about the functional significance of facilitation between agonist and antagonist muscles in humans, using the *pronator teres* and *extensor carpi radialis* muscles as examples.

The fourth section provides a useful introduction to the use of evoked potentials and surface electromyography. The authors show how these combined measures can help to evaluate and diagnose disorders of the muscles and motor neurons. There are four interesting chapters that give good examples of the use of electromyography (EMG) in combination with electrical neuromuscular stimulation (ENS) to clarify the integrity of neuromuscular function and neural pathways. This area could be of significant interest to readers from multiple disciplines. The first chapter in this section is a general review by Zaher. It is followed by a chapter by Yamada describing methods for the extraction and analysis of the single motor unit F-weave from median nervemonopolar multichannel surface EMG signals. By increasing the volume of data measured under different stimulus conditions, many single MU F-waves could be extracted, and the properties of F-waves and MUs could be analyzed successfully. The third chapter is by Chung and Grigorian, who describe the use of free run EMG and stimulated (evoked) potentials in the operating room for patient monitoring. The chapter provides a clear introduction to the use of EMG as a clinical electrodiagnostic tool, including an overview of EMG recording techniques in the operating room (OR), and discussion of the recording electrodes, EMG signal recording parameters, and a table showing muscle group selections and electrode placement. The authors explain the procedures used for monitoring EMG and Evoked Potentials for the neuromuscular junction (NMJ) including the interpretation of the signal and the use of audio over visual display for the surgeon for immediate feedback. The stimulated EMG section of the chapter provides the reader with details on monitoring segmental motor nerve root function, and an evaluation of the use of lumbosacral, cervical and thoracic pedicle screws. There is a brief introduction to somatosensory evoked potentials (SSEPs), motor evoked potentials (MEPs), dermatomal somatosensory evoked potentials (DSSEPs), and the recording techniques appropriate for each type of evoked potential. The authors list additional safety concerns for MEPs. The assessment of spinal nerve roots with SSEPs and MEPs is reviewed with the relative benefits of each technique summarized with reference to current literature. A final section on anesthesia is followed by the conclusion and suggestion that the simultaneous use of evoked potential and EMG recording can improve specificity and clinical efficacy of EMG during cervical and thoracic spinal procedures. The fourth and final chapter in this section is contributed by Farzan and colleagues. It covers both the use of EMG and MEPs for assessing neurological pathways in experiments using Transcranial magnetic stimulation (TMS) and the extension of these methods in combination with concurrent electroencephalography (TMS-EMG-EEG) to evaluate cortico-cortical connectivity between different areas of the motor cortex, such as the left and right motor cortices in the study of functional asymmetry. The authors discuss their innovative work using these methods to study cortical inhibition and modulation in non-motor areas in different disease states, such as schizophrenia and depression.

The fifth section of this first volume covers the use of EMG in combination with other technologies. The first chapter in this section is by Cao and deals with Muscle Force Analysis of the human foot, based on wearable sensors and EMG. Forces were estimated through inverse dynamics methods in the "AnyBody Modeling System", a wearable sensor system that was developed to measure rotational angles and centers of pressure (COP) in combination with EMG. The third chapter in this section, by Guerra, describes effective processing of familiar faces. The authors describe emotional processing research, with special emphasis on the contribution of EMG recordings, which has consistently shown that highly pleasant pictures are associated with (a) a pattern of accelerative changes in heart rate, (b) reduced eye-blink startle responses, (c) increases in zygomatic muscle activity, and (d) decreases in *corrugator supercilii* muscle activity. The inverse pattern is observed with highly arousing unpleasant pictures. The fourth chapter in this section is by Terzi, and covers the non invasive monitoring of the interaction between breathing and swallowing using EMG and other additional methods for capturing respiratory events.

The sixth and final section discusses new frontiers in research and technology, beginning with a chapter by Wehner that reviews man to machine applications in electromyography. Wehner describes how EMG is a detailed art, and can easily lead to erroneous conclusions if not practiced carefully. With new applications, particularly where EMG is employed as a means for humans to control electromechanical systems, care must be taken to ensure that these systems are developed with robust safety systems, and improper assumptions about EMG do not cause harm, injury, or even death. The second chapter by Panek describes water surface electromyography. In this chapter, significant attention is paid to the methodology and the issue of correct placement and fixing of electrodes in all neuro-physiological methods. In general, the approach to recording an EMG signal in a water environment is no different from the common methodology of surface EMG, but there are certain specifics that are important. Currently, great attention is paid in the literature to the issue of the different effects of water and dry environments on the nature of the EMG recording itself. The third chapter by Navallas is on scanning electromyography. The main objective of scanning EMG is to record the electrical activity of a motor unit from different locations along a scanning corridor as the needle electrode passes through the motor unit territory. A very important aspect is that, although a single recording is made at each location, all recordings must be synchronized in relation to the firing of the motor unit, equivalent to simultaneously recording from all the sites. The fourth chapter is by Okkesim and covers EMG measures in people undergoing orthodontic treatment. EMG signals were used to measure and evaluate changes in jaw muscles (*anterior temporalis* and *masseter*), in children with Class II malocclusion who received Twin-Block appliances. Power spectral density (PSD) methods were used to evaluate changes in muscle activity following 6 months of treatment. Finally, Fiorucci discusses new measurement techniques for surface EMG signals of resting eye position in the ophthalmological field. The author reviews the importance of signal detection during rest, and challenges inherent in filtering noise from the signal without removing the signal of interest. The authors describe a new type of measurement equipment and various precautions taken during signal processing. The authors conclude with import discussions about the potential of SEMG to be used as a tool to evaluate the effects of the graduation of eyeglasses and contact lenses on the eye muscles. The study provides an interesting conclusion to this first volume and provides a bridge to the second volume on clinical applications of electromyography.

Mark Schwartz, Director
Learn From the Best Program
Biofeedback Foundation of Europe

Part 1

Principles & Methods

1

A Critical Review and Proposed Improvement in the Assessment of Muscle Interactions Using Surface EMG

James W. Fee, Jr. and Freeman Miller
Alfred I. DuPont Hospital for Children
USA

1. Introduction

The purpose of this chapter is to propose a mathematical relationship between EMG excitation recorded from muscles in opposition to, or in coordination with each other. The concept of correlating co-activation between muscles with EMG parameters is not new. Cowan et al. (1998) investigated the use of the Pearson Product-Moment correlation coefficient to quantify muscle co-activation using electromyography. They concluded that this method shows promise for describing side differences in diplegics and for assessing the effects of physical therapy and other interventions. Careful reading of this work shows that only "select" intervals of the EMG data were compared. These intervals were selected on the basis of "burst activity" of one muscle. This selection is done by hand and for large quantities of data, typical of a gait laboratory, would be labor intensive. In our laboratory the authors have found the Pearson Product-Moment unable to distinguish between two noisy signals from inactive muscles and two that are fully active. Using insights from the literature review, presented below, this chapter will propose an alternative, continuous function for describing muscle interaction over any and all portions of a gait cycle.

2. Background

The history of the development of EMG's as an assessment tool follows closely the development of mathematics over the last century and a half. In an extensive review, Reaz et al.(2006) traces this history from Francesco Redi's documentation of electrical activity in a muscle in 1666, to its present use as a controlling mechanism for modern human computer interaction. Most of the mathematical analysis applied to EMG signals concerns itself with the relationship between various parameters of the signal and the forces generated in the muscle.
In its simplest form, an isometric contraction results in electrical activity in the muscle. De Luca (1997) states that while a simple equation describing this relationship would be extremely useful, such a simple relationship does not exist. In spite of this, numerous researchers have applied a countless variety of methods to the extraction of force from EMG signals.
Christensen et. al. (1986) compared the number of zero crossings with force production and found a linear relationship up to 50% of a maximum voluntary contraction. At low levels of maximum contraction the number of spikes was found to increase with increasing force

(Haas, 1926). At higher force levels, the mean rectified value of the signal was found to exhibit linearity with force (Fuglsang-Frederiksen, 1981). Other investigators turned to the frequency domain and demonstrated an inverse relationship between force and frequency (Ronager et al, 1989). At the same time it has been shown that mean power frequency increases with increasing force (Li & Sakamoto, 1996). A study in 1999 showed that the median frequency increases with force up to a point equal to 50% of the maximum contraction (Bernardi M, et al. 1999). In a review article on surface EMG and muscle force, Disselhorst-Klug, et al. (2009) conclude that muscle force can be estimated from EMG signals in geometrically well-defined situations during isometric contractions.

When limb motion and coordination are involved the relationship between (dynamic) EMG and force takes on greater dimensions of complexity. There are three basic types of data utilization involved in the study of dynamic EMG. Most common is the interest in the presence or absence of the particular muscle's activity during a portion of some movement, for example a gait cycle. A second interest is in the envelope shape of the EMG waveform over an entire movement. Lastly, there is the interest in relating the force generated by a muscle to itself (at some other part of the movement) or to some other muscle (Rechtien, et al. 1999). In order for the EMG representation of forces to be related to one another, each must be normalized to some standard value.

Burden (2002) gives an extensive review of research, performed over the last two and a half decades, on normalization methods. The author identifies eight methods of normalization. Of these eight, two are of the most interest: first, a method whereby an EMG signal is divided by the maximum of itself (Peak Task, PT), and a second (Mean Task, MT) whereby an EMG signal is divided by the mean of itself. The author reports that, with respect to other more complex methods, both the PT and the MT methods reduced inter-individual variability, and improves the sensitivity of surface electromyography as a diagnostic gait analysis tool. The use of these methods also increases the effect size and hence the power of statistical comparisons between groups in relation to the output from other methods. The drawbacks of these methods are, first in the case of PT, the selected maxima could easily be an artifact in the recording of the signal. In the second method, normalizing to the mean of the signal could easily result in the existence of normalized EMG points in excess of 100%. If these points are attenuated to 1.00 as is often the case, the normalized task EMGs may not reveal the proportion of an individual's muscle activation capacity required to perform a specific task.

To compare EMG patterns between muscles groups, it is necessary to use a time-normalization technique so that a point-by-point comparison of EMG activity is possible. Carollo JJ & Matthews (2002) suggest that this can be done by breaking the EMG pattern up into individual stride cycles, which are considered the period between successive heel-strikes in the same leg. The individual EMG stride patterns are then time normalized, expressed as a percentage of total cycle. In a review paper on muscle coordination, (Hug, 2011) finds fault with this method because of the variability of the point of toe-off (between 58 and 63% of the gait cycle). To correct this, Sadeghi et al. (2000) and Decker et al. (2007) use "curve registration" or "Procrustes analysis" methods, respectively. Curve registration relies on finding the peak points in the joint power curves and aligning gait cycles accordingly. The Procrustes method describes curve shape and shape change in a mathematical and statistical framework, independent of time and size factors. Thus the method normalizes both time and stride magnitude at the same time.

Hodges & Bui (1996) state that, in order to allow comparisons between muscles, experimental conditions and subjects or subject groups, accuracy of onset determination is crucial. Onset is most often recognized as the point where the EMG values cross and remain above a pre-chosen threshold value. The choice of this threshold value varies among researchers. Some place it at two standard deviations above the noise level (Micera et al. 1998). Lidierth (1986) added to this method by specifying that the threshold value be exceeded, and remain so, for a specific time constant. Others use a percentage of the peak EMG, and report that this percentage varies from 15 to 25% of the maximum signal (Staude, 2001). More sophisticated methods evaluate statistical properties of the measured EMG signal before and after a possible change in excitation level (Staude & Wolf, 1999).

De Luca (1997) suggests that, at least in the case of the threshold method, off time be found as the opposite of on time, that is when the amplitude falls below the same percentage of maximal contraction. He further suggests that when comparing on and off times of two muscles, that a 10ms window of error is the best that can be expected.

Having extracted a measure of force from the EMG signal by whatever means, and knowing when a muscle is active or inactive, attention turns toward the comparison of activity in two or more groups of muscles. The most elementary technique for the examination of two coordinating muscles groups is the visual inspection of the raw EMG signal together with appropriate graphics of the joint angles. Conclusions drawn from such observations are subjective at best, thus a more quantitative method is needed (Kleissen et al. 1998).

De Luca (1997) defines two parameters that are commonly used to represent the EMG signal: the average rectified value and the root mean square value:

$$\text{RMS} = 1/n\sum x^2(i)$$

Here x is a sample point with the sum taken over sample size n.

For comparison purposes Fukuda et al.(2010) state that the RMS value is prefered because it is a parameter that better reflects the levels of muscle activity at rest and during contraction, and for this reason, it is one of the most widely used in scientific studies. A slightly more complex method of analysis was reviewed by Fuglsang-Frederiksen (2000). When comparing the activation of different muscles, he found that the turns/amplitude analysis method was more useful than other methods. Turns analysis consists of counting the number of positive and negative potential changes exceeding 100υv ("turns") and their amplitudes. The turns ratio is computed by dividing the mean amplitude (of the turns) by the number of turns. The method was used by Garcia et al.(1980) as a quantitative assessment of the degree of involvement of antagonist muscles.

In a variation on the turns counting method, Jeleń & Sławińska (1996) compared the activation of two muscles using a spike counting method. This method counts the number of times the EMG signal crosses a "noise level" threshold. These authors showed that this count is in good agreement with muscle activity.

Area under the EMG curve has been used successfully to compare co-contraction. In a unique normalization scheme, reported by Poon & Hui-Chan (2009), EMG co-contraction ratios were calculated as ratios of the antagonist EMG area to the total agonist-plus-antagonist EMG areas. The authors claim this technique allowed the comparison of data obtained on different days for within- or between-subjects.

Work presented in the next section will demonstrate that the method to be outlined in this chapter is quite similar to Poon's (Poon & Hui-Chan, 2009). However a simple mathematical construct reveals that the author's ratio is not unique:

$$A / (A + a) = B / (B + b)$$

$$\text{Let: } B = 2 * A \quad \text{and } b = 2 * a$$

If "A" in the above equation is antagonist EMG area and "a" is agonist area, it is possible to conceive of another muscle group such that antagonist area "B" is twice that of "A" and agonist muscle "b" is twice the area of "a". The calculation for both muscles groups will produce the same co-contraction ratio, however a clinician, observing the muscle group's behavior, would find the two levels of co-contraction to be quite different. The authors of this chapter will assert that it is not possible to represent the co-activation of two muscles by a single parameter. One must consider the activation of both relative to the normalized value and the ratio of each to the other.

The next level of sophistication in the analysis of EMG data is the examination of the frequency content of the signal. Several parameters are obtained from the power spectrum (the Fourier transformation of the EMG signal). The mean frequency is defined as the mathematical mean of the spectrum curve, the total power is the integral under the spectrum curve, and the median frequency is defined as the parameter that divides the total power area into two equal parts. Finally the peak power is the maximum value of the total power spectrum curve.

The most commonly used parameter in the frequency domain is the median frequency. Hermens et al.(1992) report that this parameter deviates from its normal value in a number of neuromuscular disorders, therefore the parameter is often used in clinical settings. In a comparative study this parameter, like the turns ratio and the spike count, would be calculated for each muscle group and then compared using a statistic such as the ANOVA or a paired t-test (Lam, 2005). A slight variation on this is the mean power frequency which is found by dividing the summed product of the frequency and power by the summed power. Feltham et al. (2010) used this parameter to demonstrate differences in co-contraction levels between the right and left sides in children with spastic hemiparetic cerebral palsy and both arms of typically developing children. In the case of the other two variables peak power has been shown to be related to muscle fiber conduction velocity and total power to muscle force (Li & Sakamoto, 1996; Farina et al. 2004).

Among the newest methods of EMG analysis are those involving wavelet analysis, which examines both the frequency and time domain combined. A wavelet transform is a Fourier transform performed on a particular section of an EMG signal. Further, the time width (or window) of the “section” can be dependent on the frequency content of that section. That is, the window is narrowed for high frequencies and widened for low frequencies. Karlsson et al.(2009) define this as a mathematical microscope in which different parts of the signal can be observed by adjusting the focus. When testing children with cerebral palsy, Prosser et al.(2010) point out that wavelet analysis eliminates the need for amplitude normalizations. This is beneficial because many of these subjects cannot make a maximal contraction.

In a paper presented at the IEEE conference on Engineering in Medicine and Biology Dantas, et al.(2010) compared Fourier analysis with wavelet transform analysis. They point out that Fourier analysis assumes signal stationarity, which is unlikely during dynamic contractions. Wavelet based methods of signal analysis do not assume stationarity and may be more appropriate for joint time-frequency domain analysis.

The nature of the Fourier analysis is that it transforms the signal into a series of sine-cosine functions and is therefore especially well adapted for analyzing periodic signals. Herein lies its major drawback, EMG signals are not only non-stationary, but non-periodic, “fractal” and seemingly chaotic. Borg (2000) points out, that instead of decomposing and

reconstructing a signal in terms of the sines and cosines functions, wavelet analysis allows the use of an array of waveforms such as: saw tooth functions, rectangle waves (Walsh functions), or finite time pulses. In a paper published last year, Bentelas (2010) demonstrated how the Continuous Wavelet Transform (CWT) is mathematically similar to surface EMG signals with noise and is therefore the favorite candidate for analyzing these signals.
The wavelet transform method has been applied with increasing success. In a paper on the ergonomics of driving, Moshou et al. (2000) clearly demonstrate the ability to remove noise from the EMG signal. As a result, small coordinated muscle activity of the shoulder can be observed, that would otherwise have been hidden in the noise. The use of this method to investigate dynamic muscle dysfunction in children with cerebral palsy has lead to clear distinctions between this population and the normally developing group (Wakeling et al. 2007). Lauer et al. (2007) expanded on this and were able to show differences in levels of co-contraction between the less and more involved side.

3. Methodology

With the above review in mind, the authors propose a method of comparing two EMG signals. While most of the illustrations presented will be of raw or stylized raw EMG data, the method will be demonstrated to work equally as well on filtered, enveloped data. The method begins with a full wave rectification of surface EMGs recorded as gait data. The gait data presented here will be from multiple walks; each walk will have been cut into cycles beginning and ending either at toe-off or heel-strike and then pieced together end to end (i.e. toe-off to toe-off or heel-strike to heel-strike). For simplified illustrative purposes only one cycle will be presented, however all mean values will have been calculated over the entire ensemble.
The method of normalization is a combination of both the "Peak Task" and "Mean Task" methods of (Burden, 2002). Figure 1, below, is an illustration of the method. For illustrative purposes a stylized EMG signal is presented. The signal consists of two sine waves, of different

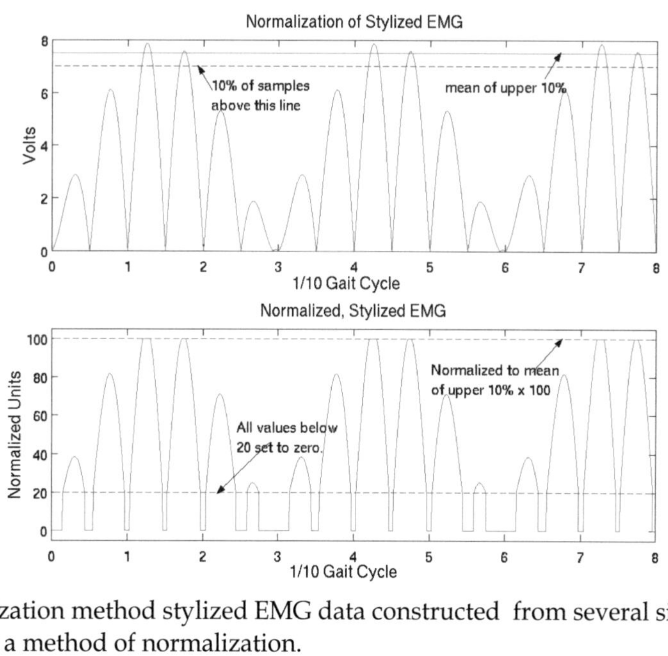

Fig. 1. Normalization method stylized EMG data constructed from several sin waves is used to demonstrate a method of normalization.

amplitude and frequency summed together. The timing of half a "wave" will be considered one tenth of a gait cycle. For the normalization process, a set of points are found such that they are the upper 1/10 of all samples in the particular gait cycles of interest. The mean of these samples (in the illustrative case 80 points are found to have a mean of 7.8 volts) is taken as the normalizing value. All points in the ensemble are then divided by this mean. The result of this division will be a signal with several points that have a value higher than unity. These will be considered artifacts and set to the value one. The signal is then multiplied by 100. After this multiplication, all values below 20 are considered to be noise and are set to zero.

The comparison of two muscle excitations requires the defining of two parameters. The first of these parameters will be called the "Excitation Index". If it can be imagined for a moment that, for a tenth of a gait cycle, the EMG were at maximum potential, the signal over that time period would be a full ten volts. The normalized value would be 100 over the entire time period (tp). The integration of this full excitation would equal the area of a rectangle (100 x tp). When two signals are involved, both maximally on for the same time period (tp), the total possible area under both signals is (200 x tp). This will be considered the "standard" Excitation. The excitation index will be defined as the sum of the integration of the two EMG signals over a tenth of a gait cycle divided by that tenth's "standard". It should be noted here, that tp is not a constant and is likely to vary over each gait cycle, as a result a "Standard Excitation" must be calculated for each tenth cycle.

The second parameter to be defined will be called the co-activation ratio. This ratio will be defined simply as the smaller of the two integrated EMG signals divided by the larger. The result will always be a number between zero and one. An illustration of the calculation of the two parameters is presented in figure 2. In this case the second EMG signal is

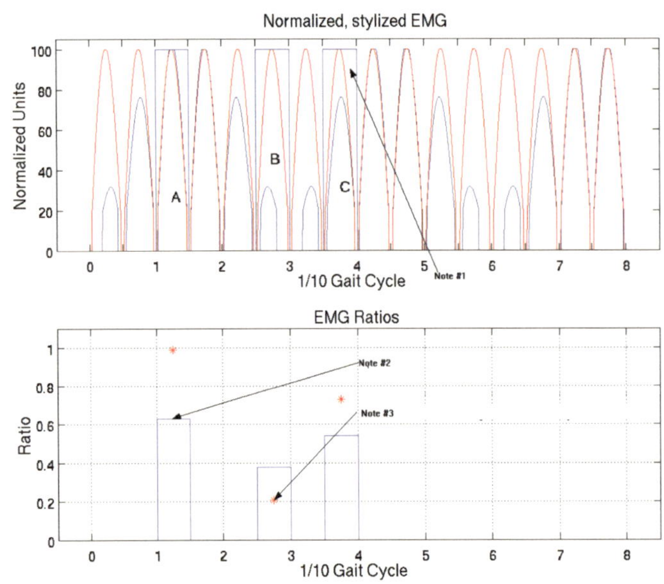

Note:
#1 Area under the rectangle equals the total area of a 1/10 gait cycle. Twice this area is the maximum integral of the combined EMG signals (The Standard Excitation (SE)).
#2 Bar Height = The ratio of the sum of the integral of both EMG signals / SE.
#3 Point Value = Ratio of the two "stylized" EMG signals in "B" above.

Fig. 2. Stylized assessment method

represented as a full wave rectified sine wave whose frequency was set to the combined frequency of the first. In the case of the A'th tenth cycle both EMG signals are almost the same, however the area of a sin wave is not equal to a square wave. The height of the bars of the graph in the lower half of the figure represents this difference in area. In the case of "A" the area under the two stylized EMG signals is 0.6 of 60% of the "Standard Excitation". The red dot represents the ratio of the two signals, slightly less than one because the two areas are almost equal. The B'th and C'th tenths can be similarly interpreted. The assessment system can be applied to the co-activation of two antagonistic muscles (better known as co-contraction) as shown in figure 3. This figure delineates the differences between co-contraction in a normally developing limb and one with hemiplegia. Clearly, in this gait cycle, there is almost no co-contraction evidenced in the normally developing subject. This is not the case in the subject with hemiplegia. A quick review of the profiles reveals that, while the highest co-contraction occurs in the eight tenth of the gait cycle, the total excitation of both muscles is less than 10% of maximum. From the mean values it can be seen that, while the excitation index is just below 9%, the co-activation ratio is just below 17% (the rounded off value). With these values presented, it is left to the clinician to decide if this co-activation is significant.

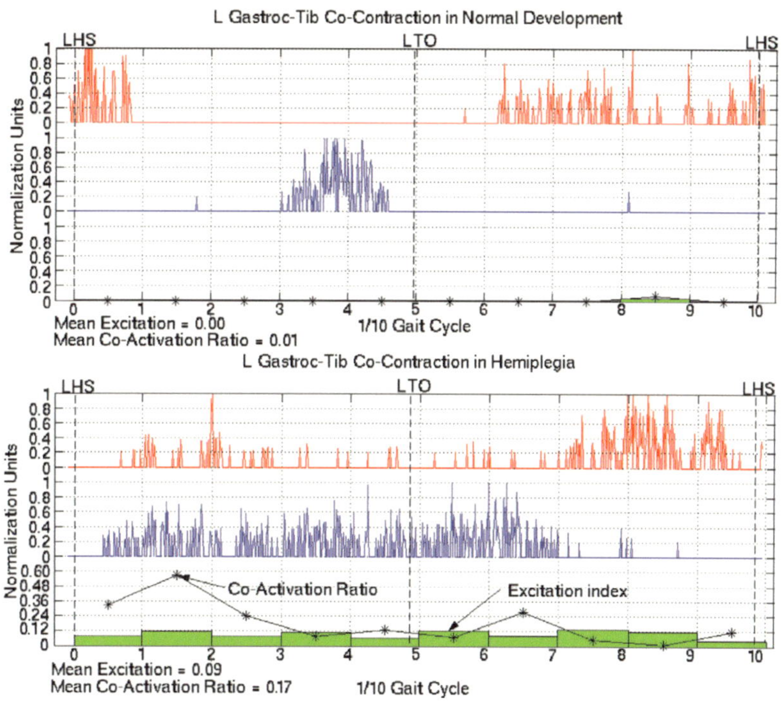

Note: Means are calculated over 14 cycles (140 points).

Fig. 3. Assessment of a Co-Contracting Muscle- This figure illustrates a clear difference between hemiplegia and normally developing gait cycles on a 1/10 cycle by cycle basis.

Turning to the original motivation for this work, Figure 4 demonstrates the use of the assessment method to explore excitation in contralateral muscles. Our hypothesis states that if "mirrored excitation" exists, it is most likely to be seen at mid-stance/mid-swing, where the muscles of the "swinging" limb should be inactive and the supporting limb's muscles should be most active. While it is not the intent of this chapter to prove or disprove our

working hypothesis, some results will be presented in order to demonstrate the efficacy and efficiency of the method of assessment outlined and advocated.
With regard to mirrored excitation, it is expected, that the excited muscle will be mirrored onto the inactive muscle. In the example below, for the normally developing subject, it can be seen that the co-activation ratio for this gait cycle is highest at mid-stance of both limbs. This is actually an atypical gait cycle, chosen so the numbers would be large enough to be seen on the graph. The mean values were in fact 0.07 on the left and 0.04 on the right. An examination of the means of these values over the 10 cycles, in the subject with hemiplegia, reveals a mean excitation index on the left of 0.14 (slightly higher than the value of the complete gait cycle) and a mean ratio of 0.44 (almost twice the value for the complete cycle). While the values at mid-stance on the right are 0.08 and 0.62 respectively. From this, one would conclude that there is an influence at left mid-stance, but without the greater excitation index at right mid-stance, information from other muscles would be needed to draw any conclusions.

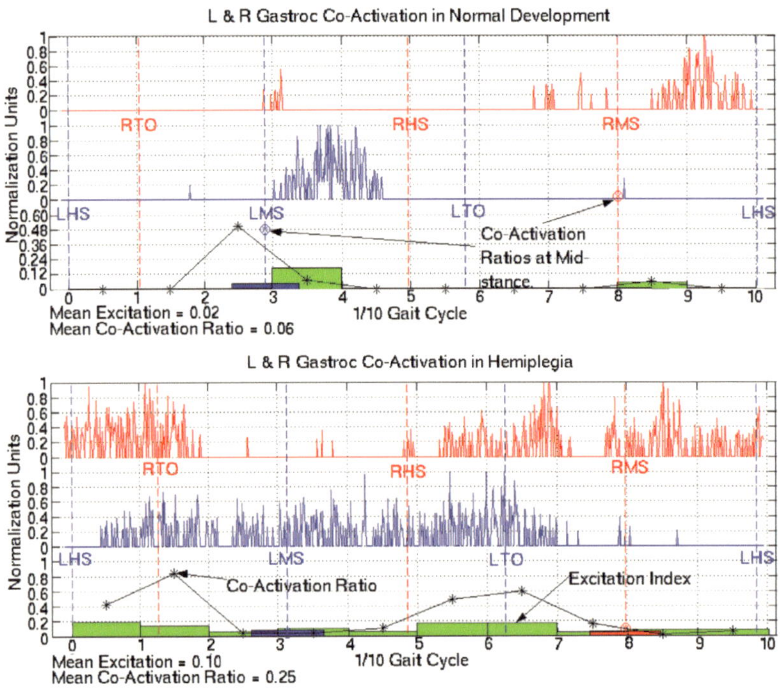

Note: Mid-stance (L & R MS) values are calculated from data taken between 1/20th cycle on either side of the mid-stance point.

Fig. 4. Left and right side co-activation.

The previous two graphics presented EMG data in raw, rectified, normalized form, with the assessment analysis being performed on this raw data. This is simply the authors' preference and should not be interpreted as the only way the analysis can be done. The next graphic, Figure 5, presents a comparison of the analysis performed on both raw and filtered data. To be noted here is the fact that both profiles, that of the excitation index and the co-activation ratio appear very much alike. The mean excitation index is slightly less (0.06 vs. 0.10) while the mean co-activation ratio is slightly greater (0.37 vs. 0.25). Each of these differences makes sense when considering what filtering does. By lowering the peak values of the EMG data, the excitation index has a smaller numerator and thus a smaller value for each 1/10 cycle. At the same time that peaks are made lower the data is spread over a larger region of time, this causes the regions with the higher peaks to take up greater area. Since the co-activation ratio is calculated by dividing the smaller number by the larger, an increase in the smaller number (in this case) is reflected by a larger ratio.

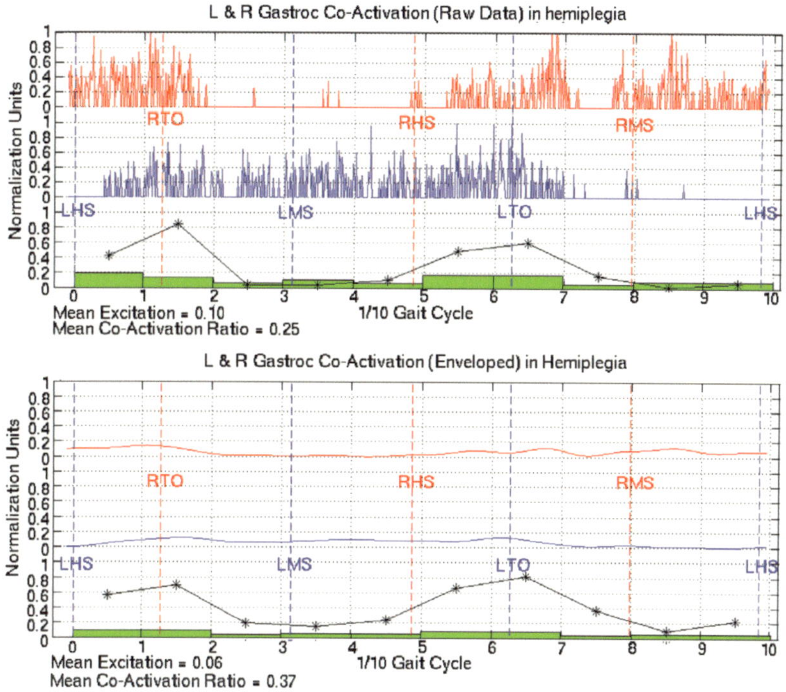

Fig. 5. Raw and filtered EMG and their resulting parameters.

The presentation of this data in a meaningful way so that different muscle groups among different subjects can be compared, is not a trivial matter. A method for plotting twenty points per muscle per gait cycle for several muscles of interest must not overwhelm the reader with data while at the same time allow a readily recognizable comparison of pertinent information. In the case of the authors, the interest is in comparing contralateral co-activation with co-contraction in both limbs. At the least this involves three muscle groups, adding to this is the desire to compare these muscle groups at particular points in each gait cycle (mid-stance) thus adding an additional two comparison groups to the representation task.

The method to be suggested here will utilize two distinct graphing methods; in the first, line graphs will present the excitation index and co-activation ratios in their pure calculated form. In the second, bar charts will compare normalized values of the excitation indices. It is felt that both are of value and both have a valid place. The bar charts provide an immediate means of comparing muscle groups within the same subject. Line graphs provide a means of comparing data across subject.

To construct the graphs, the authors calculate a mean value of each parameter over the ensemble of gait cycles recorded for each subject. From each ensemble of muscle groups to be compared, the maximum muscle excitation index is chosen and all other excitation indices are normalized on this value. Each normalized value now represents the comparative excitation of each muscle group. Since the co-activation ratio represents the comparison of activation between the two muscles of a given group, multiplying the normalized excitation index by this ratio, preserves its comparative property between the groups. The process lends itself well to a graphical representation by means of a stacked column graph. Figure 6 presents a comparison of Gastrocnemius-Anterior Tibialis interaction in seven subjects with hemiplegic cerebral palsy. The data presented represent a number of interesting interactions between the groups. In the third, fourth and sixth subject, co-contraction is the dominant muscle activity. In the other 4, the dominant activity is the co-activation between the right and left sides. In two of the subjects (#1 and #7) this dominance is seen across the entire gait cycle, in the remaining two the dominance occurs only at the points of mid-stance. While the method of presenting the normalization of means clearly has its value in the intragroup comparison for a single subject, it can give misleading results when comparisons are made across subjects. To address the issue, data is presented as it was before normalization. These two added sets of data insures that a very strong excitation, when normalized to unity, is not seen as comparable to a weak excitation that might happen to the maximum value for another subject.

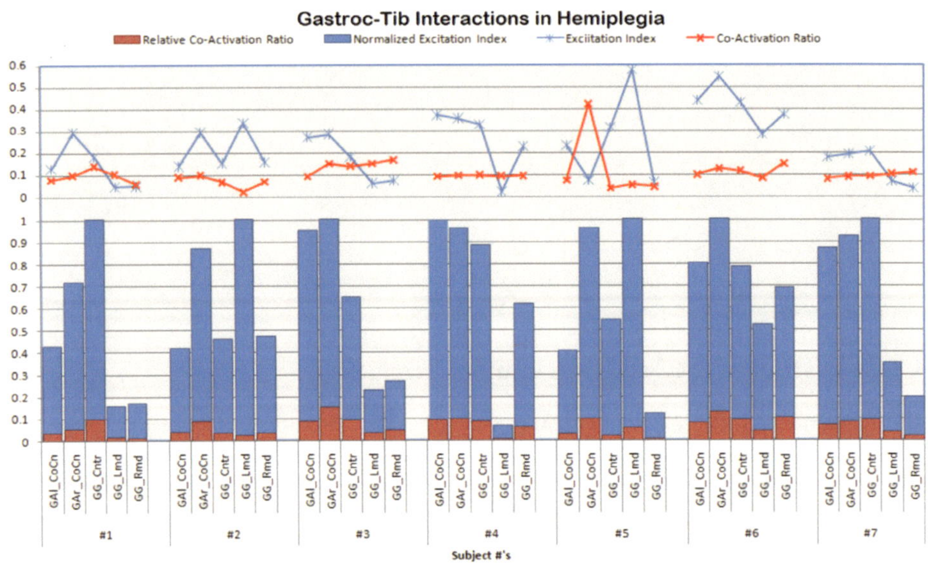

Legend: GAl = Gastroc-Tib left, GAr = Gastroc-Tib right, CoCn = Co-contraction, Cntr = contralateral co-activation (measured over the complete cycle), GG = Gastroc-Gastroc, Rmd = Right Mid-Stance, Lmd = Left Mid-Stance
Bar charts are normalized data, line graphs are actual values.

Fig. 6. Excitation indices and co-activation ratios for seven subjects

In the example presented in Figure 6, maximum excitation is almost the same for subjects 1, 2, 3, 4, and 7. Comparison of these subjects would be fairly reasonable. Comparison of these with subjects 5 and 6 becomes more problematic because their maximum excitations are clearly more intense.

As a final step Figure 7, below, provides a comparison to data from three normally developing subjects for the same muscle groups. This graph demonstrates the value of both

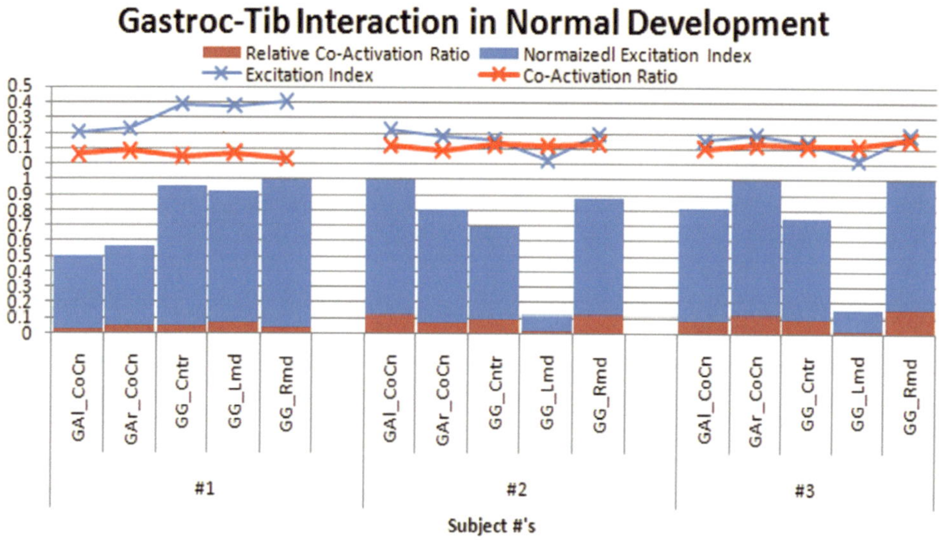

Legend: GAl = Gastroc-Tib left, GAr = Gastroc-Tib right, CoCn = Co-contraction,
Cntr = contralateral co-activation (measured over the complete cycle), GG = Gastroc-Gastroc,
Rmd = Right Mid-Stance, Lmd = Left Mid-Stance
Bar charts are normalized data, line graphs are actual values.

Fig. 7. Normalized mean excitation indices for three normally developing subjects

the bar and line graphics. While the bar graphs suggest that it may not be unusual for co-activation across the body to exist at mid-stance, the line graphs make it clear that it is not a dominant form of excitation. The most obvious difference between the normally developing subjects and those with hemiplegia are the obviously consistent indices and ratios seen in the normal developing subjects. All interaction in this data seem to be at about the same level. The slight elevation in excitation index of contralateral muscle groups of subject #1 may not be indicative of all normal subjects, a larger subject population would be necessary to identify true trends in normal developing subjects.

While the normalization method presented above may provide a good tool for visualization, the set of values calculated from tenths of a gait cycle should easily form the basis of a statistical analysis using a paired t-test or a two-way ANOVA.

4. Conclusion

It has been the purpose of this chapter to present a method whereby the co-activation of two muscles can be compared and presented to the clinician in a meaningful way. It has been shown, with the use of both stylized EMG data, and real data from ongoing experimentation, that the method presented provides two unique numbers which completely define the state of excitation of a muscle group. It has been demonstrated further that this method overcomes the pitfalls of previous attempts. Among its attributes are the method's ability to deal with both active and inactive muscle activity and to easily fit into many standard gait analysis reports.

The method begins with a normalization that combines two previously described methods. This combination of normalization on peak values and mean values of the data set itself

eliminates drawbacks of both methods. Additionally it eliminates the need for a maximal contraction which many of those in the cerebral palsy population cannot perform.
The assessment method provides two numbers, the first, the Excitation Index, measures the activation of both muscles of interest in combination. The second number, the Co-activation Ratio, provides a measure of each muscle's excitation relative to the other. In combination, the two measures completely define the comparative excitation of any two muscles of interest.
The chapter presents several graphical methods of presenting the assessment method so that it can be used to compare a single set of muscles in a gait analysis, or to compare multiple groups of muscles across a sample population.
Although the data analyzed have largely been raw, unfiltered EMG data, the method can be applied equally as well to filtered "enveloped" data. In the case of one such analysis presented, while the mean values were somewhat different for filtered data, the overall profiles of both the excitation indices and the co-activation ratios remain consistent over the gait cycle presented.
Finally the chapter has demonstrated that the method can be applied to ongoing research in the author's laboratory. The authors believe that this demonstrates the value of the method in a real application.

5. References

Bentales Y (2010) An Algorithm of Wavelets for the Pretreatment of EMG Biomedical Signals. Contemporary Engineering Sciences, Vol. 3, No. 6, (2010) pp. 285 - 294, ISSN 1313-6569.

Bernardi M, Felici F, Marchetti M, Montellanico F, Piacentini MF, & Solomonow M. (1999) Force generation performance and motor unit recruitment strategy in muscles of contralateral limbs. *J Electromyogr Kinesiol* Vol. 9, (1999) pp. 121–30, ISSN: 1050-6411.

Borg F. (2000) EMG and Wavelet Analysis – Part I. Technical Report HUR – FB 07/16/00. 1. HUR Ltd.

Burden A. (2002) How should we normalize electromyograms obtained from healthy participants? What we have learned from over 25 years of research. *Journal of Electromyogr Kinesiol.* Vol. 20, (2010) pp. 1023–1035, ISSN: 1050-6411.

Carollo JJ & Matthews D. (2002) Strategies for clinical motion analysis based on functional decomposition of the gait cycle, *Phys. Med. Rehabil. Clin. N. Am.*, Vol. 13 (2002) pp. 949–977, ISSN:1047-9651.

Christensen H & Fuglsang-Frederiksen A. (1986) Power spectrum and turns analysis of EMG at different voluntary efforts in normal subjects. *Electroencephalogr Clin Neurophysiol* Vol. 64, No. 8, (Aug., 1986), pp. 528–35, ISSN: 0018-9294.

Cowan MM, Stilling DS, Naumann S & Colborne GR. (1998) Quantification of antagonist muscle coactivation in children with spastic diplegia. *Clin. Anat.* Vol. 11 No. 5. (May, 1998), pp. 314-9, ISSN: 0897-3806.

Dantas JL, Camata TV, Brunetto MA, Moraes AC, AbrÃ£o T, & Altimari LR. (2010) Fourier and wavelet spectral analysis of EMG signals in isometric and dynamic maximal effort exercise. Proceedings of the IEEE Eng Med Biol Soc. 2010:5979-82, (2010), ISBN: 978-1-4244-4123-5

Decker L, Berge C, Renous S, & Penin X. (2007) An alternative approach to normalization and evaluation for gait patterns: Procrustes analysis applied to the cyclograms of sprinters and middle-distance runners. *J Biomech,* Vol. 40, No. 9 (Sept., 2007) pp. 2078-87, ISSN: 0021-9290.

De Luca CJ. (1997) The use of surface electromyography in biomechanics. *Journal of Applied Biomechanics,* Vol. 13, No. 2, (May, 2006), pp. 135-163, ISSN: 1065-8483.

Disselhorst-Klug C, Schmitz-Rode T, & Rau G. (2009) Surface electromyography and muscle force: limits in sEMG-force relationship and new approaches for applications. *Clin Biomech (Bristol, Avon),* Vol. 24, No. 3 (Mar., 2009) pp. 225-35, ISSN: 0268-0033.

Farina D, Merletti R, & Enoka RM (2004) The extraction of neural strategies from the surface EMG. J Appl Physiol Vol. 96 (2004) pp. 1486-1495, ISSN: 8750-7587

Feltham MG, Ledebt A, Deconinck FJ, & Savelsbergh GJ (2010) Assessment of neuromuscular activation of the upper limbs in children with spastic hemiparetic cerebral palsy during a dynamical task. *J Electromyogr Kinesiol.* 2010 Jun; Vol. 20, No. 3 (Jun, 2010) pp. 448-56, ISSN: 1050-6411.

Fuglsang-Frederiksen A (2000) The utility of interference pattern analysis. *Muscle Nerve,* Vol. 23, No. 1 (Jan, 2000) pp. 18-36, ISSN: 0148-639X.

Fuglsang-Frederiksen A. (1981) Electrical activity and force during voluntary contraction of normal and diseased muscle. *Acta Neurol Scand,* Vol. 63(Suppl. 83), (1981) pp. 1–60, ISSN: 0065-1427.

Fukuda TY, Echeimberg JO, Pompeu JE, Lucareli PRG, Garbelotti S, Gimenes RO, & Apolinário A (2010) Root Mean Square Value of the Electromyographic Signal in the Isometric Torque of the Quadriceps, Hamstrings and Brachial Biceps Muscles in Female Subjects, *J. Applied Research,* Vol. 10, No. 1 (2010) pp. 32-39, ISSN: 1537-064X.

Garcia HA, Milner-Brown HS, & Fisher MA (1980) "Turns" analysis in the physiological evaluation of neuromuscular disorders. *J Neurol Neurosurg Psychiatry* Vol. 43 (1980) pp. 1091-1097, ISSN: 0022-3050.

Haas E. (1926) Uber die Art der Tatigkeit unserer Muskeln beim Haltenverschieden schwerer Gewichte. Pflugers Archiv fur die gesamte, *Physiologie,* Vol. 212, (1926) pp. 651–6, ISSN as 0031-6768

Hermens HJ, Bruggena TAM, Batena CTM, Rutten WLC & Boom HBK (1992) The median frequency of the surface EMG power spectrum in relation to motor unit firing and action potential properties, *Electromyogr Kinesiol.* Vol. 2, No. 1, (1992) pp 15-25, ISSN: 1050-6411.

Hodges PW & Bui BH (1996) A comparison of computer-based methods for determination of onset of muscle contraction using electromyography. *Electroenceph. Clin. Neurophysiol.* Vol. 101 (1996) pp. 511–519, ISSN: 1388-2457.

Hug F (2011) Can muscle coordination be precisely studied by surface electromyography? J *Electromyogr Kinesiol.* Vol. 21, No. 1 (Feb, 2011) pp. 1-12, ISSN: 1050-6411.

Jeleń P & Sławińska U (1996) Estimation of the distribution of the EMG signal amplitude, *Acta Neurobiol Exp* (Wars). Vol. 56, No. 1 (1996) pp. 189-96, *ISSN*: 0065-1400.

Karlsson JS, Roeleveld K, Granlund C, Holtermann A & Ostlund N (2009) Signal processing of the surface electromyogram to gain insight into neuromuscular physiology. *Philos Transact A Math Phys Eng Sci.* Vol. 28, No. 367 (Jan, 2009) pp. 337-56, ISSN = 1364-503X.

Kleissen RF, Buurke JH, Harlaar J & Zilvold G (1998) Electromyography in the biomechanical analysis of human movement and its clinical application, *J. Gait Posture,* Vol. 1, No. 8(2) (Oct., 1998) pp. 143-158, ISSN: 0966-6362.

Lam WK, Leong JC, Li YH, Hu Y, & Lu WW (2005) Biomechanical and electromyographic evaluation of ankle foot orthosis and dynamic ankle foot orthosis in spastic cerebral palsy. *Gait Posture.* 2005 Nov; Vol. 22, No. 3 (Mar, 2005) pp. 189-97, ISSN: 0966-6362.

Lauer RT, Stackhouse CA, Shewokis PA, Smith BT, Tucker CA, & McCarthy J (2007) A time-frequency based electromyographic analysis technique for use in cerebral palsy. Gait Posture, Vol. 26, No. 3 (Sep, 2007) pp. 420-7, ISSN: 0966-6362.

Li W & Sakamoto K (1996) The influence of location of electrode on muscle fiber conduction velocity and EMG power spectrum during voluntary isometric contraction measured with surface array electrodes. Appl Human Sci. Vol. 15, No. 1 (Jan, 1996) pp. 25-32, ISSN: 1341-3473.

Lidierth M (1986) A computer based method for automated measurement of the periods of muscular activity from an EMG and its application to locomotor EMGs, *Electroenceph. Clin. Neurophysiol.*, vol. 64, (1986) pp. 378–380, ISSN: 0018-9294.

Micera S, Sabatini AM, & Dario P (1998) An algorithm for detecting the onset of muscle contraction by EMG signal processing, *Med. Eng. Phys.* Vol. 20 (1998) pp. 211–215, ISSN: 1350-4533.

Moshou, D, Hostens I, Papaioannou G, & Ramon H (2000) Wavelets and self-organising maps in electromyogram (EMG) analysis, in *Proceedings of the European Symposium on Intelligent Techniques (ESIT)*, ISBN 3-89653-797-0, Aachen, Germany, 14-15 September 2000

Poon DM & Hui-Chan CW (2009) Hyperactive stretch reflexes, co-contraction, and muscle weakness in children with cerebral palsy. *Dev Med Child Neurol.* Vol. 51, No. 2 (Feb, 2009) pp. 128-35, ISSN: 0012-1622.

Prosser LA, Lee SC, Barbe MF, VanSant AF & Lauer RT (2010) Trunk and hip muscle activity in early walkers with and without cerebral palsy--a frequency analysis. *J Electromyogr Kinesiol.* Vol. 20 No. 5 (Oct, 2010) pp. 851-9, ISSN: 1050-6411.

Raez MBI, Hussain MS, & Mohd-Yasin F. (2006) Techniques of EMG signal analysis: detection, processing, classification and applications. *Biol Proced Online.* (Aug 2006) ISSN: 1480-9222.

Rechtien JJ, Gelblum JB, Haig AJ, & Gitter AJ. (1999) Guidelines in electrodiagnostic medicine. Technology review: dynamic electromyography in gait and motion analysis. *American Association of Electrodiagnostic Medicine, Muscle Nerve Suppl.* Vol. 8 (1999) pp. S233-8, ISSN: 0148-639X.

Ronager J, Christensen H, & Fuglsang-Frederiksen A. (1989) Power spectrum analysis of the EMG pattern in normal and diseased muscles. *J Neurol Sci*, Vol. 94, (1989) pp. 283–94, ISSN: 0022-510X.

Sadeghi H, Allard P, Shafie K, Mathieu PA, Sadeghi S, Prince F, et al. (2000) Reduction of gait data variability using curve registration, *J. Gait Posture*, 2000 Dec; Vol. 12 No. 3 (Dec, 2000) pp. 257-64, ISSN: 0966-6362.

Staude GH (2001) Precise onset detection of human motor responses using a whitening filter and the log-likelihood-ratio test. *IEEE Trans Biomed Eng*, Vol. 48 (2001) pp. 1292–305, ISSN: 0018-9294

Staude GH & Wolf W (1999) Objective motor response onset detection in surface myoelectric signals, *Med. Eng. Phys.*, v Vol. 21 (1999) pp. 449–467, ISSN: 1350-4533.

Wakeling J, Delaney R, & Dudkiewicz I (2007) A method for quantifying dynamic muscle dysfunction in children and young adults with cerebral palsy. *Gait Posture* 2007; Vol. 25, No. 4 (Apr, 2007) pp. 580–9, ISSN: 0966-6362.

2

Location of Electrodes in Surface EMG

Ken Nishihara[1] and Takuya Isho[2]
[1]*Department of Physical Therapy, School of Health and Social Services*
Saitama Prefectural University
[2]*Department of Rehabilitation*
National Hospital Organization Takasaki General Medical Center
Japan

1. Introduction

Motor unit action potentials (MUAPs) from motoneurons are transmitted to muscles through end-plates and then propagated to the tendons. These bioelectrical signals are detected via electromyography (EMG), which is performed using electrodes.

The electrodes used in EMG are primarily surface electrodes and inserted (wire or needle) electrodes, of which surface and wire electrodes are mainly used for kinesiological studies. Surface electrodes are widely used because of noninvasive attachment, painless usage, suitability for detecting muscle activation by generation of EMG signals and simplicity, although detection is usually limited in surface muscles. Surface EMG is a practical and noninvasive procedure that has potential usage in sports and rehabilitation medicine.

The signal amplitude of surface EMG is analyzed to estimate the level of muscle contraction, while the frequency component is used to estimate performance of muscle activation. For example, a change in EMG signal amplitude is regarded as a change in the strength of muscle activation, and a shift of the surface EMG signal towards a lower mean frequency is correlated with decreasing muscle fiber conduction velocity due to muscle fatigue. However, the detected EMG signal amplitude and mean frequency are influenced by the location of surface electrodes, although the action potentials in a muscle are generated at the same time. For these reasons, the location of surface electrodes is very important for accurate evaluation of muscle activation.

In this chapter, the propagation or conduction of action potentials is illustrated to understand the EMG signal recorded by surface electrodes. Proper electrode locations are suggested with theoretical and practical methods.

2. Surface EMG signals according to the propagation of action potentials

EMG can explain the superimposed waveform of MUAPs, which are detected by electrodes. The EMG signal can be prepared by the summation of theoretically generated MUAP waveforms. The EMG signal observed by electrodes can also be estimated.

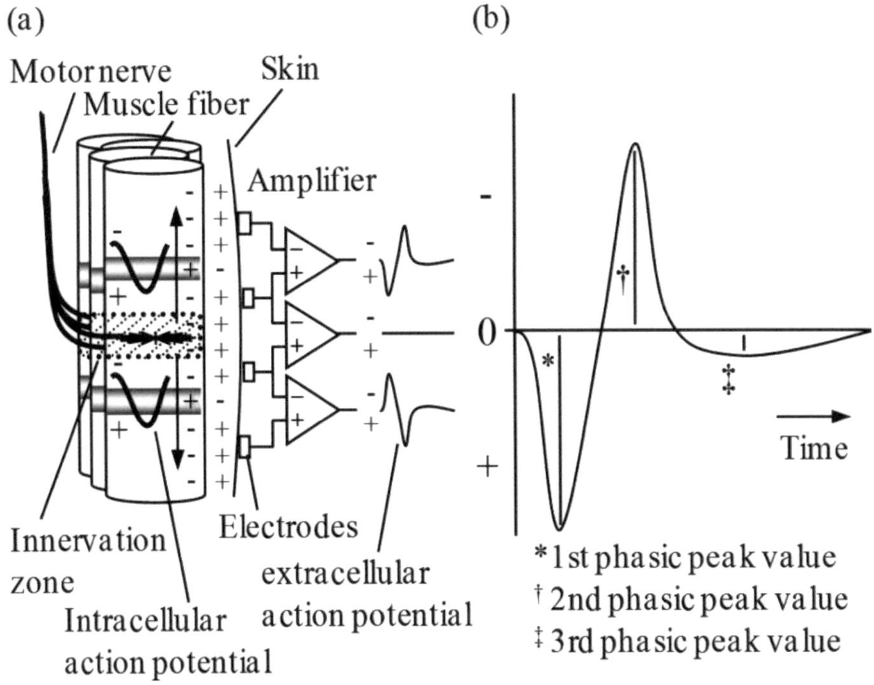

Fig. 1. Theoretical waveform of an MUAP measured using a surface electrode.
The action potential from the innervation zone (IZ) is propagated bilaterally along the muscle fibers. The direction of the waveform will reverse depending on whether the surface electrode is proximal or distal to IZ (a). The normal MUAP is triphasic, consisting of larger first- and second-phase peaks and a smaller third phase peak (b; Nishihara et al., 2010).

2.1 Detection of MUAP waveform with surface electrodes

Rosenfalck recorded action potentials during muscle contraction in individual muscle fibers of frogs, rats and humans, and performed a detailed calculation of the predicted action potentials when the signals were detected by bipolar electrodes placed on the skin surface (Rosenfalck, 1969). In humans, the basic action potential is triphasic; the first two phases are similar in amplitude, whereas the terminal phase has a peak-to-peak amplitude, which is only 5%–10% of those of the first two phases (Fig. 1).

If only a single MUAP is generated, whether the peak in each phase starts in a positive or negative direction theoretically depends on whether the recording bipolar electrode is proximal or distal to IZ (Hilfiker & Meyer, 1984; Zalewska & Hausmanowa-Petrusewicz, 2008).

The waveform of an MUAP is propagated from the end-plate to the muscle tendons. If the end-plates are concentrated in one location, then the direction of the positive or negative side of the MUAP waveform will reverse depending on whether the position of the electrode that is recording muscle activity is proximal or distal to IZ (Masuda & Sadoyama, 1991). The waveform of a MUAP will be canceled or attenuated in IZ.

When measuring a surface EMG signal during voluntary contraction, many MUAPs can interfere with each other, thus making it more complicated to identify a single whole MUAP from a raw waveform display.

2.2 Relationship between the direction of electrodes and muscle fibers

Action potentials from motoneurons are propagated along muscle fibers. Bipolar surface electrodes are usually placed in the approximated direction of muscle fibers and used with a differential amplifier, which suppresses signals common to both electrodes.
The potential at one electrode is subtracted from that at the other electrode, and then the difference is amplified. Subsequently, the common noise of both electrodes is eliminated.
Multichannel electrodes arranged along the direction of muscle fibers can be used to investigate the muscle fiber conduction velocity or propagation of the action potentials. However, many EMG channels must be used for a single muscle (Nishizono et al., 1979). Multichannel surface array electrodes or grid electrodes would facilitate the stable observation of action potentials because these electrodes are attached to a plate that fixes the electrodes in close proximity to each other (Fig. 2; Zwarts & Stegeman, 2003).

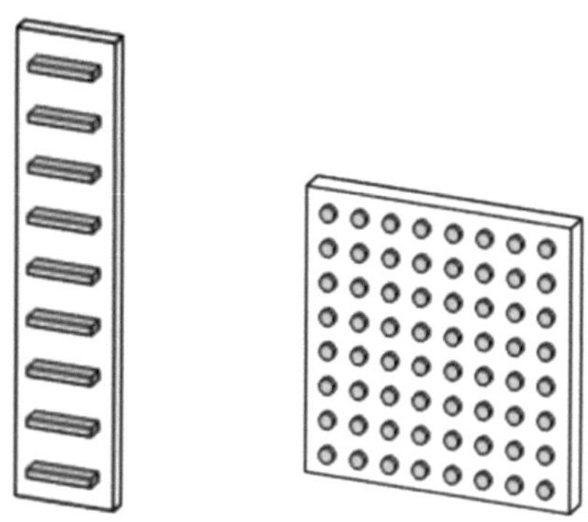

Fig. 2. Multichannel surface array electrodes (left) and grid electrodes (right).
The gray rectangles and circles represent electrodes attached to the boxes.

The propagated MUAPs are attenuated depending on their distance from the surface electrodes, the location of subcutaneous tissue, and the electrical impedance of the skin (Fig. 3). Usually, MUAPs generated at a distance from the electrode are greatly attenuated. The higher frequency components of the interfered waveform are more difficult to detect when surface electrodes are placed over subcutaneous tissue; in addition, it is difficult to identify the propagation of MUAPs. The propagation pattern from raw EMG signals may be observed during lower level of voluntary muscle contraction (Fig. 4).
The propagations are estimated by detecting time shifts of pulses, which are considered as one MUAP although they appear across EMG signals of several channels (Fig. 4). The time shifts of pulses indicate that the surface electrodes are approximately located along the direction of muscle fibers. The pulses shift maximally when the electrodes are placed along the direction of muscle fibers that are anatomically arranged in the same direction. Close to the tendons of a muscle, however, the amplitude of the EMG signal is reduced and the time shifts of pulses are unidentifiable.
Appropriate analysis techniques are needed to estimate the propagation of EMG signals in higher level of muscle contraction because many motor units are activated and the generated MUAPs interfere with the observed raw waveforms of EMG.

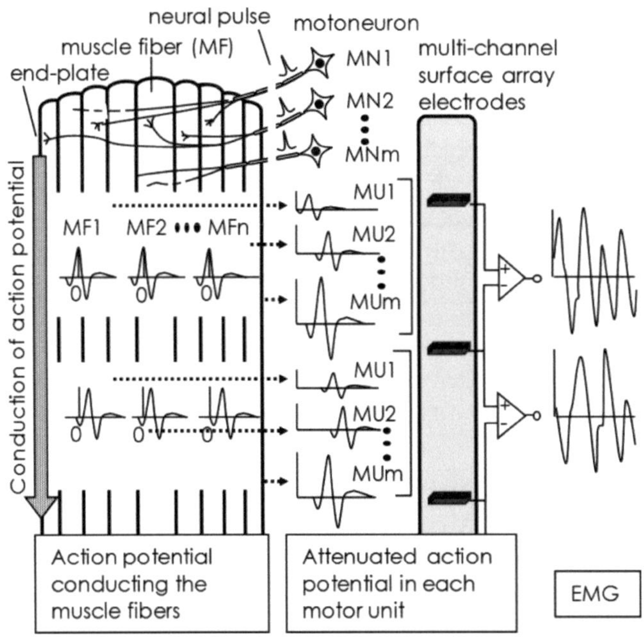

Fig. 3. Theoretical EMG signal from action potentials propagated along muscle fibers. The action potentials propagated along muscle fibers are attenuated according to the distance between the muscle fibers and the surface electrodes and are superimposed in surface EMG (Nishihara et al., 2003).

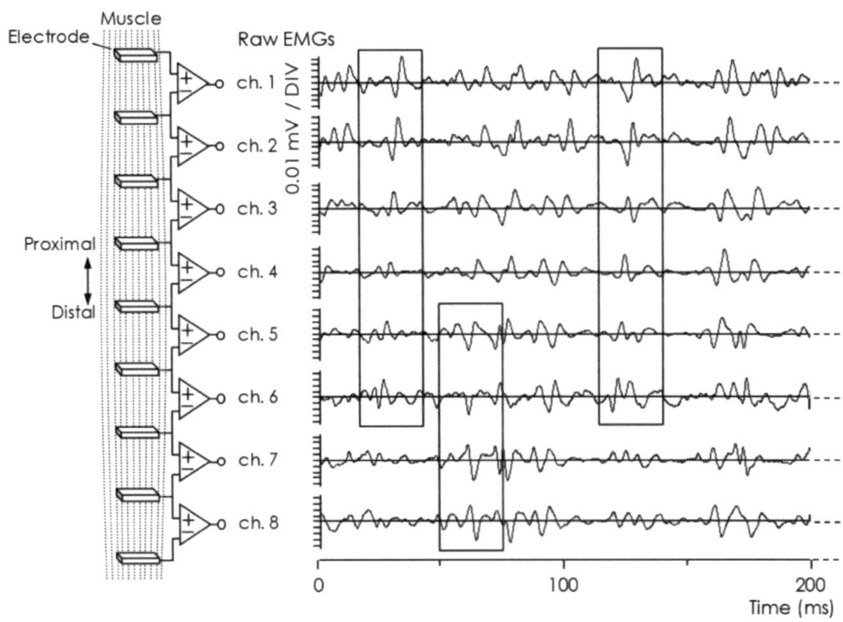

Fig. 4. Example of raw EMG signals detected by multichannel surface array electrodes. The propagations are estimated by detecting the continuous time shifts across several channels (rectangular boxes).

2.3 Cross-correlation method to estimate the propagation of action potentials

The cross-correlation method has been widely applied to estimate action potential propagation by multichannel surface EMGs using automated computer programs (Yaar & Niles, 1991). The correlation coefficient ($R\tau$) used to calculate the time shift is calculated from the reference EMG (X) and comparison EMG (Y) using the following equation (1):

$$R\tau = \frac{\sum_{i=0,j=i+\tau}^{N,N+\tau} (X_i - \overline{X}) \cdot (Y_j - \overline{Y})}{\sqrt{\sum_{i=0}^{N} (X_i - \overline{X})^2 \cdot \sum_{j=i+\tau}^{N+\tau} (Y_j - \overline{Y})^2}} \qquad (1)$$

where $R\tau$ is a normalized value ranging from −1 to +1. The peak value of $R\tau$ displaced from time 0 is the time shift reflecting the conduction time between the two EMG signals (Fig. 5). A time shift could be assumed to occur according to the muscle fiber conduction. If the surface electrodes were attached in the proper direction, the peak value of $R\tau$ would be close to 1, which is relatively high.

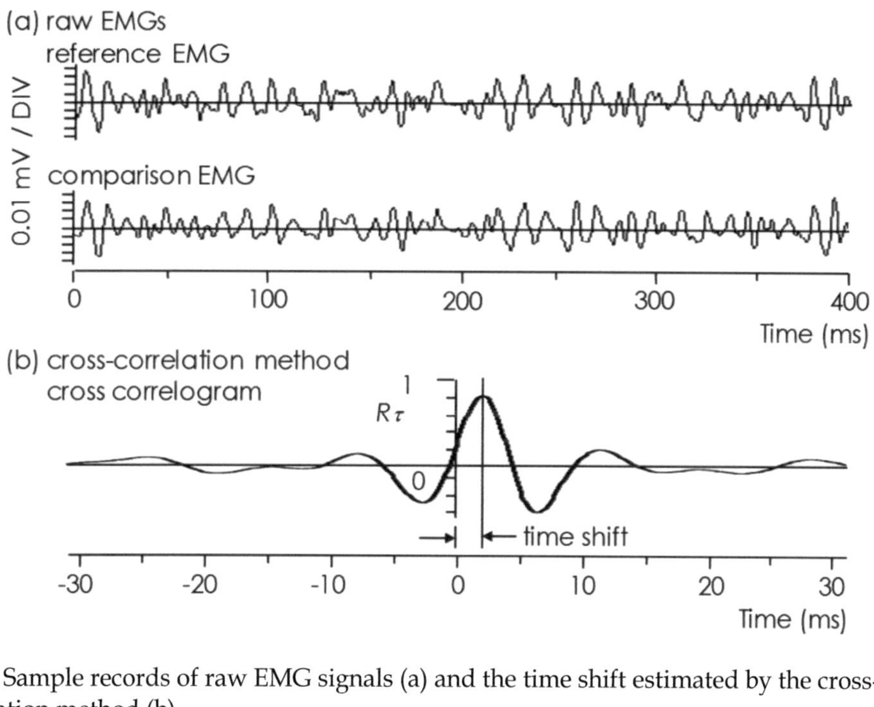

Fig. 5. Sample records of raw EMG signals (a) and the time shift estimated by the cross-correlation method (b).
The time shift estimated using the cross-correlation method by calculating the time between zero and the peak of the cross-correlogram of an EMG signal (Nishihara et al., 2003).

2.4 Peak averaging method to estimate the propagation of action potentials

The propagation pattern from a raw surface EMG signal can be observed by detecting the peaks in a surface EMG and averaging them using computer programs (Nishihara et al., 2003; Isho et al., 2011).

The smallest value at which the pulses were not detected from resting muscle EMGs was set as the threshold to avoid the detection of a noise component. When a positive peak value was larger than the set threshold in the EMG signals, the amplitude and time were registered as the peak of positive pulse. The negative peak value of the EMG signals is processed as the peak of negative pulse using the same method.

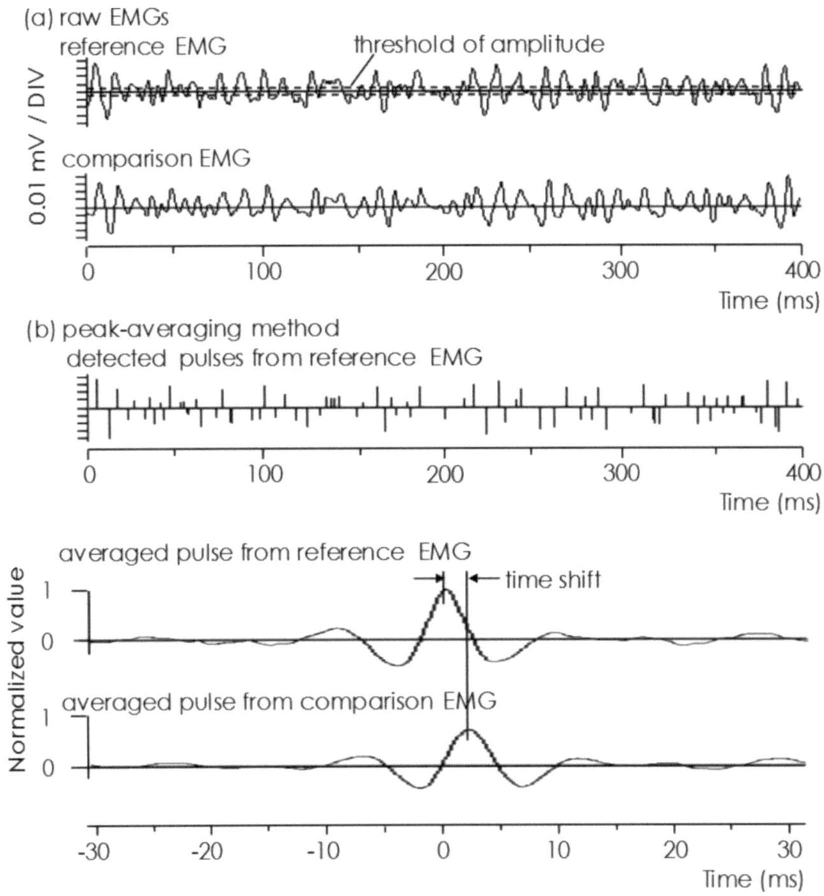

Fig. 6. Sample records of raw EMGs (a) and action potentials estimated using the peak averaging method (b).
The time shift is the time difference between the peak averaged pulses obtained using the peak averaging method (Nishihara et al., 2003).

Pulses from a reference EMG were superimposed at time 0 and averaged to minimize the irregular components of other interfering action potentials and noises. The value of the averaged pulse (*PAi*) at the point *i* on the reference EMG is obtained using the following equation (2):

$$PA_i = \frac{\sum_{j=1}^{N} \frac{1}{A_j} \cdot X_{T_j+i}}{N} \tag{2}$$

where N is the number of detected pulses in EMG with the reference electrodes, X is the reference EMG, Aj is the peak value of a detected pulse j in X, and Tj is the time at which a peak detected pulse j is obtained in X.
The peak value of PAj is 1, and its peak point of time is 0.
An averaged pulse is obtained simultaneously from a comparison EMG with an averaged time delay. The waveform of the comparison EMG is averaged with the same Aj and Tj of the detected pulse j in the reference EMG (not in the comparison EMG). Thus, the averaged pulse PBi at point i from the comparison EMG is obtained using the following equation (3):

$$PB_i = \frac{\sum_{j=1}^{N} \frac{1}{A_j} \cdot Y_{T_j+i}}{N} \qquad (3)$$

where Y is the comparison EMG.
The time shift estimated by investigating the time difference between PAi and PBi is calculated from the time difference between the peaks or cross-correlation of PAi and PBi (Fig. 6).
This method permits simple observation of the propagation of action potentials across multichannel array electrodes.

3. Surface EMG signals in IZ

Action potentials were generated in the end-plates used for signal transmission from motoneurons. These end-plates are usually concentrated in areas such as IZ. The propagation pattern was investigated using the peak averaging method, and the location of IZ was also estimated by analyzing this propagation pattern.

3.1 EMG recording

Multichannel array electrodes were attached to the medial aspect of the belly in the direction of fibers of the biceps brachii muscle and the array was secured to the skin with surgical tape. The array electrodes comprised nine wires (material: silver/silver chloride, width: 1 mm, length: 10 mm) attached at 5-mm intervals to a transparent acrylic resin box.
A weight band was attached to the wrist of the subject. Isometric elbow flexion was performed for one second to the extent of <10% maximum voluntary isometric contraction, and an EMG signal was recorded. The adequacy of the distance between the array electrodes and the tendons was checked by palpation.

3.2 Estimation of IZs

The averaged pulses from the recorded EMG signal were calculated as shown in Fig. 7. If the array electrodes are shifted towards the adjacent muscles, the time shifts are not clear, and hum components, which are easily mixed if the reference electrode is incompletely attached, are detected as pulses. This results in many dummy averaged pulses appearing in each channel. In that case, the locations of electrodes must be corrected.
The origin of the propagation is considered as IZ. If the directions of electrodes and muscle fibers are substantially different, these time shifts of averaged pulses would not be clearly shown, or the peak correlation coefficient obtained would be of a relatively low value (equation (1)).

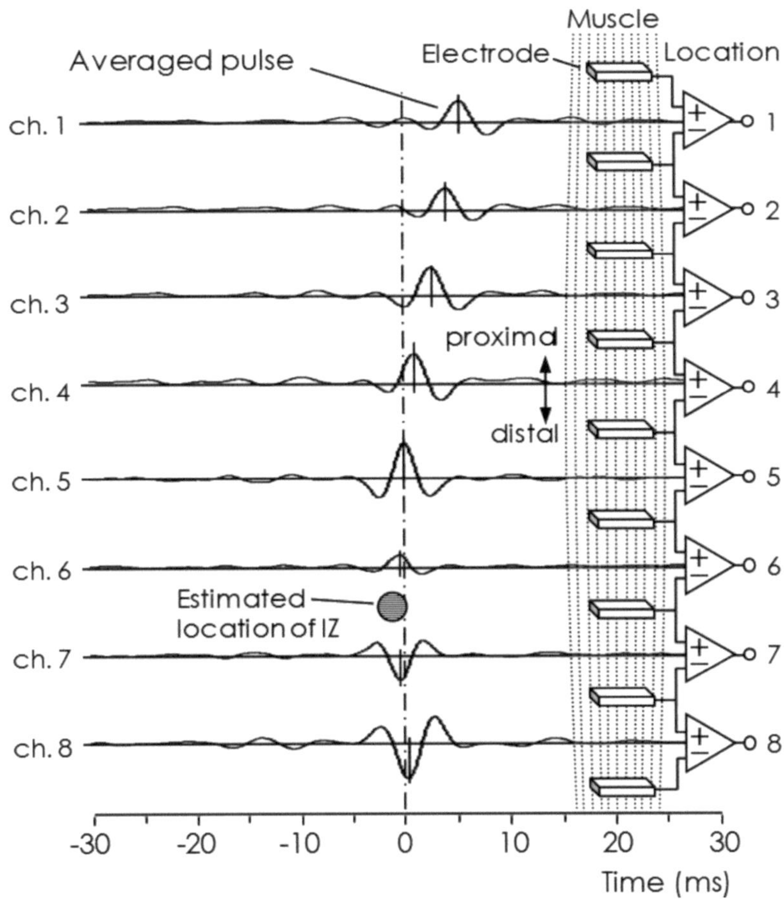

Fig. 7. Example of the generation of averaged pulses.
The EMG signal is the same as that in Fig. 4. Channel 5 was selected as the reference EMG. Detected pulses from the EMG signal are averaged, and these averaged pulses indicate the direction of propagation in muscle fibers. In this subject, the estimated location of IZ is between channels 6 and 7 (Nishihara et al., 2009).

4. IZ locations and directions of muscle fibers across several muscles

IZs are usually located around the muscle belly, or in other words, around the center of muscle fibers. However, determining the locations of IZs is difficult by the muscles. The muscles have been classified by the structures.

4.1 The structure of muscles according to the direction of muscle fibers

Muscles are classified on the basis of the direction of muscle fibers rather than the overall direction of the muscle (Fig. 8). The biceps brachii muscle is a typical example of a fusiform muscle, because it has a relatively uniform direction of muscle fibers with IZ located around its center in most cases. However, IZs were dispersed in many cases in spite of the biceps brachii muscle being used for the study in all cases (Fig. 9).

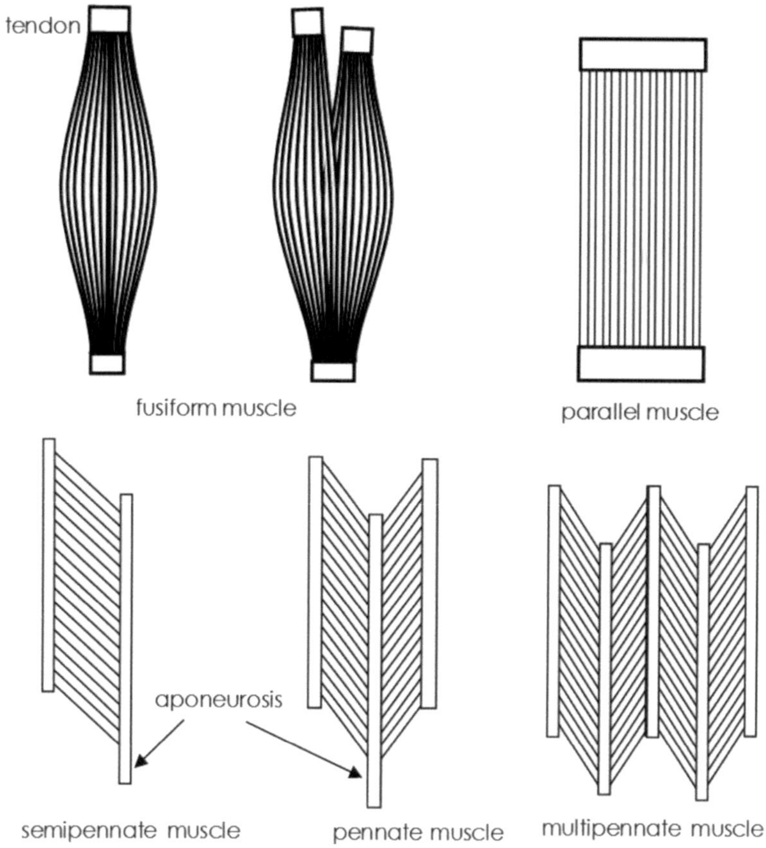

Fig. 8. Classification of muscles based on the directions of muscle fibers.

The direction of fibers is irregular in many muscles; consequently, IZs of these muscles are scattered around them (Saitou et al., 2000). Therefore, it is very difficult to attach surface electrodes in the exact direction of the muscle fibers of such muscles. In this case, the EMG signal does not comprise the waveform of generated MUAPs as illustrated in Fig. 1. The time shifts of averaged pulses from the gluteus medius muscle are not very clear compared to those from the biceps brachii muscle (Fig. 10). Clear time shifts do not appear even when the directions of array electrodes are rotated up to 30° (not shown in this figure).

The deltoid muscle is divided into three sections: anterior, intermediate, and posterior. In particular, the intermediate section of the deltoid muscle has a typical pennate structure. The direction of the muscle fibers in this section of the deltoid muscle are irregular compared to that of the biceps brachii muscle. The time shifts across the channels of the averaged pulses are not very clear; therefore, it is difficult to investigate the location of IZ (Fig. 11; Nishihara et al., 2008).

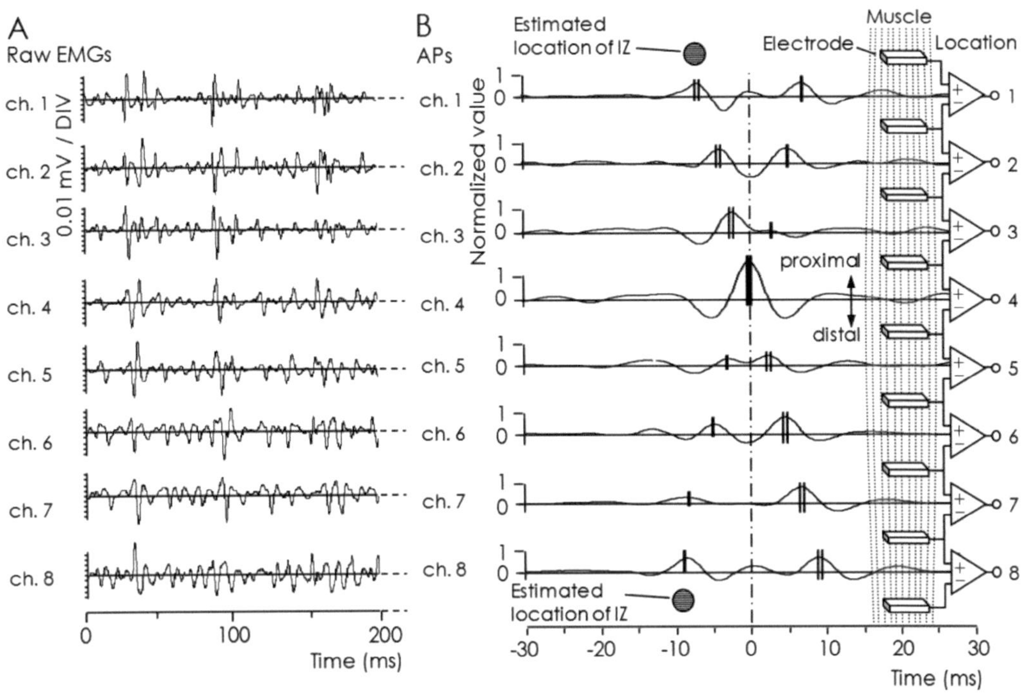

Fig. 9. An example of dispersed IZs in the biceps brachii muscle.
The calculation method is same as that described in Fig. 7. (A) Channel 4 is selected as the reference EMG. (B) The estimated locations of IZs are proximal at location 1 and distal at location 8 in this subject.

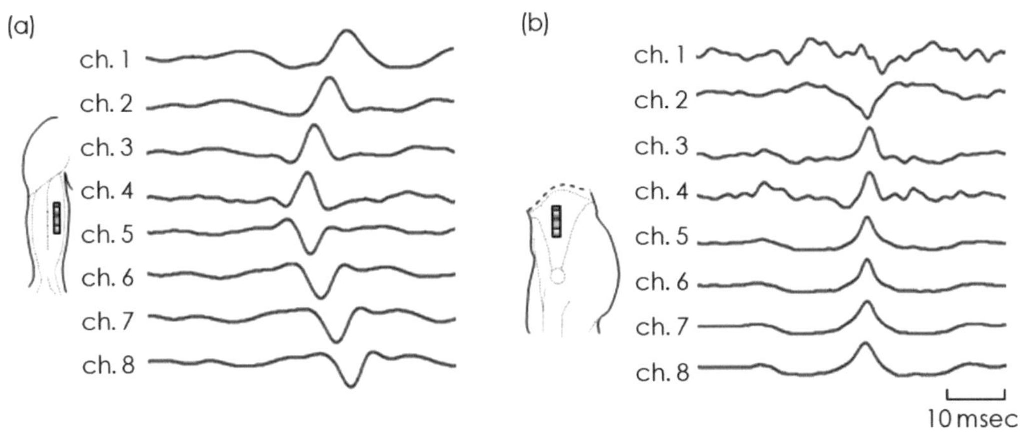

(a) The time shifts of averaged pulses across the various channels are revealed in the biceps brachii muscle. (b) However, the time shifts of averaged pulses are not revealed in the gluteus medius muscle. The gray rectangles demonstrate the locations of array electrodes, which were attached at 10-mm intervals.

Fig. 10. An example of calculating the averaged pulses of different muscles.

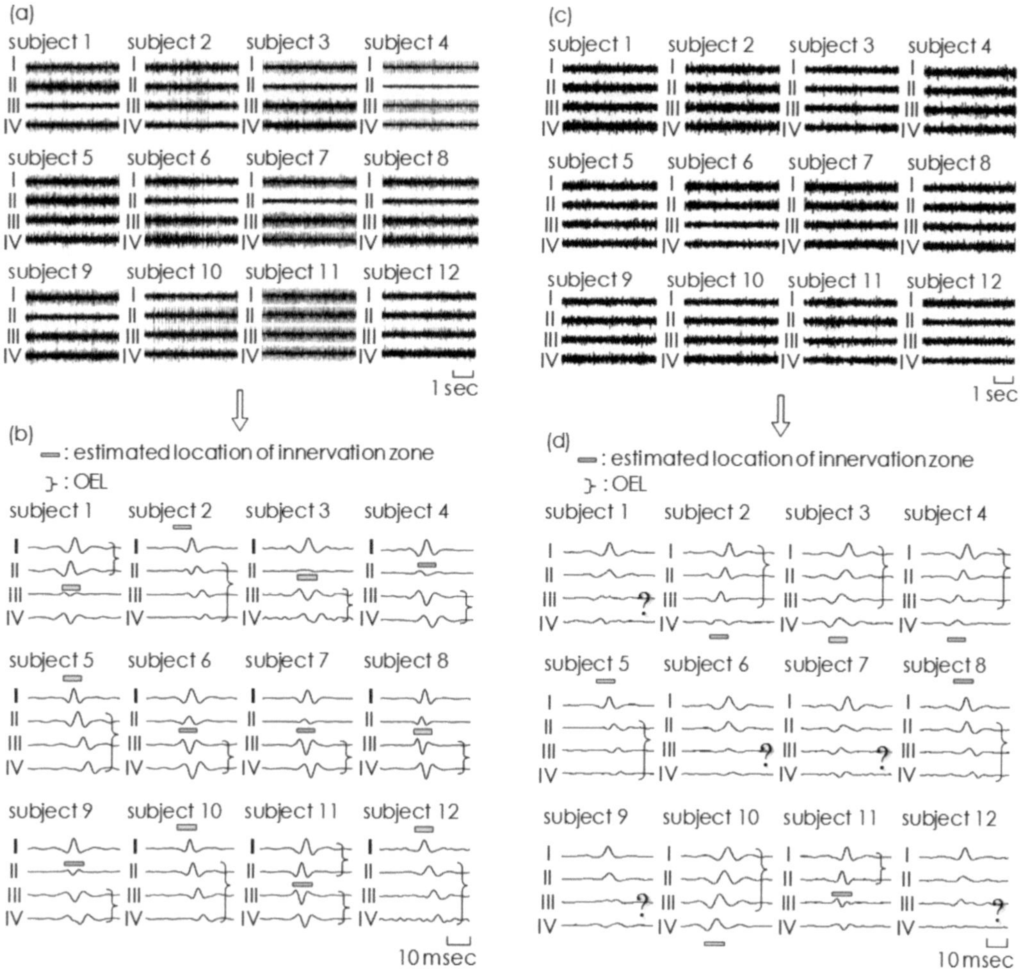

(a) Raw EMG signals of the biceps brachii muscle are shown. Particularly small amplitudes are exhibited in channel 3 in subject 1 and channel 2 in subjects 3, 4, 7, 8 and 9. (b) Calculated averaged signals of the muscles with pulse detection in EMG for channel 1 (shown in bold). (c) Raw EMG signals of the intermediate section of the deltoid muscle are shown. (d) Propagation patterns are shown for seven subjects. The propagation patterns of the other five subjects were not estimated because central peaks in the averaged signals could not be obtained for all four channels, or peaks in the averaged signals of neighboring channels did not exhibit time differences in the propagation of action potentials along electrodes. The optimum electrode location (OEL) is investigated on the basis of the location of IZ (Nishihara et al., 2008). Note the lower amplitudes of the raw EMG signals around channels of IZ locations.

Fig. 11. Analysis of EMG signals for the biceps brachii muscle (left) and deltoid muscle (right).

4.2 EMG signals near IZ

The changes in EMG signal amplitudes near IZs can be estimated if multichannel electrodes are used. For example, EMG signals with smaller amplitudes are observed using the raw EMG signals of the biceps brachii muscle as shown in Fig. 11, and the data for these channels agree with those of the channels near estimated IZs. The EMG signal amplitude can be calculated from the root mean square (RMS) of the EMG signal. The RMSs of EMG signals are obviously attenuated near IZ as shown in Fig. 12. Sufficiently large RMS values can be obtained at locations far from IZs.

IZs of the deltoid muscle are not very clear compared to those of the biceps brachii muscle (Fig. 11, d). However, this does not imply that the EMG signal of the deltoid muscle more correctly reflects the level of muscle activation than that of the biceps brachii muscle. Small RMS values are shown in some channels of subjects, although the locations of IZs are not estimated in the deltoid muscle (Fig. 12, right half). The EMG signal amplitudes may be attenuated by the different electrode directions relative to the axes of the muscle fibers rather than the small, scattered IZs in the deltoid muscle.

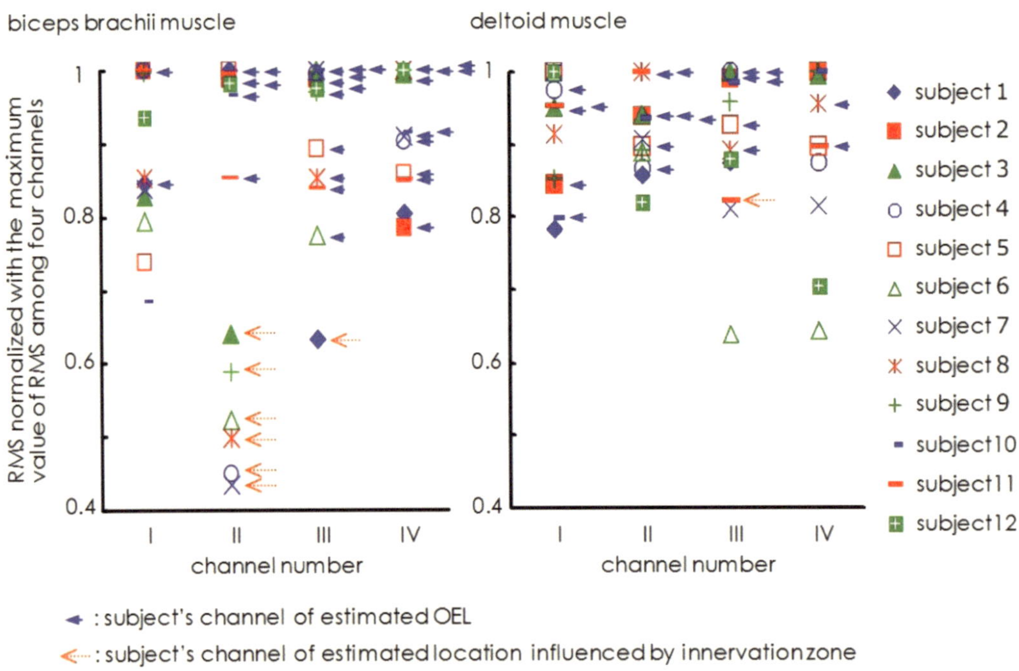

Fig. 12. RMSs of raw EMG signals for the subject channels depicted in Fig. 11.
The EMG signals shown in Fig. 11 a and c are used. The subject's channel of estimated location, which was influenced by IZ, gave particularly small values (indicated by the large arrow with dotted line) compared with the subject's channel of estimated OEL (indicated by the small arrow with solid line). Small values were recorded in the channels of subjects whose deltoid muscle was not evaluated (channels 3 and 4 of subject 6 and channel 4 of subject 12).

5. Conclusion

These results demonstrate that EMG signals are affected by location of electrodes. Proper location of electrodes can be suggested by these findings.

5.1 Identification of targeted muscle

The location of electrodes has to be carefully determined for the targeted muscle. Superficial muscle could be identified with manipulation. When the electrodes were shifted towards the adjacent muscles, the unassumed action potentials from different muscles were mixed with the EMG signal. The electrodes were also easy to place on the tendon of the muscle. In that case, low-amplitude EMG signals that do not reflect muscle activity could be observed. Muscle and tendons can be distinguished by palpation.

5.2 Identification of the direction of muscle fibers

The direction of electrodes affects the EMG signal when the direction is differing from the directions of muscle fibers. The direction of the electrodes must align with that of muscle fibers. An ideal situation would be when one whole MUAP is detected by one electrode and the next one by the other electrode. The muscle fibers need not always be in the direction of the muscle. However, if muscle fibers are diagonally directed, obtaining sufficient space to attach bipolar electrodes may prove difficult.

5.3 Attaching the reference electrode

The reference electrode must be attached firmly to eliminate noise components such as hum. The reference electrode has to be located on electrically neutral tissue such as a bony prominence. The propagation pattern is not revealed by the peak averaging method (Fig. 7) if large noise components are included in the EMG signal.

5.4 The relationship between electrode and IZ locations

Propagation has to be regarded relative to the location of electrodes because their placement can affect the signal amplitude and frequency components in surface EMG. As previously mentioned, to correctly quantify muscle activity, electrodes must be placed along the course of muscle fibers between tendons in the targeted muscle. The cutaneous area, which is useful for observing the surface EMG signal, could be very limited in this restricted rule. For this reason, the electrodes should be located near the muscle belly. However, the EMG signal is easily affected when the electrodes are located near IZs, which are concentrated in the muscle belly (Fig. 11). A stable EMG signal is necessary for the reliable investigation of voluntary muscle activation.

The channels located near the estimated IZs agree with the channels of the smallest amplitude or RMS of the EMG signals (Fig. 12). As a result, it is suggested that electrodes should be placed at a sufficient distance from IZ for detection of the surface EMG signals during voluntary muscle contraction.

Moreover, IZ is known to shift with changes in muscle length due to muscle activity. In other words, when electrodes are attached to the skin and EMG for muscle activity is recorded, the positional relationship between the surface electrodes and IZ can shift markedly. Electrodes must also be attached after considering the moving IZ during EMG recording (Nishihara et al., 2010).

5.5 Effect of muscle structure

The aforementioned rules are based on the assumption that all muscle fibers are aligned in the same direction and IZs are concentrated in the muscle belly of the targeted muscle. The anatomical structure of the targeted muscle must be investigated before attaching the electrodes. However, in muscles with irregularly oriented muscle fibers, such as pennate muscles, the proper direction of electrodes could be not determined. There are limitations to consider regarding the optimum surface electrode locations while investigating the activity of these muscles using EMG signals.

6. References

Hilfiker, P., & Meyer, M. (1984). Normal and myopathic propagation of surface motor unit action potentials. *Electroencephalography and Clinical Neurophysiology,* Vol.57, No.1, pp. 21-31, ISSN 0013-4694

Isho, T., Nishihara, K., Gomi, T. (2011). Inter-method measurement variability of muscle fiber conduction velocities during isometric fatigue contraction. Proceedings of *16th International Congress of the World Confederation for Physical Therapy,* Amsterdam, The Netherlands, June, 2011

Masuda, T., & Sadoyama, T. (1991). Distribution of innervation zones in the human biceps brachii. *Journal of Electromyography and Kinesiology,* Vol.1, No.2, pp. 107-115, ISSN 1050-6411

Nishihara, K., Hosoda, K., & Futami, T. (2003). Muscle fiber conduction velocity estimation by using normalized peak-averaging technique. *Journal of Electromyography and Kinesiology,* Vol.13, No.6, pp. 499-507, ISSN 1050-6411

Nishihara, K., Kawai, H., Gomi, T., Terajima, M., & Chiba, Y. (2008). Investigation of optimum electrode locations by using an automatized surface electromyography analysis technique. *IEEE Transactions on Biomedical Engineering,* Vol.55, No.2, pp. 636-642, ISSN 0018-9294

Nishihara, K., Chiba, Y., Moriyama, H., Hosoda, M., Suzuki, Y., & Gomi, T. (2009). Noninvasive estimation of muscle fiber conduction velocity distribution using an electromyographic processing technique. *Medical Science Monitor,* Vol.15, No.9, pp. MT113-120, ISSN 1234-1010

Nishihara, K., Chiba, Y., Suzuki, Y., Moriyama, H., Kanemura, N., Ito, T., Takayanagi, K., & Gomi, T. (2010). Effect of position of electrodes relative to the innervation zone on surface EMG. *Journal of Medical Engineering & Technology,* Vol.34, No.2, pp. 141-147, ISSN 0309-1902

Nishizono, H., Saito, Y., & Miyashita, M. (1979). The estimation of conduction velocity in human skeletal muscle in situ with surface electrodes. *Electroencephalography and Clinical Neurophysiology,* Vol.46, No.6, pp. 659-664, ISSN 0013-4694

Rosenfalck, P. (1969). Intra- and extracellular potential fields of active nerve and muscle fibers. A physico-mathematical analysis of different models. *Acta Physiologica Scandinavica,* S321, pp. 1-168, ISSN 0001-6772

Saitou, K., Masuda, T., Michikami, D., Kojima, R., & Okada, M. (2000). Innervation zones of the upper and lower limb muscles estimated by using multichannel surface EMG. *Journal of Human Ergology,* Vol.29, No.1, (May , 2000), pp. 35-52, ISSN 0300-8134

Yaar, I., & Niles, L. (1991). Muscle fiber conduction velocity Dip analysis versus cross correlation techniques. *Electromyography and Clinical Neurophysiology,* Vol.31, No.8, pp. 473-482, ISSN 0301-150X

Zalewska, E., & Hausmanowa-Petrusewicz, I. (2008). Approximation of motor unit structure from the analysis of motor unit potential. *Clinical Neurophysiology,* Vol.119, No.11, pp. 2501-2506, ISSN 1388-2457

Zwarts, M., & Stegeman, D. (2003). Multichannel surface EMG: basic aspects and clinical utility. *Muscle & Nerve,* Vol.28, No.1, (January, 2003), pp. 1-17, ISSN 0148-639X

3

The Relationship Between Electromyography and Muscle Force

Heloyse Uliam Kuriki, Fábio Mícolis de Azevedo, Luciana Sanae Ota Takahashi, Emanuelle Moraes Mello, Rúben de Faria Negrão Filho and Neri Alves
Univ. Estadual Paulista
Univ. de São Paulo
Brazil

1. Introduction

The generation of physical movement in animals involves the activation and control of muscle forces. Understanding the mechanisms behind force generation and control is essential for professionals who work to promote health. The human body can be represented as a system of articulated segments in static or dynamic balance. Within this system, movement can arise from internal forces acting outside the joint axis, causing angular displacement of these segments, or by forces external to the body. Knowledge of the contribution of muscle forces to joint position and movement is of great importance for the study of muscle activity during exercise and also for understanding the coordination of muscle activities during functional movement. However, muscles forces cannot be easily measured in vivo; rather, they must be assessed, calculated or modeled (Amadio & Duarte, 1996; Amadio & Barbanti 2000).

Closely associated with the generation of force by a muscle, is the generation of an electrical signal that can be observed by placing electrodes on the skin surface to detect underlying electrical activity displaying the associated waveform on a computer monitor. This process is called electromyography (EMG) and the waveform is the electromyogram. The assumption that there is an association between EMG and underlying muscle forces is the basis for many applications of EMG, allowing inferences regarding various aspects of muscle physiology. However, it is not possible to measure muscle force directly using EMG. Since 1952 there have been studies that show some cases where there is a linear relationship between force and EMG (Lippold, 1952), however this relationship is not always simple and linear. In recent years methods for detecting and processing EMG signals have been refined considerably, with the availability of better equipment, tools, mathematical, statistical and computational techniques. Although the determination of muscle strength using EMG measurements has also evolved, it has not yet fully exploited the technological potential available. In this chapter, we describe a practical approach to the quantitative evaluation of muscle force through analysis of the EMG signal.

2. Muscle strength

Force is a fundamental concept, understood as an agent capable of modifying the state of rest or motion of a body. Force can be defined as:

$$F=m.a \tag{1}$$

where *m* is mass and and *a,* acceleration.
Animals move and interact with the environment generating muscleforce, either voluntarily or passively. Biomechanics is a field of science dedicated to understanding human movement and the study of the muscular forces involved in human movement. It is the application of mathematical principles, laws and concepts to mechanical, biological systems. It studies the generation and performance of internal and external forces on these systems and the effects of these forces on each part of the body. These forces can be calculated indirectly by parameters of kinematics and dynamics of movement or based on the mechanical characteristics of the locomotor system and its functional structures. External biomechanics refers to externally observable characteristics of the body studied, for example, its movement in space: position, velocity, acceleration, externally applied forces, reaction forces and muscle electrical activity (Amadio & Duarte, 1996; Amadio & Barbanti, 2000).
The muscle behavior approach to biomechanics uses analytical methods that include anthropometry, kinemetry, dynamometry and electromyography. The EMG is the method of recording the electrical activity of a muscle, including information about the physiological processes that occur during muscle contraction. The biological structure of the body, movement dynamics and characteristics of the measurement techniques complicate the analysis of the motion variables and indicators of internal phenomena. The assessment of muscle strength, in particular, becomes more complex due to the mechanisms of controlling dosage or magnitude, enabling the execution of movements or of achieving internal and external balance amongst body elements. Thus, direct measures of muscle strength and interaction forces between segments are not viable. Assessments of internal forces are based on models built from the parameters of motion of the body or its segments, measures of external linkages, or both. Understanding the relationships between internal forces and movement is one of the major methodological challenges for biomechanics (Amadio & Duarte, 1996).

3. Determinant factors for the generation of muscle strength

The term muscle strength refers to the ability of a muscle to generate tension. For the generation of muscular force that produces mechanical work, the first necessary condition is nerve stimulation that triggers the process. Sensory input from muscles travels via afferent pathways to the central nervous system (CNS), where it promotes the recruitment of motor neurons that stimulates muscle fibers and results in the generation and demonstration of muscle strength. These muscle forces act through a bone system that depend on nervous, muscular, and biomechanical factors, as shown in Figure 1.
The functional unit of muscle is the motor unit (MU), which consists of an alpha motor neuron and all fibers innervated by it. Muscle fibers are the structural unit of contraction. One UM can have from 3 to 2000 muscle fibers, depending on the degree of control and strength required by the muscle: muscles that control fine movements and require precise but low strength have fewer fibers per MU, whereas the large muscles that control larger movements requiring greater strength, may contain 100 to 1000 fibers per MU (Rash, 2002).

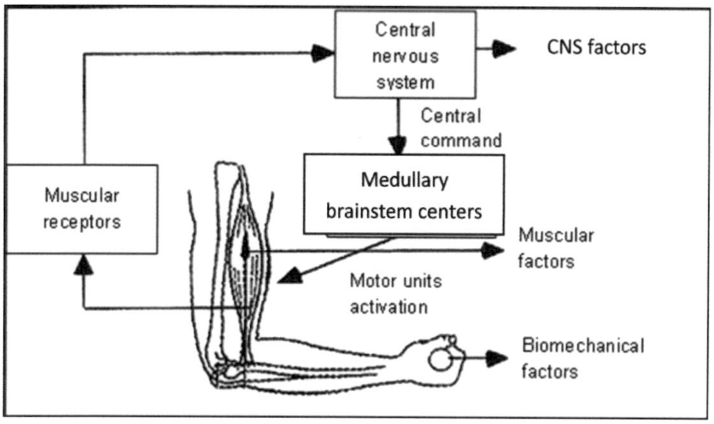

Fig. 1. Diagram illustrating the factors associated with muscle force generation.

The contraction of muscle fibers occurs when action potentials are generated in the motor neuron that supplies them. When the action potential reaching the motor neuron and axon terminal exceeds the threshold of depolarization in the postsynaptic membrane of the neuromuscular junction, it becomes a muscle action potential. Different from nerve action potentials, the muscle action potential is propagated in both directions of the muscle fiber, triggering the process of the sliding of actin filaments on myosin, the major contractile proteins of the myofibrils, thus, promoting muscle contraction (Fox & Keteyian, 2000).

During voluntary contractions, muscle force is modulated by the central nervous system, which combines recruitment with the frequency of MU activation and synchronization. MU recruitment involves the control of the number and type of fibers activated. The frequency of activation of MUs refers to the fact that the fibers do not remain contracted, relaxing after each activation, and therefore reflects the repeatability of activation. The synchronization of activation refers to the temporal coincidence of the pulses of two or more MUs firing in combination. The greater the ability to recruit MUs simultaneously, the greater the force produced by the muscle (Barbanti et al., 2002; Fox & Keteyian, 2000). These mechanisms operate in different proportions depending on the muscle. Relatively small muscles, such as those of the hand; and big muscles, like those of the legs and arms are controlled by different schemes of recruitment and activation (Basmajian & De Luca, 1985).

Muscle fibers are classified either as type I or type II, according to their metabolic and functional capabilities. As the number of MUs per muscle is variable, the ratio of fiber types varies among individuals (Rash, 2002; Fox & Keteyian, 2000). Type I fibers are recruited first during muscle contraction, and are always active regardless of exercise intensity.Type IIA fibres are recruited next, and, with higher levels of exercise demand, type IIB are recruited. Type II fibers are typically recruited during tasks involving rapid effort, high power and high intensity (Fox, Keteyian, 2000; Gerdle et al., 1991).

Muscle strength is also influenced by the contractile and elastic structure of the muscle itself. The contractile units refer to the proteins of the functional units of the muscle, the sarcomeres, containing filaments of actin and myosin. An elastic component is present in the connective tissue sheaths surrounding the muscle (epimysium), the bundles of muscle fibers (perimysium) and the interior of the muscle fiber (endomysium), which join at their ends to form tendons. During concentric muscle contraction, there is a slip of actin filaments on the myosin filament; the filament length remains constant, but the muscle length decreases.

Instead, during the eccentric contraction, muscle length is increased. And during an isometric contraction, slippage of the contractile elements occurs and elastic strain arises, i.e., muscle work is performed, although there is no movement observed (Fox & Keteyian, 2000; Nordin & Frankel, 2001). Muscle strength depends on the length of the muscle. When the actin and myosin overlap along their entire lengths, the number of crossbridges reaches its maximum, allowing the muscle to generate maximum tension. The length at which force is produced with the greatest intensity varies between different muscles within a single individual, but does not change in the same muscle across different individuals (Mohamed et al., 2002; Nordin & Frankel, 2001).

In addition to the generation ofactive tension through the sliding of the filaments, there is the phenomenon of passive tension, which arises from the stretch of connective or elastic tissue (or elastic. As muscle length shortens, these passive elements become "loosened" and their contribution to muscle tension decreases gradually as tension subsides (Mohamed et al., 2002).

In addition to neural and muscular components there are biomechanical factors, which can influence muscle action of muscle without direct relationship to power generation. Such factors include angular variations of the joint and different types and levels of resistance that may be applied. In a biomechanical system involving two muscle segments and a joint, variation of joint angle determines the degree of mechanical advantage that a limb has when generating force. The perpendicular distance between the axis of the joint and tendon line of action defines this mechanical advantage. The outer lever refers to the distance between the joint axis and the point at which resistance is applied, and changes when the joint angle is modified. There are different types of overload that can be applied to a limb such as those produced by fixed weight, elastic resistance and isokinetic [isokinetic WHAT?]. The action of a muscle, of course, responds differently to each overload imposed. This answer depends on the multiplier or reducing effect of the internal and external lever system, as well as the speed of the gesture in question. These factors are all interconnected. The angular variation of the limb is directly related to the change in muscle length.

Knowing all the variables that can influence muscle strength, we are able to propose a model for its calculation. In this chapter we base the calculation of muscle strength to the quadriceps muscle during isometric and isotonic exercises, in the position showed in figure 2.

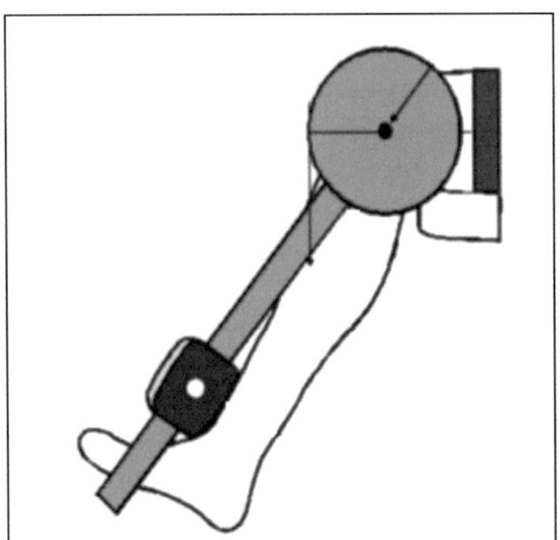

Fig. 2. Schematic diagram of the exercise. For the isometric contraction the movement occurs against a fixed resistance and for the isotonic the knee is able to execute the extension.

4. Experimental protocol

We will illustrate the lever model using the example of the quadriceps muscle. To calculate the strength of the quadriceps muscles, three steps are needed: i) a theoretical simulation of muscle force based on biomechanical models, ii) experimental testing to determine the curve of maximal isometric strength of knee extension as a function of joint angle, and iii) analysis of the internal relationship between muscle strength and the EMG signal during isometric and isotonic exercises. These steps will be detailed below:

4.1 Simulation of muscle strength

The adoption of an appropriate biomechanical model of the knee joint is essential to measure the forces transmitted by these muscles to the skeletal system. In the muscle model of Hill (Hof & Van Den Berg, 1981) force is described to be made up of three components: i) a parallel elastic component (PEC), which represents the elasticity of the passive elements of the muscles and ligaments ii) a contractile component (CC), which determines the behavior of active elements of the muscle, and iii) elastic components connected in series (SEC). These components should not be construed as if each one corresponds to a separate constituent of the muscle structure. Figure 3 shows a representation of the Hill model. The length of the elements is expressed by the relation:

$$x = l l0 \quad (2)$$

where l is the length at a given moment, and l_0 is the length in the resting position.

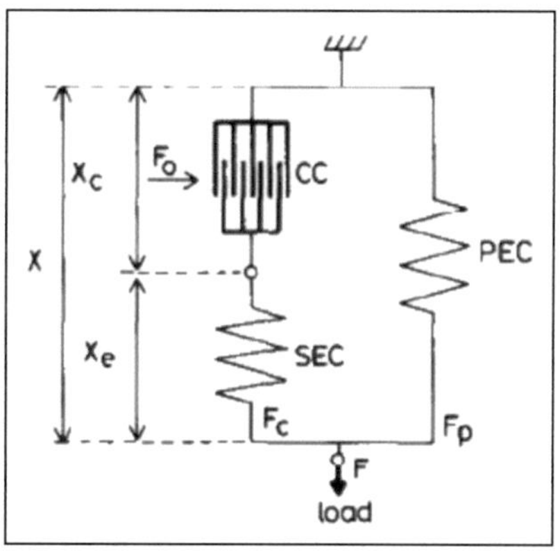

Fig. 3. Schematic diagram of Hill model.

The modeling of the motor unit will be discussed in a later section of this chapter. First we describe the contribution of contractile and passive components to force generation. The intensity of each component depends on the length of the muscle in a non-linear and non-monotonic way, as shown in Figure 3. Passive elastic force (curve 1, fig. 4) is exerted by the elastic components and contractile force is generated by the contractile proteins (curve 2, fig. 4). The sum of these two components produces the curve 3, which represents the overall strength of the muscle as a function of its length. The curve illustrates that maximum force is generated when the muscle is stretched to approximately 1.2 to 1.3 times its resting length. This position often coincides with the length of the muscle in a relaxed state. It appears that the anatomical architecture of the musculoskeletal system is organized for the benefit of the force-length relationships of the muscular system (Basmajian & De Luca, 1985).

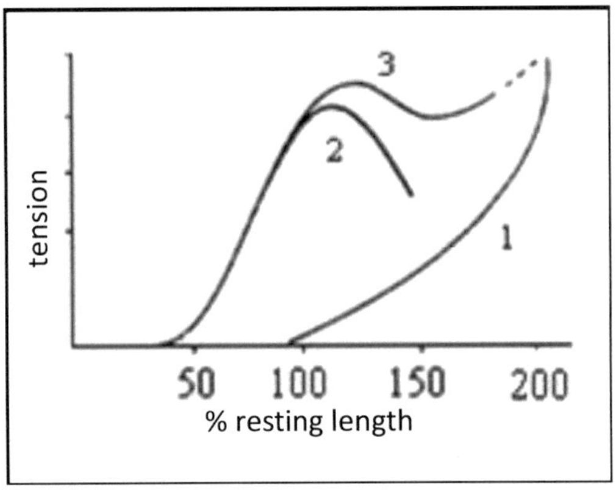

Fig. 4. Force-length curve for an isolated muscle.

In addition to length-dependent characteristics of strength, there are also speed-dependent properties. The ability to generate muscle force depends on the speed and type of contraction. Thus, movements in concentric, eccentric and isometric contractions illustrate important differences in force behavior (Figure 5) (Barbanti et al., 2002). The ability of a muscle to generate force is higher in an isometric situation (contraction velocity equal to zero) than in a concentric contraction, and this capacity decreases as the speed of contraction increases. The velocity of shortening that a muscle can produce is at its maximum when the external load is zero, but as the load increases, muscle shortening slows until the external load is equal to the maximum force that the muscle can exert (isometric contraction). If the load continues to increase even more, the muscle will contract eccentrically. During an eccentric contraction, the muscle can develop tension higher than in isometric contraction, and in this case the force increases with speed of muscle contraction (Barbanti et al., 2002; Nordin & Frankel, 2001).

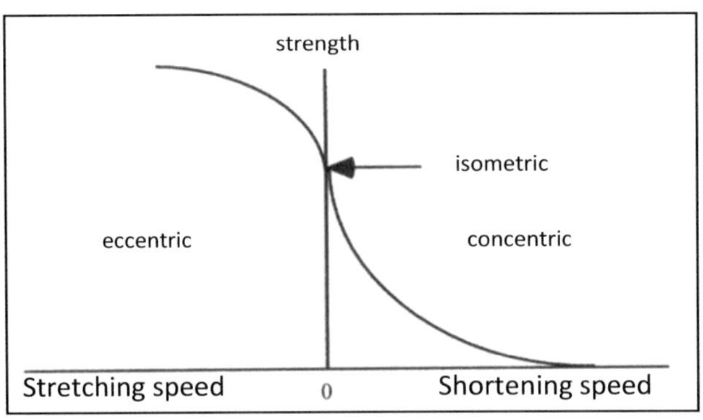

Fig. 5. Force-velocity curve for an isolated muscle.

An equation that describes the curves shown in figures 3 and 4 can be derived from the Hill model shown in figure 3. The force *F* that represents the total force generated by the muscle is given by:

$$F = Fc + Fp \tag{3}$$

where F_c is the contractile component in series and in the passive state (CC and SEC) and F_P is the force provided by parallel components (PEC).
As previously discussed, the force generated by the parallel components grows exponentially, so can be expressed by:

$$Fp(x) = Fpoep(x-1) \quad (4)$$

where x is the total length of the muscle, F_{P_0} and p the parameters of the exponent.
This relationship represents the properties of muscle, tendon, ligament and joint when a muscle is not active. Normally passive forces have significant values when the muscle is close to the greatest or smallest possible length . Contractile force, as discussed, depends on speed, and can be described by the following equations:

$$Fc= F0fxc-nvcb1+vcb, \text{ for } v_c 0 \quad (5)$$

$$Fc\leq(1+c)F0f(xc), \text{ for } v_c <0 \quad (6)$$

where v_c is the velocity of shortening of the muscle and x_c is the length of the contractile component shown in Figure 3, $f(x_c)$ is a function of normalization to values between 0 and 1 and F_0 is the F_c value when $f(x_c)$ is maximum. The F_c values decrease with increasing v_c for v_c>0 and the rate of decrease depends on the parameter b, while n defines the concavity of the curve. For values of v_c>0, the force F_c is greater than in the isometric case, where the difference is given by the parameter c.
Through these equations, it can be seen that the Hill model provides a very close representation of experimentally observed muscle behavior.
The muscle strength in the isometric activity, that is, when v_c is equal zero, can be seen from equations 4, 5 and 6. These equations can then be rewritten to reflect isometric contraction.

$$Fc = F0f(xC) \quad (7)$$

Then

$$F= F0fxC+ Fpoep(x-1) \quad (8)$$

In this last equation it can be observed that in isometric activity, muscle strength depends on the length of the muscle, and that the diagram from figure 2 is represented by $x = x_e + x_C$. Thus, it can be appreciated that during so-called isometric contractions there is actually considerable variation in the lengths of the contractile elements of the muscle(x_C).

4.2 Calculation of muscle strength (biomechanical models)

Several biomechanical models have been constructed to represent the performance of the musculoskeletal system in various situations of interest to sports, clinicians or others. The representations include two-dimensional approaches, to complex computer simulations that produce quantitative and three-dimensional visual representations. Currently available computing resources, including those intended for graphic animation, allow for the development of powerful tools for motion analysis. There are softwares that enable the user to develop detailed musculoskeletal models with representations of bones, muscles, ligaments and other structures. It is also possible to input experimental data regarding motion to some of these softwares, through direct or inverse dynamics, and to calculate muscle forces and visualize the geometric changes of the musculoskeletal system.

The relation between strength applied externally by a limb and the muscle strength is, however, not obvious. To illustrate, we will consider the calculation of quadriceps strength during leg extension (concentric contraction) in the sitting position, with an external resistance applied perpendicular to the leg. To calculate the strength, we use a simple two-dimensional model of the quadriceps. The free body diagram is shown in figure 6, where L_p is the length of the leg, L_{cm} the longitudinal position of the center of mass, F_{pl} the force applied to the tibial tuberosity through the patellar ligament, F_c the contact tibio-femoral force, γ the angle between the patellar ligament and the axis of the leg, θ the angle of the knee joint, W_p the weight of the leg and F_a the external force applied perpendicular to the limb.

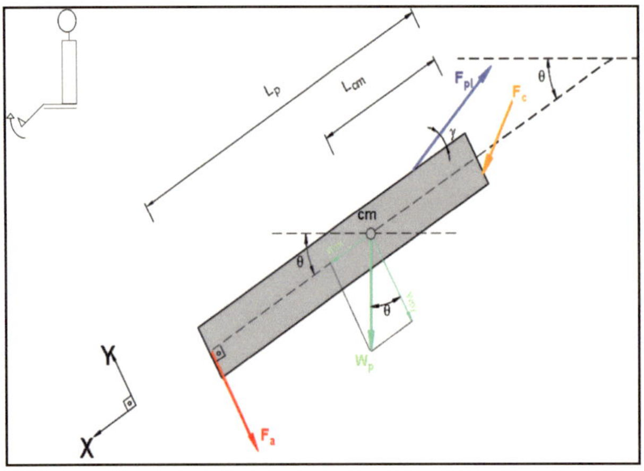

Fig. 6. Free body diagram representing the leg of a sitting person in a movement of concentric contraction of the quadriceps.

Through geometrical considerations illustrated in the free body diagram and calculation of torque, in which $\Sigma\tau = I\alpha$, and τ the torque, I the moment of inertia and α the angular acceleration, an equation can be written that defines the strength of the quadriceps muscle as a function of joint angle θ.

$$Fq = LpF\alpha + LcmWp\cos\theta + I\alpha RBm \quad (9)$$

In this equation, Fq is the force exerted by the quadriceps, I is the moment of inertia of the leg, α is the angular acceleration during exercise and Bm is the moment arm of force of the patellar ligament in relation to the point of tibiofemoral contact, around which the femur rotates. It must be recognizeded that the point of rotation changes as a function of the angle θ, and consequently the moment arm also changes. The relationship between the strength of the patellar ligament and the force exerted by the quadriceps is called R ($R = F_{pl}/F_q$) and also varies with the joint angle θ.

Figure 7 shows the strength of the quadriceps calculated for different forces applied perpendicular to the leg, considering a female individual, typical for the anthropometric model adopted (De Leva, 1996), with mass of 61.9 kg and height of 1.73 m. In these simulations using the values of R and Bm obtained by Van Eijden et al. (1986) and Kellis and Baltzopoulos (1999), respectively, the experimental condition assumed that the angular velocity was constant - W = ct and α = 0. The model was developed considering that the external force is always applied perpendicular to the limb and, therefore, remains constant. It can be observed that, while the leg moves a certain weight through the range of motion, the quadriceps displays variable strength. With this simple model, it is only possible to assess the strength of the muscle group, not each component part, (in this case, the vastus medialis, vastus lateralis, vastus intermedius and rectus femoris muscles).

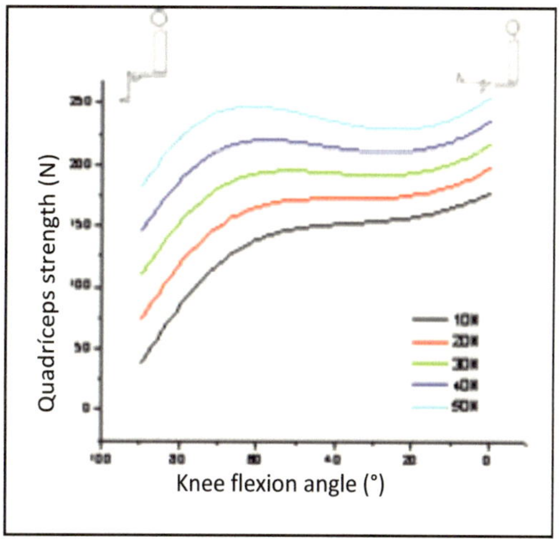

Fig. 7. Simulation of the quadriceps muscle strength in knee extension exercise in sitting position.

The maximum force that a limb is able to apply externally varies with angular position. This is because the geometrical arrangement determines the degree of mechanical advantage, and also because changes in muscle length alter the efficiency of muscle force generation, in addition to the the different contributions of different components of the muscle group. Figure 8 shows the maximum force applied externally by a leg during isometric contraction of the quadriceps. In the same graph the corresponding force generated by the quadriceps

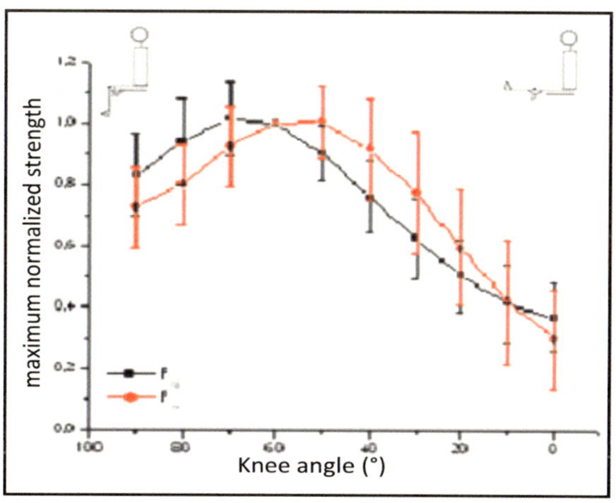

Fig. 8. Values of the applied force and muscle strength normalized as a function of the knee joint angle (average of 10 individuals).

muscle group is shown, calculated by the model (equation 9). The values are normalized by the strength at a 60º angle and were obtained from 10 female volunteers, with a mean age of 20.4 ± 1.6 years, mean weight of 51.15 ± 6.72 kg and mean height of 1.66 ± 0.05 m, during cued isometric contractions, with the maximum force defined as the greatest force exerted across three repetitions.

4.3 General considerations on the assessment of muscle strength

In the preceding sections, we have discussed aspects related to muscle force generation, presenting briefly the main factors - nerve, muscle and biomechanical - that determine the ability to generate muscle force. We have qualitatively discussed the participation of active and passive elements of muscle and shown that the force generated by a muscle can be represented by the Hill model. To understand the role of muscle force generation in movement, it is necessary to refer to biomechanical models. This was then demonstrated using a simple model of the quadriceps, in which we calculated the force exerted by this muscle when the leg applies an external force. Then, results were presented showing the maximum strength of the quadriceps as a function of joint angle in isometric contractions.
Starting from the theories of force generation in muscle fibers, it is not easy to understand the internal force exerted by a muscle, when it involves a complex articulation, such as the quadriceps. One very important consideration for health professionals involves the participation of each portion of the muscle in force generation as a function of angular position. For example, figure 9 shows how the different portions of quadriceps acting on the knee extension.

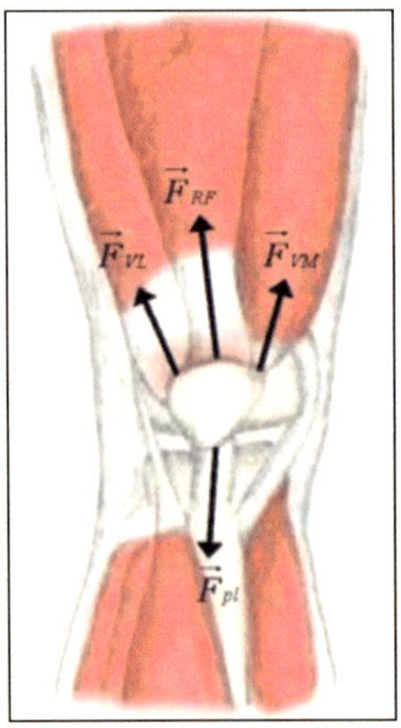

Fig. 9. Illustrative schema of how the forces of each portion of the quadriceps acts during the contraction.

The EMG signal is recorded by electrodes in response to muscle activity. As previously mentioned, skeletal muscle cells are formed by the muscle fibers, which constitute the structural contractile units. Each fiber, if excited, has the ability to stretch or contract. The activation of the muscle fiber by nerve endings induces two waves of depolarization that travel at a speed of 3 to 6m/s. The internal tissue is electrically conductive. Thus, electrical signals related to depolarization of the fiber can be recorded by electrodes on the skin or muscle.

Two events occur simultaneously during muscle contraction: one electrical and one mechanical. Depolarization releases calcium ions, which starts the process of contraction in the main body of the muscle fiber. But this contraction is much slower than the cycle of depolarization, which occurs over approximately 2 ms. Maximum forces are achiveved between 20 to 150ms after depolarization and then decaying gradually due to reabsorption of calcium. Consequently, it cannot be said that there is a direct relationship between EMG and force.

In muscle contraction, the degree of force can be controlled by changes in the number of recruited MUs or by changes in the frequency of recruitment. To increase the strength of a muscle the number of fibers recruited must increase one by one in order of size (size principle). After recruitment of all fibers, force can be further increased by increasing the frequency of activation. The EMG signal is a record of action potentials produced during a muscle contraction. The action potential motor unit (APMU) is the temporal and spatial summation of individual action potentials of all fibers of a MU. However, the catchment area of an electrode will often include more than one MU, because the muscle fibers of different MUs are interwoven throughout the muscle. Any portion of the muscle may contain fibers belonging to 20-50 MUs. An electrode located in this field will detect the algebraic sum of several APMUs within its catchment area. In order to maintain muscle contraction, the nervous system sends a sequence of stimuli, so that the MUs are activated repeatedly, resulting in a train of APMUs. The EMG signal is the superposition of the resulting space-time relationship of these trains, considering the number of MUs involved for maintenance and activation of muscle contraction.

4.4 Relationship between EMG and force

The relationship between force and surface EMG during voluntary contractions is not well understood. Some authors have concluded , for various muscles, that the magnitude of the EMG signal is directly proportional to muscle strength for isometric and/or isotonic contractions with constant speed, but others claim that this relationship is not linear (Bilodeau et al., 2003; Gerdle et al., 1991; Gregor et al., 2002; Herzog et al., 1998; Karlsson & Gerdle, 2001; Moritani & Muro, 1987; Onishi et al., 2000). In most cases, the EMG increases non-linearly with increasing force of muscle contraction (Guimaraes et al., 1994; Madeleine et al., 2000; Lawrence & De Luca, 1983; Solomonow et al., 1990). Theoretical analyses suggest that the amplitude of the signal in isometric contraction should increase with the square root of the force generated if the motor units are activated independently (Basmajian & De Luca, 1985; Lawrence & De Luca, 1983). This variety of different interpretations among researchers not surprising, given the inherent limitations of surface EMG. The measured force of muscle contraction is a result of the global activity of the underlying muscle fibers, and surface EMG provides information about the electrical activity of motor units located in the region near the electrode; in most experiments, the catchment area of the electrode does not extend sufficiently to detect the signal generated across the entire muscle volume (De Luca, 1997; Siegler et al., 1985).

Factors that prevent the direct quantification of muscle force from EMG signals include cross-talk, variations in the location of the recording electrodes and the involvement of synergistic muscles in force generation.

The electrical cross-talk of adjacent muscles is often considered as a possible factor that complicates the determination of the relationship between EMG and force. Its influence would manifest most prominently when the measured strength of the muscle increases. The presence of cross-talk is more dominant in smaller muscles where the electrodes (especially the surface) must be placed close to the adjacent musculature. The complexity of cross-talk is also determined by the anisotropy of muscle tissue and homogeneity of the tissues adjacent to the muscle. Often it is not possible to identify precisely the source of contamination of the physiological signal.

The degree of synergistic action of other muscle groups and the amounts of co-contraction between antagonistic muscle groups can change the contribution of muscle strength in research on the net force measured in the joint (Lawrence & De Luca, 1983). Ideally, in order to improve the EMG-force relationship, the muscle chosen should be the muscle uniquely responsible for generating the force measured (Bigland-Ritchie, 1981).

The relative location of fast and slow muscle fibers inside the muscle, and their distribution and location relative to the electrode are also factors to be considered. The amplitude of the action potential generated by a single muscle fiber is proportional to its diameter. Fast fibers generally have larger diameters and display a greater range of action potentials than slow fibers, and consequently generate a higher signal amplitude. However, the amplitude of the action potential, is a function of the distance between the active fibers and the recording electrodes, and the greater the distance, the lower the measured amplitude. The largest motor units, containing the largest diameter of fast twitch fibers are preferentially recruited at high force levels, according to the size principle (Henneman et al., 1965; Henneman & Olson, 1965). Thus, the relative location of fast muscle fibers in relation to the electrodes, determines how the electrical activity of these motor units affects the surface EMG signal (Basmajian & De Luca, 1985). It has been reported that muscles with homogeneous composition of fibers, such as the soleus of the cat, display a linear force-EMG relationship (Guimarães, 1994).

Figure 10 shows, as an example, an EMG signal picked up during a ramp isometric contraction (with slow growth to isometric force) in the vastus lateralis (VL), vastus medialis (VM) and rectus femoris (RF) muscles. The EMG signal shown –was passed througha third-order Butterworth filter, and band passed between 20 to 500 Hz during signal acquisition – but was otherwise unprocessed and therefore, it is called raw. The load shown in the figure refers to the external resistance applied to the leg. The signal intensity in the three muscles clearly increases with increasing external force. The questions that arise are: What is the relationship between force and EMG signal for each muscle? What treatment should be given to the EMG signal? What is the involvement of each muscle to form the resultant force? The following discussion seeks to bring some clarity to these issues.

In general, most studies involving the relationship between EMG and force aim to develop a noninvasive method to measure muscle strength during different actions. In experimental biomechanics there are different ways process of raw EMG signal and thus extract parameters related to the level of muscle contraction. Debate continues regarding the best signal processing techniques to use (Siegler et al., 1985). For example, one can find examples in the literature, in which strength has been related to the intensity, or to the median or mean frequency of the EMG signal.

Among the most used EMG parameters for such analysis, is the time series analysis, in which the the effective value of the signal, is derived from the root mean square - RMS (Basmajian & De Luca, 1985; Bigland-Ritchie, 1981; Bilodeau et al. 2003; Gerdle et al. 1991;

Gregor et al. 2002; Guimaraes et al. 1994; Herzog et al. 1998; Lawrence & De Luca, 1983; Madeleine et al., 2000; Onishi et al., 2000; Solomonow et al., 1990). This is a method to quantify the signal amplitude, recommended to assess the level of muscle activity, since the parameter is not affected by the superposition of APMU (Acierno et al., 1995; Basmajian & De Luca, 1985; De Luca, 1997). We have reported a positive correlation between this approach to parameter analysis and the strength of the quadriceps muscle in an isometric ramp task, suggesting that the coinciding increase in RMS and strength reflects two main mechanisms: the recruitment of new motor units and an increase in the frequency of active units firing (Bilodeau et al. 2003; Karlsson & Gerdle, 2001; Gerdle et al., 1991).

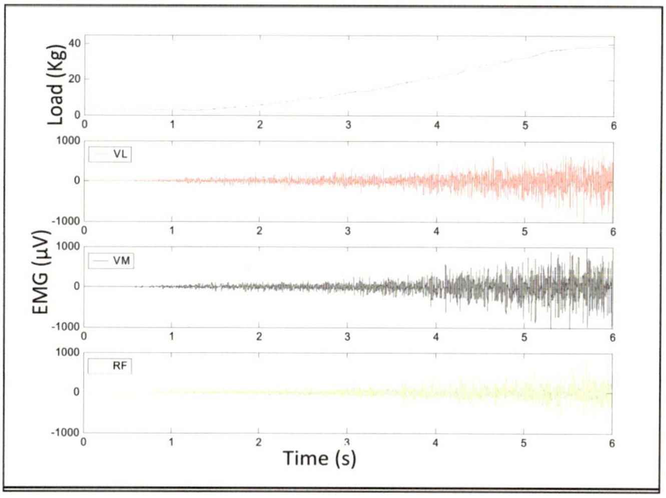

Fig. 10. EMG of the vastus medialis (VM), vastus lateralis (VL) and rectus femoris (RF) during a ramp contraction.

The normalization of the signal is a very important aspect in signal analyses displaying this relationship. A prominent feature of signal RMS is its variability, which makes it inherently difficult to compare signal amplitude across different individuals or even across different sessions within the same individual. To enable these comparisons, normalization processes are needed. The normalization process can be accomplished using a variety of reference methods. The most common example, which is standard in isometric exercises, is to express muscle contractions as a percent of the EMG amplitude observed in maximal voluntary isometric contraction (MVIC). It should however, be noted that in isotonic exercises, this process may lead to distortions, given that the muscle acts differently when changing the angular position of the limb, especially during maximal contraction. It is therefore essential to remember, that during isotonic exercise, there is an effect of changes in muscle length in electromyographic activity, as pointed out by Mohamed et al. (2002).

5. EMG x force analysis for the quadriceps

In this section we present an analysis of the EMG-force relationship for the quadriceps. This muscle is composed of four portions: rectus femoris (RF), vastus medialis (VM), vastus lateralis (VL) and vastus intermedious (VI); and the force applied to the patella is the result of the forces generated by each portion, therefore:

$$FVL+FVM+FRF+FVI=Fq \tag{10}$$

Where FVL is the force exerted by the VL, FVM is the force of VM, FRF is the force of RF, FVI is rhe force of VI and Fq is the resultant force of the quadriceps muscle group.
In figure 11 the forces that act on the quadriceps are illustrated. FVI is not presented because it is a deep muscle. (fig. 11.b).

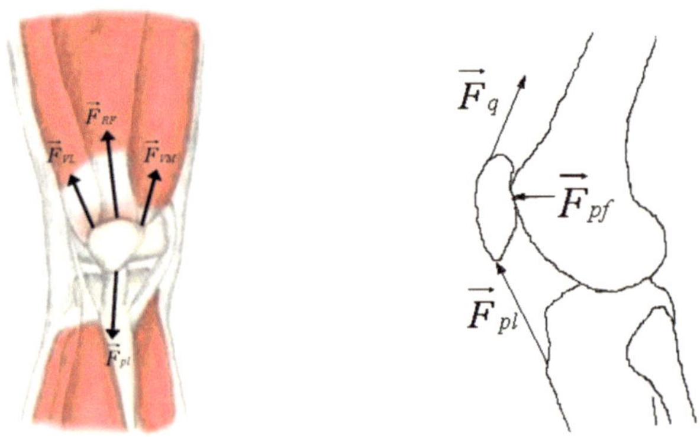

(a) (b)

Fig. 11. a) schematic representation of the forces involved in quadriceps action. b) Forces acting on the patella, whose fixation point varies with the knee angle. Fpl is the patellar tendon force, Fq is the resultant quadriceps force and Fpf is the tibiofemoral contact force.

Each muscle's contribution is different and depends on various factors. The EMG assessed during voluntary contractions provides a way to verify differences in the activation behavior of the different quadriceps portions (Pincivero et al., 2003). Studies have demonstrated that contraction of different muscle portions contraction is dependent on the contraction intensity. During isometric contractions of low to moderate intensity, the VL recruitment is significantly higher than VM and RF; the highest activation of the VM occurs close to maximum force levels, when EMG becomes equivalent to that of the VL and RF (Pincivero et al., 2003). However, we highlight that different studies show methodological variations, so it is difficult to compare results. It should be also considered that each muscle has distinct physiological and structural properties, and these morphological characteristics are altered with changes in muscle length. Each portion can present its greater length (where the greater force is generated) at different joint angles.
The physiological and structural properties and the morphological characteristics, altered with the change in muscle length, differ for each of the agonist muscles, in this case, the four portions that make up the quadriceps muscles. Taking into account that the magnitude of the overall strength of the quadriceps is the sum of the contribution of each component muscle, we can define an α relationship between the strength modules of each muscle and the overall strength of the muscle group.

$$\alpha VL=FVLFq \rightarrow FVL=\alpha VLFq \tag{11}$$

$$\alpha VM=FVMFq \rightarrow FVM=\alpha VMFq \tag{12}$$

$$\alpha RF=FRFFq \rightarrow FRF=\alpha RFFq \tag{13}$$

$$\alpha VI = FVIFq \rightarrow FVI = \alpha VIFq \tag{14}$$

It can be assumed that the intensity of EMG is related to the magnitude of the force generated (F), because the EMG signal is generated regardless of the direction and sense of strength. You can also define a function β representing the relationship between EMG and F for any muscle, such as:

$$\beta\theta,F,v,w = EMGF \tag{15}$$

Where $\beta(\theta, F, v, \omega)$ is the function that correlates EMG with the quadriceps total force.
In this expression we consider the explicit dependence of β with four variables: θ, the angular position; ω, the angular displacement speed of the member, given by w=dθdt; F, the intensity of muscle strength; and v, the velocity contraction which is related to the temporal variation of force (v∝dFdt). The dependence on these variables was noted in the previous discussions, experimental verification of the authors and the literature studies. The ability to generate muscle force depends on its length, and it varies with the angular position, justifying the dependence on θ and ω. The experimental results show that, even holding other variables constant, there is a dependence on the level of force F. It is also noted that the contraction velocity v is an important factor. The speed of contraction is related to the time necessary for the force range up to the level considered.
Based on the above discussion, it can be said that in an experimental situation in which the quantities θ, F, v and ω are known and held constant, there is a direct relationship between EMG and force given by β. Thus, for example, to the VL, we have:

$$EMGVL = \beta VL(\theta,F,v,w)FVL \tag{16}$$

Substituting eq.(16) in eq.(11):

$$EMGVL = \beta VL(\theta,F,v,w)\alpha VLFVL \tag{17}$$

Defining the product by α per $\beta(\theta, F, v, \omega)$ as $r(\theta, F, v, \omega)$, this product represents the function that correlates the overall strength of the quadriceps with the EMG signal portion of each muscle. Thus, to the VL, we have:

$$EMGVLFq = rVL(\theta,F.v,w) \tag{18}$$

In the same way, we can definethe r_{VM}, r_{RF} and r_{VI} for the other muscles. Although already discussed, it is important to emphasize that the angle θ is the variable that dependes on the initial condition of the muscle, including both length and tension. The value of the function r depends on the level of force, and this reflects recruitment strategies and types of fiber used by the muscle during low and high levels of force. Also very important are the dependencies of this function on muscle velocity and angular velocity of the limb. The first is related to the temporal variation of the force, while the second is related to the temporal variation of the angle.

5.1 Force and EMG in isometric contraction

The study of muscle strength using EMG has been applied more frequently and with greater success in isometric or in limited sectors of dynamic contractions that approximate the isometric condition (De Luca, 1997; Herzog et al. 1998 ; Lloyd & Besier, 2003).

In the particular case of isometric exercise, the function that correlates the overall strength of the quadriceps with the EMG signal can be expressed by equation 19, when the angle θ is constant and consequently w=dθdt=0. Thus, for the VL, we have:

$$EMGVLFq=rVL(\theta cte,F,v) \tag{19}$$

Although θ does not vary in the isometric case, the relationship between EMG and force must be different for each angle, and depends on the level of strength and speed of contraction. It is well documented that in isometric conditions the magnitude of EMG provides a reasonable estimate of the force exerted by the muscle. Basmajian and De Luca (1985) concluded that the relationship between the intensity of EMG signal and muscle force measured during an isometric contraction has considerable inter-subject variation and, moreover, the dependence of the type of muscle is almost linear for the small muscles of the hand and non-linear for larger limb muscles - this distinction in behavior may possibly reflect the difference in the properties of firing rate and recruitment of small and large muscles, as well as other anatomical and electrical considerations, including a dependence on the level of training.

The examples showed in this text are result of an evaluation with ten female subjects with no history of pain in the knee joint, 20.4 ± 1.6 years, 51.15 ± 6.72 kg and 1.66 ± 0.05 m. For the experiment was used a leg extension chair, a system of surface EMG with Ag/AgCl electrodes placed in the bellies of the VMO, VL and RF, with a gain of 20 times, CMRR greater than 80dB and impedance of 1012 Ω. Were also used a load cell type strain-gauge with a capacity of 5000N and an electrogoniometer.

Figure 12 shows a normalized EMG signal as a function of force. EMG data are normalized by the value obtained at maximal contraction and the force is normalized by the maximum

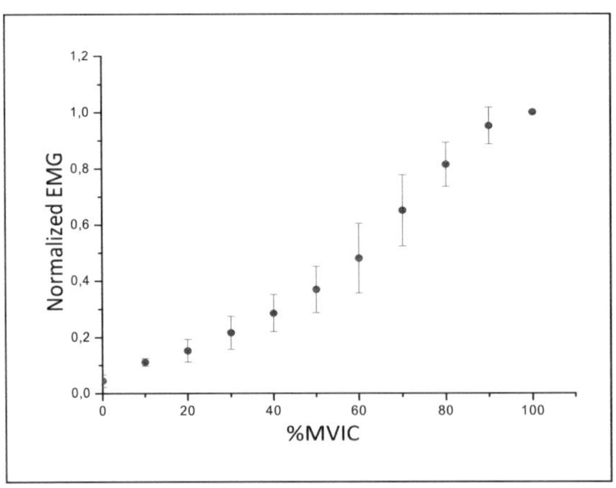

Fig. 12. Normalized EMG values of the vastus lateralis, measured isometrically in ramp at 20° of knee flexion.

force (MVIC). The illustrated values are the average of 10 subjects, and the EMG was obtained from the VL muscle. There is a positive correlation between EMG and force, as noted by Karlsson and Gerdle (2001), Gerdle et al. (1991) and Bilodeau et al. (2003). There are two regions that are clearly close to linear. A change in the slope of the force-EMG relationship is associated with a change in recruitment strategy; after full recruitment the frequency of activation is varied (Merletti & Parker, 2004).

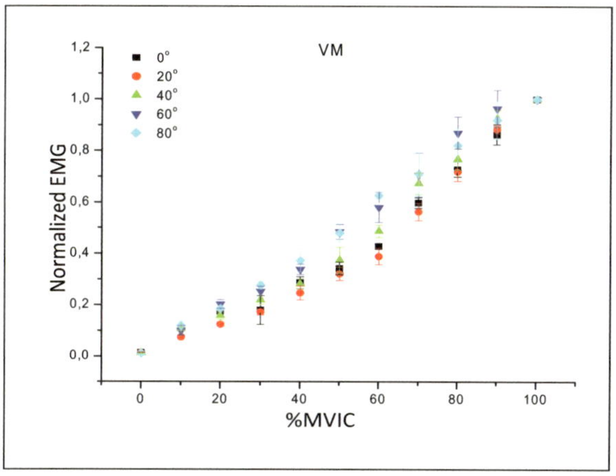

Fig. 13. Normalized EMG values of the vastus medialis, assessed isometrically in ramp at 0, 20°, 40°, 60° and 80° of knee flexion.

The same behavior is observed across different angles and muscles, but with different slopes, as shown in figure 13. In this figure, the data are for the VM muscle of a single volunteer. Although there is great variability, the dependence of the EMG values on the joint angle is clearly illustrated. This same behavior, with the same curves is observed in all subjects studied. Even in isometric exercise, keeping θ constant and ω=0, and the experimental care to keep v constant, the function $r(\theta_{ct}, F, v_{ct}, \omega=0)$ which relates the force with EMG still varies with the level of strength, which in fact can be seen in figure 12.

5.2 EMG in MVIC

The maximum isometric contraction is always taken as an individual reference, especially for the normalization of EMG signals. In Figure 8, we showed that the maximum force that the individual can exert with the leg, in isometric contractions of the quadriceps, as well as the maximum force of quadriceps, varies with joint angle. Figure 14 shows the corresponding normalized EMG signal from an individual, for the three portions analyzed. It appears that the EMG signal as well as the relationship between EMG and force, when the individual generates full force, and the maximum force all change as a function of joint angle. Therefore, the results of studies in which normalization has been performed at different angles are not easily comparable.

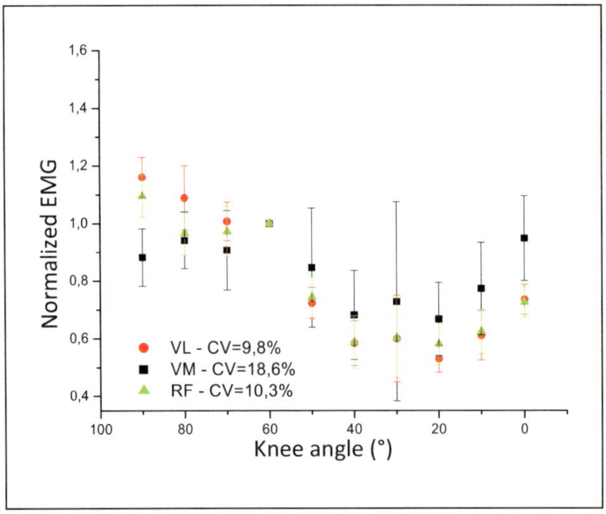

Fig. 14. EMG values during MVIC as a function of joint angle, for an individual, where VL: vastus lateralis, VM: vastus medialis and RF: rectus femoris.

5.3 Comparison of EMG with the force calculated by the model

As shown in the Hill model, even when there is an isometric contraction, there is a change in muscle length. This is important; in equation 20, it can be seen that there is a dependency between the EMG-force relationship and contraction velocity. These two aspects are equivalent, because the change in muscle length predicted by the Hill model in the isometric case, has a direct correlation with contraction velocity. The results presented in this section were all obtained at about the same rate of growth of the force ramp, i,e., at the same contraction velocity, so the function β for each angle is the same.

The graphs in figures 12 and 13 show EMG normalized according to MVIC versus isometric force normalized across the maximum force. Here we can see that force is that which was applied externally, that is, the force that the leg applies in the experimental system, rather than the quadriceps force, as shown in equation 19. Although a linear relationship is shown, this is not a causal relationship. When considering the strength of the quadriceps as the model predicts, we must also consider individual variations such as size and weight of the leg, and these may be more or less significant for the different component muscles.

The same EMG data from figures 12 and 13, when plotted as a function of the quadriceps muscle strength normalized by the maximum - as shown in Figures 15 and 16, show a change in slope, which differs from angle to angle. This is because, for the same applied force, the force that develops in the quadriceps is different for every angle, as already mentioned.

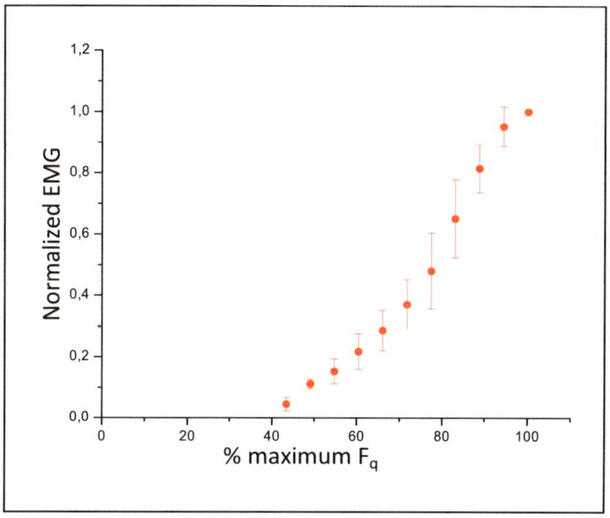

Fig. 15. Normalized EMG values of vastus lateralis in function of the percentage of quadriceps force, asssessed isometrically in ramp, in 20° of knee flexion.

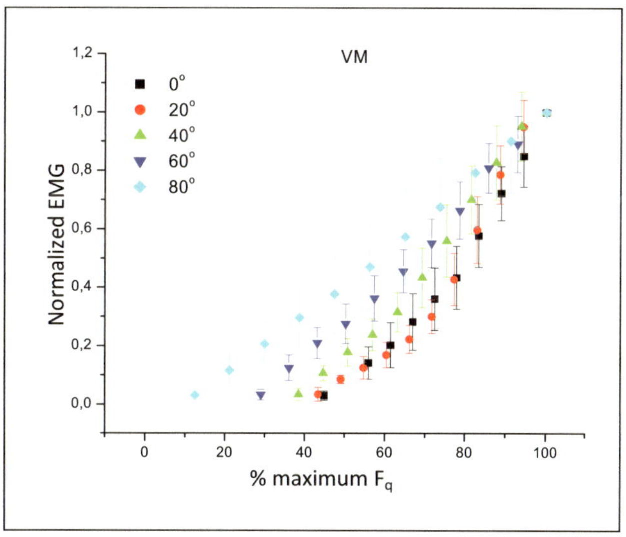

Fig. 16. Normalized EMG values of vastus medialis in function of the percentage of quadríceps force, assessed isometrically in ramp, in 0, 20°, 40°, 60° and 80° of knee flexion.

In the literature, the EMG has been compared to the applied force or torque. As in the preceding discussion, even if a coherent relationship is shown, it cannot be considered causal, because the EMG is generated by the muscle strength and is not related to the biomechanical parameters of the joint.

5.4 Isotonic contractions

In dynamic contractions, the relationship between EMG and force has a greater complexity due to experimental and physiological characteristics. A movement implies change in joint angle over which the muscle acts. Angular displacement can change the muscle geometry, and then the relative positions between the active motor units and surface electrodes may change (Basmajian & De Luca, 1985; Doorenbosch & Harlaar, 2004).

The complexity of the EMG-force relationship in an isotonic contraction can be understood through the function $r(\theta, F, \nu, \omega)$, where θ, F, ν e ω are varied simultaneously. Therefore, to quantitatively assess the strength of isotonic contractions, in addition to the experimental care with the placement of the electrodes and movement of the skin, should be restricted to the situation that is closest to an isometric contraction. In fact, it is desirable to minimize the effect of each variable. Thus, we recommend the use of low levels of force, and control of the application of force during movement in order to limit variation in this parameter (F~ct), which is important to ν exert little influence on r, and impose a lower angular velocity (w~0).

6. Other instrumental tools and applications

To obtain the data presented in this chapter, the relationship between electromyography and strength in the quadriceps muscle was evaluated through conventional measures, using a differential EMG electrode placed on the skin. As discussed above, there is a limitation in these measures arising from the fact that the EMG signal recorded is the sum of action potentials occurring in the area of the electrode.. Studies show that the use of electrode arrays significantly improves the ability to estimate force with EMG measures. An interesting example of such analysis can be seen in Staudenmann et al. (2006) who employed multivariate statistical analysis of principal components.

Although this chapter has discussed the measurement of muscle strength by measuring EMG, it can be said that most applications of EMG are related to some aspect of muscle force generation, because the signal is generated when muscle contractile elements are activted. In this respect, it is pertinent to mention other methods, such as: i) the use of PCA (principal component analysis) to identify the pulse trains of action potentials on a surface electromyography signal collected with multiple electrodes (Nakamura et al., 2004); ii) application of multivariate statistical techniques and multidimensional visualization in 3D space - Viz3D (Artero, 2005), to identify differences between isometric activities carried out against a rigid obstacle and with a weight of equivalent inertial load (Mello, 2007); iii) applications in studies of muscle coordination, techniques that allow, through measures of EMG, set parameters for determining the action of various muscles; and iv) studies of the relationship between force sensation and muscle stretching (Branco et al., 2006).

The magnitude of force or torque has also been compared with the spectral variables of the EMG signal (Bernardi et al., 1996, Bilodeau et al., 2003; Gerdle et al., 1991; Hermans et al., 1999; Karlsson & Gerdle, 2001; Moritani & Muro, 1987; Onishi et al., 2000). The calculation of these parameters should involve the application of appropriate techniques to obtain the power spectrum of the EMG signal. The parameters obtained in the frequency domain involves more complex procedures than those for the time domain, being the spectral distribution obtained by the fast Fourier transform or discrete Fourier transform (Bendat Piersol, 1986). Recent studies show the technique of wavelet transform as a very interesting tool for analysis in the frequency domain.

7. Conclusion

In this chapter, we have explored the relationship between EMG signals and muscle strength calculated using biomechanical models. In the literature, a common approach has been to adjust the intensity of EMG using equations derived from the Hill model. It has also been shown that the application of EMG to measure the force requires a process of calibration parameters for each individual. This process of calibration and standardization should be conducted having enough control of the variables that influence the relationship between EMG and force, as specified in equation 13.

The relationship between electrical activity and isometric muscle strength has been the focus of research since the 1950s. However, we still lack consensus regarding a precise methodology that can be widely used to quantify muscle strength based on EMG. The use of EMG as a metric for determining the force is both fascinating, and challenging. It is fascinating because of the possibilities for making a quantitative measure of strength in an individual while performing a gesture, through noninvasive surface electrodes. It is challenging in view of the complexity and variability inherent in biological signals, especially in dynamic situations. However, the application of current equipment for collecting and processing the signal remains the motivation for the use of EMG as a metric measure of force. The study of this issue, using methodologies that combine calibration processes or normalize instrumental resources, including arrays of electrodes, and signal processing using multivariate statistical techniques (PCA), can provide great advances.

8. References

Acierno, SP; Baratta, RV; Solomonow, M. (1995). *A practical guide to electromyography for biomechanists*, Bioengineering Laboratory/LSUMC Department of Orthopaedies, Louisiana.

Amadio, AC, Duarte M. (1996). *Fundamentos biomecânicos para análises do movimento humano.* Laboratório de Biomecânica/EEFE-USP, São Paulo.

Amadio, AC, Barbanti, VJ. (2000). *A biodinâmica do movimento humano e suas relações interdisciplinares*, Estação Liberdade, ISBN 85-7448-019-3, São Paulo.

Artero AO. (2005). *Estratégias para apoiar a detecção de estruturas em visualizações multidimensionais perceptualmente sobrecarregadas*, Instituto de Ciências Matemáticas e de Computação/ICMC, USP, São Carlos.

Barbanti, VJ et al. (2002). *Esporte e atividade física: interação entre rendimento e saúde* (1), Manole, ISBN 8520413889, São Paulo.

Basmajian, JV; De Luca, CJ. (1985). *Muscles alive: their functions revealed by electromyography* (5), Williams and Wilkins, ISBN 068300414X, Baltimore.

Bendat, JS; Pierson, AG. (1986). Decomposition of wave-forces into linear and nonlinear components. *Journal of Sound and Vibration*, Vol.106, No.3, May.1986, pp.391-408, ISSN 0022-460X.

Bernardi, M et al. (1996). Motor unit recruitment strategy changes with skill acquisition. *European Journal Applied Physiology*, Vol. 74, No. 1, Aug. 1996, pp. 52-59, ISSN 1439-6319.

Bigland-Ritchie, B. (1981). EMG/force relations and fatigue of human voluntary contractions. *Exercise Sport and Science Reviews*, Vol.9, pp.75-117, ISSN 1538-3008.

Bilodeau, M. et al. (2003). EMG frequency content changes with increasing force and during fatigue in the quadriceps femoris muscle of men and women. *Journal of Electromyography and Kinesiology*, Vol.13, No.1, Feb. 2003, pp.83-92, ISSN 1050-6411.

Branco VR. Et al. (2006). relação entre a tensão aplicada e a sensação de desconforto nos músculos isquiotibiais durante o alongamento. Revista Brasileira de Fisioterapia, Vol.10, No.4, Dez.2006, pp.465-472, ISSN 1413-3555.

De Leva, P. (1996). Adjustments to Zatsiorsky-Seluyanov´s segment inertia parameters. *Journal of Biomechanics*, Vol.29, No.9, Sept. 1996, pp.1223-1230, ISSN 0021-9290.

De Luca, CJ. (1997). The use of surface electromyography in biomechanics. *Journal of Applied Biomechanics*, Vol.13, No.2, May. 1997, pp.135-163, ISSN 1065-8483.

Doorenbosch, CAM.; Harlaar, J. (2004). Accuracy of practicable EMG to force model for knee muscles: short communications. *Neuroscience Letters*, Vol.368, No.1, Sept. 2004, pp.78-81, ISSN 0304-3940.

Fox, E.; Foss, ML.; Keteyian, SJ. (2000). Bases fisiológicas do exercício e do esporte (6), Guanabara-Koogan, ISBN 8527705303, Rio de Janeiro.

Gerdle, B. et al. (1991). Dependence of the mean power frequency of the electromyogram on muscle force and fibre type. *Acta Physiologica Scandinavica*, Vol.142, No.4, Aug. 1991, pp.457-465, ISSN 0001-6772.

Gregor, SM. et al. (2002). Lower extremity general muscle moment patterns in healthy individuals during recumbent cycling. *Clinical Biomechanics*, Vol.17, No.2, Feb. 2002, pp.123-129, ISSN 0268-0033.

Guimarães, AC. et al. (1994). EMG-force relationship of the cat soleus muscle studied with distributed and non-periodic stimulation of ventral root filaments. *Journal of Experimental Biology*, Vol.186, No.1, Jan.1994, pp.75-93, ISSN *0022-0949*.

Hermans, V.; Spaepen, AJ.; Wouters, M. (1999). Relation between differences in electromyographic adaptations during static contractions and the muscle function. *Journal of Electromyography and Kinesiology*, Vol.9, No.4, Aug. 1999, pp.253-261, ISSN 1050-6411.

Henneman, E.; Somjen, G.; Carpenter, DO. (1965). Functional significance of cell size in spínal motoneurons. *Journal of Neurophysiology*, Vol.28, May. 1965, pp.560-580, ISSN *0022-3077*.

Henneman, E.; Olson, CB. (1965). Relations between structure and function in the design of skeletal muscles. *Journal of Neurophysiology*, Vol.28, May. 1965, pp.581-598, ISSN *0022-3077*.

Herzog, W. et al. (1998). EMG-force relation in dynamically contracting cat plantaris muscle. *Journal of Eletromyography and Kinesiology*, Vol.8, No.3, June 1998, pp.147-155, ISSN 1050-6411.

Hof, AL.; Van Den Berg, JW. (1981). EMG to force processing I: an electrical analogue of the hill muscle model. *Journal of Biomechanics*, Vol.14, No.11, pp.747-758.

Karlsson, S.; Gerdle, B. (2001). Mean frequency and signal amplitude of the surface EMG of the quadriceps muscles increase with increasing torque – a study using the continuous wavelet transform. *Journal of Eletromyography and Kinesiology*, Vol.11, No.2, Apr. 2001, pp.131-140, ISSN 1050-6411.

Kellis, E.; Baltzopoulos, V. (1999). The effects of the antagonist muscle force on intersegmental loading during isokinetic efforts of the knee extensors. *Journal of Biomechanics*, Vol.32, No.1, Jan. 1999, pp.19-25, ISSN 0021-9290.

Lawrence, JH.; De Luca, CJ. (1983). Myoelectric signal versus force relationship in different human muscles. *Journal of Applied Physiology*, Vol.54, No.6, June. 1983, pp.1653-1659, ISSN. *8750-7587.*

Lippold, OCJ. (1952). The relation between integrated action potentials in a human muscle and its isometric tension. *The Journal of Physiology*, Vol. 117, pp. 492-499, ISSN *1469-7793.*

Lloyd, DG.; Besier, TF. (2003). An EMG-driven musculoskeletal model to estimate muscle forces and knee joint moments in vivo. *Journal of Biomechanics*, Vol.36, No.6, June 2003, pp.765-776, ISSN 0021-9290.

Mohamed, O.; Perry, J.; Hislop, H. (2002). Relationship between wire EMG activity, muscle length and torque of the hamstrings. *Clinical Biomechanics*, Vol.17, No.8, Oct. 2002, pp.569-576, ISSN 0268-0033.

Moritani, T.; Muro, M. (1987). Motor unit activity and surface electromyogram power spectrum during increasing force of contraction. *European Journal of Applied Physiology*, Vol.56, No.3, May 1987, pp.260-265, ISSN 1439-6319.

Madeleine, P. et al. (2000). Mechanomyography and electromyography force relationships during concentric, isometric and eccentric contractions. *Journal of Electromyography and Kinesiology*, Vol.10, No.1, Feb. 2000, pp.33-45, ISSN 1050-6411.

Mello EM. (2006). *Estudo da atividade mioelétrica em exercícios isométricos com diferentes contrações*, Programa de Pós-Graduação Interunidades Bioengenharia, USP, São Carlos.

Merletti, R.; Knaflitz, M.; De Luca, CJ. (1990). Myoelectric manifestations of fatigue in voluntary and electrically elicited contractions. *Journal of Applied Physiology*, Vol.69, No.5, Nov. 1990, pp.1810-1820, ISSN *8750-7587.*

Nakamura H. et al. (2004). The application of independent component analysis to the multi-channel surface electromyographic signals for separation of motor unit action potential trains: part I - measuring techniques. *Journal of Electromyography and Kinesiology*, Vol.14, No.4, Aug. 2004, pp. 423-432, ISSN 1050-6411.

Nordin, M.; Frankel, VH. (2001). *Biomecânica básica do sistema musculoesquelético* (3), Guanabara-Koogan, ISBN 852770823X, Rio de Janeiro.

Onishi, H. et al. (2000). Relationship between EMG signals and force in human vastus lateralis muscle using multiple bipolar wire electrodes. *Journal of Electromyography and Kinesiology*, Vol.10, No.1, Feb.2000, pp.59-67, ISSN 1050-6411.

Pincivero, DM. et al. (2003). Knee extensor torque and quadriceps femoris EMG during perceptually-guided isometric contractions. *Journal of Electromyography and Kinesiology*, Vol.13, No.2, Apr. 2003, pp.159-167, ISSN 1050-6411.

Rash, GS. (2002). *Electromyography fundamentals.* Gait and Clinical Movement Analysis Society. Disponível em:<www.gcmas.org>. Acesso em: 17/10/05.

Siegler, S. et al. (1985). Effect of myoeletric signal processing on the relationship between muscle force and processed EMG. *American Journal of Physical Medicine*, Vol.64, No.3, pp.130-149, ISSN 0002-9491.

Solomonow, M. et al. (1990). The EMG-force relationship of skeletal muscle dependence on contraction rate, and motor units control strategy. *Electromyography and Clinical Neurophysiology*, Vol.30, No.3, Apr. 1986, pp.141-152, ISSN. 0301-150X.

Staudenmann D. et al. (2006). Improving EMG-based muscle force estimation by using a high-density EMG grid and principal component analysis. IEEE TRANSACTIONS

ON BIOMEDICAL ENGINEERING, Vol.53, No.4, Apr. 2006, pp.712-719, ISSN 0018-9294.

Van Eijden, TMGJ. et al. (1986). A mathematical model of the patellofemoral joint. *Journal of Biomechanics*, Vol.19, No.3, pp.219-229, ISSN 0021-9290.

Whiting, WC.; Zernicke, RF. (2001). *Biomecânica da lesão muscuesquelética* (1). Guanabara-Koogan, ISBN 852770630X, Rio de Janeiro.

4

Electromyography in Myofascial Syndrome

Juhani Partanen
University Hospital of Helsinki
Department of Clinical Neurophysiology
Finland

1. Introduction

Myofascial syndrome is a muscular pain syndrome with regional symptoms, often in limb girdle or neck and back area. It is common and causes much disability and inability to work. Myofascial pain may be activated by precision work, repetitive strain or recent injury. Typical findings in symptomatic muscles are taut bands and painful trigger points (TrPs), where pressure elicites a typical spreading of pain (Cummings & Baldry, 2007). Microdialysis of TrPs has detected local elevation of contraction, and inflammatory and pain metabolites (Shah et al., 2008). Reduced high-energy phosphate levels but no signs of myositis have observed in painful muscles in histological studies (Bengtsson et al., 1986).

2. Electromyography of trigger points

There are several studies of EMG in TrPs. There is no sustained spontaneous activation of motor unit potentials (MUPs) (spasticity) or any signs of denervation i.e. fibrillation potentials or motor unit potential alterations typical for nerve sprouting (Couppé et al., 2001).

2.1 Spontaneous electrical activity at the endplate

When EMG in TrPs is compared to EMG in painless points of the same or other muscle, there are some differences. TrPs show more numerous local findings of spontaneous electrical activity (SEA) than control points (Couppé et al., 2001). SEA may consist of endplate activity which is reflected in two forms, often activated together: endplate noise (EPN) (miniature end plate potentials MEPPs) and end plate spikes (EPS). In EPN there are either small, discrete high-frequency depolarizations rarely exceeding 100 µV (MEPPs) or just "sea shell" noise, depending on the orientation and localization of the needle electrode with respect to the source (Wiederholt, 1970). It was also claimed that EPN is more prevalent in TrPs within the end plate zone and more prevalent in active than latent TrPs (Simons et al., 2002). End plate spikes are larger in amplitude than MEPPs, exceeding even several hundred microvolts. EPSs are usually observed together with EPN (Fig. 1).

EPSs have a characteristic irregular firing pattern with numerous short intervals less than 30 ms. Thus it is easy to distinguish EPSs from other spontaneous EMG patterns or MUPs. In addition, EPSs have a characteristic wave form with initial negativity or with a short (less than 0,3 ms) initial positivity. Rarely, EPSs with a typical firing pattern but a large polyphasic waveform may be observed (Partanen, 1999).

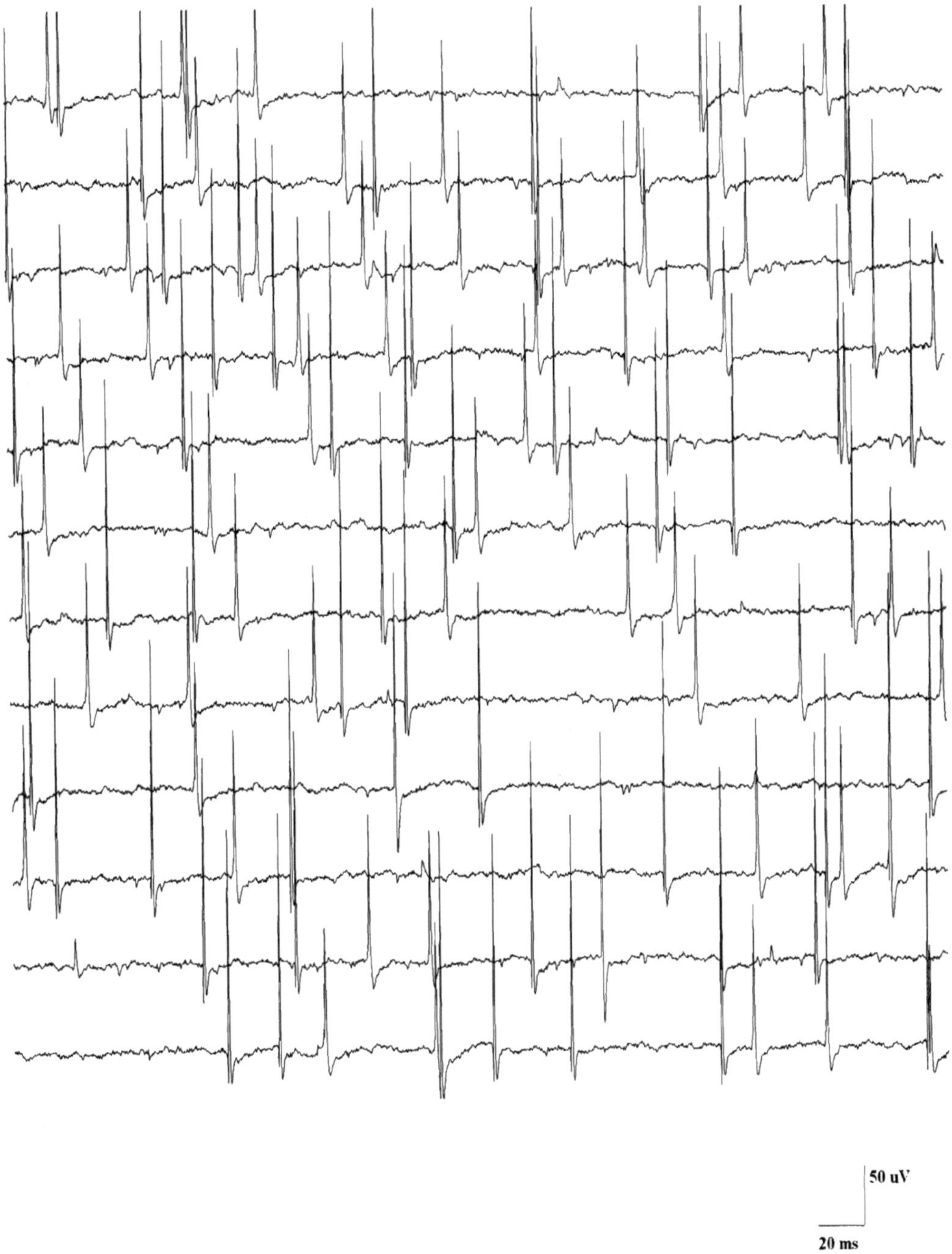

Fig. 1. Several sequences of end plate spikes in an active spot of a normal relaxed muscle. Most of them have a negative onset but some have a short initial positive component. Observe also the end plate noise in the background. From Pathophysiology, with permission.

2.2 Complex repetitive discharge

Another spontaneous waveform, which is repeatedly found in taut bands is complex repetivite discharge (CRD) (Fig. 2). It was originally described by Janet Travell in TrPs

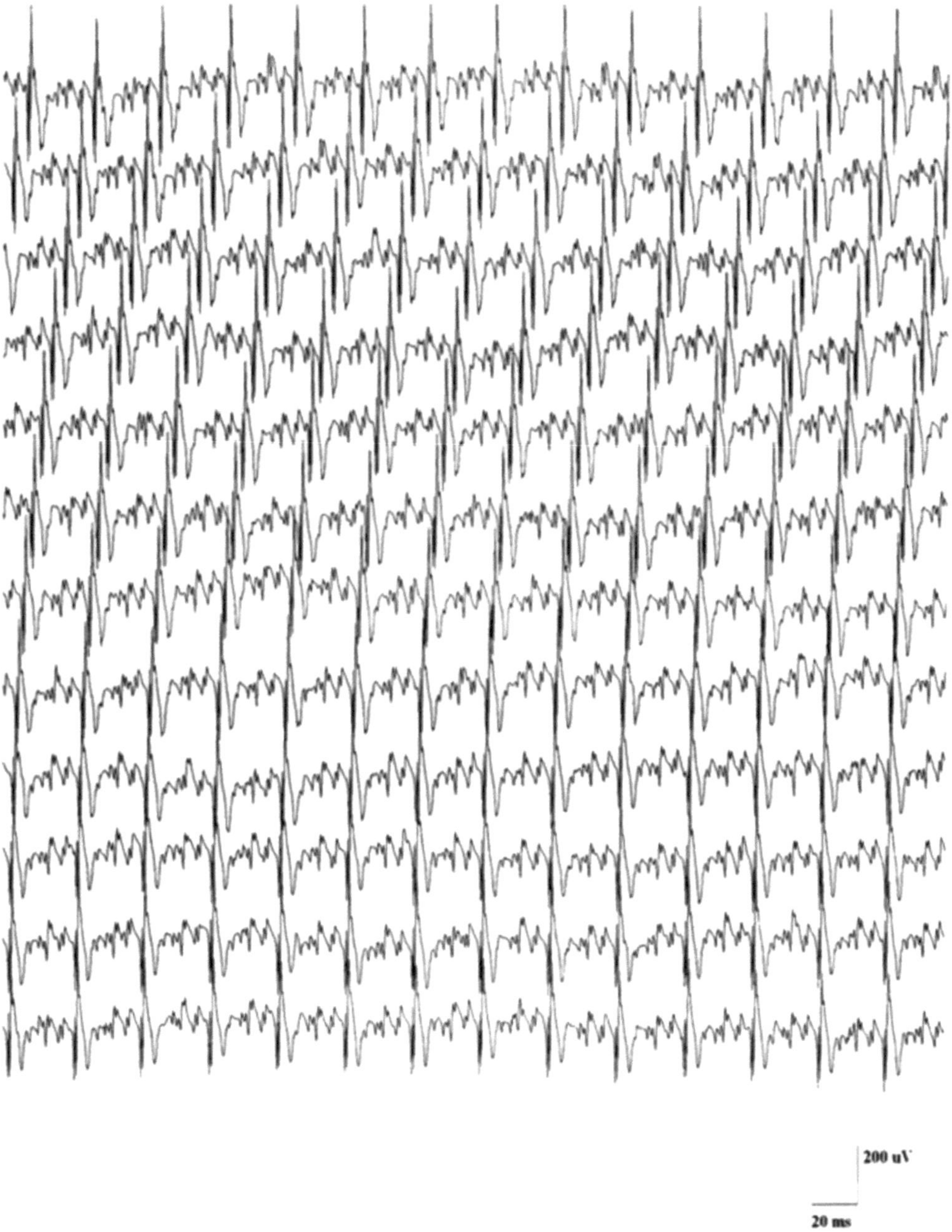

Fig. 2. Complex repetitive discharge (33 Hz) in a taut band of the levator scapulae muscle of a patient suffering from myofascial syndrome. Otherwise the needle EMG was normal. From Pathophysiology, with permission

(Travell, 1957) but later on it was depicted in about 15% of patients suffering from myofascial syndrome (Ojala et al., 2006). CRD has been observed in several types of chronic neuropathy or myopathy (Emeryk et al., 1974a), but in these cases CRD is accompanied by other pathological alterations in EMG. In myofascial syndrome CRD is observed in muscles with otherwise normal EMG (Ojala et al., 2006).

3. Prevailing hypotheses of the origin of EPN, EPS and CRD

EPN and MEPPs are observed to originate from the postsynaptic surface of the neuromuscular junction. MEPPs are activated by spontaneous leakage of small amounts of acetycholine (exocytosis) from the nerve terminal. MEPPs are local, non-propagated discrete depolarizations of muscle membrane. MEPPs should be found mainly at the end plate zone of the muscle, where neuromuscular junctions are localized. EPSs are supposed to be elicited by summation of a number of MEPPs, if the sum potential exceeds the critical level to fire an action potential (Buchthal & Rosenfalck, 1966). Another explanation is a nerve potential activated by the irritation caused by the EMG needle electrode. The nerve potential then travels to the nerve terminal and activates a postsynaptic action potential which is recorded with the same EMG needle as an EPS (Dumitru, 1995). CRD is supposed to arise when an action potential is circulating in muscle fibres, leaping from one fibre to another with ephaptic conduction, forming eventually a vicious cycle with sustained circulation of action potentials (Trontelj & Stålberg, 1983). The participation of motor neurone and even "spindelisation" of extrafusal muscle fibres due to changed innervation was also discussed (Emeryk et al., 1974b).

4. Discussion of the discrepancies of prevailing hypotheses for EPS and CRD and suggestions for new explanations

Even if mechanical irritation of nerve terminal may cause marked increase of the frequency of MEPPs, there are no data demonstrating that this may cause activation of postsynaptic action potentials of the muscle fibre, recorded as EPSs. The mechanical irritation of the terminal motor nerve branch by the needle electrode may cause injury potential and rarely rhythmic spontaneous activity but sustained irregular firing has not been described in experimental studies (Wall et al., 1974). Thus the firing pattern of EPSs clearly differs from the known patterns of injury potentials (Macefield, 1998). CRDs are not found in totally denervated muscles (personal observation). Thus, evidently CRD needs the presence of intramuscular motor axons. In fact, CRD in myofascial syndrome may represent activation of a spinal reflex arch, instead of an ephaptic circuit of muscle fibres (see Heading 7).
The third explanation for EPSs is that they are action potentials of intrafusal muscle fibres. There are several points which suggest this possibility, for example activation of EPSs by passive stretching of the muscle (Partanen, 1999; Partanen & Nousiainen, 1983).

5. Multi-channel recordings of EPSs

Different patterns of propagation of EPSs may be observed with multi-channel recording of EPSs in relaxed human muscles, using 3-5 EMG needles in parallel with the muscle fibres (Fig 3).

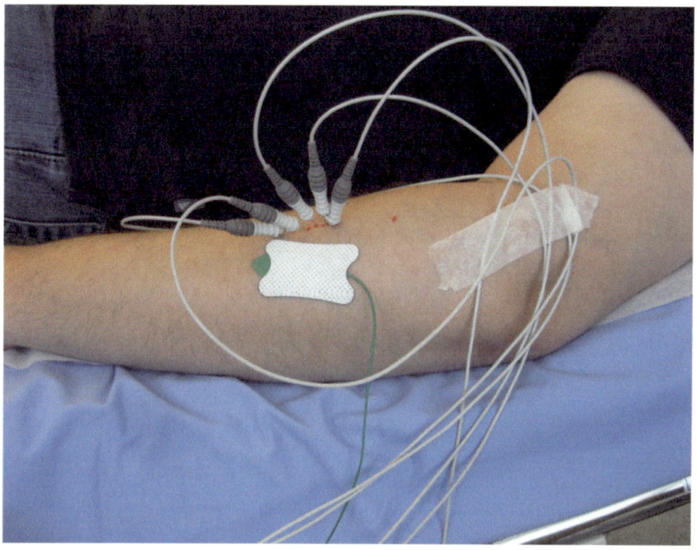

Fig. 3. A five-channel recording of the extensor carpi radialis muscle. The EMG needles are lying in parallel with the muscle fibres and the interelectrode distance is 3 mm.

The first type of EPSs does not propagate at all: there are local large potentials (Fig. 4). The second type of EPSs propagates for a short distance (a few mm) (Fig. 5) and third type propagates like a motor unit potential (Fig. 6-7). The first type may reflect activity of intrafusal nuclear bag fibres, which show this non-propagating junctional potential pattern in experimental recordings (Barker et al., 1978). The second type of EPS with a short propagation

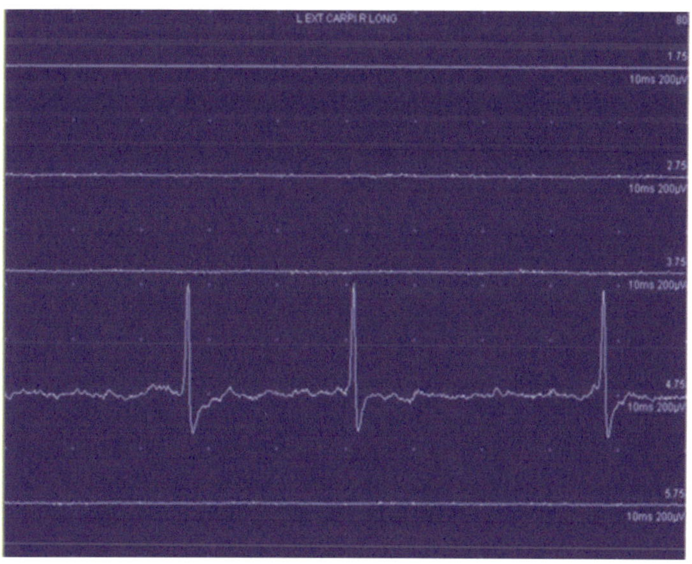

Fig. 4. An end plate spike sequence in channel 4. It does not propagate at all. It was not possible to find synchronous potentials in any of the other channels. End plate spikes may represent activation of a nuclear bag muscle fibre. Calibration 10 ms, 200 μV.

distance is in concert with the activity of nuclear chain fibres (Barker et al., 1978) and the third type corresponds to the activity of beta motor units (Partanen, 1999; Partanen & Palmu, 2009).

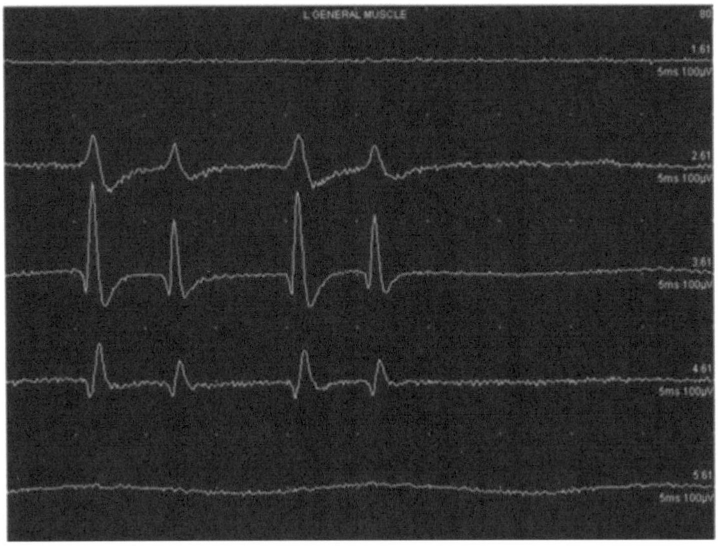

Fig. 5. Sequence of end plate spikes propagating from channel 2 to channel 4 (note the development of positive onset). This sequence may represent activation of nuclear chain muscle fibres. Calibration 5 ms, 100 μV.

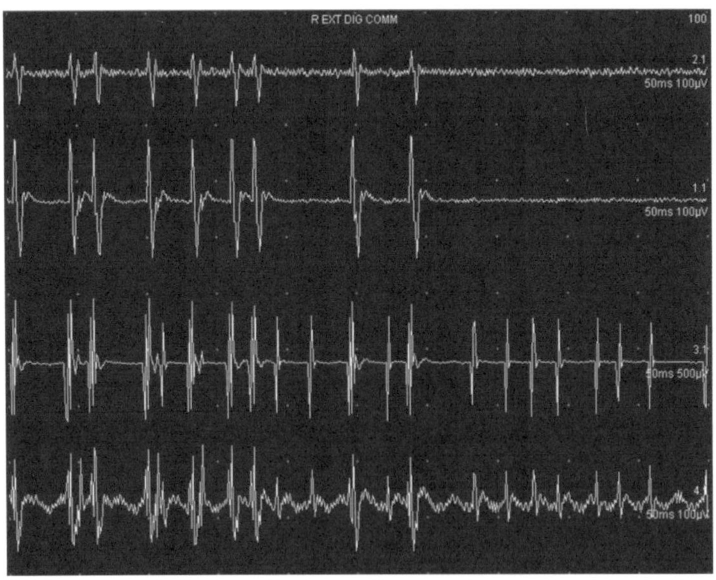

Fig. 6. Two sequences of end plate spikes. One is propagating to all channels and may represent beta motor unit potentials. The other propagates only from channel three to channel four and may represent activation of nuclear chain fibres. Calibration 50 ms, 100 μV, except Ch 3, 500 μV.

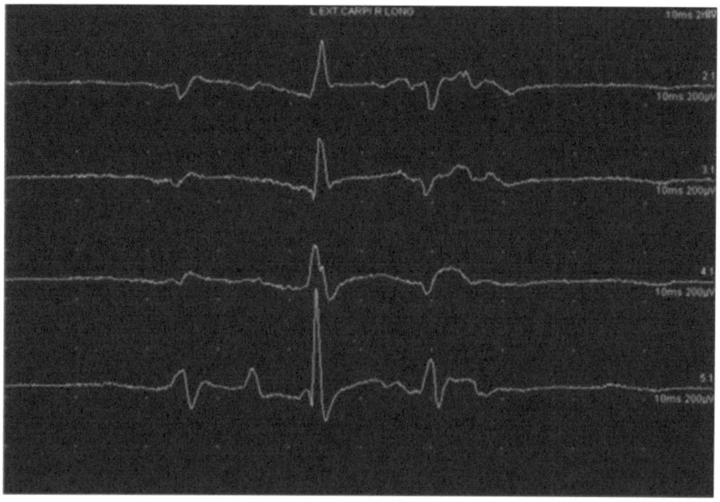

Fig. 7. Propagation of voluntarily activated motor unit potentials to all channels. Because of the slow firing of motor unit potentials compared to end plate spikes, they do not recur in this time window. Calibration 10 ms, 200 μV.

6. The "integrated hypothesis" for myofascial syndrome

The "integrated hypothesis" for myofascial syndrome comprises a local energy crisis of muscle tissue caused by strain. This leads to accumulation of irritative metabolites and thus activation of local nerve terminals with sustained contraction of postsynaptic muscle fibre. This is followed by rigor and a contraction knot, and development of a taut band, as well as activation of pain and sympathetic nerve fibres (Simons et al., 1999; Cummings & Baldry, 2007).

7. Discussion of the discrepancies of "integrated hypothesis" and suggestion of a new explanation for myofascial syndrome

The capillaries of extrafusal muscle tissue offer an effective perfusion, which is able to transport all irritative metabolites out of the muscle tissue. Thus the local inflammation of muscle without any signs of myositis seems improbable. On the other hand the capillaries of muscle spindles are different. There is a blood/spindle barrier and a non-permeable capsule around the spindle (Banks & Barker, 2004). Thus metabolites released into the capsular periaxial space of muscle spindle are readily concentrated. Sustained fusimotor activation of muscle spindle caused by for example precision work may achieve increased release of contraction metabolites intrafusally. This may activate release of inflammatory metabolites and finally pain metabolites. Only Ia-afferents of the muscle spindle activate alpha motor neurons (myotatic reflex). II- III- and IV-afferents activate intrafusal muscle fibres via gamma- and beta efferent pathways. III- and IV-afferents have been observed inside the muscle spindle (Paintal, 1960, Stacey, 1969). If inflammatory and pain metabolites are concentrated intrafusally, III- and IV-afferents, which comprise also chemical and pain receptors, may activate gamma- and beta-efferent activity via spinal reflex pathway. Beta efferent activation may be seen as CRD in EMG of taut bands for a limited time. Thus taut bands may be formed by extrafusal muscle fibres of beta motor units in metabolic exhaustion and rigor. Myotatic reflex (twitch) is present in taut bands (Shah et al., 2008) and this reflex is evidently activated by intact Ia afferent- alpha efferent reflex arch (Partanen et al., 2010).

8. Final comments

Needle EMG in myofascial syndrome is usually normal. In 15 % of patients CRD may be observed in some of the trigger points in taut bands (Ojala et al., 2006). This finding seems to be specific for myofascial syndrome, if there are no other EMG alterations. It remains to be seen if a thorough study of as many trigger points as possible increases the possibility to find CRD in a greater percentage of patients. The search may be justified because dry needling is also one of the treatments of myofascial syndrome (Cummings & Baldry, 2007). Incidence of end plate activity is increased in trigger points but this fact is not useful for diagnostics, because end plate activity is often observed in painless points as well. MEPPs with EPSs may represent intrafusal activity. In neuromuscular junctions of alpha motor units only MEPPs but not EPSs may be seen (Partanen et al., 2010). The different hypotheses discussed here can be tested and they help to comprehend the context "myofascial syndrome", which is not accepted by all physicians. At present the diagnosis of myofascial syndrome is clinical: there are no specific laboratory or imaging studies or other means to confirm the diagnosis (Dommerholt & Huijbregts, 2011).

9. References

Banks, R. W., & Barker, D. (2004). The muscle spindle, In: *Myology* (3rd edition), Engel, A., & Franzini-Armstrong , C., pp. 489-509, McGraw-Hill, Medical Publishing Division, New York

Barker, D., Bessou P., Jankowska, E., Pagès, B., Stacey, M.J. (1978). Identification of intrafusal muscle fibres activated by single fusimotor axons and injected with fluorescent dye in cat tenuissimus spindles. *J. Physiol*, Vol 275, pp. 149-165

Bengtsson, A., Henriksson, K. G., & Larsson, J. (1986). Reduced high-energy phosphate levels in the painful muscles of patients with primary fibromyalgia. *Arthritis & Rheumatism*, Vol.29, No.7, (July 1986), pp. 817-821

Buchthal, F., & Rosenfalck, P. (1966). Spontaneous electrical activity of human muscle. *Electroencephalography and Clinical Neurophysiology*, Vol.20, No.4, (April 1966), pp. 321-336

Couppé, C., Midttun, A., Hilden, J., Jørgensen, U., Oxholm, P., & Fuglsang-Frederiksen, A. (2001). Spontaneous needle electromyographic activity in myofascial trigger points in the infraspinatus muscle: a blinded assessment. *Journal of Musculoskeletal Pain*, Vol.9, No.3, pp. 7-17

Cummings, M., & Baldry, P. (2007). Regional myofascial pain: diagnosis and management. *Best Pract Res Clin Rheumatol.*, Vol.21, No.2, (April 2007), pp. 367-387

Dommerholt, J., & Huijbregts, P. (2011). *Myofascial trigger points: pathophysiology and evidenceinformed diagnosis and management*, Jones and Bartlett Publishers, Sudbury, Mass.

Dumitru, D. (1995). *Electrodiagnostic Medicine*, pp. 29-64, 218-221, Hanley & Belfus, Philadelphia

Emeryk, B., Hausmanowa-Petrusewicz, I., & Nowak, T. (1974a). Spontaneous volleys of bizarre high-frequency potentials (b.h.f.p.) in neuro-muscular diseases. Part 1. Occurrence of spontaneous volleys of b.h.f.p. in neuro-muscular diseases. *Electromyogr Clin Neurophysiol*, Vol.14, No.3, (June-July 1974), pp. 303-312

Emeryk, B., Hausmanowa-Petrusewicz, I., & Nowak T. (1974b). Spontaneous volleys of bizarre high-frequency potentials (b.h.f.p.) in neuro-muscular diseases. Part II. An analysis of the morphology of spontaneous volleys of bizarre high-frequency potentials in neuro-muscular diseases. *Electromyogr Clin Neurophysiol*, Vol.14, No.4, (August-September 1974), pp. 339-354

Macefield, V. G. (1998). Spontaneous and evoked ectopic discharges recorded from single human axons. *Muscle & Nerve*, Vol.21, No.4, (April 1998), pp. 461-468

Ojala, T. A., Arokoski, J. P. A., & Partanen, J. V. (2006). Needle-electromyography findings of trigger points in neck-shoulder area before and after injection treatment. *J. Muskuloskel. Pain*, Vol.14, pp. 5-14

Paintal, A. S. (1960). Functional analysis of group III afferent fibres of mammalian muscles. *J Physiol* Vol.152, pp. 250-270

Partanen, J. (1999). End plate spikes in the human electromyogram. Revision of the fusimotor theory. *J Physiol*, Paris, Vol.93, No.1-2, (January-April 1999), pp. 155-166

Partanen, J. V., & Nousiainen, U. (1983). End-plate spikes in electromyography are fusimotor unit potentials. *Neurology*, Vol.33, No.8, (August 1983), pp. 1039-1043, Cleveland

Partanen, J. V., Ojala, T. A., & Arokoski, J. P. A. (2010). Myofascial syndrome and pain: A neurophysiological approach. *Pathophysiology*, Vol.17, (February 2010), pp. 19-28

Partanen, J. V., & Palmu, K. (2009). Different ways of propagation of human end plate spikes in electromyography. *Muscle Nerve*, Vol.40, (2009), pp. 720-721

Shah, J. P., Danoff, J. V., Desai, M. J., Parikh, S., Nakamura, L. Y., Phillips, T. M., & Gerber, L. H. (2008). Biochemicals associated with pain and inflammation are elevated in sites near to and remote from active myofascial trigger points. *Arch Phys Med Rehabil*, Vol.89, No.1, (January 2008), pp. 16-23

Simons, D. G., Hong, C. Z., & Simons, L. S. (2002). Endplate potentials are common to midfiber myofascial trigger points. *Am J Phys Med Rehabil*, Vol.81, No.3, (March 2002), pp. 212-222

Simons, D. G., Travell, J. G., & Simons, L. S. (1999) *Myofascial Pain and Dysfunction: The Trigger Point Manual*, Vol.1, *Upper Half of Body*, (2nd edition), Williams & Wilkins, Baltimore

Stacey, M. J. (1969). Free nerve endings in skeletal muscle of the cat. *J Anat*; Vol.105, pp. 231-254.

Travell, J. (1957). Symposium of the mechanisms and management of pain syndromes. *Proc Rudolf Virchow Med Soc*, Vol.16, pp. 128-136

Trontelj, J., & Stålberg, E. V. (1983). Bizarre repetitive discharges recorded with single fibre EMG. *J Neurol Neurosurg Psychiatry*, Vol.46, No.4, (April 1983), pp. 310-316

Wall, P. D., Waxman, S., & Basbaum, A. I. (1974). Ongoing activity in peripheral nerve: injury discharge. *Exp Neurol*, Vol. 45, pp. 576-589

Wiederholt, W. C. (1970). End-plate noise in electromyography. *Neurology*, Vol.20, No.3, (March 1970), pp. 214-224, Minneapolis

5

Clinical Implications of Muscle-Tendon & -Force Interplay: Surface Electromyography Recordings of *m. vastus lateralis* in Renal Failure Patients Undergoing Dialysis and of *m. gastrocnemius* in Individuals with Achilles Tendon Damage

Adrian P. Harrison[1], Stig Molsted[1], Jessica Pingel[2],
Henning Langberg[2] and Else Marie Bartels[3]
[1]*IBHV, Faculty of Life Sciences, Copenhagen University*
[2]*Institute for Sports Medicine, Bispebjerg Hospital, Copenhagen NV*
[3]*The Parker Institute, Frederiksberg Hospital, Frederiksberg*
Denmark

1. Introduction

The Surface Electromyography (sEMG) technique offers a safe, quick, pain-free, non-invasive and repeatable means of assessing the important physiological processes that cause muscles to generate force and produce movement, yet it has many limitations that must be understood, considered, and removed where possible (Hermens et al., 1999). Thus, it has been said of electromyography that;

"EMG is a tempting muse .. it is too easy to use and consequently too easy to abuse"
(De Luca CJ 1993 – Wartenweiler Memorial Lecture).

An sEMG signal comprises what is otherwise termed a compound muscle action potential (CMAP) being the sum of any number of motor unit action potentials within a given recording area. However, just such an sEMG signal, which provides an insight into the level of activity of a given skeletal muscle, can be altered/affected in many ways by what have been defined as causative, intermediate and deterministic factors (De Luca, 1997). The causative factors include such parameters as the configuration of the recording electrodes (size, distance apart etc.), skin thickness and subcutaneous tissue composition and depth, blood flow, muscle fibre diameter and orientation as well as the number of active motor units within the muscle of choice and their firing rate one with another, that is to say their synchronization (De Luca, 1997). Added to these parameters are the intermediate factors which include the choice of using a differential electrode filter, the risk of cross-talk from adjacent muscles or underlying tissue, the occurrence of spatial filtering as a consequence of fibre depth, the volume of the muscle that is detectable, and the conduction velocity of muscle fibres. Finally, there are the deterministic factors which comprise the number of active motor units within a muscle as well as their detectability, their recruitment and stability, plus the action potentials resulting from such active motor units and their amplitude and duration. These then, when combined, give rise to an sEMG or compound muscle action potential which has a given amplitude and any number of spectral variables. It is the analysis of such sEMG signal data and its interpretation in terms of muscle force (RMS conversion), the activation of a muscle (On *versus* Off), any signs of fatigue and hints relating to the biochemical processes in a muscle that make this such a tempting, yet complex field to study (see Fig. 1 & 2).

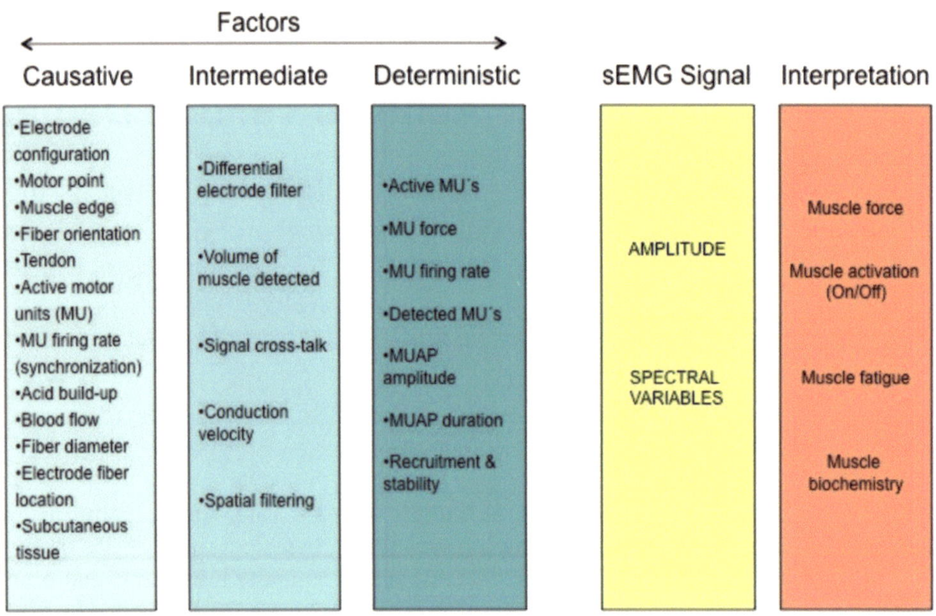

Fig. 1. The factors "causative", "intermediate" and "deterministic" and their effect on both sEMG signal amplitude and spectral variables, and the interpretation one can make of a recorded sEMG signal (after De Luca, 1997).

In spite of the large number of variables that influence the sEMG signal (De Luca,1997; Farina et al., 2004; Hogrel, 2005), studies on correlations between intrinsic muscle parameters and recorded signals are becoming more numerous (Gerdle et al., 1997; Karlsson & Gerdle, 2001; Kupa et al.,1995; Larsson et al., 2002 & 2006; Tygesen & Harrison, 2005).

In rats, EMG parameters have been shown to be a useful tool to predict muscle excitability (Harrison & Flatman, 1999), and in sheep the technique has been used to follow postnatal muscle development (Tygesen & Harrison, 2005). sEMG recordings have also been related to the morphological state of muscles, for example i) muscle fibre composition (identified using MHC isoforms or mATPase activity)in humans (Gerdle et al., 1997; Larsson et al., 2002 & 2006) and in rats (Kupa et al., 1995) and, ii) muscle fibre diameter in humans (Gerdle et al., 1997; Larsson et al., 2006) and in rats (Kupa et al., 1995).

With the non-invasiveness of sEMG recordings comes the possibility, for clinicians and physiologists alike, to determine whether structural and functional changes have occurred in muscles over a period of time.

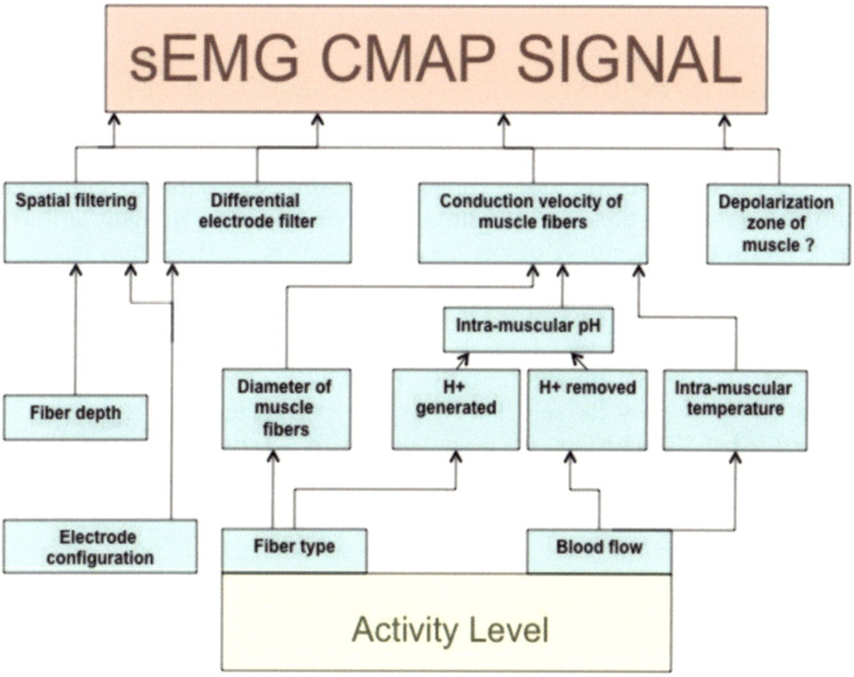

Fig. 2. Factors affecting the sEMG signal during a period of sustained contraction. In the case of "conduction velocity", "intramuscular pH" and "H+ generated" a clear association between changes in these parameters over time during a period of sustained contraction has been established. It is less clear, however, as to whether and with what degree "depolarization zone of muscle" is changed during a period of sustained contraction (after De Luca, 1997).

Recorded parameters such as signal Area and Corrected Peak relate to muscle force production, and over time they can be used to give an idea of an individual's fatigue resistance, along with an RMS analysis of the recorded signal, whereas Leading Slope and Trailing Slope are more closely related to the speed of contraction and relaxation in a given muscle, providing information about an individual's physical capabilities, as well as the fibre-type composition of specific muscles (De Luca, 1997).

It is relevant to measure sEMG prior to and after strength training. An increase in muscle strength after a period of strength training can be due to an improvement in neuro-muscular communication and/or an increase in the cross-sectional area of muscle fibres. In cases where no response to strength training is observed, the limiting factor may be due to affected neuro-muscular function. Indeed, CKD are associated with neuropathies (Krishnan et al., 2005), which could well affect the sEMG signal and any response to strength training. Thus the sEMG serves as a control/explanatory factor together with muscle strength measurements and CSA fibre measurements when looking for an indicator of strength training success in individuals.

The sEMG of a person with good muscle function would therefore be characterized by a signal with the following characteristics; relatively high frequency, large corrected peak, relatively stable RMS - at least initially, and fast leading and trailing slopes.

1.1 Understanding & interpreting sEMG signals

1.1.1 sEMG parameters

sEMG signals can be characterized either by temporal analysis (e.g. peak amplitude, root mean square or average rectified values), by spectral analysis (e.g. mean frequency, median frequency), or by propagation analysis (e.g. muscle fibre conduction velocity).
Amplitude estimations are used frequently in sEMG research. The amplitude of a voluntary signal is stochastic (random) and can therefore be reasonably represented by a Gaussian distribution function. The amplitude of a sEMG signal is highly influenced by the distance and the conductivity of the tissue between the active fibres as well as the recording electrodes, their properties and placement. The root mean square, that is to say the square root of the average power of the sEMG signal for a given period of time, is a technique that allows for rectification of the raw "bipolar" signal, converting it to a "monopolar" amplitude that is easier to present and interpret (Hermens et al., 1999). The average rectified value takes the rectified signal one step further and represents the area under the rectified sEMG signal over a period of time. It is generally thought that the root mean square is more appropriate when assessing voluntary contractions as it represents the signal power, unlike the average rectified value, which has no specific physical meaning (De Luca, 1997).

1.1.2 sEMG issues

As motor units are recruited and potentially increase their firing rate during sustained muscle activation, increasing numbers of motor unit action potentials (MUAP´s) may contribute to an sEMG signal at any one point in time. It would be logical then to predict that the magnitude of the sEMG signal should increase almost linearly with activation rate. However, the sEMG signal underestimates the actual activation signal sent from the spinal cord to a particular muscle since increasing MUAP overlap and signal cancellation typically occurs, and this reduces the sEMG signal. This loss of sEMG signal has been shown to arise from the linear summation of overlapping positive and negative phases of motor unit potentials which serve to cancel one another out and thereby reduce the amplitude of the signal (Day & Hullinger, 2001; Keenan et al., 2005; Keenan et al., 2006).
In general terms, the sEMG parameters "area" and "amplitude" relate to the force of contraction, yet no simple equation exists to describe their relation. Indeed, the fact that the amplitude increases as muscle force increases only serves to provide a qualitative indicator. Quantitatively, exactly how much the force varies between two tasks cannot at present be answered with any certainty. One should be very cautious then when using the sEMG signal as an absolute measure of the force developed by a muscle as there are occasions when this relation can become non-linear (De Luca, 1997; Turker, 1993). Apart from the fact that the amplitude is highly influenced by both extrinsic and intrinsic parameters, two other factors have an enormous effect on the relation between force and amplitude. The first is that of the number of motor units detected by the recording electrodes is almost always less that the number of active motor units in an active muscle. The second is the issue of relative placement of active motor units with regard to the recording electrodes, such that if a newly recruited motor unit is located in close proximity to a recording electrode, that motor unit will contribute more than an average unit of energy to the recorded signal. Conversely, if a newly recruited motor unit is located at a distance from the recording electrode, the force in that muscle will most likely increase whilst the amplitude of the sEMG signal will not alter dramatically (De Luca, 1997).

Spectral analysis of the sEMG signal has been used to study muscle fatigue (Komi & Tesch, 1979; Linssen et al., 1991; Milnerbrown & Miller, 1986; Moritani et al., 1982), and changes in motor unit recruitment (Bernardi et al., 1996; Bernardi et al., 1999; Solomonow et al., 1990). Spectral analyses have also been used to estimate the activation of type I and type II muscle fibres during a contraction (Gerdle et al., 1988; Gerdle et al., 1991; Tesch et al., 1983), as well as to predict the actual muscle fibre type composition (Kupa et al., 1995). Interpretation of the most commonly used spectral descriptors (mean frequency and median frequency) is facilitated by the use of the power spectral density function. The mean frequency has a smaller estimation of variance than the median frequency, yet the median frequency is less sensitive to noise and more sensitive to fatigue (Hermens et al., 1999; Merletti et al., 1992). Thus these different characteristics should be considered when analyzing an sEMG signal. For example, under conditions of a high signal:noise ratio the mean frequency is preferable due to the low variance, but under conditions where the signal:noise ratio is low, one should consider using the median frequency because of its relative insensitivity to noise (Hermens et al., 1999).

In propagation analysis, the muscle fibre conduction velocity is measured using two electrodes with the same alignment as the muscle fibres. By measuring the inter-electrode distance, the muscle fibre conduction velocity can be calculated as the ratio between the distance and the time delay between the two recorded signals. In most cases the underlying tissue poses very little local variation, so in terms of both detected signals the filtering effects can be assumed to be similar. This gives the muscle fibre conduction velocity parameter an advantage compared to temporal and spectral analysis, where the filtering effect of underlying tissue may distort the travelling signal (Hermens et al., 1999; Hogrel, 2005). The muscle fibre conduction velocity is to some degree proportional to the muscle fibre diameter. Thus in general muscles with large diameter fibres, such as those belonging to higher threshold motor units, will possess a greater average muscle fibre conduction velocity, which will in turn shift the frequency spectrum towards the high frequency range (De Luca, 1997).

To illustrate use of sEMG in a clinical setting, we will give an account of two chosen studies which together will show where sEMG has its strength and which considerations have to be made when using sEMG in these settings.

2. Uremic study

2.1 Introduction

Patients with end-stage renal disease (ESRD; uremia) have limited physical fitness, which can lead to subsequent problems, namely cardiac dysfunction and depression (Gutman et al., 1981; Painter, 1988, Kouidi et al., 1997; Shalom et al., 1984), as well as muscle abnormalities, which severely affect their daily life, whether it be work- or recreation-related (Nakao et al., 1982). Yet, whilst muscle weakness is a common complaint amongst dialysis patients, it remains an unexplained phenomenon.

Muscle atrophy with uremia has been shown to be fibre-specific, in that the disease is mainly associated with a loss of type II fibres and predominantly the type IIB fibres, which are fast-twitch and glycolytic in nature (Fahal et al., 1997). Atrophy of type I (slow-twitch, oxidative fibres) also occurs in some patients (Molsted et al., 2007; Moore et al., 1993). Yet despite these changes, exercise training has been shown to significantly alleviate the loss of physical capacity that occurs in dialysis patients with end-stage renal disease (Shalom et al., 1984; Painter, 1988; Eidemak et al., 1997; Kouidi et al., 1998; Molsted et al., 2004).

Whilst these patients suffer an array of medical problems that plagues them and the quality of their life (QoL), they are interested in receiving any form of help that will improve their condition and help them to lead a more normal life. It is for this reason that studies have been attempted to assess the causes behind the observed muscle atrophy and physical weakness that they incur. It should be mentioned though that these studies are not without problems. Patients arriving for a period of dialysis are usually very weak and can become easily confused, and after their dialysis most cannot wait to get out into the World and use the time and energy they have had temporarily restored upon them. This necessitates that any experimental design must be simple and easy to understand, it should not be painful, and most of all it must be relatively quick - time being of the essence after a period of dialysis. Thus it has been our experience that whilst studies of nerve conduction have not been accepted by patients with end-stage renal disease, being seen as both time consuming and painful, our sEMG recordings have been well tolerated.

2.2 Patients

Patients were recruited from Rigshospitalet, Denmark. Inclusion criteria were; ages above 18 years, undergoing haemodialysis for a minimum of three months, and being able to climb stairs. Exclusion criteria were inability to participate in the intervention due to physical health, blindness, lower limb amputation, diabetic retinopathy, severe cognitive reduction, and treatment with the anti-coagulation drug Fondaparinux. All patients gave their informed consent and the protocol was approved by the local ethical committee (H-D-2008-124).

2.3 Training programme

The included patients participated in a training programme consisting of heavy load resistance training three times a week for a period of 16 weeks. The exercise sessions varied in time from the last dialysis, since some patients were dialyzed three times a week, others only twice a week.

The exercise began with 5 minutes of warm-up. Three exercises were performed at each exercise session: leg press, leg extension and leg curl. During the intervention period the load was increased and repetition maximum (RM) decreased from 15 to 6 RM. An individual patient's progress during the interventions was adjusted according to changes of 1-6 RM.

2.4 sEMG recordings, measurements and analyses

The study used both a single and a double differential electrode configuration, with electrodes (N-00-S & R-00-S; Blue Sensor R, Medicotest A/S, Ølstykke, Denmark) configured as described previously (Harrison et al., 2006). sEMG recordings were taken *via* an ML 131 amplifier connected to a PowerLab 4/25T A/D converter (AD Instruments, Chalgrove, Oxfordshire, UK) with a further connection to a Mac PowerBook Air with Chart v. 5.5.6 Software, Peak Parameters, and Spike Histogram extensions. Input impedance was 200 MΩ differential, and a high- and a low-pass filter of 3 Hz and 500 Hz, respectively, were used. Sampling speed was set to 40,000 per second.

Recordings, which were taken from the vastus lateralis of the left leg, followed the guidelines laid out in the *European Recommendations for Surface ElectroMyoGraphy* as detailed by the SENIAM project (Hermens et al., 1999). Differential recordings of sEMG signals were made *via* surface electrodes from the *vastus lateralis*, as described in detail previously. Information of any expected electromyography performance results were not divulged, and patients were not allowed to follow their sEMG recordings on the computer screen in real time. The recorded sEMG signal was assessed as described previously (Harrison et al., 2006) in terms of signal frequency (Hz) and peak-to-peak amplitude (V), using Chart analysis software (AD Instruments, Chalgrove, Oxfordshire, UK).

2.5 Statistics

Data distribution was tested using a Q-Q plot. Due to the discovery that the data was not normally distributed, statistical analysis of any effects was performed using non-parametric tests. A Wilcoxon Signed Ranks Test was applied to measure significant differences between pre-training (Baseline) and post-training (Re-test) values. Data are presented as means plus and minus the standard error of the means (SEM). All tests were two-tailed and significance was deemed to be at $P \leq 0.05$.

2.6 Results

A clear and significant improvement in the amplitude of the recorded sEMG signal was noted in the uremic patients when values taken pre-training were compared with those obtained post-training (see Fig. 3).

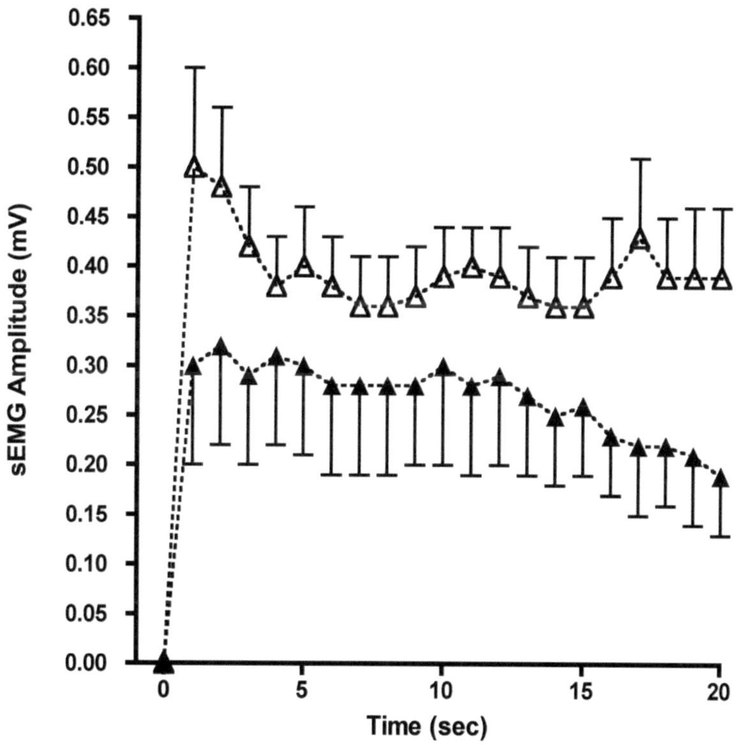

Fig. 3. The recorded sEMG signal from *m. Vastus lateralis* of uremic patients taken prior to (▲) and after a 16 week programme of strength training (△). Recordings, which represent a 20 second period of sustained leg lift, were taken at a sampling rate of 40,000 data samples per second, using an impedance of 200 MΩ and a high- and low-pass filter of 3 Hz and 500 Hz, respectively. Values represent the Mean ± SEM of 8 patients.

In contrast, to the sEMG amplitude values, measurements of the sEMG signal frequency from these uremic patients were not significantly altered by a 16 week period of strength training (see Fig. 4). Indeed, if anything one gets the impression, at least initially, that a lower firing frequency is employed by these patients during a period of sustained leg extension and contraction of *m. Vastus lateralis.*

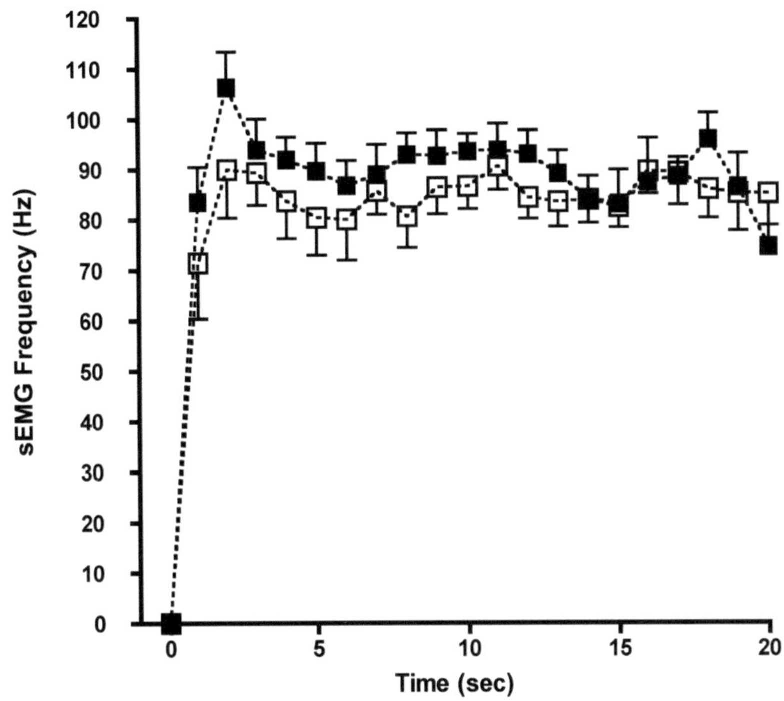

Fig. 4. The recorded sEMG signal from *m. Vastus lateralis* of uremic patients taken prior to (■) and after a 16 week programme of strength training (□). Recordings, which represent a 20 second period of sustained leg lift, were taken at a sampling rate of 40,000 data samples per second, using an impedance of 200 MΩ and a high- and low-pass filter of 3 Hz and 500 Hz, respectively. Values represent the Mean ± SEM of 8 patients.

Our investigation of muscle performance in the uremic patients also included a sEMG recording of *m. Vastus lateralis* taken during a period of dynamic contraction (see Fig. 5).

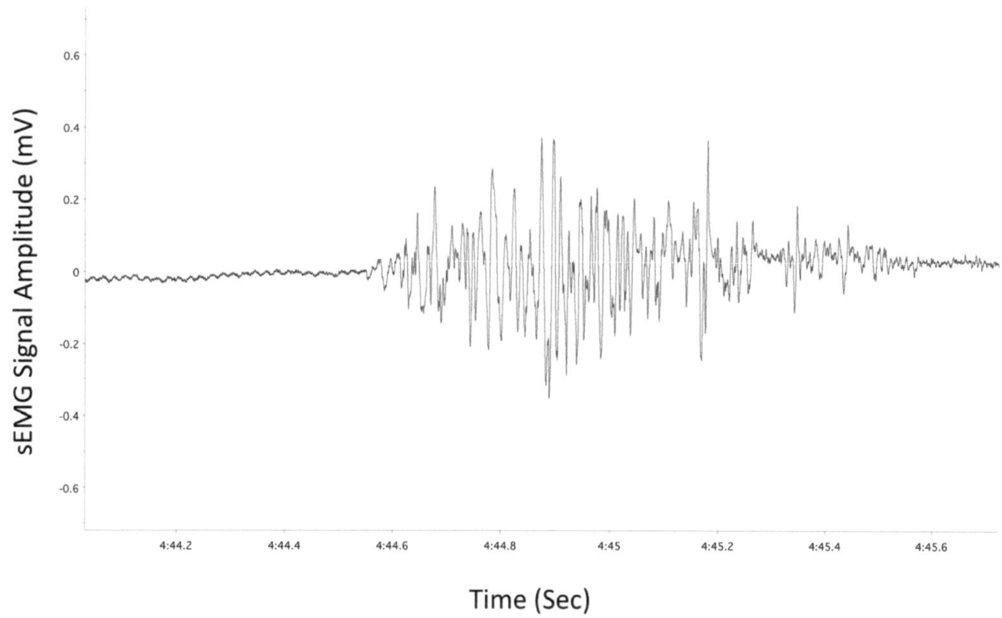

Fig. 5. The results of a dynamic muscle strength test involving a knee extension with 1 RM. This figure illustrates a sEMG recording taken from *m. Vastus lateralis* at a recording speed of 40,000 data samples per second. Note the burst of power as the leg is extended. This sEMG signal was analyzed in terms of its peak-to-peak amplitude (mV) and its inherent frequency (Hz).

Both the dynamic and the isometric sEMG signal were analyzed in terms of their inherent frequency and their amplitude. Recordings taken after a period of 16 weeks of strength training "Re-test" were then compared with "Baseline" pre-training levels, and the results are shown below in Table 1.

Dynamic 1RM 1. Sec			
Parameter	*Baseline*	*Re-test*	*P*
Frequency (Hz)	71 ± 11	71 ± 6	NS
Amplitude (mV)*	309 ± 81	571 ± 71	0.017
Dynamic 1RM 1. sec/kilo			
Frequency/kilo (Hz/Kg)	1.3 ± 0.2	0.9 ± 0.1	NS (0.093)
Amplitude/kilo (mV/Kg)*	6.2 ± 2.4	7.2 ± 1.1	NS

Isometric 50% 1RM 20 sec			
Parameter	*Baseline*	*Re-test*	*P*
Frequency Peak (Hz)	107 ± 6	102 ± 5	NS
Amplitude Peak (mV)*	350 ± 104	568 ± 86	NS
Frequency Mean (Hz)	89 ± 5	85 ± 5	NS
Amplitude Mean (mV)*	273 ± 83	396 ± 54	NS
Isometric 50% 1RM 20 sec/kilo			
Frequency Peak/kilo (Hz/Kg)	3.7 ± 0.5	2.6 ± 0.4	0.017
Amplitude Peak/kilo (mV/Kg)*	14.8 ± 6.6	14.2 ± 2.3	NS
Frequency Mean/kilo (Hz/Kg)	3.0 ± 0.3	2.2 ± 0.3	0.017
Amplitude Mean/kilo (mV/Kg)*	11.6 ± 5.2	10.1 ± 1.7	NS

Table 1. The response of *m Vastus lateralis* to a period of 16 weeks of strength exercise training in uremic patients. Data are presented as uncorrected values *versus* values corrected for the weight lifted (per kilo) by the patients. Note that sEMG correction for individual variation in terms of the weight lifted has a huge effect on the results, highlighting the fact that signal analysis can affect the interpretation of the recordings. Values represent the Mean ± SEM of n=8 haemodialysis patients. * indicates x 1000.

2.7 Discussion

The first large-scale studies of the physical capacity of patients with chronic renal failure were performed at the end of the 1970´s as reviewed by Laville & Fouque (1995). It was noted that 50% of patients requiring dialysis had stopped their professional activity as a result of chronic renal failure, attributed to coronary (15% of patients), cardiovascular (23%), and bone or muscle (24%) related conditions (Evans et al., 1985).

In a recent study involving patients on haemodialysis, *in vivo* measurements of muscle function were made using sEMG (Harrison et al., 2006). The sEMG frequency recorded prior to dialysis was generally found to be abnormal, when compared with a normal range of *2nd dorsal interosseous* muscles of the hand and on the thigh *m. Vastus lateralis*. This study also revealed a clear benefit of haemodialysis in terms of sEMG frequency of the *2nd dorsal interosseous* muscle (Harrison et al., 2006). Moreover, these authors found that the *in vivo* analysis of sEMG changes with a session of haemodialysis seemed to be limited to relatively fast-twitch muscles, a finding that was supported by a study of isolated rat *extensor digitorum longus* muscle, in which changes in the uremic environment were shown to exert a rapid loss of contractile force (Harrison et al., 2006).

In the present study, the combined graphs and table show that a period of exercise training results in an improved sEMG amplitude with very little change to the signal frequency. This finding, which indicates that a period of exercise training in these patients results in the ability to lift more weight (kilos), may be due to enhanced spatial summation (Henneman et al., 1965) - that is to say an increased and more synchronized recruitment of motor units. However, a considerable degree of individual variation is masked by this data set, and upon correction of the sEMG amplitude and frequency data for the weight in kilos used under training, a different interpretation is arrived at. Suddenly, signal analysis designed to remove an element of individual variation from the data now reveals that a period of exercise training induces an increase in sEMG signal frequency, and not an alteration in sEMG amplitude. It has to be said though, that this form of signal analysis reveals a finding that is more consistent with what is known to occur during the initial period following commencement of exercise training. What is observed is an improvement in neuro-muscular recruitment and activation "coordination" that typically precedes fibre and vascular changes "hypertrophy". Indeed, this conclusion is supported by the fact that looking at the histology of the fibres, we have not found any significant changes in fibre, cross-sectional area with the 16 week period of strength training in biopsies taken from *m. Vastus lateralis* in these patients (data not shown).

Of course recordings of sEMG from muscles of such patients are not without problem, and the interpretation of such data should not be made without careful consideration. In Figures 1 & 2 we identified a number of factors that can affect sEMG recordings, and in terms of uremic patients perhaps the most important would be as follows;

Fig. 1: **Causative** - active motor units, motor unit firing rate (synchronization) & fibre diameter
Intermediate - volume of muscle detected (fibre diameter) & conduction velocity
Deterministic - active motor units, detected motor units, motor unit action potential amplitude, motor unit action potential duration, recruitment & stability

Fig. 2: Diameter of muscle fibres, conduction velocity of muscle fibres & blood flow

In uremic patients one finds that ion imbalances and the build up of toxic compounds, confounded by other health issues and the effects of medication, affect neuro-muscular recruitment and activation. The effect is that neural conduction velocity is impaired, that fewer motor units tend to be active, and when active they often reveal action potentials that are of long duration and consequently of small amplitude. More long-term changes with uremia also include an atrophy of muscle fibres and a reduction in vascularisation, which will affect causative factors as well as intermediate factors, and furthermore reduce the blood flow to the contracting muscle fibres.

With strength training, it seems that a natural loss of synchronization and recruitment of motor units as the uremia progresses can be reversed. As mentioned earlier, we have not seen any changes in fibre size, and it therefore seems that the improved sEMG signal, which is supported by an improved physical function determined with a sit-to-stand test (data not shown), is due not to an increase in the number or size of active fibres, but rather a better control of those already working fibres.

3. Tendinopathy study

3.1 Introduction

The Achilles tendon is one of the most frequently injured tendons of the body due to trauma and overuse - very often in young or middle-aged, physically active subjects (Alfredson et al., 2000; Cook 2009). This arises, most likely, from muscle force in the gastrocnemius being trained to develop an extremely rapid and high level of force without being compensated by equally rapid changes in the Achilles tendon (Olesen et al., 2006; Holm et al., 2009). Although adaptation of tendons has been demonstrated (Langberg et al., 2007; Couppé et al., 2009), this adaption is slower than the development of a stronger muscle, and the tendon does not possess the dimensions necessary to accommodate such rapid increases in force production, and the result will very often be damage to the tendon structure or partial/complete rupture (Hess, 2010).

A number of systemic diseases are also known to be associated with general defects in matrix metabolism and structure that compromise tendon strength and elasticity, moreover the term 'spontaneous tendon rupture' is being used on a more regular basis in both the sports- and work-environments (Järvinen et al., 2001). Indeed, despite the fact that the Achilles tendon is the strongest tendon in the human body, there are increasing numbers of cases of overload of the Achilles tendon, both associated with sports as well as to work-related situations. It is estimated that the most common healthcare problem in Denmark is muscular-skeletal, accounting for approximately 15 % of all diseases (Ekholm et al., 2006). In spite of the extent of the problem not much is at present known about the etiology and pathogenesis of chronic tendon pain. The cause of the lack of knowledge within the area is primarily due to several limiting factors. First, that the early development of tendinopathy is unsymptomatic (Fredberg & Stengaard-Pedersen, 2008). Second, the establishment of a human tendinopathy model is deemed unethical. A few animal studies have been performed using an overuse protocol developed by Soslowsky and colleagues (Scott et al., 2007; Perry et al., 2005; Soslowsky et al., 2002), where rats ran with a velocity of 17m/minute, 5 days/week, 1 hour/day, either uphill or downhill for a period of between 2-16 weeks. In such experiments, a decreased collagen fiber organization and increased numbers of cell nuclei were observed (Soslowsky et al., 1996; Glazebrook et al., 2008). Yet, exactly how the tendon manages the active tension transfer from muscle to bone and if this tension transfer is affected by tendinopathy remains unclear. Thus, a form of assessment or a technique that could detect potentially damaging changes in a tendon very early on, and in so doing prevent muscle dysfunction, would be of great benefit.

It is with this point in mind, that we have investigated Achilles tendon parameters in combination with the contractile profile of *m. Gastrocnemius* in a number of healthy sports subjects, as a way of increasing the current knowledge of the ways in which tendon adapts to the mechanical loading associated with running/jogging. Our approach has been to better understand the active participation of tendons in the tension transfer from muscle to bone, and in order to achieve this goal we have returned to the topic of recording artefacts to see if they might not be used to some advantage.

3.2 Subjects

Healthy subjects were recruited from www.forsøgsperson.dk. Inclusion criteria were; no current tendon injury issues, regular training and ability to complete 60 minutes running on a treadmill. In total 8 subjects were examined (5 males; 3 females). The average age was 31 years (24-40) and average weight of was 74 kg (54-85). All had a BMI between 19 and 25, i.e. normal weight. All participants gave their informed consent and the protocol was approved by the Copenhagen and Frederiksberg Municipalities ethical committee (H-2-2010-121).

3.3 sEMG recordings, measurements and analyses

The study used both a single and a double differential electrode configuration, with electrodes (N-00-S & R-00-S; Blue Sensor R, Medicotest A/S, Ølstykke, Denmark) configured as described previously (Harrison et al., 2006). sEMG recordings were taken *via* an ML 131 amplifier connected to a PowerLab 4/25T A/D converter (AD Instruments, Chalgrove, Oxfordshire, UK) with a further connection to a Mac PowerBook Air with Chart v. 5.5.6 Software, Peak Parameters and Spike Histogram extensions. Input impedance was 200 M□ differential, and a high- and a low-pass filter of 3 Hz and 500 Hz, respectively, were used. Sampling speed was set to 40,000 per second.

Recordings were taken from the vastus lateralis of the left leg, following the guidelines laid out in the *European Recommendations for Surface ElectroMyoGraphy* as detailed by the SENIAM project (Hermens et al., 1999). Differential recordings of sEMG signals were made *via* surface electrodes from the *vastus lateralis*, as described in detail previously. Information of any expected electromyography performance results were not divulged, and subjects were not allowed to follow their sEMG recordings on the computer screen in real time. The recordings were carried out during 60 minutes treadmill running at a velocity of around 10 km/hour. The recorded sEMG signal was assessed as described previously (Harrison et al., 2006) in terms of signal frequency (Hz) and peak-to-peak amplitude (V), using Chart analysis software (AD Instruments, Chalgrove, Oxfordshire, UK).

3.4 Statistics

Data are presented as means plus and minus the standard error of the means (SEM). All tests were two-tailed and significance was deemed to be at $P \leq 0.05$.

3.5 Results

The results, (see Fig. 5 & 6), show that for lateral and medial *m.Gastrocnemius,* there is a pattern of sEMG signal parameter change over a 60 minute run/jog. After a few minutes of adjustment to a steady running/jogging rhythm, the sEMG mean amplitude becomes fairly stable, only showing signs of fatigue during the last ten minutes. It is likely that there is a fibre type distribution difference between the lateral and medial heads of *m.Gastrocnemius* as the lateral head increases slightly in sEMG frequency, while the amplitude decreases as the run/jog proceeds, whilst the medial head shows the reverse trend.

Of more importance from our perspective is the measurement of the sEMG to tendon artefact peak (ΔmSec), which remains very stable and uniform throughout the entire run/jog (see Fig. 6 & 7).

3.6 Discussion

In a recent paper written by De Luca and colleagues (2010) the authors address the issue of inevitable noise contamination of sEMG signals taken from muscles. Such noise originates from the skin-electrode interface, the electronics used to amplify the recorded signal, and a number of external sources (see Figs. 1 & 2). De Luca and colleagues focused on the low-frequency part of the recorded sEMG spectrum and proposed a number of approaches that can be taken to refine the recorded signal in a clinical setting (De Luca et al., 2010).

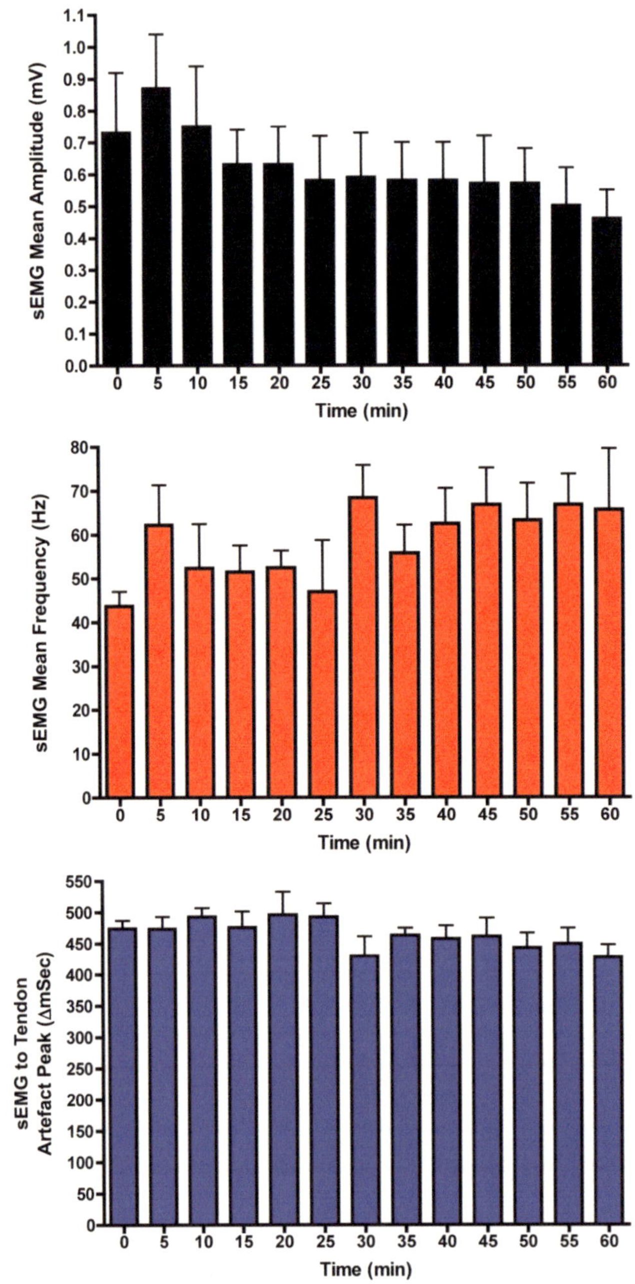

Fig. 6. The mean recorded sEMG signal from *m. Gastrocnemius* (Lateral Head) of healthy subjects - Upper Panel: Amplitude (mV), Middle Panel: Frequency (Hz) and Lower Panel: sEMG to Tendon Artefact Peak (ΔmSec). Recordings, which represent 5 minute interval means of a 60 minute run/jog at 11-13 km/hr, were taken at a sampling rate of 40,000 data samples per second, using an impedance of 200 MΩ and a high and low pass filter of 3 Hz and 500 Hz, respectively. Values represent the Mean ± SEM of 8 subjects.

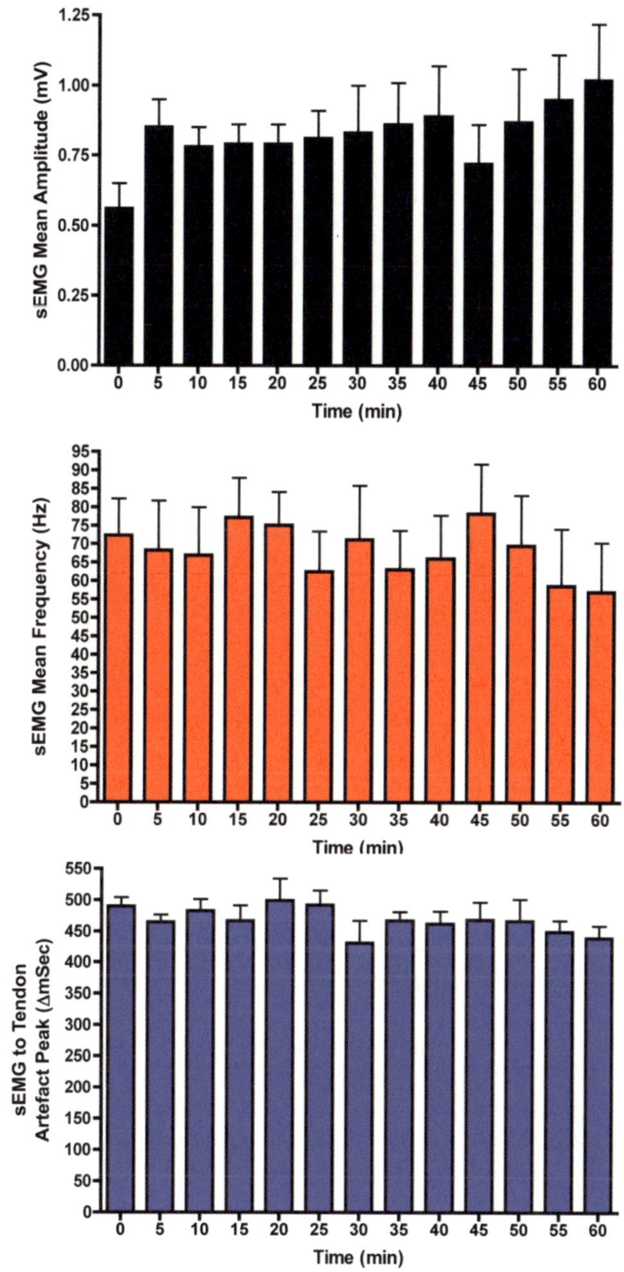

Fig. 7. The mean recorded sEMG signal from *m. Gastrocnemius* (Medial Head) of healthy subjects - Upper Panel: Amplitude (mV), Middle Panel: Frequency (Hz) and Lower Panel: sEMG to Tendon Artefact Peak (ΔmSec). Recordings, which represent 5 minute interval means of a 60 minute run/jog at 11-13 km/hr, were taken at a sampling rate of 40,000 data samples per second, using an impedance of 200 MΩ and a high and low pass filter of 3 Hz and 500 Hz, respectively. Values represent the Mean ± SEM of 8 subjects.

However, a good working knowledge of the artefacts one can encounter when recording a sEMG signal in a clinical setting can also provide a recording opportunity, which researchers may wish to exploit rather than eradicate. Typically, one finds that movement artefacts represent a large proportion of the recorded signal at low spectrum frequencies (60% or more) (De Luca et al., 2010). Here, one may envisage that just such a movement artefact could be of importance and use when assessing muscle:tendon interactions. Indeed, our results, obtained with healthy controls, show that just such a recorded movement artefact taken from the Achilles tendon of individuals whilst running/jogging can be used successfully in connection with a sEMG signal recording from both heads of *m. Gastrocnemius*.

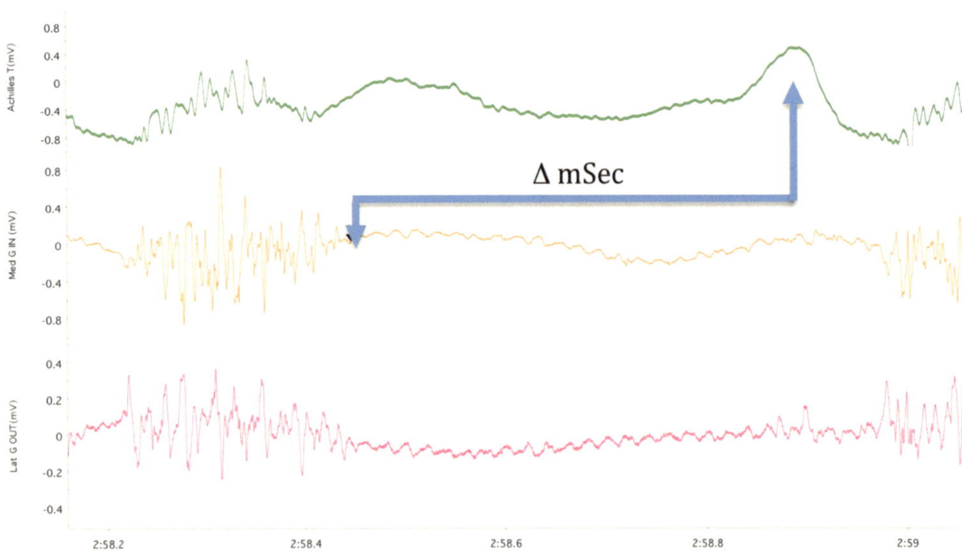

Fig. 8. The results of a 10 km/hr jog on Achilles tendon (upper panel) and both the medial head (middle panel) and lateral head (lower panel) of *m. Gastrocnemius*. The sEMG recording was from the right leg and at a recording speed of 40,000 per second per channel. Note, that after the synchronized bursts of power in the medial and lateral heads of Gastrocnemius a rise in the Achilles tendon signal to a maximum follows, after a delay of some 430 mSec, and this is again followed by a rapid fall back to resting levels. This deflection in the Achilles tendon trace is, however, merely a recording artefact representing the movement of the tendon under tension relative to the electrodes on the skin. The sEMG signal was analyzed in terms of its peak-to-peak amplitude (mV) and its inherent frequency (Hz).

The Achilles tendon is one of the most frequently injured tendons of the body due to trauma and overuse - very often in young or middle-aged, physically active subjects (Alfredson et al., 2000; Cook 2009). However, a recent study has shown that many inactive and often obese people develop tendinopathy (Gaida et al., 2008). Furthermore, one could easily imagine that tendinopathy in such individuals will result in these patients becoming even more inactive and therefore even more overweight. The question that then arises is how does muscle force affect the tendon tissue, when the tissue is overloaded either chronically as with obesity, or very frequently as with elite athletes. Muscle force in the gastrocnemius can be trained to develop an extremely rapid and high level of force, which may not always be met by equally rapid changes in the Achilles tendon (Olesen et al., 2006; Holm et al., 2009). Although adaptation of tendons has been demonstrated (Langberg et al., 2007; Couppé et al., 2009) the tendon does not possess the dimensions necessary to accommodate such rapid increases in force production, with the result that damage, often to the tendon structure or partial/complete rupture, occurs. Thus, an understanding of the active participation of tendons in the tension transfer from muscle to bone may lead to more optimal and effective treatment of tendinopathy - perhaps through further studies of the sEMG to tendon artefact peak.

Recent *in vivo* studies utilizing ultrasound imaging have shown that the human Achilles tendon undergoes a pattern of rapid lengthening and shortening during the stance phase of running (Lichtwark et al., 2007). Such a change in the tendon has a clear benefit in terms of the return of elastic energy stored in the Achilles tendon to the muscle, making the muscle:tendon unit largely free of metabolic costs. Another advantage of this change is that the Achilles tendon enables *m. Gastrocnemius* fascicles to remain nearly isometric for a large part of each stance (Ishikawa et al., 2007). Combined these changes greatly enhance the efficiency of this muscle:tendon interface.

Creep is defined as the lengthening of an elastic structure held under constant tension, or in other words an increasing lengthening per contraction cycle (Ker et al., 2000). To date, some scientists believe that tendon is capable of creep during periods of constant loading (Ker et al., 2000; Maganaris et al., 2002). However, increased lengthening for a given force as explained by creep would necessitate a reduction in tendon stiffness. Moreover, just such a creep, should it exist in human tendon, must most likely be detectable during the course of a run. In just such an experiment Farris and colleagues (2011) recently documented that the loading experienced during a single bout of running had no effect on the stiffness of the Achilles tendon, and that its properties remained stable throughout the period of activity - a finding that argues strongly against the existence of creep in loaded human tendons.

Looking at our results (see Fig. 6 & 7) for the sEMG to tendon artefact peak, we find that throughout a 60 minute run/jog there are no signs of a change in the time interval between the onset of muscle contraction with the initiation of the sEMG signal in both the lateral and medial heads of *m. Gastrocnemius* in healthy subjects. This confirms the findings of Farris et al., (2011), lending weight to the fact that Achilles tendon properties remain stable throughout a period of activity. Keeping this in mind, the tendon artefact would seem to be a useful tool, rather than something that should be filtered out of the recording, enabling the assessment of tendon inflammation and/or damage at an early stage, thus avoiding muscle dysfunction.

Indeed, the sEMG to tendon artefact peak has been found to be very consistent between individuals in the healthy subject group. The delta mSec value indicates the elasticity of the tendon as it interacts with the contracting muscle, absorbing the muscle force and transferring it gradually and smoothly over to the bone and the ankle joint. This should not be confused with creep, which is a change in tendon length once loaded. Rather the recorded artefact illustrates the development of tension/loading within a healthy tendon as muscle contraction proceeds and tendon loading approaches a maximum. Consequently, if an Achilles tendon is damaged and seriously inflamed, one would expect it to have less elasticity and a lower maximum load upon muscle contraction, which would be observed as a much lower delta value. Preliminary data with a few subjects with tendon injuries supports this idea (data not shown).

As stated earlier, recordings of sEMG from leg muscles of healthy subjects, as well as from injured individuals with tendinopathy, are not without problem, and the interpretation of such data should not be made without careful consideration. In Figures 1 & 2 we identified a number of factors that can affect sEMG recordings, and in terms of running/jogging and tendinopathy perhaps the most important would be as follows;

Fig. 1: **Causative** - motor point, tendon, active motor units, motor unit firing rate, acid build-up & blood flow
Intermediate - conduction velocity
Deterministic - active motor units, motor unit firing rate, detected motor units, motor unit action potential amplitude, motor unit action potential duration, recruitment & stability

Fig. 2: Intra-muscular temperature, conduction velocity of muscle fibres & blood flow

In the individuals examined in this section, without doubt the biggest issues to be addressed in terms of a stable sEMG recording are those of lead movement and the release of sweat, which affects electrode adhesion and stable localization. We have sought to reduce lead movement and signal noise arising from the recording cables swinging and moving during running/jogging by asking participants to wear net stockings which serve to hold the cables in place close to the leg and thereby prevent lead movement noise. The second issue of sweat accumulation under the recording electrodes as individuals begin to warm up during the 60 minute run/jog is not so easily solved. We have chosen to use a self-adhesive and elastic tape to ensure that the recording electrodes do not move appreciably, and have cooled the environment in which the run/jog takes place. Nevertheless, in some instances these precautions are not adequate and a degree of sEMG signal noise is unavoidable.

Among the other confounding factors affecting the sEMG signal are parameters closely associated with the level and duration of the exercise itself. As metabolites are used by contracting fibres there is an inevitable acidification close to the muscle membrane which has the advantage of initially improving blood flow through the displacement of K^+, which serves to induce vasodilatation. However, it is known that a build up of H^+ ions close to muscles results in a loss of excitability. Thus a period of exercise over time will affect such parameters as the number of active motor units, the blood flow, and the intra-muscular temperature - the later having an impact on the conduction velocity of muscle fibres.

4. General discussion

As already stated at the start of this manuscript, surface electromyography as a technique offers a safe, quick, pain-free, non-invasive and repeatable way of assessing the physiological processes which cause muscles to generate force and produce movement. It is for this reason that it must be seen as *"a tempting muse"*. As to the critique that *"it is too easy to use and consequently too easy to abuse"* this is surely unfair. It seems to us that if sEMG is being abused as a technique then it is because those using the technique do not fully understand the factors comprising the recorded signal and, as a consequence, do not take the time to assess their results in a critical fashion. One would rarely make a diagnosis of an illness based on just one symptom - the patient has a fever so it must be malaria - and in just the same way, sEMG should be used as a technique alongside other forms of assessing physical function e.g. circulation, muscle strength, Quality of Life etc.

The strength of ones scientific judgement lies surely with a detailed knowledge of any particular technique. In this way, a working understanding of the sEMG signal, its low and high frequency spectrum, and the causes of noise and artefacts, can only serve to reduce the risk of abuse of this technique. Used alongside other assessment tools for judgment of an individual's health, sEMG will support and help towards validation of a diagnosis, and hopefully give directions towards the optimal form of treatment. In the case of tendinopathy, the described tendon artefact suddenly changes from being an artefact - which is something often considered as disturbance - to becoming the reliable measure for tendon condition.

One should not, however, ignore the fact that surface electromyography has a number of limitations that must be understood and corrected for, if meaningful measurements are to be obtained (De Luca, 1993; Hermens et al., 1999, Seniam 1999). In a memorial lecture at the International Society for Biomechanics in 1993, Carlo J. De Luca clearly outlined the inherent problems associated with surface electromyography and provided recommendations for electrode configuration, placement, signal sampling and recording (De Luca, 1993). Later a complete set of guide lines were given by the SENIAM initiative (Hermens et al., 1999). In the examples given here, these guidelines were followed closely in both studies.

Besides the technical aspects of ensuring an accurate sEMG signal recording from a muscle, one should also consider the biological aspects that affect signal parameters, most of which are beyond the recorders control. Here one should pay particular attention to factors that might cause muscle fatigue/weakness as a result of a progressive illness (e.g. uremia) or as the consequence of a period of exercise (e.g. running/jogging).

The aetiology of muscle fatigue is a particularly important question, as the losses in force, velocity and power that define fatigue often lead to serious limitations in muscle and whole body performance (Fitts, 1994). Fatigue results from the effects of multiple factors, which makes unequivocal identification of causative agents a difficult task. It is, however, known that force production is inhibited by a build-up in both P_i and H^+, two products that are known to change with a period of intense exercise with P_i increasing from 5 to 30 or 40 mM, and intracellular pH declining from 7.0 to 6.2 (Thompson & Fitts 1992; Fitts, 1994). Moreover, such changes not only affect force production in fast-twitch muscles, they also reduce cross-bridge interactions due to a changed ionic environment (Metzger & Moss, 1990), leading to a fatigue-induced drop in tension. In uremic patients, a clear reduction in phosphate is often noted after dialysis (48% reduction $P<0.01$) from a value of 1.85 mmol/l (normal adult range of 0.8-1.5 mmol/l). It is also known that alterations in sarcolemma function induce muscle fatigue by preventing cell activation (Sjøgaard, 1990). Indeed, it has been shown that exposure of muscles to a high extracellular K^+ concentration gives rise to depolarization of muscle fibres and results in a loss of contractility (Fitts, 1994), particularly when this is associated with a simultaneous reduction in extracellular Na^+ concentration (Nielsen & Overgaard, 1996).

In an earlier study by the authors investigating recorded interference EMG signals in the hand muscle *2nd dorsal interosseous* of uremic patients under a period of voluntary contraction, it was shown that a significant increase in the deterministic factor "mean signal frequency" occurred when one compared post- to pre-dialysis values (Harrison et al., 2002). These findings, which indicate an inhibitory effect of the uremic state prior to dialysis on the number of recordable events from this particular muscle, are unlikely to be affected by such problems as detection volume of the recording electrodes or by cross-talk from adjacent muscles, as the size and position of this muscle would exclude such issues. It therefore seems realistic to assume, that a haemodialysis session removes some form of inhibition at the level of; 1) the motor nerve e.g. K^+ or so called "middle molecules" with a molecular weight range of 500-2000 Daltons (Bostock et al., 2004), 2) the motor endplate, and 3) the muscle fibre, or any combination of these three. Moreover, the aforementioned study found that one of the largest changes in plasma values in patients undergoing dialysis was that of inorganic phosphate.

The exact mechanism of P_i on force production remains to be elucidated but one might speculate that the increased myoplasmic P_i may decrease force production by direct action on cross-bridge function, or change the distances in the filament lattice due to different ion binding to the filaments (Naylor et al., 1985; Bartels et al., 1985), alternatively increased P_i may inhibit the ATP driven sarcoplasmic Ca^{2+} uptake, such that less Ca^{2+} would be available for release, leading to a decline in force (Duke & Steele, 2000).

In the case of studies involving uremic patients this change in distribution of ions over the cell membrane between dialyses may very well affect the measured sEMG, showing most effect of training right after dialysis. Since each patient is assessed against themselves, this should not affect the overall effect of training, although the true maximal effect may be higher than that seen here.

Likewise, the changes seen in the runners/joggers over a 60 minute exercise period may very well be due to changes in ion balance over the muscle cell membrane. However, whilst this is a valid point with regard to muscle measurements, it has no importance in terms of the use of bipolar recording electrodes to assess tendon function, since this constitutes an artefact, which is independent of a change in frequency and/or amplitude.

5. Conclusions

What can be safely concluded from these results are that direct sEMG recordings can be used as part of an assessment package for weak patient groups with musculo-skeletal problems due to the following two facts. First, that sEMG is quick and painless, making the method well tolerated by weaker patient groups like the uremic patients. Although the method at present is not very specific, it may still be preferential if a clear procedure for measurements and interpretation of data can be set up. The areas to consider are the noise issues, cross-talk between fibres and muscle selection, electrode placement etc. Second, that sEMG is cheap and easily available in a clinical setting, as long as clear guidelines about measurements, data handling and interpretation for the selected setting are available.

Moreover, sEMG represents a trustworthy and reliable means of gaining an insight into muscle function/dysfunction, particularly when used in conjunction with other diagnostic tools.

In the case of uremic patients, sEMG correlates well with such forms of functional assessment as the "stand chair test" and the "Quality of Life Questionnaire – KDQOL-SF-36" (Heaf et al., 2010), and during periods of exercise training there is a significant effect on sEMG frequency and amplitude, indicating a clear improvement in coordination.

As for tendinopathy, it can be concluded from the present results that the application of non-invasive surface electromyography on both heads of *m. Gastrocnemius* during a period of jogging on a treadmill not only shows the initial phase of muscle synchronization as an athlete warms up, and the relative contributions made by the medial and lateral heads of this muscle, it also gives an insight into Achilles tendon activity when combined with a differential recording above the point of insertion to the calcaneous. Furthermore, used with understanding and alongside other diagnostic tools, this technique has the potential to extend our understanding of the active participation of tendons in the tension transfer from muscle to bone.

6. Acknowledgement

We thank Birgitte Holle for her skilled technical assistance in connection with the sEMG recordings, and Prof. Per Aagaard, the Institute of Sports Science and Clinical Biomechanics,

University of Southern Denmark for his most valuable critique of our clinical data. We are also most grateful to the Oak Foundation in terms of the financial support offered (EMB) in connection with this work.

7. References

Alfredson, H.; Ljung, B.O.; Thorsen, K. & Lorentzon, R. (2000) In vivo investigation of ECRB tendons with microdialysis technique - no signs of inflammation but high amounts of glutamate in tennis elbow. *Acta Orthopedica Scandinavica,* Vol. 71, pp. 475-479.

Allison, G.T. & Purdam, C. (2009). Eccentric loading for Achilles tendinopathy - strengthening or stretching? *British Journal of Sports Medicine*, Vol. 43, pp. 276-279.

Bartels, E.M. & Elliott, G.F. (1985). Donnan potentials from the A- and I-bands of glycerinated and chemically-skinned muscles, relaxed and rigor. *Biophysical journal,* Vol. 48(1), pp. 61-76.

Bernardi,M.; Solomonow,M.; Nguyen, G.; Smith, A & Baratta, R. (1996). Motor unit recruitment strategy changes with skill acquisition. *European Journal of Applied Physiology and Occupational Physiology*, Vol. 74, pp 52-59.

Bernardi, M.; Felici, F.; Marchetti, M.; Montellanico, F.; Piacentini, M.F. & Solomonow, M. (1999). Force generation performance and motor unit recruitment strategy in muscles of contralateral limbs. *Journal of Electromyography and Kinesiology,* Vol. 9, pp. 121-130.

Cook, J. (2009). In search of the tendon holy grail: predictable clinical outcomes. *British Journal of Sports Medicine*, Vol. 43, p. 235.

Couppé, C.; Hansen, P.; Kongsgaard, M.; Kovanen, V.; Suetta, C.; Aagaard, P.; Kjaer, M. & Magnusson, S.P. (2009) Mechanical properties and collagen cross- linking of the patellar tendon in old and young men. *Journal of Applied Physiology,* Vol. 107, pp. 880-886.

Day, S.J. & Hullinger, M. (2001). Experimental simulation of cat electromyogram: Evidence for algebraic summation of motor-unit action-potential trains. *Journal of Neurophysiology,* Vol. 86, pp. 2144-2158.

De Luca, C.J. (1997). The use of surface electromyography in biomechanics. *Journal of. Applied Biomechanics,* Vol. 13, pp. 135–163.

De Luca, C.J.; Gilmore, L.D.; Kuznetsov, M. & Roy, S.H. (2010). Filtering the surface EMG signal: Movement artifact and baseline noise contamination. *Journal of Biomechanics,* Vol. 43, pp. 1573-1579.

Ekholm, O.; Kjøller, M.; Davidsen, M.; Hesse, U.; Eriksen, L.; Christensen, A.I. & Grønbæk, M. (2006). Sundhed og sygelighed i Danmark 2005 & udviklingen siden 1987. *København: Statens Institut for Folkesundhed.*

Farina, D.; Merletti, R.; Enoka, R.M. (2004). The extraction of neural strategies from the surface EMG. *Journal of Applied Physiology,* Vol. 96, pp. 1486–1495.

Farris, D.J.; Trewartha, G. & McGuigan, M.P. (2011). The effects of a 30-min run on the mechanics of the human Achilles tendon. *European Journal of Applied Physiology.* DOI: 10.1007/s00421-011-2019-8.

Fredberg, U. & Stengaard-Pedersen, K. (2008). Chronic tendinopathy: tissue pathology, pain mechanisms, and etiology with a special focus on inflammation. *Scandinavian Journal of Medicine and Science in Sports,* Vol. 18(1), pp. 3-15.

Gaida, J.E.; Cook, J.L. & Bass, S.L. (2008). Adiposity and tendinopathy. *Disability and Rehabilitation,* Vol. 30(20-22), pp. 1555-1562.

Gerdle, B.; Karlsson, S.; Crenshaw, A.G. & Friden, J. (1997). The relationships between EMG and muscle morphology throughout sustained static knee extension at two submaximal force levels. *Acta Physiologica Scandinavica,* Vol. 160:, pp. 341–351.

Gerdle, B.; Wretling, M.L. & Henriksson-Larsen, K. (1988). Do the fibre-type proportion and the angular velocity influence the mean power frequency of the electromyogram. *Acta Physiologica Scandinavica* Vol. 134, pp. 341-346.

Gerdle, B.; Henriksson-Larsen, K., Lorentzon, R. & Wretling, M.L. (1991). Dependence of the mean power frequency of the electromyogram on muscle force and fibre type. *Acta Physiologica Scandinavica,* Vol. 142, pp 457-465.

Glazebrook, M.A.; Wright, J.R. Jr; Langman, M.; Stanish, W.D. & Lee, J.M. (2008). Histological analysis of Achilles tendons in an overuse rat model. *Journal of Orthopedic Research* Vol. 26, pp. 840-846.

Harrison, A.P. & Flatman JA. (1999). Measurement of force and both surface and deep M wave properties in isolated rat soleus muscles. *American Journal of Physiology - Regulative Integrative and Comparative Physio*logy, Vol. 277, pp. R1646–R1653.

Harrison, A.P.; Flatman, J.A.; Nielsen, A.H.; Eidemak, I.; Mølsted, S. & Unmack, M.A. (2002). Integrated surface electromyography (EMG) analysis in m. vastus lateralis and m. 2. dorsal interosseous in uremic patients. *Journal of Muscle Research and Cell Motility,* Vol. 23, p. 29.

Harrison, A.P.; Nielsen, A.H.; Eidemak, I.; Molsted, S. & Bartels, E.M. (2006). The uremic environment and muscle dysfunction in man and rat. *Nephron Physiology* , Vol. 103(1), pp. 33-42.

Heaf, J.G.; Mølsted, S.; Harrison, A.P.; Eiken, P.A.; Prescott, L. & Eidemak, I. (2010). Vitamin D, Surface Electromyography and Physical Function in Uraemic Patients. *Nephron,* Vol. 115, pp. c244-c250.

Henneman, E.; Somjen, G. & Carpente, D.O. (1965). Functional significance of cell size in spinal motor neurons. *Electroencephalography and Clinical Neurophysiology,* Vol. 19, pp. 533-580.

Hermens, H.J.; Freriks, B.; Merletti, R.;, Stegeman, D.; Blok, J.;, Rau, J.,; Disselhorstklug, C. & Hâgg, G. (1999). SENIAM 8 - european recommendations for surface electromyography. *Roessingh Research and Developmen*t b.v., Enschede, The Netherlands, 1999.

Hess, G.W. (2010). Achilles tendon rupture: a review of etiology, population, anatomy, risk factors, and injury prevention. *Foot Ankle Speciality.* Vol. 3(1), pp. 29-32.

Hogrel, J,Y. (2005). Clinical applications of surface electromyography in neuromuscular disorders. *Clinical Neurophysiol*ology, Vol. 35, pp. 59–71.

Holm, L.; van Hall, G.; Rose, A.J.; Miller, B.F.; Doessing, S.; Richter, E.A. & Kjaer, M. (2009). Contraction intensity and feeding affect collagen and myofibrillar protein synthesis rates differently in human skeletal muscle. *American Journal of Physiology Endocrinology and Metab*olisme, Vol. 298, pp. E257-E269.

Ishikawa, M.; Pakaslahti, J. & Komi, P.V. (2007). Medial gastrocnemius muscle behavior during human running and walking. *Gait and Posture,* Vol. 25, pp. 380-384.

Järvinen, T.A.; Kannus, P.; Paavola, M.; Järvinen, T.L.; Józsa, L. & Järvinen, M. (2001). Achilles tendon injuries. *Current Opinion in Rheumatology,* Vol. 13(2), pp. 150-155.

Karlsson, S. & Gerdle, B. (2001). Mean frequency and signal amplitude of the surface EMG of the quadriceps muscles increase with increasing torque — a study using the continuous wavelet transform. *Journal of Electromyography and Kinesiology,* Vol. 11, pp. 131–140.

Keenan, K.G.; Farina, D.; Maluf, K.S.; Merletti, R. & Enoka, R.M.(2005). Influence of amplitude cancellation on the simulated surface electromyogram. *Journal of Applied Physiology,* Vol. 98, pp. 120-131.

Keenan, K.G.; Farina, D.; Merletti, R. & Enoka, R.M. (2006). Amplitude cancellation reduces the size of motor unit potentials averaged from the surface EMG. *Journal of Applied Physiology,* Vol. 100, pp. 1928-1937.

Ker, R.F.; Wang, X.T. & Pike, A.V.L. (2000). Fatigue quality of mammalian tendons. *Journal of Experimental Biology*, Vol. 203, pp. 1317-1327.

Komi, P.V. & Tesch, P. (1979). EMG frequency-spectrum, muscle structure, and fatigue during dynamic contractions in man. *European Journal of Applied Physiology and Occupational Physiology,* Vol. 42, pp. 41-50.

Krishnan, A.V.; Phoon, R.K.S.; Pussell, B.A.; Charlesworth, J.A.; Bostock, H. & Kiernan, M.C. (2005). Altered motor nerve excitability in end-stage kidney disease. *Brain,* Vol. 128, pp. 2164-2174

Kupa, E.J.; Roy, S.H.; Kandarian, S.C. & Deluca, C.J. (1995). Effects of muscle-fiber type and size on EMG median frequency and conduction-velocity. *Journal of Applied Physiology*, Vol. 79, pp. 23–32.

Langberg, H.; Ellingsgaard, H.; Madsen, T.; Jansson, J.; Magnusson, S.P.; Aagaard, P. & Kjaer, M. (2007). Eccentric rehabilitation exercise increases peritendinous type I collagen synthesis in humans with Achilles tendinosis. *Scandinavian Journal of Medicine and Science in Sports,* Vol. 17, pp.61-66.

Larsson, B.; Andersen, J.L.; Kadi, F.; Bjork, J. & Gerdle, B. (2002). Myosin heavy chain isoforms influence surface EMG parameters: a study of the trapezius muscle in cleaners with and without myalgia and in healthy teachers. *European Journal of. Applied Physiology,* Vol. 87, pp. 481–488.

Larsson, B.; Kadi, F.; Lindvall, B. & Gerdle, B. (2006). Surface electromyography and peak torque of repetitive maximum isokinetic plantar flexions in relation to aspects of muscle morphology. *Journal of Electromyography and Kinesiology,* Vol. 16, pp. 281–290.

Lichtwark, G.A.; Bougoulais, K. & Wilson, A.M. (2007). Muscle fascicle and series elastic element length changes along the length of the human gastrocnemius during walking and running. *Journal of Biomechanics,* Vol. 40, pp. 157-164.

Linssen, W.H.J.P.; Stegeman, D.F.; Joosten, E.M.G.; Binkhorst, R.A.; Merks, M.J.H.; Terlaak, H.J. & Notermans, S.L.H. (1991). Fatigue in type-I fiber predominance - a muscle force and surface EMG study on the relative role of type-I and type-II muscle-fibers. *Muscle & Nerve,* Vol. 14, pp. 829-837.

Maffulli, N. & Longo, U.G. (2008). How do eccentric exercises work in tendinopathy? An Editorial. *Rheumatology,* Vol. 47, pp. 1444-1445.

Maganaris, C.N. & Paul, J.P. (2002). Tensile properties of the in vivo human gastrocnemius tendon. *Journal of Biomech*anics, Vol. 35, pp. 1639-1646.

Merletti, R.; Knaflitz, M. & De Luca, C.J. (1992). Electrically evoked myoelectric signals. *Critical Reviews in Biomedical Engineering,* Vol. 19, pp. 293-340.

Meyer, A.; Tumilty, S. & Baxter, G.D. (2009). Eccentric exercise protocols for chronic non-insertional Achilles tendinopathy: how much is enough? A Review. *Scandinavian Journal of Medicine and Science in Sports,* Vol. 19, pp. 609-615.

Milnerbrown, H.S. & Miller, R.G. (1986). Muscle membrane excitation and impulse propagation velocity are reduced during muscle fatigue. *Muscle & Nerve,* Vol. 9, pp. 367-374.

Molsted, S.; Eidemak, I.; Sorensen, H.T. & Kristensen, J.H. (2004). Five months of physical exercise in hemodialysis patients: Effects on aerobic capacity, physical function and self-rated health. *Nephron,* Vol. 96(3), pp. c76-c82.

Molsted, S.; Eidemak, I.; Sorensen, H.T.; Kristensen, J.H.; Harrison, A.P. & Andersen, J.L. (2007). Myosin heavy-chain isoform distribution, fibre-type composition and fibre size in skeletal muscle of patients on haemodialysis. *Scandinavian Journal of Urology and Nephrology,* Vol. 41(6), pp. 539-545.

Moritani, T.; Nagata, A. & Muro, M. (1982). Electro-myographic manifestations of muscular electromyography. *Medicine and Science in Sports and Exercise,* Vol. 14, pp. 198-202.

Morrissey, D.; Roskilly, A.; Twycross-Lewis, R.; Isinkaye, T.; Screen, H.; Woledge, R. & Bader, D. (2011). The effect of eccentric and concentric calf muscle training on Achilles tendon stiffness. *Clinical Rehabilitation* , Vol. 25, pp. 238-247.

Naylor, G.R.S.; Bartels, E.M.; Bridgman, T.D. &.Elliott, G.F (1985). Donnan potential changes in rabbit psoas muscle in rigor. *Biophysical Journal,* Vol. 48(1), pp. 47-60.

Olesen, J.L.; Heinemeier, K.M.; Langberg, H.; Magnusson, S.P.; Kjaer, M. & Flyvbjerg, A. (2006). Expression, content, and localization of insulin-like growth factor I in human achilles tendon. *Connective Tissue Research,* Vol. 47, pp. 200-206.

Perry, S.M.; McIlhenny, S.E.; Hoffman, M.C. & Soslowsky, L.J. (2005). Inflammatory and angiogenic mRNA levels are altered in a supraspinatus tendon overuse model. Journal of Shoulder and Elbow Surgery, Vol. 14(1 Suppl S), pp. 79S-83S.

Scott, A.; Cook, J.L.; Hart, D.A.; Walker, D.C.; Duronio, V. & Khan, K.M. (2007). Tenocyte responses to mechanical loading in vivo: a role for local insulin-like growth factor 1 signaling in early tendinosis in rats. *Arthritis and Rheumatology,* Vol. 56, pp. 871-881.

Simpson, M.R. & Howard, T.M. (2009). Tendinopathies of the Foot and Ankle. *American Family Physician,* Vol. 80, pp. 1107-1114.

Solomonow, M.; Baten, C.; Smit, J.; Baratta, R.; Hermens, H.; Dambrosia, R. & Shoji, H. (1990). Electromyogram power spectra frequencies associated with motor unit recruitment strategies. *Journal of Applied Physiology,* Vol. 68, pp. 1177-1185.

Soslowsky, L.J.; Carpenter, J.E.; DeBano, C.M.; Banerji, I. & Moalli, M.R. (1996). Development and use of an animal model for investigations on rotator cuff disease. *Journal of Shoulder Elbow Surgery,* Vol. 5, pp. 383-392.

Soslowsky, L.J.; Thomopoulos, S.; Esmail, A.; Flanagan, C.L.; Iannotti, J.P.; Williamson, J.D. 3rd & Carpenter, J.E. (2002). Rotator cuff tendinosis in an animal model: role of extrinsic and overuse factors. *Annals of Biomedical Engineering,* Vol. 30, pp. 1057-1063.

Tesch, P.A.; Komi, P.V.; Jacobs, I.; Karlsson, J. & Viitasalo, J.T. (1983). Influence of lactate accumulation on EMG frequency-spectrum during repeated concentric contractions. *Acta Physiologica Scandinavica,* Vol. 119, pp. 61-67.

Turker, K.S. (1993). Electromyography - some methodological problems and issues. *Physical Therapy,* Vol. 73, pp. 698-710.

Tygesen, M.P. & Harrison, A.P. (2005). Nutritional restriction in utero programs postnatal muscle development in lambs. *Animal Science Journal,* Vol. 76, pp. 261–271.

Van der Worp, H.; van Ark, M.; Roerink, S.; Pepping, G.-J.; van den Akker-Scheek, I. & Zwerver, J. (2011). Risk factors for patellar tendinopathy: a systematic review of the literature. *British Journal of Sports Medicine,* Vol. 45, pp. 446-452.

Part 2

Signal Processing

6

Nonlinear Analysis for Evaluation of Age-Related Muscle Performance Using Surface Electromyography

Hiroki Takada[1], Yasuyuki Matsuura[1],
Tomoki Shiozawa[2] and Masaru Miyao[3]
[1]*University of Fukui, Fukui*
[2]*Aoyama Gakuin University, Shibuya, Tokyo*
[3]*Graduate School of Information Science, Nagoya University, Nagoya*
Japan

1. Introduction

Several electromyographic methods are currently used, but needle electromyography (nEMG) and surface electromyography (sEMG) are most often applied. To physiologically evaluate electromyographic wave patterns for the detection of abnormalities, the wave patterns obtained with nEMG or sEMG have been macroscopically examined, and subjectively judged by physicians.

- nEMG findings are used for the evaluation of whether a disorder is neurogenic or myogenic, and if it is both neurogenic and myogenic, they provide important information about whether it is acute, subacute, or chronic (KIMURA, 1989). However, the probe is a needle electrode, which is percutaneously inserted into muscular tissues.
- sEMG findings are used for various evaluations, such as the classification of trembling for the diagnosis of involuntary motion, the diagnosis or differential diagnosis of dystonia and spasm, and the identification of involuntary constrictor muscles (KIZUKA et al., 2006).
- sEMG is further used for the determination of the electric potential through a nerve conduction examination (evoked EMG). In evoked EMG, the electrostimulation of peripheral nerves is percutaneously performed (KIMURA, 1989).

The examination methods described, except for method B), are invasive and cause severe pain in patients. Generally, "smoothing" and "integration" refer to two ways of quantifying EMG energy over time; smoothing refers to continuously averaging out the peaks and valleys of a changing electrical signal. On the other hand, integration refers to measuring the area under a curve over a period of time. These methods are used to examine the relative degree of muscular contraction, and are also employed to provide a parameter for the evaluation of muscular training conditions (Aukee, 2002). However, the results obtained are affected by the location of the measuring electrodes and the shape and size of the probes. That is, EMG findings are macroscopically and subjectively evaluated, as described above, and no algorithm for the quantification of the degree of muscular abnormalities or recovery has been established. In this study, we apply and discuss the measurement parameters that have been developed for evaluating the average rectified sEMG (ARS) data obtained from perineal muscles during biofeedback training (BFT) for the treatment of dysuria (Tries & Eisman, 1995) (Fig. 1), and we evaluated the effects of this training (SHIOZAWA et al., 2007). Kegel (1948; 1951) was the first to use BFT for the treatment of urinary incontinence (UI), and it was observed that if the pelvic floor muscles are hypotonic, bladder suspension surgery is less effective for treating stress-related incontinence. In order to improve the contractability of the pubococcygeus portion of the levator ani muscle, Kegel invented the pressure perineometer (KEGEL, 1951). In the U.S.A., at least 13 million community-living adults and more than 50% of all residents in nursing facilities suffer from UI (FANTL et al., 1996). The direct medical expenditure incurred for the care of these people is estimated to be >$15 billion annually, in addition to the $35.2 billion incurred annually for nursing home residents (PEEK et al., 1995). There is a consensus that in most cases, behavioral treatment modalities, including biofeedback, should be used before invasive modalities such as surgery.

A biofeedback instrument has three tasks (PEEK et al., 1995): i) To monitor (in some way) a physiological process of interest, ii) To measure (objectify) what is monitored, and iii) To present what is monitored or measured as meaningful information. The contributions of many previous researchers and practitioners can be cited as the forerunners of biofeedback.

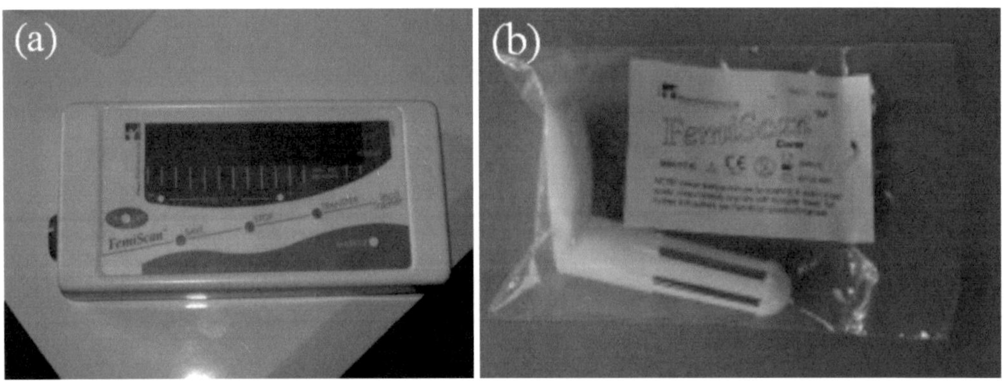

Fig. 1. A biofeedback system (FemiScan Co. Ltd., Finland). The main body (a), and a disposable electrode that can be inserted into perineal muscles (b).

Edmund Jacobsen commenced research at Harvard in 1908, and throughout the 1920s and 1930s worked to develop progressive muscle relaxation as an effective behavioral technique for the alleviation of neurotic tensions and many functional medical disorders (JACOBSEN, 1938). He used crude electromyographic equipment to monitor the levels of muscle tension in his patients during the course of treatment. The classification of and historical perspectives on biofeedback applications can be found in Gaarder and Montgomery (GAARDER and MONTGOMERY, 1981), Gatchel and Price (GATCHEL and PRICE, 1979), and Basmajian (BASMAJIAN, 1989).

Recently, the rapid atrophy of the muscles used for bending at the hip joint during walking (flexor muscles around the hip joint) with age has drawn attention. The flexor muscles around the hip joint consist of the femoral rectus and abdominal muscles. It has been indicated that a lack of these muscles is responsible for the falling of the elderly. In this study, we examined the ARS of the femoral rectus muscles performed during the BFT of the dominant leg, using the measurement parameters mentioned above, and evaluated changes with age.

2. Sensor output signal evaluation system

The sensor output signal evaluation (SOSE) system was developed in 2006 (Shiozawa et al., 2006a). The SOSE system can evaluate the exponential curve-fitting in BFT.

2.1 Participants

The subjects consisted of 31 healthy adults aged 20-73 years (mean, 44.3±19.9 years). All of the subjects were Japanese and lived in Nagoya and its environs. The following were the exclusion criteria for the subjects: subjects working in a night shift, subjects with a dependence on alcohol, subjects who consumed alcohol and caffeine-containing beverages after waking up and within two hours of eating a meal, subjects who may have had a previous history of bone, joint, or nerve problems, and special strength training exercises were not usually done. The subjects were not prescribed drugs for any disease.

2.2 Design

The subject sat back on a four-legged stool, and electromyographic electrodes were applied at an interval of several centimeters to the center of the femoral rectus muscles in the dominant left or right leg (Fig.2). The subjects were instructed to kick a fixed belt by moving the bottom of the lower leg forward (kicking motion).

2.2.1 Biofeedback training

Temporal data were obtained using sEMG, and they are expressed here as $\{y(t)\}$. Generally, sEMG data are recorded by a computer at 2 kHz. Here, the integral calculation was performed every 0.1 s using the following equation:

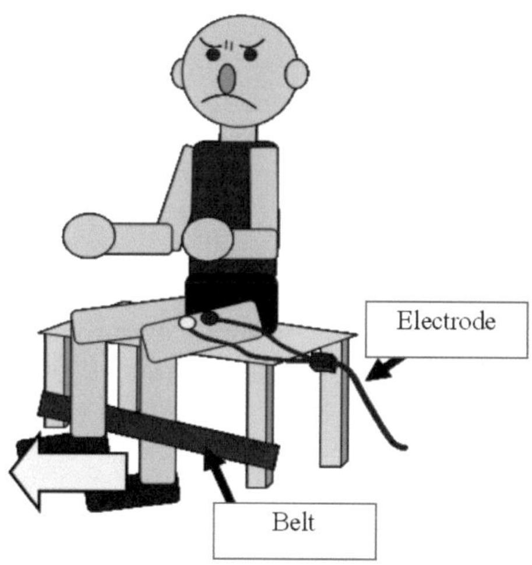

Fig. 2. Biofeedback training instruction signal. The BFT instruction signal produced by superimposing the ARS on the target instruction signal.

$$x(t) = \sum_{k=0}^{199} \left| y(t + 0.0005k) \right| , \tag{1}$$

and the ARS $\{x(t)\}$ was calculated in real time and outputted. The subject was told to observe the outputted wave patterns and the rectangular waves $f(t)$ of a 10-s cycle superimposed on the same display (Fig. 3), and then perform intermittent continuous contractions of the femoral rectus muscles corresponding to the patterns (BFT).
The subjects performed BFT for 2 min. We ensured that the body sway was not affected by environmental conditions; using an air conditioner, we adjusted the *temperature* to 25 °C in the exercise room, which was large, quiet, and *bright*. All subjects were tested from 10 am to 5 pm in an exercise *room*. All subjects gave consent in writing after a sufficient explanation of this study.

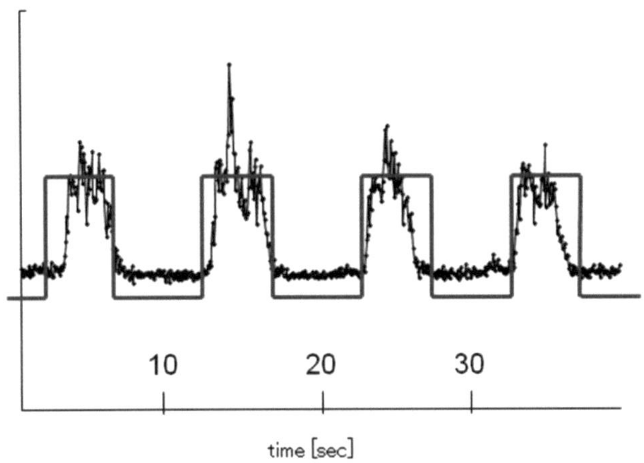

Fig. 3. Biofeedback training instruction signal. BFT instruction signal produced by superimposing the ARS on the target instruction signal.

2.2.2 Materials
A special electromyographic transformation box (AP-U027, TEAC Co.) was connected to a commercially available portable and versatile amplifier and recorder (Polymate AP1532, TEAC Co.), and electromyographic electrodes (bipolar) with preamplifiers were used.

2.2.3 Procedure
First, the electromyographic wave patterns obtained over 5 seconds at the maximum effort of the kicking motion (maximum voluntary contraction (MVC) (CARLO and DELUCA, 1997) were integrated in real time using a computer, and the ARS data on the display were shown to the subject. Next, the threshold line at 75% of the mean ARS (mV) during the muscular contraction period was shown to the subject, who was requested to perform muscular training aiming at the threshold line for 1 min 20 s. In other words, BFT was performed at 75% of the MVC. During BFT, data were recorded in a notebook computer (AP Monitor, NoruPro) at a sampling rate of 2 kHz. The low frequency cut-off filters were used at 16 Hz, and an alternating current-eliminating filter was also used.

2.3 Algorithm in the SOSE system

The initial 20 s of the sEMG data recorded over a total of 1 min 20 s were excluded, because the subjects may have required this time to adjust to the training. The sEMG data of the 6-cycle rectangular waves that occurred over the remaining minutes of training (target value) $f(t)$ and the ARS were analyzed in accordance with the Double-Wayland algorithm (TAKADA et al., 2006a) and our own mathematical algorithms of the sensor output signal evaluation system. Fig. 4 shows a revision of the flow chart in SHIOZAWA et al. (2006a). Taking a mean of the ARS (MARS) as a threshold H for determining continuous muscular contractions, the time sequences above the threshold H were regarded as continuous muscular contractions. Based on whether differences such as $x(t) - x(t - 0.1)$ and $(x(t + 0.1) - x(t))(x(t) - x(t - 0.1))$ were positive or negative, a maximal series for the continuous muscular contractions was extracted as shown in Fig. 5.

a. The value of the MARS during the muscular relaxation period (x^a) and the measurement parameters in the other terms (SHIOZAWA et al., 2006b; SHIOZAWA et al., 2006c; TAKADA et al., 2006b) indicating the shape of the ARS were determined every cycle, and the ARS values obtained from the femoral rectus muscles were evaluated.
b. Maximum amplitude (x^b): This maximum value was examined and recorded.
c. Duration of continuous muscular contraction (x^c): The duration between the first and last maximal values in a cycle exceeding the MARS sEMG was measured (Fig. 5).
d. The time constant of the exponential decay curve fit to the maximal points during the muscular contraction period in the BFT (x^d): All maximal values between the first and last maximal values exceeding the MARS in a cycle were extracted as $\{x_m(t)\}$ and fit to the exponential decay curve $\hat{x}_m(t) = C\exp[-x^d t]$. On a semi-log graph, the time constant (x^d) was estimated using the mean least square method, which minimized the sum of the squared residuals;

$$L = \sum_t \{\log \hat{x}_m(t) - \log x_m(t)\}^2 . \tag{2}$$

In order to estimate the time constant (x^d), the following simultaneous equation should be solved.

$$\frac{\partial L}{\partial \log C} = 0, \frac{\partial L}{\partial x^d} = 0 \tag{3}$$

The numerical sequences of the 4 measurement parameters were determined at a repetition number of 6. The relationship between the age (z) of the subjects who had undergone sEMG and the value $x^i(z)$ (i = a,b,c,d) estimated in the 5th cycle was statistically examined to evaluate correlations between each measurement parameter and age (Appendix).

2.4 Practical study of the SOSE system

The numerical sequences of each of the measurement parameters at a repetition number of 6 were obtained by sEMG performed during BFT. The relationship between the age (z) of the subjects who had undergone sEMG and the value $x^i(z)$ (i = a,b,c,d) was examined in 5th cycle. Fig. 6 shows the $x^i(z)$ of all 50 subjects. The linear regression analysis using the least-square method, demonstrated that the coefficients by which age (z) was multiplied were 0.071, -0.268, -0.006, and -0.010 for (a), (b), (c), and (d), respectively, and the parameters,

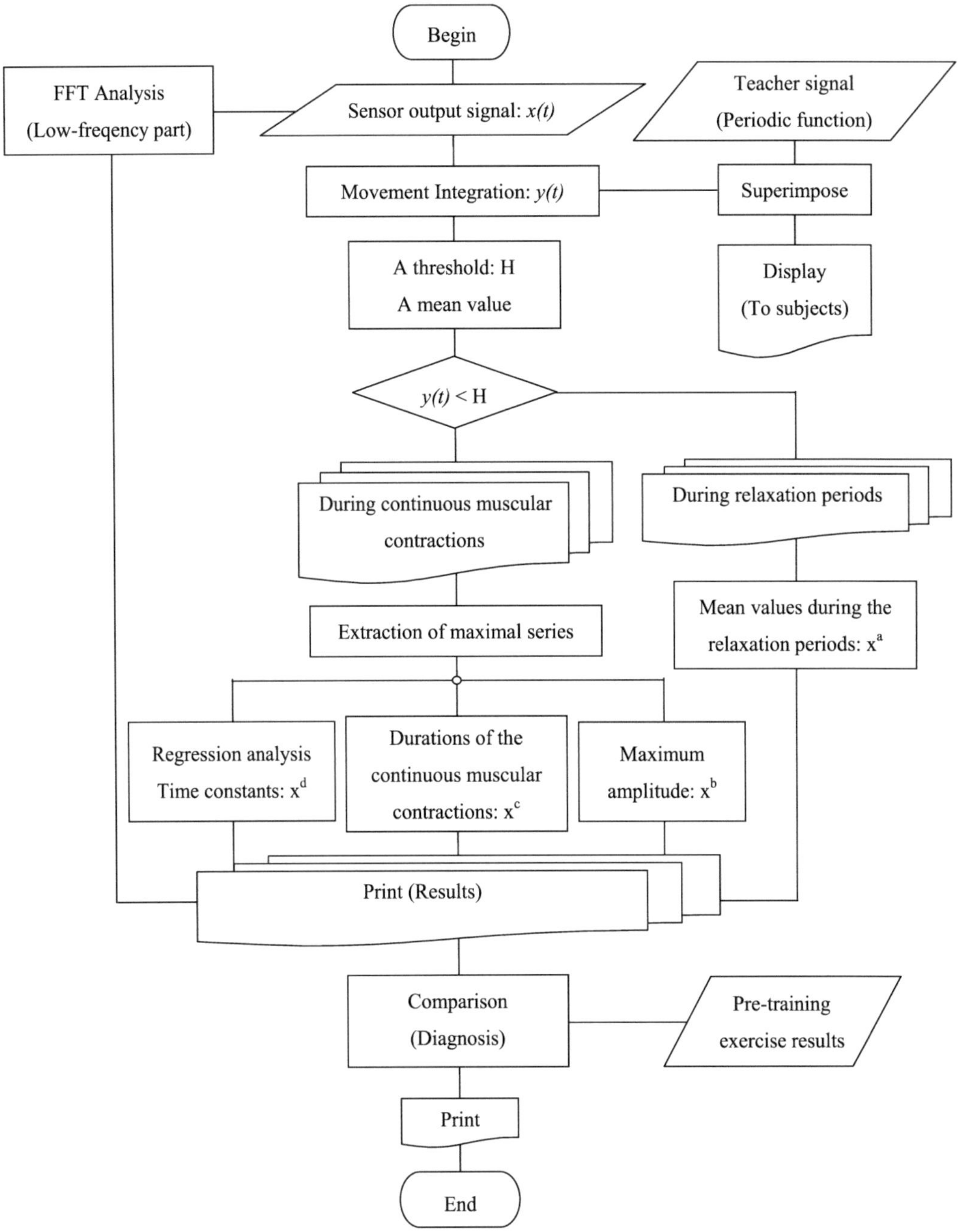

Fig. 4. A part of the flow chart of our mathematical algorithm of the sensor output signal evaluation system.

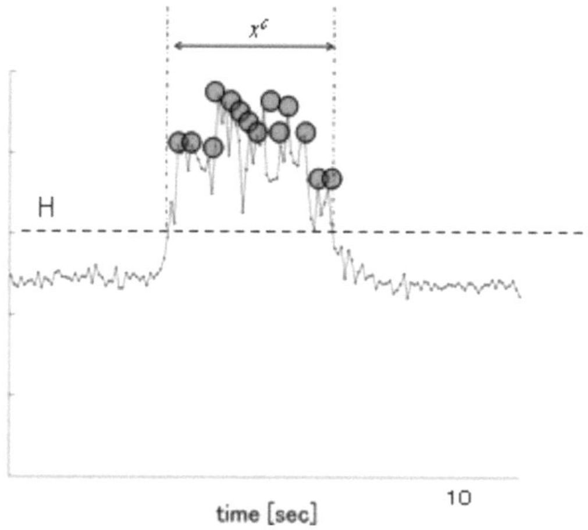

Fig. 5. A series of maximal values of the ARS during the muscular contraction periods in the BFT were extracted by our mathematical algorithm of the sensor output signal evaluation system.

except for (a), decreased with age. Since the linear regression coefficients varied with the measurement parameters, correlations between these parameters and age could not be judged using only the coefficients by which age (z) was multiplied. When using the t-test to evaluate the null hypothesis ($\hat{b}=0$) for the regression coefficient ($\hat{b}$), the test values (A.3) were 1.105, 0.238, 1.621, and 3.245 for (a), (b), (c), and (d), respectively, and the only parameter exceeding $t_{48}(0.975)$ was the time constant of the exponential decay curve fit to the maximal points of the muscular contraction period in the BFT (x^d).
We examined correlations between the parameters of the ARS and age. Regression equations (A.1) for each parameter (i = a,b,c,d) were determined, and the null hypothesis ($\hat{b} = 0$) for the regression coefficient ($\hat{b}$) was examined using the t-test. Since the test value (A.3) was larger than the two-sided 5% point, t_{48} (0.975), in the t distribution with a latitude of 48, the null hypothesis was rejected in the case of i = d. Therefore, the time constant of the exponential decay curve fit to the maximal points during the continuous muscular contraction period (x^d) is significantly dependant on age ($p<0.05$).

2.5 Problem

The analysis of sEMG data is generally performed by the fast Fourier transformation (FFT), which is a linear analytical method. A Fourier series expansion of the function $f(t)$, showing target levels (instruction signals) for BFT, is possible, and the following expansion equation (MATSUMOTO and MIYAHARA, 1990) is useful for evaluating the differences between the ARS and the rectangular waves:

$$f(t)=1+\sum_{k=1}^{\infty}\frac{2}{k\pi}\{1+(-1)^{k+1}\}\sin\frac{2\pi k}{T}t\,. \tag{4}$$

Higher-order terms (high-frequency components) are included in this expansion equation, but the coefficients are small due to the presence of the order in the denominator. Accordingly, the high-frequency power was considered to be theoretically irrelevant for the

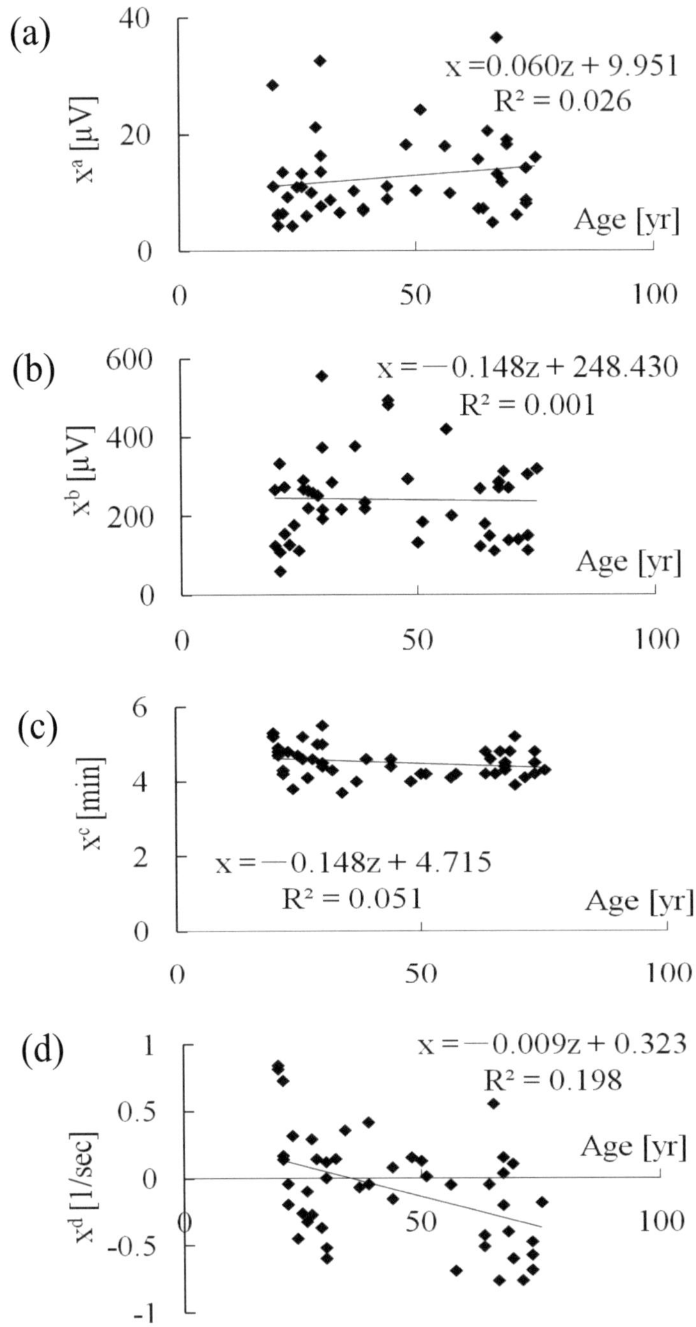

Fig. 6. Relationships between the measurement parameters of the ARS and age and their linear regressions. R^2 shows the coefficient of determination. MARS during the muscular relaxation period, x^a (a). Maximum amplitude, x^b (b). Duration of continuous muscular contraction, x^c (c). Time constant of the exponential curve fit to the maximal points of the continuous muscular contraction period, x^d (d).

evaluation shown in Eq. (4). Since muscular conditions always vary, signals should be regarded as non-steady (BEYER, 1987). Since a spectral estimation by the Fourier analysis is based on the assumption that the signals to be analyzed are steady and linear, this linear analysis of sEMG data is inappropriate.

Myopotentials are induced by changes in the firing patterns of nerve impulses. Several muscle fibers controlled by a motor nerve are collectively called a motor unit (MU), and several MUs can be excited by nerve impulses, causing an MU action potential. The MU action potential measured on the skin's surface is a superficial myopotential, and it is observed at a site spatially distant from the local region where the MU action potential waves are generated. In sEMG, a very large number of MU action potential waves are superimposed, and the activity states of whole muscles are observed by this method (YOSHIDA et al., 2004). Therefore, sEMG signals should be considered nonlinear, or more generally, sEMG shows a time series produced by stochastic processes. Recently, it has been recognized that sEMG data can be examined by nonlinear analytical methods, such as the recurrence plot and the Wayland algorithm (YOSHIDA et al., 2004; TAKADA et al, 2006c). However, the measurement parameters used in the present study, such as the time constant of the exponential decay curve fit to the maximal points of the continuous muscular contraction period (x^d), are used as a linear analytical method for sEMG. In the next section, we discuss the reason why we have succeeded in findings a linear index showing a correlation with age.

3. Solution & recommendations

The complexity of the bio-signal or the degree of visible determinism generating those signals can be measured by our Double-Wayland algorithm (TAKADA et al, 2006a), which is introduced in this section.

3.1 Double-Wayland algorithm

The translation error is a statistical index that measures the smoothness of flow in an attractor generating a time series. In addition, randomness can be evaluated by the Double-Wayland algorithm by comparing the translation errors in the temporal differences of the time series (differenced time series) with the results of the Wayland algorithm in each embedding space (Wayland et al., 1993).

An attractor is reconstructed from a time series. The attractor is constructed by means of embedding the time series data proposed by Takens (1981) in the phase space. Embedding is a method that draws an orbit in phase space supposing a vector whose elements are the values for when the time elapses from t to Δt, $2\Delta t$, ..., $(N\text{-}1)\Delta t$ as a point in N dimensional phase space (embedding space). N and Δt are referred to as the embedding dimension and the sampling time, respectively. The delay coordinates $\{\mathbf{x}(t)\}$ can reconstruct a continuous trajectory without crossing into an embedding space that has a high dimension. If we only resample the time series at every delay time τ when the auto-correlation coefficient $\rho(\tau)$ is regarded as zero, components of the delay coordinate $\mathbf{x}(t) = (\mathbf{x}(t), \mathbf{x}(t+\tau), ..., \mathbf{x}(t+(N\text{-}1)\tau))$ cannot linearly correlate with each other. In this study, the auto-correlation function $\rho(t)$ was estimated from the time series data (Matsumoto et al., 2002) and regarded as zero when $\rho(t)$ decreased below $1/e \cong 0.37$ for the first time ($t \geq 0$).

The Wayland algorithm assumes that the difference vectors $\mathbf{v}(t) = \mathbf{x}(t+\tau) - \mathbf{x}(t)$ in the embedding space characterize the nonlinear variations of the trajectories and estimate the translation error in an m-dimensional embedding space ($m = 1, 2, ..., 10$). Here, τ was estimated at 73-76 times the sampling time. A linear correlation between adjacent vectors $\mathbf{x}(t)$ and $\mathbf{x}(t+\tau)$ is eliminated by resampling the time series with respect to each embedding delay τ.

i. A series of delay coordinate vectors $\{\mathbf{x}(t)\}$ is embedded in each space.
ii. M onset periods t_0 are randomly selected.
iii. The values of

$$E_{\text{trans}}(t_0) = \frac{1}{K+1}\sum_{i=0}^{K}\frac{|\mathbf{v}(t_i) - \overline{\mathbf{v}}|}{|\overline{\mathbf{v}}|} \tag{5}$$

are standardized by the average of the difference vectors at $K+1$ points $\{\mathbf{x}(t_i)\}_{i=0}^{K}$.

$$\overline{\mathbf{v}} = \frac{1}{K+1}\sum_{i=0}^{K}\mathbf{v}(t_i) \tag{6}$$

is obtained at every onset period, where the K points nearest to $\mathbf{x}(t_0)$ are selected as $\{\mathbf{x}(t_i)\}_{i=0}^{K}$.

iv. The median of the M values of Eq. (5) is extracted.
v. Q medians are obtained by repeating the above steps. The translation error E_{trans} is estimated by the expectation value of these Q medians.

The Double-Wayland algorithm includes the following additional steps.

vi. Translation errors, E_{trans}', are derived from temporal differences in the time series data (differenced time series) $\{\mathbf{x}(t+\tau) - \mathbf{x}(t)\}$ by the Wayland algorithm outlined above.
vii. If a differential equation system that included stochastic factors was the generator of the time series, the flow would not be smooth. In such a case, a significantly higher number of translation errors might be estimated in the last step than in step (v).

In this study, we set the conditions of the coefficients M, K, and Q to be 51, 3, and 10, respectively (Wayland et al., 1993).

If a time series is produced from a chaos process, the translation vectors point in almost the same direction unless the time implementation τ is too large, since deterministic aspects remain in time development. The minimum translation error would be estimated in such an embedding space that has no false intersection along the orbit and best reflects the degree of freedom. Hereby, the optimum embedding dimension to capture the chaos process can be obtained.

The differenced time series produced in the stochastic process often reconstitutes an indifferentiable orbit in embedding space. This indicates that the translation error estimated from the differenced time series exceeds the translation error estimated from the time series data. Accordingly, we weighed the translation error estimated from the time series data against the error estimated from the differenced time series in m dimensional phase space.

In general, the threshold of the translation error for classifying the time series data as deterministic or stochastic is 0.5, which is half of the translation error resulting from a random walk (MATSUMOTO et al., 2002). The abovementioned E_{trans} is compared with the translation error (E_{trans}') estimated from the differenced time series.

3.2 Non-linear analysis of the sEMG in the BFT

Using the Double-Wayland algorithm, translation errors were estimated from the sEMG measured during a continuous muscle contraction period and during BFT. We compared the translation errors E_{trans} and E_{trans}' in each embedding space (Figs.7). Intermittent muscle the differenced sEMG's of the younger subjects. E_{trans}' would be less than E_{trans} if the degree of determinism involved in the generator were reduced. The form of a rectangular wave as a teacher signal might reduce the nonlinearity involved in the generator of sEMG for the young. Moreover, we employed the method of surrogate data to ascertain the cause of the correlation between age and a linear index for the ARS. According to the Fourier shuffle algorithm, 20 surrogate sequences were generated from each ARS during the 3 s continuous muscle contraction period and the 3 s of BFT shown in Fig. 7. Using the Wayland algorithm, translation errors were estimated from the surrogate sequences. The embedding delay was estimated as 0.064 ± 0.003 s and 0.290 ± 0.135 s from the surrogate data of the ARS during the continuous muscle contraction period and BFT, respectively. A significant difference was observed between the translation errors, E_{trans}, estimated during the continuous muscle contraction period and the BFT ($p < 0.01$). The E_{trans} calculated during the continuous muscle contraction period was greater than that taken after this period. BFT could enhance the linearity in the generator of sEMG.

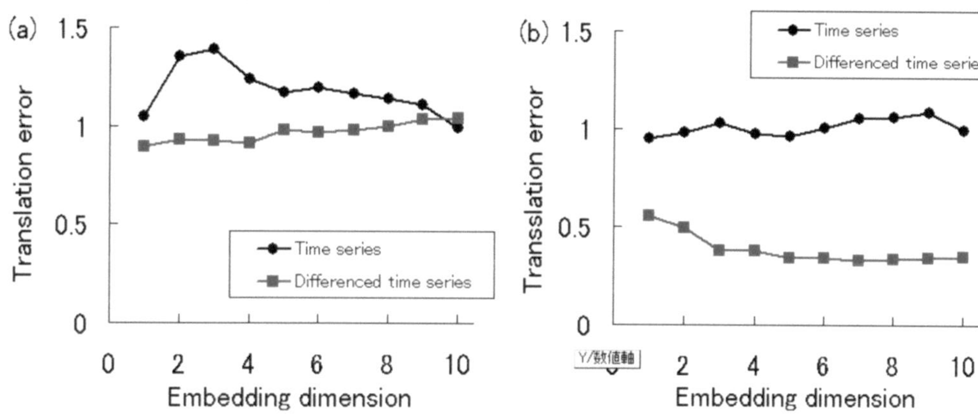

Fig. 7. Results of the calculations involved in sEMG using the Double-Wayland algorithm. Translation errors, E_{trans} and E_{trans}', were estimated from sEMG data measured during a continuous muscle contraction period for 3 s (a) and during 3 s of BFT (b) (TAKADA et al., 2010).

3.3 Stability of the sEMG in the BFT

Since there were differences in not only the unit of measurement but also the numerical order between the parameters, they were normalized using the intermediate values $\bar{x}^i$ for each cycle, and the reproducibility (stability) of the measurements was evaluated using the standard deviation $\sigma[x^i/\bar{x}^i]$. The normalized value is 1 when the measurement is equal to the intermediate value. When the reproducibility (stability) of repeated measurements is high, the deviations from this value are small, and the standard deviation is close to 0.

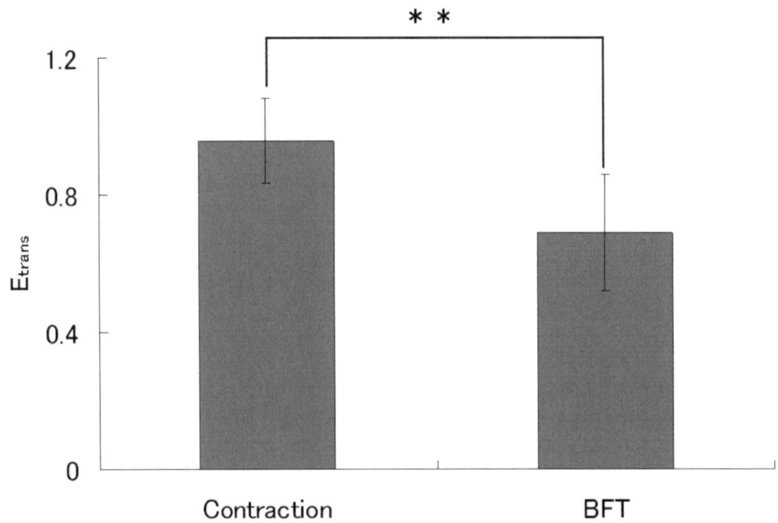

Fig. 8. Result of the surrogate data analysis. In 10 dimensional embedding space, translation errors were estimated from the surrogate data of the ARS during the continuous muscle contraction period and the BFT.

The intermediate values of the parameters and the standard deviations (σ) of normalized measurements were determined for each subject, and the medians of σ in the age groups are compared in Table 1. The duration of continuous muscular contraction (x^c) alone showed $\sigma < 0.1$ for any age group.

Age group	*N*	*Mean during relaxation*	*Maximal amplitude*	*Duration of continuous muscular contraction*	*Time constant*
≤25	*8*	*0.24*	*0.13*	*0.06*	*1.51*
≤45	*9*	*0.21*	*0.14*	*0.08*	*0.55*
≤65	*6*	*0.33*	*0.14*	*0.08*	*1.84*
65 <	*8*	*0.07*	*0.06*	*0.06*	*0.89*

N expresses the number of subjects in each age group.

Table 1. Standard deviations of normalized indices $x/\bar{x}$ [8]

4. Future research directions

The decline in translation errors, E_{trans}', was not always seen in the middle-aged and the elderly. Poor muscular control might enhance the instability of the temporal variations involved in the ARS, which should be maintained as a constant during a muscular contraction in BFT. The relationship between age and the decline in the translation errors, E_{trans}', should be investigated in future work.

We will employ a time series analysis, such as a surrogate method, to ascertain the cause of the correlation between age and a linear index of ARS.

5. Conclusion

Recently, there has been an increasing focus on the rapid reduction of the muscles that are required for bending the hip joint during walking with age. Atrophy of the flexor muscles has been implicated in falling in the elderly. In this study, we examined the ARS of the femoral rectus muscles during BFT of the dominant leg. To this end, we developed parameters for the measurement of the shapes in the ARS, and evaluated the changes in these parameters as the muscles age. A statistical analysis indicated that it was necessary to include the time constant of the exponential decay curve fit to the maximal points during prolonged muscular contraction to evaluate changes with age using the ARS during BFT. A reduction in the function of muscular control due to aging can be detected by performing sEMG during BFT using this time constant. Using our Double-Wayland algorithm, we have also confirmed the stationarity of the ARS during the muscle contraction period.

6. Appendix

The relationship between each of the above measurement parameters and age was examined. $x_j^i(z_j)$ of subject j ($j = 1, 2, \cdots, 50$) was plotted, and a linear regression analysis of these 50 points was performed by the least-square method (MATSUMOTO and MIYAHARA, 1990). The regression equation of each measurement parameter was determined.

$$x^i = \hat{a} + \hat{b}\, z \tag{A.1}$$

$$\text{s.t.} \quad \hat{a} = \frac{1}{50}\left(\sum_{j=1}^{50} x_j^i - \hat{b}\sum_{j=1}^{50} z_j\right), \tag{A.2.1}$$

$$\hat{b} = \frac{1}{S_{zz}}\sum_{j=1}^{50} x_j^i\left(z_j - \frac{1}{50}\sum_{j=1}^{50} z_j\right). \quad (i = \text{a, b, c, d}) \tag{A.2.2}$$

Here, S_{zz} denotes a variance of age. The dependence of each measurement parameter on age was statistically evaluated by a two-sided t-test with the null hypothesis that the regression coefficient $\hat{b} = 0$.

$$\left|\hat{b} - 0\right| \Big/ \sqrt{S_E / 48 S_{zz}} \tag{A.3}$$

If the above value is larger than $t_{48}(1-\alpha/2)$, the null hypothesis is rejected, and the measurement parameter is considered to be correlated with age (SHIMIZU and TAKADA, 2001). Here, S_E denotes the residual sum of squares by the least-square method, and $t_{48}(1-\alpha/2)$ represents the t distribution at a probability of $1-\alpha/2$ and a latitude of 48. In this study, since the significance level (α) was defined as 0.05, $t_{48}(1-\alpha/2)$ was approximately 2.010.

7. Acknowledgment

This work was supported in part by a ground-based study proposal for the fiscal year of 2005-2007 (17659189) and the Hori Information Science Promotion Foundation.

8. References

Aukee, P., Penttinen, J., Immonen, P. & Airaksinen, O. (2002) Intravaginal surface EMG probe design test for urinary incontinence patients. *Acupunt. Electro-Ther. Res. Int. J.*, Vol.27, 2002, pp.37–44, 0360-1293.

Basmajian, S. (1989) *An anthology of visual poetry and collage*, Sober Minute Press, 0921280009, Toronto.

Beyer, W.H. (eds.) (June 30,1987) *CRC Standard Mathematical Tables and Formulae* (28th ed.), CRC Press, ISBN 0849306280,Boca Raton, FL.

Bosco, C. & Komi, P. V. (1980) Influence of aging on the mechanical behaviour of leg extensor muscles. *European Journal of Applied Physiology*, Vol.45, Dec 1980, pp.209-219, 1439-6319.

Carlo, J. & Deluca, C.J. (1997) The use of surface electromyography in biomechanics. *Journal of Applied Biomechanics*, Vol.13, July 1993, pp.135–163, 1065-8483.

Chang, T., Schiff, S.J., Sauer, T., Gossard, J.P. & Burke, R.E. (1994) Stochastic Versus Deteriministic Variability in Simple Neuronal circuits: I. Monosynaptic Spinal Cord Reflexes, *Biophysical Journal*, Vol.67, No.2, Aug 1994, pp.671-683, 0006-3495.

Chang, T., Sauer, T. & Schiff, S.J. (1995) Tests for nonlinearity in short stationary time series, *Chaos*, Vol.5, No.1, Mar 1995, pp.118-126, 1054-1500.

Fantl, J.A., Newman, D.K., Colling, J., Delancey, J., Keeys, C.,Loughery, R., Mcdowell, J., Norton, P., Ouslander, J., Schnelle, J., Staskin, D., Tries, J., Urich, V., Vitousek, S.H., Weiss, B.D., & Whitmore, K. (Mar 1996) *Urinary Incontinence in Adults : Acute and Chronic Management.* Clinical practice guideline. Rockville, MD: Agency for Health Care Policy and Research, Public Health Service, US Department of Health and Human Services.

Gaarder, K.R. & Montgomery, P.S. (Jun, 1981) *Clinical Biofeedback-Procedural Manual for Behavioral Medicine*, Williams & Wilkins, 0683034014, London.

Gatchel, R. J. & Price, K. P. An introduction and historical overview, In: Gatchel, R.J. and Price, K.P.(eds.), Mar 1979. *Critical Applications of Biofeedback: Appraisal and Status*, Pergamon Press, 0080229786, New York.

Hanayama, K. (2001) Evaluation of muscle fatigue with muscle fiber conduction velocity, Clinical Electroencephalography, Vol.43, No.3, pp.144-147, 0009-9155.

Jacobsen, E.(Dec, 1938) *Progressive relaxation*, University of Chicago Press, 0226390586, Chicago.

Kegel, A.H. (1948) Progressive resistance exercise in the functional restoration of the perineal muscles. *American Journal of Obstetrics and Gynecology*, Vol.56, Aug 1948, pp.238-248, 0002-9378.

Kegel, A.H.(1951) Physiologic therapy for urinary stress incontinence. *Journal of the American Medical Association*, Vol.146, 1951, pp.915-917, 0098-7484.

Kiryu, T. (1997) Monitoring local muscle fatigue using surface electromyography. *Journal of the Society of Biomechanisms*, Vol.21, No.2, Feb 1997,pp.75-80, 0285-0885.

Kimura, J. (Jun 15, 1989) *Electrodiagnosis in Diseases of Nerve and Muscles: Principles and Practice* (2nd), Oxford University Press, pp.209-304, 0803653425, Philadelphia.

Kizuka, T., Masuda, T., Kiryu, T. & Sadoyama, T. (Mar 2006) *Practical usage of surface electromyography*, Tokyo Denki University Press, pp.65-92, 4501325100, Tokyo.

Matsumoto, H. & Miyahara, Y. (Jun 1999) *Introduction to mathematical statistics*, Gakujutsu Tosho, pp.106-108, 4873611741, Tokyo.

Matsumoto, T., Tokunaga, R., Miyano, T. & Tokuda, I. (Nov 2002) *Chaos and time series*, Baihukan, pp.49–64, 4563014974, Tokyo.

Peek, C. J. (Jan 1, 1995) A primer of biofeedback instrumentation, In: *Biofeedback a Practitionaer's Guide*, Schwartz, M.S., pp.597-629, Guilford Press, 0898628067, New York.

Shimizu, Y. & Takada, H. (2001) Verification of air temperature variation with form of potential, *Forma*, Vol.16, No.4, 2001, pp.339-356, 0911-6036.

Shiozawa, T., Takada, H. & Miyao, M. (2006a) Sensor output signal evaluation system, Japan Patent P2006-111387.

Shiozawa, T., Takada, H., Miyao, M. & Kawasaki, H.(2006b) Propositions of evaluating indices of muscle performancs detected by using surface electromyography and evaluation of stability of the indices, *Proceedings of the 21th Symposium on Biological and Physiological Engineering 2006*, Kagoshima(Japan), Nov 2006.

Shiozawa, T., Takada, H., Miyao, M., Takada, M., Kawasaki, H. & Watanabe, Y. (2006c) Evaluation of muscle performances detected by using surface electromyography, *Japanese Journal of Ergonomics*, Vol.42, Jun 2006, pp.S440-S441. 0549-4974.

Shiozawa, T., Takada, H. & Miyao, M. (2007) Sensor output signal evaluation system, PCT Patent Publication No. WO 2007/129452.

Takada, H., Morimoto, T., Tsunashima, H., Yamazaki, T., Hoshina, H. & Miyao, M. (2006a) Applications of Double-Wayland Algorithm to Detect Anomalous Signals, *Forma*, Vol.21, No.2, 2006, pp.159-167, 0911-6036.

Takada, H., Shiozawa, T., Miyao, M., Takada, M. & Kawasaki, H. (2006b) Mathematical analysis of skeletal muscle electromyogram and the aging, *Japanese Journal of Ergonomics*, Vol.42, Jun 2006, pp.S444-S445. 0549-4974.

Takada, H., Shiozawa, T., Miyao, M., Nakayama, M. & Kawasaki, H.(2006c) Theoretical consideration to set the amplitude of teacher signal in the biofeedback training, *Proceedings of the 21th Symposium on Biological and Physiological Engineering 2006*, Kagoshima(Japan), Nov 2006.

Takada, H., Shiozawa, T., Takada, M., Miyao, M. & Kawasaki, H.(2007) Propositions of evaluaing indices of muscle performances detected by using surface electromyography and the aging, *Bulletin of Gifu University of Medical Science*, Vol.1, Mar 2007, pp.91-95, 1881-9168.

Takada, H., Shiozawa, T., Miyao, M. Matsuura, Y. & Takada, M. (Oct 6, 2010) Consideration of indices to evaluate age-related muscle performance by using surface electromyography. In: *Advances in computational biology*, Arabnia, H. R., pp.585-591, Springer, 9781441959126, New York

Takens, F. (1981) Detecting strange attractors in turbulence, *Lecture Notes in Mathematics*, Vol.898, 1981, pp.366-381, 0075-8434.

Theiler, J., Eubank, S., Longtin, A., Galdrikian, B. & Farmer, J.D. Testing for nonlinearity in time series: The method of surrogate data, Physica D, 58, pp.77-94, 1992, 0167-2789.

Tries, J. & Eisman, E. (Jan 1, 1995) Urinary incontinence—evaluation and biofeedback treatment. In: *Biofeedback a Practitionaer's Guide*, Schwartz, M. S., pp.597-629, Guilford Press, 0898628067, New York.

Wayland, R., Bromley, D., Pickett, D. & Passamante, A. (1993) Recognizing determinism in a time series, *Phys. Rev. Lett.*, Vol.70, No.5, Feb 1993, pp.580–582, 0031-9007.

Yoshida, H., Ujiie, H., Ishimura, K. & Wada, M. (2004) The estimation of muscle fatigue using chaos analysis, *Journal of the Society of Biomechanisms*, Vol.28, No.4, 2004, pp.201-212, 0285-0885.

Young, A. (1997) Ageing and physiological functions. *Philos Trans R Soc Lond B*, Vol.352, Dec 1997, pp.1837–1843, 0264-3839.

7

The Usefulness of Wavelet Transform to Reduce Noise in the SEMG Signal

Angkoon Phinyomark, Pornchai Phukpattaranont and Chusak Limsakul
Department of Electrical Engineering, Prince of Songkla University, Songkhla, Thailand

1. Introduction

This chapter presents a usefulness of wavelet transform (WT) algorithm in pre-processing stage of surface electromyography (sEMG) signal analysis particularly in application of noise reduction. The successful pre-processing stage based on wavelet decomposition and denoising algorithm is proposed in this chapter together with the principle, theory, up-to-date literature review and experimental results of the wavelet denoising algorithms. Main application of this algorithm is sEMG control systems, notably prosthetic devices or computers.

SEMG signal is one of the useful electrophysiological signals. It is measured by surface electrodes that are placed on the skin superimposed on the muscle. Rich useful information has occurred in the muscles subjacent to the skin as a mixture of the whole motor unit action potentials (MUAPs). Such information is also useful in a wide class of clinical and engineering researches which may lead to providing the diagnosis tools of neuromuscular and neurological problems and to providing the control systems of assistive robots and rehabilitation devices (Merletti & Parker, 2004). Generally, in order to use the sEMG as a diagnosis signal or a control signal, a feature is often extracted before performing classification stage due to a lot of information obtained from raw sEMG data and a low computational complexity required in the embedded devices (Boostani & Moradi, 2003). However, the sEMG signals that originate in a wide class of human muscles and activities are definitely contaminated by different types of noise (De Luca, 2002; Reaz et al., 2006). This becomes a main problem to extract certain features and thus the reach to high accurate classification. In the last decade, many research works have been interested in developing better algorithms and improving the existing methods to reduce noises and to estimate the useful sEMG information (De Luca et al., 2010; Mewett et al., 2004; Phinyomark et al., 2011).

Generally, noises contaminated in the sEMG signal can be categorized into four major types: ambient noise, motion artifact, inherent instability of the sEMG signal, and inherence in electronic components in the detection and recording equipment (De Luca, 2002). The first three types have specific frequency band and do not fall in the energy band of the sEMG signal. For instance, power-line interference has the frequency component at 50 Hz (or 60 Hz), and motion artifact and instability in nature of sEMG signal have most of their energy in the frequency range of 0 to 20 Hz. Usage of conventional filters, i.e. band-pass filter and band-stop filter, can reduce noises in these types (De Luca et al., 2010). However, the last noise type is a central concern in analysis of the sEMG signal. It is an inherent noise that is generated by electronic equipment. The frequency components of this noise are random in nature and range in the usable energy of sEMG frequency band from 0 to several thousand Hz. It causes difficulty in elimination using the conventional filters. Moreover, using high-quality electronic components, intelligent circuit design and construction techniques, noises can be only reduced but it cannot be entirely eliminated (De Luca, 2002). Hence, it may cause a problem in extracting the robust features (Phinyomark et al., 2008; Zardoshti-Kermani, 1995).

Wavelet transform and adaptive filter are used in advanced filtering methods that are commonly used as a powerful tool to remove random noise in non-stationary signals. Nonetheless, the drawback of adaptive filter is the complexity of devising an automatic procedure. Its performance depends on a reference input signal which is difficult to apply in the real-world applications. On the other hand, wavelet transform method does not require any reference signals. The pre-processing stage based on wavelet denoising algorithm for sEMG upper- and lower- limb movement recognitions have been a huge success over the past few years (Hussain et al., 2007, 2009; Khezri & Jahed, 2008; Phinyomark et al., 2010a, 2011; Ren et al., 2006). To achieve the best performance in wavelet denoising algorithm, five wavelet parameters must be addressed. Hence, in this chapter, we have evaluated all wavelet denoising parameters for improving the classification performance of sEMG control systems. As a result, the improvement of classification accuracy of the sEMG recognition system has been presented and a robustness of the system has also been improved.

The rest of this chapter is as follows: Section 2 presents various types of electrical noises in sEMG signals and discusses how to simulate these artificial noises. In Section 3, principle and theory of wavelet transform algorithm in both general and denoising viewpoints are described. Extensive review and careful survey of up-to-date wavelet denoising methods in numerous biomedical signals and applications are summarized in Section 4 and recent trend of wavelet denoising algorithms in the sEMG signal analysis is discussed in Section 5. In Section 6, the experimental results of using wavelet denoising algorithms with real sEMG signals are presented and discussed. Lastly, conclusion and future trends of using wavelet transform to reduce noise in the sEMG signal are proposed in Section 7.

2. Electrical noises in the SEMG signal

2.1 Different types of the noises

Noises contaminated in the sEMG signal can be categorized into four main types: ambient noise, motion artifact, sEMG signal inherent instability, and inherence in electronic components in the detection and recording equipments (De Luca, 2002; Kale & Dudul, 2009; Reaz et al., 2006). More details about source and characteristics of each noise type are explained in the following discussion:

1. Ambient noise: This kind of noise originates from electromagnetic radiation sources such as electrical-power wires, light bulbs, fluorescent lamps, radio and television transmission, computers, etc. Essentially any electromagnetic device or device that is plugged into the A/C power supply generates and may contribute ambient noises. Moreover, our body surfaces are persistently flooded with electric-magnetic radiation and it is practically impossible to avoid exposure to it on the surface of the earth. The dominant frequency of the ambient noise arises from the 50 Hz (or 60 Hz) radiation from power sources. Generally, the main concern noise in this type is also called "Power-line noise or 50 Hz interference". The amplitude of the ambient noise is one to

three orders of magnitude greater than the sEMG signal. Therefore, in analysis of the sEMG signal in various research works have implemented a notch filter (band-stop filter) at this frequency (Mewett et al., 2004). Theoretically, this type of filter would only remove the unwanted power-line frequency; however, practical implementations also remove portions of the adjacent frequency components. Because the dominant energy of the sEMG signal is located in the 50-100 Hz range, the use of notch filter is not advisable (De Luca, 2002). One of our previous studies (Phinyomark et al., 2009a), the effect of this kind of noises with the sEMG feature extraction was investigated. The robust features for this kind of noise, notably Willison amplitude, have been found in order to avoid the implementing a notch-filter.

2. Motion artifact: This kind of noise causes irregularities in the signal. When motion artifact is putted into the data, the sEMG information may be skewed. There are two main sources of motion artifact: 1) the interface between the detection surface of electrode and skin 2) the movement of the cable connecting electrode to the amplifier. The dominant energy of the electrode motion artifact has been concerned in the frequency range from 0 to 20 Hz. The second type of noise source, cable motion artifact typically has a frequency range of 1 to 50 Hz. However, both of these sources can be essentially reduced by proper design of the electronics circuitry and set-up. Moreover, some research works suggest implementing a high-pass filter into the measurement instrumentation with a corner frequency of 10 Hz (Clancy et al., 2002) or 20 Hz (De Luca et al., 2010).
3. SEMG signal inherent instability: Amplitude of the sEMG signal is quasi-random in nature. This kind of noise is affected by the random in nature of the firing rate of the motor units which, in most conditions, fire in the frequency components between 0 and 20 Hz. Because of the unstable nature of these components of the sEMG signal, it is advisable to consider them as unwanted noise and remove them from the sEMG signal. Nevertheless, it can be removed using a high-pass filter with a cut-off frequency of 20 Hz which has already been implemented in the removing of motion artifact.
4. Inherence in electronic components in the detection and recording equipments: All electronics equipments generate electrical noise. This noise has the frequency components that range from 0 Hz to several thousand Hz. The problem is that this kind of noise cannot be eliminated. It can only be reduced by using high-quality electronic components, intelligent circuit design and construction techniques. Therefore, this kind of noise is becoming a major problem in analysis of the sEMG signal. Our previous studies, we have paid more interest in reducing the effect of noise in this group (Phinyomark et al., 2008, 2009b, 2009c, 2009d, 2009e, 2009f, 2009g, 2009h, 2010a, 2010b, 2010c, 2011).

Note that during the recording of the sEMG signal, the subject is generally instructed to relax. However, regardless of relaxation, muscles always show a basic level of electrical activity. It has been suggested that this residual sEMG activity may establish a significant part of the total noise level (Huigen et al., 2002). All of these noises also mentioned to the background noise.

2.2 Simulation of noises in SEMG signal analysis

From the above explanation, we can notice that first three types of noises have the specific frequency band and do not fall in the dominant energy band of the sEMG signal. Thus usage of the conventional filters such as band-pass filter, high-pass filter and notch filter can eliminate noises in this group (De Luca et al., 2010). However, noise of the last type is a main concern in analysis of the sEMG signal. It ranges in the usable energy of sEMG frequency band from 0 to several thousand Hz; therefore, it causes difficulty in elimination using the conventional filters. Moreover, using high-quality electronic components, intelligent circuit design and construction techniques, noise in this group can be only reduced but it cannot be entirely eliminated (De Luca, 2002; Kale & Dudul, 2009; Reaz et al., 2006).

To prepare the noisy sEMG signals, random noise is considered to be used as a representative noise, an agent of the fourth noise type. Usually, white Gaussian noise (WGN) is used as a representative random noise in the sEMG signal analysis (Boostani & Moradi, 2003; Kale & Dudul, 2009; Laterza & Olmo, 1997; Law et al., 2011; Wellig & Moschytz, 1998; Zardoshti-Kermani et al., 1995). This noise is also called artificial random noise or simulated random noise. The WGN is a random signal with a flat power spectral density and a normal amplitude distribution. To more clearly understand, the flat power spectral density means that the signal contains equal power within a fixed bandwidth at any center frequency and the normal amplitude distribution means that the signal contains random values that tend to cluster around a single mean value. Usually the WGN is set to a zero mean and a unit standard deviation (Kale & Dudul, 2009; Phinyomark et al., 2009c, 2010a, 2011). In order to evaluate performance of the denoising algorithms, different levels of the WGN are used in the preparation of noisy environment. Zardoshti-Kermani et al. (1995) estimated the WGN with root-mean-square (RMS) amplitude on each muscle position varying from 0% to 50% of the overall average RMS amplitude of the whole muscle activities. The estimated signal-to-noise ratios (SNRs) were varied from 1:3 to 7:1 which depended on level of muscle contraction. Subsequently, Andrade et al. (2006) and Law et al. (2011) estimated the WGN with amplitude ranging from 20% to 100% and from 2% to 40% of the absolute maximum amplitude, respectively. On the other hand, Boostani and Moradi (2003) estimated the WGN with one tenth of the peak-to-peak amplitude range of the sEMG signal. In our previous studies, noisy sEMG signals were simulated by adding synthetic WGNs which resulted in different SNRs. The SNRs ranged from 20 dB (low noise level) to 0 dB (high noise level) with the increasing step of 5 dB SNR (Phinyomark et al., 2009c, 2010a, 2011). In addition, some research studies have used our criterion for simulated noisy EMG environments; for instance, Huang et al. (2010) designed a robust EMG sensing interface for pattern classification by using the simulated WGN in range of 20-0 dB SNRs.

Other three important types of noises that normally are used and considered in the simulated noisy EMG environment are power-line noise, movement artifact, and baseline noise. Firstly, power-line interference is used to evaluate ability of both denoising algorithms and robust sEMG features (Boostani & Moradi, 2003; Phinyomark et al., 2009a). This kind of noise is easy to simulate because its frequency component appears at only one frequency point, 50 or 60 Hz. Secondly, movement artifact can be estimated by the volunteer movement which can be monitored by using an accelerometer sensor (De Luca et al., 2010). The accelerometers were attached in the proximity of the sEMG sensors, such as on the top or the distal. When the subjects move their muscles and a movement at the electrode-skin interface is occurred, the g value from the accelerometer can be shown that event (De Luca et al., 2010). Thirdly, noise that is considered in analysis of the sEMG signal is baseline noise. However, this kind of noise can be problematic only when the sEMG signal is very low SNR (Clancy et al., 2002) such as in the assessment of antagonist muscle co-activation or in the classification of low-level muscle contraction (Baratta et al., 1998; Law et al., 2011).

3. Principle and theory of wavelet transform in denoising viewpoint

3.1 Wavelet decomposition

Wavelet transform (WT) is a time-scale representation technique, which expresses a signal into a two-dimensional function of time and scale (pseudo-frequency). The WT uses the correlation with translation and dilation of a wavelet function to yield this transformation. It represents a signal as a sum of wavelets with different locations and scales that allows to use long time intervals for low-frequency information and to use shorter regions for high-frequency information. The WT can be categorized into two main types: continuous wavelet transform (CWT) and discrete wavelet transform (DWT). Calculating wavelet coefficients at every possible scale as implemented in CWT is a fair amount work and it generates an awful lot of data. Usually in denoising viewpoint, the researchers obtain such an analysis from DWT. The definition of DWT is given by:

$$C(a,b) = \sum_{n \in Z} x(n) g_{j,k}(n) \qquad (1)$$

where $C(a,b)$ are dyadic wavelet coefficients, a is dilation or scale ($a=2^{-j}$), b is translation ($b=k\times2^{-j}$), $x(n)$ is the input signal, and $g_{j,k}(n)$ is discrete wavelet ($g_{j,k}(n)=2^{j/2}\times g(2^{j}n-k)$ where $j \in N$ and $k \in Z$). When the input signal is decomposed to a certain level using the DWT, a set of wavelet coefficients is correlated to the high-frequency components (low-scale) while the other wavelet coefficients are correlated to low-frequency components (high-scale). In details, as shown in Fig. 1, in the first step, the original signal (S) is passed through two complementary filters, a low-pass filter and a high-pass filter, and emerges as two signals, approximations and details. The first-level approximation coefficient array (cA1) is obtained from a low-pass filter which includes down-sampling and the first-level detail coefficient array (cD1) is passed through a high-pass filter with down-sampling. The low-pass and high-pass filtering processes are similar to convolving the signal with a scaling function and a wavelet function, respectively. For many signals, generally, the low-frequency content (cA) is the most important part and the high-frequency content (cD), on the other hand, impacts flavor or nuance (noises). Hence, the second-level approximation coefficient array (cA2) and the second-level detail coefficient array (cD2) are obtained by inputting the cA1 into the filters. This is similar to dilating the original scaling function and wavelet function prior to convolving with the cA1. The process is repeated until the desired final level approximation and detail coefficient arrays are obtained. As shown in Fig. 1, it has 3 decomposition levels. When the decomposition is taken as a whole, the denoising process can be employed. If any modification process is not required, the reconstruction process will be instantaneously done. The reconstructed signal (S'), final level approximation and all level details, are true components of the original signal. This is called the perfect reconstruction. The reconstruction process is performed by up-sampling each coefficient array prior to refiltering.

The DWT provides a great advantage over the Fourier analysis and the short-time Fourier transform (STFT) analysis. Although the traditional Fourier analysis performs greatly for the stationary signals, it has a serious drawback if the interesting signals contain non-stationary or transitory characteristics. The STFT and the DWT, on the other hand, map a signal into a two-dimensional function of time and frequency by using a windowing technique. Both of them thus perform greatly for the non-stationary signals. The DWT shares some similarities to the STFT as we described above, except that the fixed window size in the STFT is no more flexible for many signals.

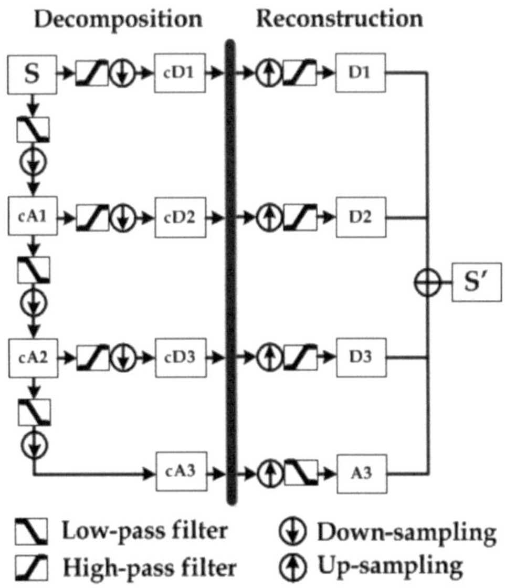

Fig. 1. Wavelet decomposition and reconstruction process.

3.2 Wavelet denoising

The undesired wavelet coefficients containing random noise can be discarded before performing the reconstruction process. The cleaner signal will be obtained from that process. To grab this outcome, thresholding is used in wavelet domain to remove or to shrink some coefficients of DWT detail sub-signals of the measured signal. Usually, the denoising method that applies thresholding in wavelet domain has been proposed by Donoho (1995). The Donoho's method for noise reduction works well for a wide class of one-dimensional and two-dimensional signals. The basic idea of wavelet-based denoising procedure is illustrated in Fig. 2. It consists of three main steps: decomposition, modification of detail coefficients and reconstruction. The first and the last main steps are the general DWT procedure as we described in the Section 3.1. The middle main step is added into the general DWT procedure that involves three parameters: threshold selection rule, threshold rescaling method and thresholding function. In other words, two main points must be addressed: how to choose the threshold value and how to perform the thresholding. In addition, two parameters in decomposition step must be evaluated that are wavelet function and decomposition level.

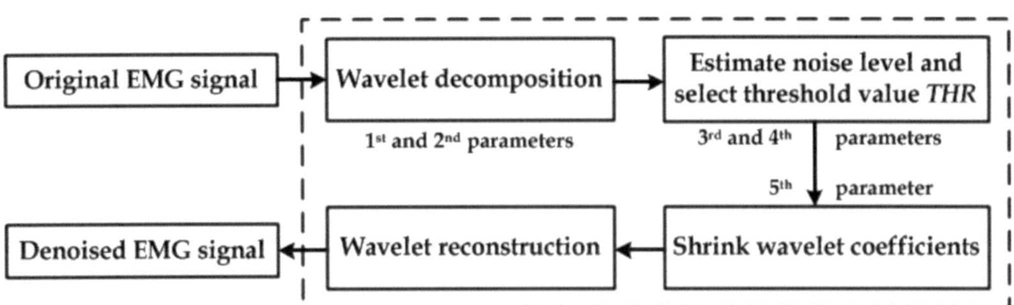

Fig. 2. Wavelet denoising procedure.

In details, the first step in producing a wavelet denoising is to choose a wavelet function (first parameter) to be used in signal decomposition. Different types of wavelet are available which each type has different sub-types. The second step, the selection of a suitable decomposition level (second parameter) must be selected with a candidate wavelet function. The third step, the threshold value *THR* (third parameter) to be applied in the wavelet domain is calculated by the product of the standard deviation of the noise energy σ and the small factor that depends on the length N of the data sample (Donoho and Johnstone, 1994). There are many modified versions of threshold selection rule. In order to rescale the threshold value *THR* obtained from the third step; the estimation of the noise energy σ (fourth parameter) is specified in this step. The fifth step, after threshold *THR* is smoothed, the thresholding is based on a threshold value *THR* which is used to compare with all the detailed coefficients. Ordinarily, two types of thresholding functions (fifth parameter) are often used: hard thresholding and soft thresholding (Donoho and Johnstone, 1994). The choice of threshold values and thresholding functions plays an important role in the global performance of a wavelet processor for noise reduction. Wavelet-based denoising algorithm is based on the underlying model. It is basically of the following form:

$$s(n) = x(n) + \sigma e(n)\,, \tag{2}$$

where $s(n)$ is the measured or noisy signal, $x(n)$ is the original or clean signal and $e(n)$ is a Gaussian white noise $N(0,1)$, σ is the strength of the noise, and time n is equally spaced.

4. Review and theory of modified wavelet denoising methods

From the last section, the application of wavelet-based denoising algorithm requires the selection of five processing parameters named "wavelet denoising parameters", including: (1) the type of wavelet basis function, (2) the decomposition level, (3) threshold selection rule (4) threshold rescaling method, and (5) thresholding function. Throughout the extensive review and careful survey of up-to-date wavelet denoising methods in a wide class of biomedical signals and applications, theory and definition of all methods are summarized in the following.

4.1 Wavelet basis functions

Wavelet function or mother wavelet can be categorised into two main types: orthogonal and biorthogonal wavelets. Orthogonal wavelet is entirely defined by the scaling filter (a low-pass finite impulse response (FIR) filter). For analysis with this wavelet, the high-pass filters are calculated as the quadrature mirror filter of the low-pass filters and reconstruction filters are defined as the time reverse of the decomposition filters. In biorthogonal wavelet, decomposition and reconstruction filters are defined as the separate filters. Commonly, there are 6 wavelet families: Daubechies wavelets (10 sub-types), Symlets wavelets (7 sub-types), Coiflet wavelets (5 sub-types), BiorSplines wavelets (15 sub-types), ReverseBior wavelets (15 sub-types) and Discrete Meyer wavelet. All of wavelet functions are presented in Table I. It is important for choosing the right wavelet function (Kania et al., 2007; Tan et al., 2007). The right filter determines perfect reconstruction and performs better analysis.

Wavelet family	Wavelet subtypes
Daubechies	db1 or haar, db2, db3, db4, db5, db6, db7, db8, db9, db10
Symlets	sym2, sym3, sym4, sym5, sym6, sym7, sym8
Coiflet	coif1, coif2, coif3, coif4, coif5
BiorSplines	bior1.1, bior1.3, bior1.5, bior2.2, bior2.4, bior2.6, bior2.8, bior3.1, bior3.3, bior3.5, bior3.7, bior3.9, bior4.4, bior5.5, bior6.8
ReverseBior	rbio1.1, rbio1.3, rbio1.5, rbio2.2, rbio2.4, rbio2.6, rbio2.8, rbio3.1, rbio3.3, rbio3.5, rbio3.7, rbio3.9, rbio4.4, rbio5.5, rbio6.8
Discrete Meyer	dmey

Table 1. List of 53 wavelet functions from 6 wavelet families.

4.2 Decomposition levels

Next step is the selection of the number of decomposition level of the signal. The decomposition level can be varied from 1 (the first level of decomposition) to $J=\log_2 N$ (the maximum depth of decomposition) where N is the length in samples of time-domain signal.

4.3 Threshold selection rules

Threshold selection rule refers to "how to choose the threshold value". Generally, most of research works have used universal threshold selection rule proposed by Donoho. It has been shown that its denoising capability is better than other classical methods such as SURE method, Hybrid method, and minimax method (Phinyomark et al., 2009f). The definition and description of four mainly threshold selection rules are summarized in Table 2. Hence, in our studies, we have interested in numerous modified versions of universal rule (rule 1 in Table 2). Six modified universal rules have been proposed as described in the following. In this chapter, we provide the specific name to each rule as follows.

Thresholding rule	Description
Rule 1: Universal	It uses a fixed form threshold (Donoho & Johnstone, 1994) which can be defined as $THR_{UNI} = \sigma\sqrt{2\log(N)}$, where N is the length in samples of time-domain signal and σ is standard deviation of noise. The parameter σ can be estimated using median parameter which can be calculated as $\sigma = \text{median}\left(\left\|cD_j\right\|\right)/0.6745$ where cD_j is the detail wavelet coefficients at scale level j and 0.6475 is a normalization factor.
Rule 2: SURE	Threshold is selected using the rule of Stein's Unbiased Estimate of Risk (SURE). It gets an estimate of the risk for a particular threshold *THR*, where risk is defined by SURE (Stein, 1981). Minimizing the risk in *THR* gives a selection of the threshold.
Rule 3: Hybrid	This rule attempts to overcome limitation of SURE. It is a mixture of the universal and the SURE rules. The exact conditions of this algorithm are described in Donoho and Johnstone (1995).
Rule 4: Minimax	This method was also proposed in Stein (1981) work. It used a fixed threshold chosen to yield minimax performance for mean square error against an ideal procedure.

Table 2. Four main threshold selection rules.

1) Length Modified Universal rule (LMU): It was modified by Donoho to be used with soft-thresholding function (Donoho, 1995). It is defined as

$$THR_{\mathrm{LMU}} = \frac{\sigma\sqrt{2\log(N)}}{\sqrt{N}}. \tag{3}$$

2) Scale Modified Universal rule (SMU): It was modified by Donoho to be used with level dependent method (Donoho, 1992). It can be expressed as

$$THR_{\mathrm{SMU}} = \sigma\sqrt{2\log(N)} \cdot 2^{\frac{j-J}{2}}, \tag{4}$$

where j is scale level from 1 to J and J is the maximum level.
3) Global Scale Modified Universal rule (GSMU): It was modified by Zhong and Cherkassky (2000) to be used in denoising of image. It is given by

$$THR_{\mathrm{GSMU}} = \sigma\sqrt{2\log(N)} \cdot 2^{\frac{-J}{2}}. \tag{5}$$

4) Scale Length Modified Universal rule (SLMU): It was modified by Donoho (1992). It is a combination between LMU and SMU rules. It is shown as

$$THR_{\mathrm{SLMU}} = \frac{2\sigma\sqrt{2\log(N)}}{\sqrt{N} \cdot 2^{\frac{J-j}{2}}}. \tag{6}$$

5) Log Scale Modified Universal rule (LSMU): It was modified by Song and Zhao (2001). It takes the different thresholds at different scales. It can be defined as

$$THR_{\mathrm{LSMU}} = \frac{\sigma\sqrt{2\log(N)}}{\log(j+1)}. \tag{7}$$

6) Log Variable Modified Universal rule (LVMU): It was modified by Zhang and Luo (2006). It uses the constant d to adapt the value of threshold THR. Experiment of Zhang and Luo (2006) showed that the constant d is associated to the wavelet function and the SNR. It should be ranging between 0 and 3. In our study, we used d = 3. The equation can be defined as

$$THR_{LVMU} = \frac{\sigma\sqrt{2\log(N)}}{\log[e+(j-1)^d]}. \tag{8}$$

4.4 Threshold rescaling methods

All threshold selection rules can be smoothing their thresholds by using rescaling methods. In threshold rescaling, three categories can be identified: global (GL), first-level (FL) and level dependent (LD) (Elena et al., 2006; Johnstone & Silverman, 1997). In the first one, standard deviation of noise (σ) can be adapted to three categories (GL, FL and LD). While the second one, length of wavelet coefficients (N) can be adapted to only GL and LD thresholding. To identify the threshold rescaling methods, GL defines σ as the estimated standard deviation of all wavelet coefficients and N as the length of the total wavelet coefficients. FL defines σ_1 as the estimated standard deviation of the first-level detail coefficients (cD_1). LD defines σ_j as the estimated standard deviation for every possible decomposition levels and N_j as the length of the wavelet coefficients at decomposition level j.

4.5 Thresholding functions

After threshold values are determined, shrinking can be done using wavelet thresholding functions. In this chapter, after extensive review of the available literatures, fifteen wavelet thresholding functions were described in the following.

1) Hard function (HAD): It is the simplest function. All wavelet's detail coefficients whose absolute values are lower than threshold are set to be zero and other wavelet's detail coefficients are kept (Donoho & Johnstone, 1994). It is defined as

$$cD_j = \begin{cases} cD_j, & if\ |cD_j| > THR_j \\ 0, & otherwise \end{cases}. \tag{9}$$

2) Soft function (SOF): It is an expanded version of HAD (Donoho & Johnstone, 1994). It can be done by first zeroing all wavelet's detail coefficients whose absolute values are lower than threshold same as HAD. Then, non-zero coefficients are shrunk towards zero. SOF function is determined by

$$cD_j = \begin{cases} \operatorname{sgn}(cD_j)(\left|cD_j\right| - THR_j), & if\ |cD_j| > THR_j \\ 0, & otherwise \end{cases}, \tag{10}$$

where $\operatorname{sgn}(x)$ is a sign function that extracts the sign of a real number x.

3) Mid function (MID): It is an extension of SOF (Percival & Walden, 2000), small wavelet's coefficients are zeroed, and then large wavelet's coefficients are not affected. However, intermediate wavelet's coefficients are reduced. MID function can be expressed as

$$cD_j = \begin{cases} cD_j, & \left|cD_j\right| > 2THR_j \\ 2\operatorname{sgn}(cD_j)(\left|cD_j\right| - THR_j), & THR_j < \left|cD_j\right| \le 2THR_j \\ 0, & otherwise \end{cases}. \tag{11}$$

4) Hyperbolic function (HYP): It is attempted to address the limitation of SOF. It is described in Vidakovic (1999) work and its equation is defined same as modulus squared function (Guoxiang & Ruizhen, 2001) that is given by

$$cD_j = \begin{cases} \operatorname{sgn}(cD_j)\sqrt{(cD_j^2 - THR^2)}, & if\ |cD_j| > THR \\ 0, & otherwise \end{cases}. \tag{12}$$

5) Modified hyperbolic function (MHP): It combines the advantage of HAD and SOF functions. It resembles the variance pattern of HAD and the removing of bias problem of SOF. It is modified by Poornachandra et al. (2005) and is shown as

$$cD_j = \begin{cases} (k \cdot cD_j)\left[1 + (\frac{cD_j^2}{6})\right], & if\ |cD_j| > THR_j \\ 0, & otherwise \end{cases}, \tag{13}$$

where k is the scaling function and, in our studies, we used 1 for the constant k.
6) Non-negative Garrote function (NNG): It combines Donoho and Johnstone's thresholding function with Breiman's NNG. The equation is modified by Gao (1998) as

$$cD_j = \begin{cases} cD_j - \frac{THR_j^2}{cD_j}, & if\ |cD_j| > THR_j \\ 0, & otherwise \end{cases}. \tag{14}$$

7) Compromising of HAD and SOF function (CHS): It estimates wavelet's coefficients by weighted average of HAD and SOF (Guoxiang & Ruizhen, 2001). For $0<a<1$, when a is 0, it changed into HAD and when a is 1, it changed into SOF. In our study, we used 0.5 for the constant a. It can be expressed as

$$cD_j = \begin{cases} \text{sgn}(cD_j)(|cD_j| - \alpha THR_j), & if\ |cD_j| > THR_j \\ 0, & otherwise \end{cases}. \tag{15}$$

8) Weighted Averaging function (WAV): It estimates coefficients by weighted average of HYP and HAD (Zhang & Luo, 2006). It is given by

$$cD_j = \begin{cases} (1-\alpha)\text{sgn}(cD_j)\sqrt{(cD_j^2 - THR_j^2)} + \alpha(cD_j), & if\ |cD_j| > THR_j \\ 0, & otherwise \end{cases}, \tag{16}$$

where $0<a<1$. If a is 0, Eq. (16) will change to HYP and Eq. (16) will change to HAD, if a is 1. We used 0.5 for the constant a.
9) Adaptive Denoising function (ADP): It is modified based on SOF (Tianshu et al., 2002). It is given by

$$cD_j = cD_j - THR_j + \frac{2THR_j}{1 + e^{2.1cD_j/THR_j}}. \tag{17}$$

10) Improved function (IMP): It is attempted to address the deficiency of HAD and SOF (Su & Zhao, 2005). It can be defined as

$$cD_j = \begin{cases} \text{sgn}(cD_j)(|cD_j| - \beta^{(THR_j - |cD_j|)} \cdot THR_j), & if\ |cD_j| > THR_j \\ 0, & otherwise \end{cases}, \tag{18}$$

where $\beta \in \Re^+$ and $\beta>1$. In our study, we used 15 from the suggestion of Su and Zhao work (2005).
11) Custom function (CUT): Idea of this function is similar to that of NNG function, in the sense that CUT and NNG are continuous and can adapt to the signal characteristics. Denote $0 < \gamma < THR_j$ and $0 < a < 1$. In our studies, we used the same threshold as in Yoon and Vaidyanathan (2004) work with $a = 1$ and $\gamma = THR_j/2$. The equation can be expressed as

$$cD_j = \begin{cases} cD_j + \mathrm{sgn}(cD_j)(1-\alpha)THR_j\,, \; if\;|cD_j| \geq THR_j \\ 0\,, if\;|cD_j| \leq \gamma, \\ \alpha \cdot THR_j \left(\dfrac{|cD_j|-\gamma}{THR_j-\gamma}\right)^2 \left\{(\alpha-3)\left(\dfrac{|cD_j|-\gamma}{THR_j-\gamma}\right)+4-\alpha\right\}, otherwise \end{cases} . \tag{19}$$

12) Firm function (FIM): It remedies the drawbacks of HAD and SOF functions. Gao and Bruce (1997) generalize a general FIM function using double threshold values. The THR_2 is defined by universal rule but THR_1 is scoped to range between 0 and THR_2. According to the previous experiments, Gao and Bruce (1997) suggested that when THR_1 equals $2/3THR_2$, the denoised results would be better. FIM can be expressed as follows

$$cD_j = \begin{cases} 0, & if\,|cD_j| \leq THR_1 \\ \mathrm{sgn}(cD_j)\left[\dfrac{THR_2\left(|cD_j|-THR_1\right)}{(THR_2-THR_1)}\right], & if\,THR_1 < |cD_j| < THR_2 \\ cD_j, & if\,|cD_j| > THR_2 \end{cases} . \tag{20}$$

13) Modified firm function (MFM): It is a modified version of general FIM function. A higher order polynomial is used to replace the linear function in the interval [THR_1, THR_2]. This modification enables to get a differentiable thresholding function. The expression (Gao & Bruce, 1997) can be defined as

$$cD_j = \begin{cases} 0, & if\,|cD_j| \leq THR_1 \\ \mathrm{sgn}(cD_j)\left(r_2 - r_1|cD_j|\right)\left(|cD_j|-THR_1\right)^2, & if\,THR_1 < |cD_j| < THR_2 \\ cD_j, & if\,|cD_j| > THR_2 \end{cases} , \tag{21}$$

$$\text{where } r_1 = \frac{(THR_1+THR_2)}{(THR_2-THR_1)^3} \text{ and } r_2 = \frac{2THR_2^2}{(THR_2-THR_1)^3} .$$

14) Qian function (QIN): It is a compromise shrinkage between HAD and SOF by constant parameter Q. Where Q is 1, it is equivalent to SOF and it is equivalent to HAD, when Q is ∞. QIN with $Q = 2$ is suggested from the experiments in (Qian, 2001). It is given by

$$cD_j = \begin{cases} cD_j \dfrac{\|cD_j\|^Q - THR^Q}{\|cD_j\|^Q}, & if\,|cD_j| > THR \\ 0, & otherwise \end{cases} . \tag{22}$$

15) Yasser function (YAS): YAS shrinks the wavelet's detail coefficients which are lower than threshold value instead of set to be zero. Moreover, it has a constant parameter γ in

order to apply a nonlinear function to the threshold value. When γ is 3, the good results in speech signal are obtained (Ghanbari & Karami-Mollaei, 2006), which can be expressed as

$$cD_j = \begin{cases} cD_j, & \text{if } |cD_j| > THR \\ \operatorname{sgn}(cD_j)\dfrac{|cD_j|^{\gamma}}{THR^{\gamma-1}}, & \text{otherwise} \end{cases} \quad . \tag{23}$$

5. Review of wavelet denoising in SEMG signal analysis

Selection of suitable wavelet denoising parameters is critical for the success of sEMG signal filtration in wavelet domain, because there is currently no known method to calculate the combination of the above wavelet denoising parameters that gives the best results. Therefore, many works have tried to find the optimal wavelet denoising parameters which lead to maximum filtration performance. All research studies about wavelet denoising parameters in analysis of the sEMG signals have been discussed in this section (Guo et al., 2004a, 2004b, 2005; Hussain et al., 2007, 2009; Jiang & Kuo, 2007; Khezri & Jahed, 2008; Li et al., 2010; Liu & Luo, 2008; Luo et al., 2007; Moshou et al., 2000; Ren et al., 2006; Yang & Luo, 2004; Zhang & Luo, 2006; Zhang et al., 2010) as summarized in Table 3.

In details, the sEMG signal analysis based on WT has been firstly proposed in 2000 by Moshou et al. (2000). Wavelet-based denoising is used to separate coordinated muscle activity of the shoulder of a driver related to certain movements that appear during driving a car. The denoised signals show clearly the real muscle activity bursts that mean the small activity peaks covered by the screen of noises are now observable. In Moshou et al. (2000) work, the simplest thresholding function, HAD, is used with a decomposition using db5 at 5 decomposition levels. Afterwards, Guo et al. (2004a, 2004b, 2005) compared four classical threshold selection rules: Universal, SURE, Hybrid and Minimax, and two classical thresholding functions: HAD and SOF, with real sEMG signal acquired from normal walking on the flat. They used the sym5 at 3 decomposition levels in their application. Evaluation criterion of both Moshou et al. (2000) and Guo et al. (2004a, 2004b, 2005) works is based on the observation of the sEMG waveforms between noisy sEMG signal and denoised sEMG signal. Jiang and Kuo (2007) compare the similar wavelet denoising parameters as Guo et al. (2004a, 2004b, 2005), but the acquired sEMG signals are changed from the normal walking activity to the mouse clicking activity; in addition, the simulated signals at 16-dB SNR have also been deployed. In Jiang and Kuo (2007) work a new evaluating function is proposed which is called signal-to-noise estimator (SNE). They prove that this evaluating function works well for the simulated signals but it does not work for the real sEMG signals. Subsequently, Jiang and Kuo concluded that the denoised sEMG signal is insensitive to the selection of wavelet denoising parameters. Furthermore, the db2 at 6 decomposition levels is used in their work due to the suggestion of previous study (Wellig & Moschytz, 1998). Zhang and Luo (2006) pay attention to apply wavelet denoising technique with control of the upper-limb prostheses. Some classical threshold selection rules and thresholding functions are employed (Liu & Luo, 2008; Luo et al., 2007; Yang & Luo, 2004). In addition, in one of their works, Zhang and Luo (2006) propose the new modified threshold selection rule and thresholding function. The sym8 at 4 decomposition levels is performed in denoising and extracting procedures. However, the results in Zhang, Luo and Liu works (Liu & Luo, 2008; Luo et al., 2007; Yang & Luo, 2004; Zhang & Luo, 2006) are also only observed from the figures as same as employed in Moshou et al. (2000) and Guo et al. (2004a, 2004b, 2005) works.

Reference	Application	Wavelet denoising parameters				
		1	2	3	4	5
Moshou et al. (2000)	Identifying car driver fatigue and movement	db5	5	-	-	HAD, SOF
Guo et al. (2004a, 2004b, 2005)	Lower limb prosthesis control	sym5	3	Universal, SURE, Hybrid, Minimax	-	HAD, SOF
Jiang & Kuo (2007)	MUAP detection	db2	6	Universal, SURE, Hybrid, Minimax	-	HAD, SOF
Zhang & Luo (2006)	Upper limb prosthesis control	sym8	4	LVMU	-	HAD, SOF, WAV
Yang & Luo (2004)	Upper limb prosthesis control	sym8	4	Hybrid	-	SOF
Khezri & Jahed (2008)	Upper limb prosthesis control	Daubechies Symlets Coiflet Biorthogonal	6	Hybrid Bayes Shrink	-	SOF
Hussain et al. (2007)	Detecting muscle fatigue	db2, db6, db8, dmey	4	-	-	HAD
Hussain et al. (2009)	Determining muscle contraction (walking speed)	db2, db4, db5, db6, db8, sym4, sym5, dmey	4	Universal	-	HAD
Li et al. (2010)	Upper limb prosthesis control	-	4	-	-	SOF
Zhang et al. (2010)	-	sym2	5	Minimax	-	SOF

Table 3. Applications of wavelet denoising algorithms with the sEMG signal. Note that wavelet denoising parameters: (1) the type of wavelet basis function, (2) the decomposition level, (3) threshold selection rule (4) threshold rescaling method, and (5) thresholding function.

Later, Khezri and Jahed (2008) proposed a usefulness of classical threshold selection rule, called Hybrid, to estimate the denoised upper-limb sEMG signals. It improved the accuracy of the sEMG classification compared with the one without denoising pre-processing stage and Bayes Shrink threshold selection rule. Following that, in one of our works (Phinyomark et al., 2009f), we compared Hybrid with three other classical threshold selection rules. The results showed that Universal yields better denoising performance than the others including Hybrid. Moreover, Hussain et al. (2007, 2009) suggested that pre-processing stage using the

Universal threshold selection rule and HAD thresholding function was able to improve the classification of the lower- and upper- limb activities, respectively. All of these introduced literatures work well for the surface EMG signal. On the other hand, for the intramuscular EMG signal, Ren et al. (2006) developed a technique for extracting and classifying motor unit action potentials (MUAPs) for needle EMG signal decomposition. In that technique, noise reduction based on threshold estimation calculated in the WT was proposed. The needle EMG signal is decomposed by the WT at ninth level with the db5. HAD thresholding is implemented with the semi-automatic threshold estimator, which is defined as $THR = \sigma \cdot \lambda$ where λ is set to be between 8 and 15 by the user in accordance with the SNR and σ is the noise energy estimated from the minimum value of the second moment feature in time domain. However, this threshold estimator is not suitable for surface EMG signal because in the MUAP detection, useful MUAP components have most of their energy in low-frequency components. Therefore, threshold obtained by this estimator has a large value (most high frequency components could be set to zeros). On the contrary, some high frequency components are still important for surface EMG signal, thus proposed technique in Ren et al. work (2006) is not included in our study. However, even though the results from most of previous works are not presented using the quantitative results, the improving ability in those applications based on wavelet denoising algorithm has been definitely established (Hussain et al., 2009; Khezri & Jahed, 2008; Ren et al., 2006; Zhang et al., 2010). In order to more clearly understand the effectiveness of wavelet denoising algorithm over conventional filters, discussion and illustration have been presented in review of Zhang et al. (2010).

6. Experimental results with real sEMG signals

The sEMG data that are used to demonstrate and evaluate the wavelet denoising parameters in our study were recorded from two forearm muscles and six upper-limb movements. Two forearm muscles are flexor carpi radialis muscle and extensor carpi radialis longus muscle and six upper-limb movements are hand open, hand close, wrist extension, wrist flexion, pronation, and supination. The sEMG signals were recorded by two pairs of surface electrodes (3M red dot 25 mm. foam solid gel). Each electrode was separated from the other by 20 mm. A band-pass filter of 10-450 Hz bandwidth and an amplifier with 60 dB gain were used. Sampling rate was set at 1000 samples per second using a 16 bit A/D converter board (IN BNC-2110, National Instruments Corporation). The sample size of each EMG data is 256 ms for the real-time constraint that the response time should be less than 300 ms (Englehart et al., 2001).

To evaluate the ability of wavelet denoising algorithm, two criteria are usually used based on: (1) the difference between signal values implied by a wavelet denoising method and the original signal values; and (2) the difference between classification accuracy obtained from the denoised signal and classification accuracy obtained from the raw signal (Phinyomark et al., 2010b). However, most studies have focused to evaluate the quality of wavelet denoising method based on the first criterion. In this chapter, we have evaluated the ability of wavelet denoising methods with only the first criterion; however, the relationship between the first criterion and the second criterion has been discussed.

The first criterion is error measure. One of the most popular methods is mean square error (MSE) that is also employed in our study. However, there are a lot of error measures; for instances, mean absolute error (MAE), mean absolute percentage error (MAPE), mean error (ME), mean percentage error (MPE), root mean square error (RMSE), percentage root-mean-square difference (PRD), signal-to-noise ratio output (SNR_{out}), and improved signal-to-noise ratio (ISNR). Due to the similarity of these measured indices, normally only one of these indices is selected to use in evaluating study. Definition of the MSE can be expressed as

$$MSE = \frac{\sum_{i=1}^{N}(f_i - fe_i)^2}{N}, \tag{24}$$

where f_i represents the estimated sEMG signal from the original signal and fe_i is estimated sEMG signal from the noisy signal. The performance of wavelet denoising method is better when these indices including MSE are smaller. It means that useful information in the sEMG signal is remained and undesirable parts of the sEMG signal are removed. To guarantee the best wavelet denoising method achieved and optimized for estimating of useful sEMG signals, more than one times of additional noises should be done and in each time the level of noises shoud be varied from low noise level to high noise level; for example, 20-0 dB SNRs. The effect of different noise levels could be observed through this procedure. Example of the original sEMG signal and the sEMG signal with the WGN at 5 dB SNR are shown in Fig. 3. The SNR can be calculated by

$$SNR = 10\log\frac{P_{clean}}{P_{noise}}, \tag{25}$$

where P_{clean} is power of the original sEMG signal and P_{noise} is power of the WGN.

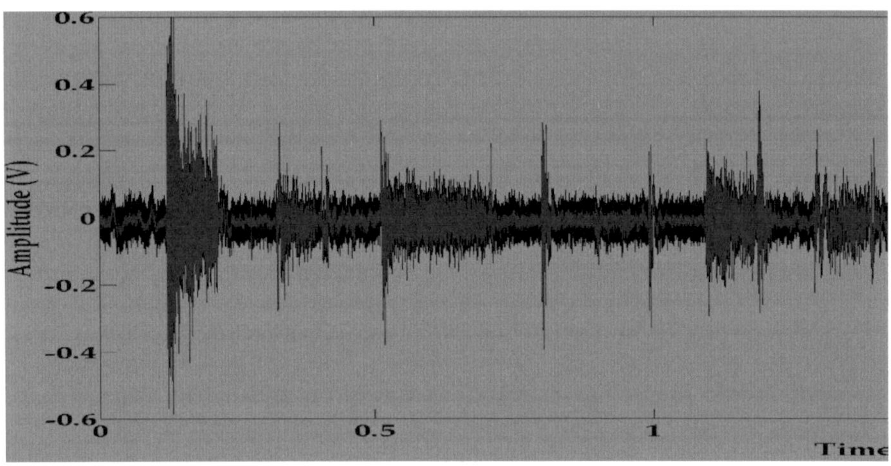

Fig. 3. Original sEMG signal (gray line) and noisy sEMG signal at 5 dB SNR (black line) with random and repeatable six upper-limb movements.

6.1 Wavelet basis functions

Firstly, the selection of an optimal wavelet function was done. The MSE calculated from 53 wavelet functions (in Table 1) were employed. The results are respectively shown in Fig. 4(a) and Fig. 4(b) at two levels of noises, low and high noise levels. The figure is plotted in log-lin type of a semi-log graph, defined by a logarithmic scale on the y axis, and a linear scale on the x axis. From the figure, the results of wavelet functions in high and low levels of noises have the similar trend. As SNR increases, the MSE of each wavelet function also increases. The smallest MSE is db1, bior1.1 and rbio1.1. Their MSEs are 0.00407, 0.01242, 0.04090, 0.12739 and 0.41242 at SNR value of 20, 15, 10, 5 and 0 dB, respectively. It produces the best denoising wavelets. The db2, db7, sym2, bior5.5 and rbio2.2 provide marginally better performance than the rest candidates. Furthermore, the various orders of Daubechies (db1-db10), Symlets (sym2-sym8), BiorSplines (bior1.1-bior1.5, bior4.4, bior5.5, and bio6.8), Coiflet (coif1-coif2), and ReverseBior (rbio1.1-rbio3.9, rbio6.8) can be used to reduce noises. The most terrible wavelet function is bior3.1. Its MSE is as much as seven of the minimum MSE. The third order of decomposition of BiorSplines (Bior3.3, bior3.5, bior3.7, and bior3.9) and Discrete Meyer (dmey) are worse performance. Its MSE is as much as two of the minimum MSE. Moreover, in high noise, the second order of decomposition of BiorSplines (bior2.2-bior2.8) and the fifth order of decomposition of ReverseBior (rbio5.5) are not good. Therefore, these functions are not recommended to use for denoising sEMG signal.

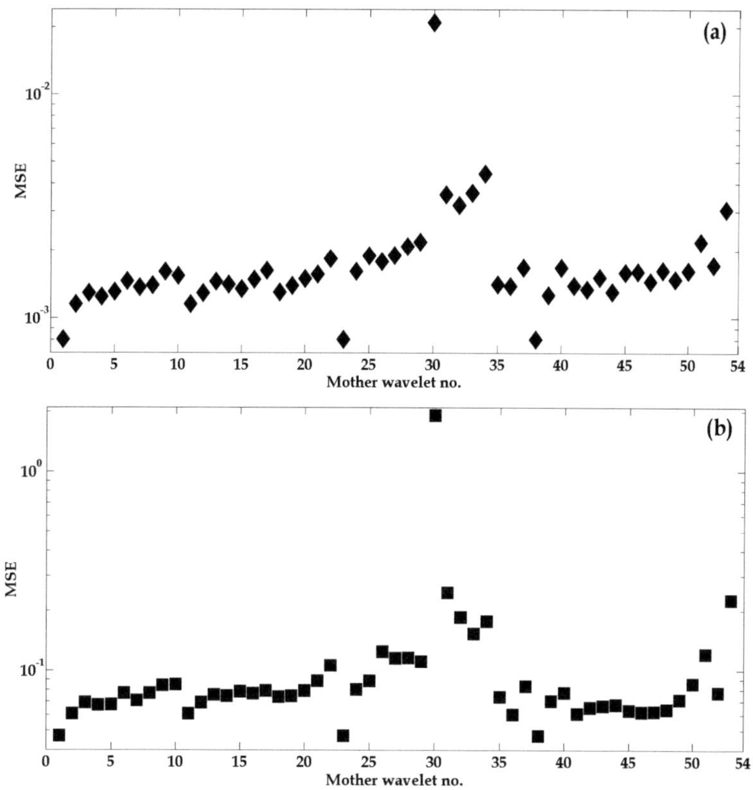

Fig. 4. MSE calculated from all wavelet functions (mother wavelet no. refer to the wavelets in Table I, i.e. #1-Daubechies order 1, #2-Daubechies order 2, …, #11-Symlets order 2, …,#18-Coiflet order 1, …, #53-Discrete Meyer) (a) at 20 dB SNR (b) at 0 dB SNR. Note that decomposition level is 4, threshold selection rule is Universal, threshold rescaling method is GL for *N* parameter and LD for σ parameter, and thresholding function is SOF.

If we consider only optimal wavelets for denoising, we can conclude that db1, bior1.1 and rbio1.1 are the best ones. However, the ability of these functions in classification viewpoint is poor. Hence, for real-world application, these wavelet functions are not recommended.

The db2, db7, sym2, bior5.5 and rbio2.2 are prospective to have good performance in both denoising and classification performance. At this point we recommend wavelet functions in this group to be used in future works. Note that we are not reported the classification results in this work because the suitable wavelet functions depend on the classifier types (such as neural network, fuzzy logic, neuro-fuzzy classifier, probabilistic classifier, etc.). One of the useful results in classification viewpoint is presented in Englehart (1998) work. In Englehart study, wavelet coefficients are extracted from upper-limb sEMG signals and are subjected to dimensionality reduction method. As a result, classification errors are reported. Within the Daubechies, Coiflet and Symlet families, the best performance is db18, coif4 and sym8, respectively. Interesting trend is the improvement of classification performance that it tends to increase with the order of wavelet function. Hence, if balance between class separability and robustness is considered, the db7, sym5 and coif4 are some compromise wavelets.

6.2 Decomposition levels

Secondly, the selection of an optimal decomposition level was done. Fig. 5(a) and Fig. 5(b) present the effects of decomposition levels for five wavelet functions. When decomposition levels are more than seven, the MSE rapidly increases. Therefore, in Fig. 5(a) and Fig. 5(b), only first eight levels are shown. We found that the third and the fourth levels are better than other levels for low level of noises (20-10 dB SNRs). On the other hand, the fourth and the fifth levels are better than the others for high level of noises (10-0 dB SNRs). The effect of wavelet function with an optimal wavelet function is a little bit. The decomposition level 4 is suggested to be used as a compromise level between high and low level of noises.

6.3 Threshold selection rules

Thirdly, the selection of an optimal threshold selection rule was done. For the classical threshold selection rules, Universal rule is better than other classical methods as can be observed in Fig. 6. Hence, modified versions of Universal threshold selection rule are proposed and also evaluated. The MSE of LSMU rule is the lowest, followed closely by LVNU, SMU and Universal rules. GSMU rule have slightly larger error, and LMU and SLMU rules have a large error. However, in classification viewpoint, GSMU rule is the best threshold selection rule (Phinyomark et al., 2009f).

6.4 Threshold rescaling methods

Fourthly, the selection of an optimal threshold rescaling method was done. From our previous study (Phinyomark et al., 2009f), the optimal rescaling method is dependent on type of threshold selection rules. However, the general trend can be observed. For the threshold rescaling of N parameter, the GL is better than the LD. For the threshold rescaling of σ parameter, the suitable rescaling method is dependent on the level of noises. At very high noise, the LD is better than the FL. On the other hand, at medium to low noise, the FL is better than the LD.

6.5 Thresholding functions

Fifthly, the selection of an optimal thresholding function was done. In Fig. 7, the MSEs of 15 thresholding functions and no denoising case with only WT are presented. At medium and high levels of noises, SNR is lower than 10 dB, all functions are better than WT except MFM. However, at low level of noises, 15 dB SNR, CUT, FIM and MFM are worse than WT. In addition, HAD, MHP, CUT and MFM are worse than WT at very low noise, 20 dB SNR.

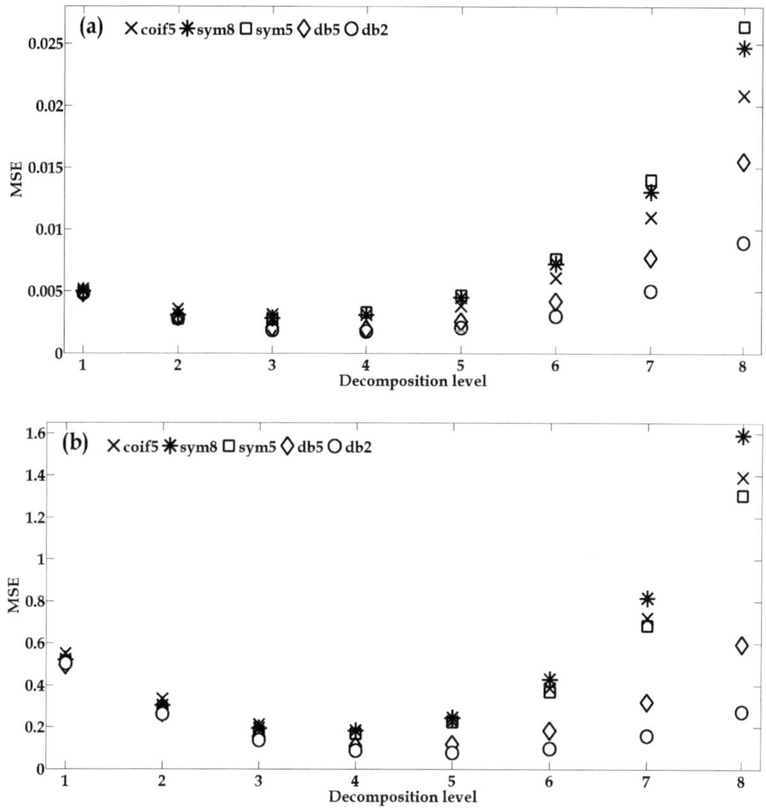

Fig. 5. MSE of five wavelet functions with eight decomposition levels (a) at 20 dB SNR (b) at 0 dB SNR. Note that threshold selection rule is Universal, threshold rescaling method is GL for N parameter and LD for σ parameter, and thresholding function is SOF.

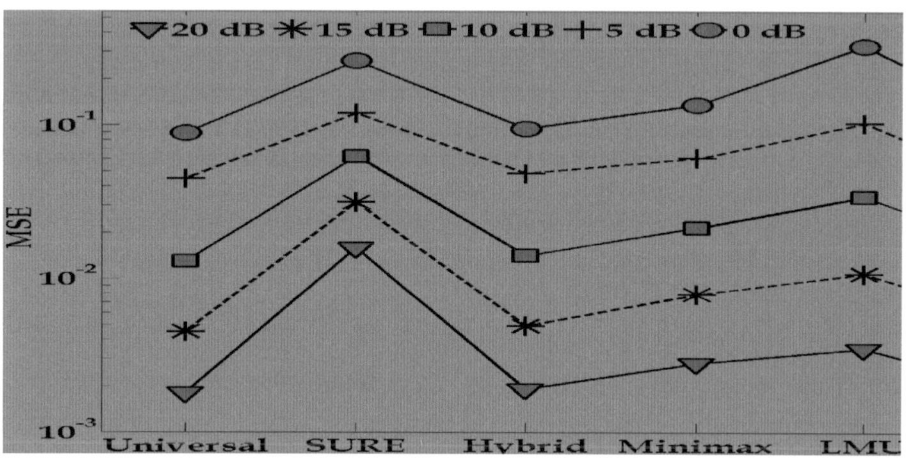

Fig. 6. MSE of four classical and six modified threshold selection rules at 20-0 dB SNR. Note that wavelet function is db2, decomposition level is 4, threshold rescaling method is GL for N parameter and LD for σ parameter, and thresholding function is SOF.

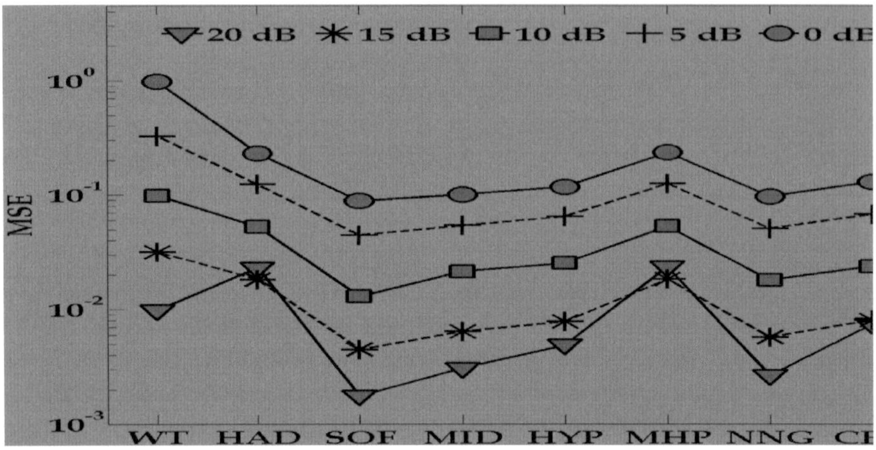

Fig. 7. MSE of WT and fifteen modified universal thresholding rules at 20-0 dB SNR. Note that wavelet function is db2, decomposition level is 4, threshold selection rule is Universal, and threshold rescaling method is GL for N parameter and LD for σ parameter.

As SNR increases, the MSE of each function as well increases. From the experimental results, the MSE of ADP is lowest, followed closely by SOF and IMP. It means that ADP is the best thresholding function in denoising viewpoint. MSE of WT is seven times the MSE of ADP at low noise and is three times the MSE of ADP at high noise. Moreover, in classification viewpoint, ADP is also the best thresholding function (Phinyomark et al., 2010b); whereas, the classification performance of SOF is not good.

7. Conclusion and future trends

Noises contaminated in the sEMG signals are an unavoidable problem during recording data; whereas noises are a main problem in analysis of the sEMG signal both in clinical and engineering applications. Random noises that have their frequency components fall in the energy band of the sEMG signal are the major problem. Conventional filters do not effectively remove random noises but wavelet denoising algorithm is not problematical in this way. Hence, numerous wavelet denoising methods have been proposed during the last decade. Suggestion of five wavelet denoising parameters in a compromise between two viewpoints, denoising and classification, is presented in the following:

- wavelet function: db2, db7, sym2, sym5, coif 4, bior5.5 and rbio2.2;
- decomposition level: 4;
- threshold selection rule: GSMU;
- threshold rescaling methods: LD for N parameter and FL or LD for σ parameter; and
- thresholding function: ADP.

Recommendation above can be useful to apply for many sEMG applications. However, for analysis of intramuscular EMG signal, re-evaluation of wavelet denoising parameters should be done because the purpose in interpretation is different (Ren et al., 2006). However, the pre-processing stage based on wavelet denoising algorithm is recommended to be implemented in analysis of sEMG signal, especially in multifunction myoelectric control system.

8. Acknowledgment

This work was supported in part by the Thailand Research Fund (TRF) through the Royal Golden Jubilee Ph.D. Program (Grant No. PHD/0110/2550), and in part by NECTEC-PSU Center of Excellence for Rehabilitation Engineering, Faculty of Engineering, Prince of Songkla University through Contact No. EMG540014S.

9. References

Andrade, A. O.; Nasuto, S.; Kyberd, P.; Sweeney-Reed, C. M. & Van Kanijn, F. R. (2006). EMG Signal Filtering based on Empirical Mode Decomposition. *Biomedical Signal Processing and Control*, Vol.1, No.1, (January 2006), pp. 44-55, ISSN 1746-8094

Baratta, R. V.; Solomonow, M.; Zhou, B. H. & Zhu, M. (1998). Methods to Reduce the Variability of EMG Power Spectrum Estimates. *Journal of Electromyography and Kinesiology*, Vol.8, No.5, (1991), pp. 279–285, ISSN 1050-6411

Boostani, R. & Moradi, M. H. (2003). Evaluation of the Forearm EMG Signal Features for the Control of a Prosthetic Hand. *Physiological Measurement*. Vol.24, No.2, (February 1980), pp. 309-319, ISSN 0967-3334

Clancy, E. A.; Morin, E. L. & Merletti, R. (2002). Sampling, Noise-reduction and Amplitude Estimation Issues in Surface Electromyography. *Journal of Electromyography and Kinesiology*, Vol.12, No.1, (1991), pp. 1–16, ISSN 1050-6411

De Luca, C. J. (2002). Surface Electromyography: Detection and Recording, In: *DelSys Incorporated*, 10.05.2011, Available from http://www.delsys.com/Attachments_pdf /WP_SEMGintro.pdf

De Luca, C. J.; Gilmore, L. D.; Kuznetsov, M. & Roy, S. H. (2010). Filtering the Surface EMG Signal: Movement Artifact and Baseline Noise Contamination. *Journal of Biomechanics*, Vol.43, No.8, (January 1968), pp. 1573-1579, ISSN 0021-9290

Donoho, D. L. (1992). Wavelet Analysis and WVD: A Ten Minute Tour, In: *Progress in Wavelet Analysis and Applications*, Meyer, Y. & Roques, S., pp. 109–128, Frontières Ed.

Donoho, D. L. (1995). De-noising by Soft-thresholding. *IEEE Transactions on Information Theory*, Vol.41, No.3, (1955), pp. 613-627, ISSN 0018-9448

Donoho, D. L. & Johnstone, I. M. (1994). Ideal Spatial Adaptation by Wavelet Shrinkage. *Biometrika*, Vol.81, No.3, (October 1901), pp. 425-455, ISSN 0006-3444

Donoho, D. L. & Johnstone, I. M. (1995). Adapting to Unknown Smoothness via Wavelet Shrinkage. *Journal of the American Statistical Association*, Vol.90, No.432, (March 1888), pp. 1200-1224, ISSN 0162-1459

Elena, M. M. ; Quero, J. M. & Borrego, I. (2006). An Optimal Technique for ECG Noise Reduction in Real Time Applications. *Proceedings of CinC 2006 Computers in Cardiology*, pp. 225-228, ISBN 978-1-4244-2532-7, Valencia, Spain, September 17-20, 2006

Englehart, K. (1998). *Representation and Classification of the Transient Myoelectric Signal*. Ph.D. Thesis, University of New Brunswick, Fredericton, N.B., Canada.

Englehart, K.; Hudgins, B. & Parker, P. A. (2001). A Wavelet-Based Continuous Classification Scheme for Multifunction Myoelectric Control. *IEEE Transactions on Biomedical Engineering*, Vol.48, No.3, (1953), pp. 302-311, ISSN 0018-9294

Gao, H. Y. (1998). Wavelet Shrinkage Denoising Using the Non-negative Garrote. *Journal of Computational and Graphical Statistics*, Vol.7, No.4, (1992), pp. 469-488, ISSN 1061-8600

Gao, H. Y. & Bruce, A. G. (1997). WaveShrink with Firm Shrinkage. *Statistica Sinica*, Vol.7, No.4, (January 1991), pp. 855-874, ISSN 1017-0405

Ghanbari, Y. & Karami-Mollaei, M. R. (2006). A New Approach for Speech Enhancement based on the Adaptive Thresholding of the Wavelet Packets. *Speech Communication*, Vol.48, No.8, (May 1982), pp. 927–940, ISSN 0167-6393

Guo, X. ; Yang, P. ; Li, Y. & Yan, W. L. (2004a) The SEMG Analysis for the Lower Limb Prosthesis Using Wavelet Transform. *Proceedings of IEMBS 2004 26th Annual International Conference of the IEEE Engineering in Medicine and Biology Society*, pp. 341-344, ISBN 0-7803-8439-3, San Francisco, CA, USA, September 1-5, 2004

Guo, X.; Yang, P.; Li, L. F. & Yan, W. L. (2004b) Study and Analysis of Surface EMG for the Lower Limb Prosthesis. *Proceedings of ICMLC 2004 3rd International Conference on Machine Learning and Cybernetics*, pp. 3736-3740, ISBN 0-7803-8403-2, Shanghai, China, August 26-29, 2004

Guo, X.; Yang, P.; Liu, H. C. & Yan, W. L. (2005). Research and Analysis on the Effect of Joint Angle on EMG in Thigh Muscles. *Proceedings of CNIC 2005 1st International Conference on Neural Interface and Control Proceedings*, pp. 139-142, ISBN 0-7803-8902-6, Wuhan, China, May 26-28, 2005

Huang, H.; Zhang, F.; Sun, Y. L. & He, H. (2010). Design of a Robust EMG Sensing Interface for Pattern Classification. *Journal of Neural Engineering*, Vol.7, No.5, (March 2004), pp. 056005-1-056005-10, ISSN 1741-2560

Huigen, E.; Peper, A. & Grimbergen, C. A. (2002). Investigation into the Origin of the Noise of Surface Electrodes. *Medical and Biological Engineering and Computing*, Vol.40, No.3, (January 1963), pp. 332-338, ISSN 0140-0118

Hussain, M.S.; Reaz, M. B. I.; Ibrahimy, M. I.; Ismail, A. F. & Yasin, F. M. (2007). Wavelet based Noise Removal from EMG Signals. *Informacije MIDEM*, Vol.37, No.2, (1971), pp. 94-97, ISSN 0352-9045

Hussain, M. S. ; Reaz, M. B. I. ; Yasin, F. M. & Ibrahimy, M. I. (2009). Electromyography Signal Analysis Using Wavelet Transform and Higher Order Statistics to Determine Muscle Contraction. *Expert Systems*, Vol.26, No.1, (July 1984), pp. 35-48, ISSN 0266-4720

Jiang, C. F. & Kuo, S. L. (2007). A Comparative Study of Wavelet Denoising of Surface Electromyographic Signals. *Proceedings of EMBS 2007 29th Annual International Conference of the IEEE Engineering in Medicine and Biology Society*, pp. 1868-1871, ISBN 978-1-4244-0787-3, Cite Internationale, Lyon, France, August 22-26, 2007

Johnstone, I. M. & Silverman, B. W. (1997). Wavelet Threshold Estimators for Data with Correlated Noise. *Journal of the Royal Statistical Society: Series B (Statistical Methodology)*, Vol.59, No.2, (1934), pp. 319-351, ISSN 1369-7412

Kale, S. N. & Dudul, S. V. (2009). Intelligent Noise Removal from EMG Signal Using Focused Time-Lagged Recurrent Neural Network. *Applied Computational Intelligence and Soft Computing*, Vol.2009, Article ID 129761, (2008), 12 pages, ISSN 1687-9724

Kania, M.; Fereniec, M. & Maniewski, R. (2007). Wavelet Denoising for Multi-lead High Resolution ECG Signals. *Measurement Science Review*, Vol.7, No.4, (2001), pp. 30-33, ISSN 1335-8871

Khezri, M. & Jahed, M. (2008). Surface Electromyogram Signal Estimation based on Wavelet Thresholding Technique. *Proceedings of EMBS 2008 30th Annual International Conference of the IEEE Engineering in Medicine and Biology Society*, pp. 4752-4755, ISBN 978-1-4244-1814-5, Vancouver, British Columbia, Canada, August 20-25, 2008

Laterza, F. & Olmo G. (1997). Analysis of EMG Signals by Means of the Matched Wavelet Transform. *Electronics Letters*, Vol.33, No.5, (March 1965), pp. 357-359, ISSN 0013-5194

Law, L. F.; Krishnan, C. & Avin, K. (2011). Modeling Nonlinear Errors in Surface Electromyography due to Baseline Noise: A New Methodology. *Journal of Biomechanics*, Vol.44, No.1, (January 1968), pp. 202-205, ISSN 0021-9290

Li, Y. ; Tian, Y. & Chen, W. (2010). Multi-pattern Recognition of sEMG based on Improved BP Neural Network Algorithm. *Proceedings of CCC 2010 29th Chinese Control Conference*, pp. 2867-2872, ISBN 978-1-4244-6263-6, Beijing, China, July 29-31, 2010

Liu, Z. & Luo, Z. (2008). EMG De-noising by Multi-scale Product Coefficient Hard Thresholding. *Journal of Huazhong University of Science and Technology (Natural Science Edition)*, Vol.36, No.1, (1972), pp. 134-136, ISSN 1671-4512

Luo, Z. Z. ; Zhang, Q. J. & Jiang, J. P. (2007). Improving Method for Surface Electromyography Denoising based on Wavelet Transform. *Journal of Zhejiang University (Engineering Science)*, Vol.41, No.2, (1956), pp. 213-216, ISSN 1008-973X

Merletti, R. & Parker, P. (2004). *ELECTROMYOGRAPHY Physiology, Engineering, and Noninvasive Applications*, John Wiley & Sons, ISBN 0-471-67580-6, USA

Mewett, D. T. ; Reynolds, K. J. & Nazeran, H. (2004). Reducing Power Line Interference in Digitised Electromyogram Recordings by Spectrum Interpolation. *Medical and Biological Engineering and Computing*, Vol.42, No.4, (January 1963), pp. 524-531, ISSN 0140-0118

Moshou, D.; Hostens, I.; Papaioannou, G. & Ramon, H. (2000). Wavelets and Self-organising Maps in Electromyogram (EMG) Analysis. *Proceedings of ESIT 2000 European Symposium on Intelligent Techniques*, pp. 186-191, Aachen, Germany, September 14-15, 2000

Percival, D. B. & Walden, A. T. (2000). *Wavelet Methods for Time Series Analysis*, Cambridge University Press, ISBN 0-521-64068-7, USA

Phinyomark, A. ; Limsakul, C. & Phukpattaranont, P. (2008). EMG Feature Extraction for Tolerance of White Gaussian Noise. *Proceedings of I-SEEC 2008 International Workshop and Symposium Science Technology*, pp. 178-183, Nong Khai, Thailand, December 15-16, 2008

Phinyomark, A. ; Limsakul, C. & Phukpattaranont, P. (2009a). EMG Feature Extraction for Tolerance of 50 Hz Interference. *Proceedings of ICET 2009 4th PSU-UNS International Conference on Engineering Technologies*, pp. 289-293, ISBN 978-86-7892-227-5, Novi Sad, Serbia, April 28-30, 2009

Phinyomark, A. ; Limsakul, C. & Phukpattaranont, P. (2009b). A Novel EMG Feature Extraction for Tolerance of Interference. *Proceedings of ANSCSE 13 13th International*

Annual Symposium on Computational Science and Engineering, pp. 407-413, Bangkok, Thailand, March 25-27, 2009

Phinyomark, A. ; Limsakul, C. & Phukpattaranont, P. (2009c). A Novel Feature Extraction for Robust EMG Pattern Recognition. *Journal of Computing*, Vol.1, No.1, (December 2009), pp. 71-80, ISSN 2151-9617

Phinyomark, A. ; Limsakul, C. & Phukpattaranont, P. (2009d). Evaluation of Wavelet Function Based on Robust EMG Feature Extraction. *Proceedings of PEC 7 7th PSU-Engineering Conference*, pp. 277-281, Hat Yai, Thailand, May 21-22, 2009

Phinyomark, A. ; Limsakul, C. & Phukpattaranont, P. (2009e). Evaluation of Mother Wavelet Based on Robust EMG Feature Extraction Using Wavelet Packet Transform. *Proceedings of ANSCSE 13 13th International Annual Symposium on Computational Science and Engineering*, pp. 333-339, Bangkok, Thailand, March 25-27, 2009

Phinyomark, A. ; Limsakul, C. & Phukpattaranont, P. (2009f). A Comparative Study of Wavelet Denoising for Multifunction Myoelectric Control. *Proceedings of ICCAE 2009 International Conference on Computer and Automation Engineering*, pp. 21-25, ISBN 978-1-4244-3564-7, Bangkok, Thailand, March 8-10, 2009

Phinyomark, A. ; Limsakul, C. & Phukpattaranont, P. (2009g). An Optimal Wavelet Function Based on Wavelet Denoising for Multifunction Myoelectric Control. *Proceedings of ECTI-CON 2009 6th International Conference on Electrical Engineering/Electronics, Computer, Telecommunications and Information Technology*, pp. 1098-1101, ISBN 978-1-4244-3388-9, Pattaya, Thailand, May 6-9, 2009

Phinyomark, A. ; Limsakul, C. & Phukpattaranont, P. (2009h). EMG Denoising Estimation Based on Adaptive Wavelet Thresholding for Multifunction Myoelectric Control. *Proceedings of CITISIA 2009 3rd IEEE Conference on Innovative Technologies in Intelligent Systems and Industrial Applications*, pp. 171-176, ISBN 978-1-4244-2886-1, Monash University, Sunway Campus, Malaysia, July 25-26, 2009

Phinyomark, A. ; Limsakul, C. & Phukpattaranont, P. (2010a). Optimal Wavelet Functions in Wavelet Denoising for Multifunction Myoelectric Control. *ECTI Transactions on Electrical Eng., Electronics, and Communications*, Vol. 8, No.1, (2003), pp. 43-52, ISSN 1685-9545

Phinyomark, A. ; Limsakul, C. & Phukpattaranont, P. (2010b). EMG Signal Estimation Based on Adaptive Wavelet Shrinkage for Multifunction Myoelectric Control. *Proceedings of ECTI-CON 2010 7th International Conference on Electrical Engineering/Electronics, Computer, Telecommunications and Information Technology*, pp. 351-355, ISBN 978-1-4244-5607-9, Chiang Mai, Thailand, May 19-21, 2010

Phinyomark, A. ; Phukpattaranont, P. & Limsakul, C. (2010c). EMG Signal Denoising via Adaptive Wavelet Shrinkage for Multifunction Upper-limb Prosthesis. *Proceedings of BMEiCON 2010 3rd Biomedical Engineering International Conference*, pp. 35-41, Kyoto, Japan, August 27-28, 2010

Phinyomark, A. ; Phukpattaranont, P. & Limsakul, C. (2011). Wavelet-based Denoising Algorithm for Robust EMG Pattern Recognition. *Fluctuation and Noise Letters*, Vol.10, No.2, (March 2001), pp. 157-167, ISSN 0219-4775

Poornachandra, S.; Kumaravel, N.; Saravanan, T. K. & Somaskandan, R. (2005). WaveShrink Using Modified Hyper-shrinkage Function. *Proceedings of IEEE-EMBS 2005 27th Annual International Conference of the Engineering in Medicine and Biology Society*, pp. 30-32, ISBN 0-7803-8741-4, Shanghai, China, January 17-18, 2006

Qian, J. (2001). Denoising by Wavelet Transform, In: *Department of Electrical Engineering, Rice University*, 11.05.2011, Available from: http://www.daimi.au.dk/~pmn/spf02/CDROM/pr1/Litteratur/Denoising%20by%20wavelet%20transform.pdf

Reaz, M. B. I.; Hussain, M. S. & Mohd-Yasin, F. (2006). Techniques of EMG Signal Analysis: Detection, Processing, Classification and Applications. *Biological Procedures Online*, Vol.8, No.1, (May 1998), pp. 11-35, ISSN 1480-9222

Ren, X.; Hu, X.; Wang, Z. & Yan, Z. (2006). MUAP Extraction and Classification based on Wavelet Transform and ICA for EMG Decomposition. *Medical and Biological Engineering and Computing*, Vol.44, No.5, (1963), pp. 371-382, ISSN 0140-0118

Song, G. & Zhao, R. (2001). Three Novel Models of Threshold Estimator for Wavelet Coefficients. *Proceedings of WAA 2001 2nd International Conference on Wavelet Analysis and Its Applications*, pp. 145-150, ISBN 3-540-43034-2, Hong Kong, China, December 18-20, 2001

Su, L. & Zhao, G. (2005). De-noising of ECG Signal Using Translation-invariant Wavelet De-noising Method with Improved Thresholding. *Proceedings of IEEE-EMBS 2005 27th Annual International Conference of the Engineering in Medicine and Biology Society*, pp. 5946-5949, ISBN 0-7803-8741-4, Shanghai, China, January 17-18, 2006

Tan, H. G. R.; Tan, A. C.; Khong, P. Y. & Mok, V. H. (2007). Best Wavelet Function identification System for ECG Signal Denoise Applications. *Proceedings of ICIAS 2007 International Conference on Intelligent and Advanced Systems*, pp. 631-634, ISBN 978-1-4244-1355-3, Kuala Lumpur, Malaysia, November 25-28, 2007

Tianshu, Q.; Shuxun, W.; Haihua, C. & Yisong, D. (2002). Adaptive Denoising based on Wavelet Thresholding Method. *Proceedings of ICOSP 2002 6th International Conference on Signal Processing*, pp. 120-123, ISBN 0-7803-7488-6, Beijing, China, August 26-30, 2002

Vidakovic, B. (1999). *Statistical Modeling by Wavelets*, John Wiley & Sons, ISBN 978-0-471-29365-1, USA

Wellig, P. & Moschytz, G. S. (1998). Analysis of Wavelet Features for Myoelectric Signal. *Proceedings of ICECS 1998 IEEE International Conference on Classification. Electronics, Circuits and Systems*, pp. 109-112, ISBN 0-7803-5008-1, Lisboa, Portugal, September 7-10, 1998

Yang, Q. Y. & Luo, Z. Z. (2004). Surface Electromyography Disposal based on the Method of Wavelet De-noising and Power Spectrum. *Proceedings of ICIMA 2004 IEEE International Conference on Intelligent Mechatronics and Automation*, pp. 896-900, ISBN 0-7803-8748-1, Chengdu, China, August 26-31, 2004

Yoon, B. J. & Vaidyanathan, P. P. (2004). Wavelet-based Denoising by Customized Thresholding. *Proceedings of ICASSP 2004 IEEE International Conference on Acoustics, Speech, and Signal Processing*, pp. ii-925-ii-928, ISBN 0-7803-8484-9, Montreal, Canada, May 17-21, 2004

Zardoshti-Kermani, M.; Wheeler, B. C.; Badie, K. & Hashemi, R. M. (1995). EMG Feature Evaluation for Movement Control of Upper Extremity Prostheses. *IEEE Transactions on Rehabilitation Engineering*, Vol.3, No.4, (March 1993), pp. 324-333, ISSN 1063-6528

Zhang, Q. J. & Luo, Z. Z. (2006). Wavelet De-noising of Electromyography. *Proceedings of ICMA 2006 IEEE International Conference on Mechatronics and Automation*, pp. 1553-1558, ISBN 1-4244-0465-7, Luoyang, China, June 25-28, 2006

Zhang, X.; Wang, Y. & Han, R. P. S. (2010). Wavelet Transform Theory and its Application in EMG Signal Processing. *Proceedings of FSKD 2010 7th International Conference on Fuzzy Systems and Knowledge Discovery*, pp. 2234-2238, ISBN 978-1-4244-5931-5, Qingdao, China, August 10-12, 2010

Zhong, S. & Cherkassky, V. (2000). Image Denoising Using Wavelet Thresholding and Model Selection. *Proceedings of ICIP 2000 International Conference on Image Processing*, pp. 262-265, ISBN 0-7803-6297-7, Vancouver, BC, Canada, September 10-13, 2000

8

Nonlinear Analysis of Surface Electromyography

Paul S. Sung
Korea University, Seoul, Republic of Korea

1. Introduction

Electromyography (EMG) detects electrically or neurogically activated muscle cells on the basis of waveform characteristics from a recorded signal. EMG is useful for evaluating and recording movement abnormalities. The EMG signals can also detect neuromuscular activation level and recruitment order in addition to analyze the biomechanics of human or animal movement (De Luca, 1984; Furey, 1963). The EMG signals are generated based on superimposed motor action potentials during active movement. The myoelectric signals are the instantaneous algebraic summation of all electrical discharges produced by a contraction of the muscle fibers. Muscle fatigue is quantified using surface EMG signals based on the power spectrum which is the Fourier transform of EMG time series (Knowlton *et al.*, 1951; Mannion & Dolan, 1994; Mannion *et al.*, 1997c). Normal electrical source is a muscle membrane potential of approximately -90 mV, and measured EMG potentials range between less than 50 μV and up to 20 to 30 mV, depending on the muscle under observation (Herzog *et al.*, 1987; Nigg *et al.*, 1988). Typical repetition rate of muscle motor unit firing is approximately 7–20 Hz, depending on the size of the muscle, previous axonal damage, and other factors (Hoffmann, 1968; Rack & Ross, 1975). Therefore, the EMG range can be utilized in many clinical and biomechanical applications as a diagnostics tool for identifying neuromuscular diseases, assessing low back pain (LBP), kinesiology, and disorders of motor control. EMG signals are also used as a control signal for prosthetic devices such as prosthetic hands, arms, and lower limbs. It is unknown how the median frequency (MF) of an individual depends on posture, extent of physical activity prior to measurements, and other attributing factors. Such factors may influence the shift of the MF in the fatigue measurement, which is not a consistent indicator for injuries to low back muscles. Subjects with LBP have less endurance and thus smaller MF during sustained muscle contractions (Mannion *et al.*, 1997a; Roy *et al.*, 1997). The MF of the EMG signal is used to characterize physiological aspects of skeletal muscles. The signal from surface EMG is the instantaneous algebraic summation of action potentials from muscle fibers, and its power spectrum can be estimated from a fast Fourier transform of the signal.

Fourier transform is a linear analysis of a signal and gives the power spectrum $P(f)$ (Hobbie, 1997). A linear system is described mathematically by equations with oscillatory or exponentially growing solutions. In contrast, EMG time series have an irregular pattern so that the signal must be interpreted as "noise." The noise is due to the interaction between a particular muscle and all other biomechanical "units" of the body. In many cases, the power spectrum follows an algebraic dependence $P(f) \sim 1/f\alpha$. The case $\alpha=0$ corresponds to "white noise" while $\alpha=2$ characterizes diffusive Brownian motion. Therefore, the MF of the EMG power spectrum is sensitive to physiological manifestations of muscular dysfunction as an alternative assessment tool to identify muscle fatigue (Mannion *et al.*, 1997b; Roy *et al.*, 1997). However, there is a lack of research that compares this tool with other nonlinear measurements based on pain level or dysfunction.

During a fatiguing contraction, a compression of the power spectrum of the EMG signal to lower frequencies is typically observed (Lindstrom *et al.*, 1974). This phenomenon is measured during a contraction as a decrease in the MF of the EMG signal. Individuals with better endurance than others exhibit a less precipitous decay rate of the MF (Mannion *et al.*, 1997b). Thus, it would be necessary to compare the results between Shannon entropy levels of the EMG and MF of the spectral quantities following intervention to enhance outcome measurements.

Other results indicated that subjects with LBP show less fatigue than healthy subjects (Humphrey *et al.*, 2005; Mannion *et al.*, 2001). Thus, despite considerable efforts by many researchers, a link between MF and musculoskeletal pain/dysfunction remains elusive. Moreover, the surface EMG is not a scientifically acceptable tool for the diagnosis of pain/dysfunction, and further studies are recommended to assess the specificity and sensitivity of surface EMG (Pullman *et al.*, 2000). Therefore, a clinical diagnosis and evaluation of LBP is still elusive, and the efficacy of therapeutic intervention and assessment for LBP cannot be tested reliably.

The power spectrum analysis provides an objective and noninvasive assessment of muscle function since EMG changes are associated with fatigue (De Luca, 1984; Mannion *et al.*, 1997a). However, contradictory results have been reported in studies using EMG as an outcome measure. The power spectrum has a limited dynamic range, and the change of the MF does not reflect such long-time correlations. New methods must be designed to capture biologically important characteristics from noisy time series. Researchers using nonlinear time series analysis have developed several mathematical tools to reveal the presence of power-law time correlations.

Investigations of physiologic time series have led to the understanding that some degree of noise is necessary for the proper functioning of biological systems (Belair *et al.*, 1995b; Glass, 2001; Strogatz, 2001). These systems must respond to external stimuli that may vary both in strength and time scale by many orders of magnitude. The "degree of irregularity" of time series can be quantified by computing the (information) entropy of the signal. The time-dependent entropy from the surface EMG signal and the entropy of the signal is lower for subjects with LBP than for healthy subjects. Furthermore, the entropy increases rapidly for short times [$t < 10$ ms], reaches a plateau value for intermediate times [10ms $< t <$ 500 ms], and then increases diffusely for long times [approximately 500 ms] (Belair *et al.*, 1995a). This behavior suggests that the plateau value is relevant for the physiology of skeletal muscles (Chialvo, 2002; Goldberger *et al.*, 2002a). In this chapter, some of these methods to surface EMG time series are discussed, and the potential use of these methods as a diagnostic tool for LBP are explored.

Therefore, the purpose of this chapter is to explore the potential use of nonlinear time series analysis as a tool for the clinical diagnosis of LBP or neuromuscular dysfunction, especially low back muscle fatigue. Of particular interest is a comparison between methods based on the power spectrum and nonlinear time series analysis of EMG signals. In order to compare quantities derived from the EMG signals, it is important to compare the different types of analyses including nonlinear time series between subjects with and without musculoskeletal dysfunction/pain. Specifically, it is important to record and analyze the EMG signals for a group of subjects with LBP and a control group of healthy subjects using spectral analysis and methods from nonlinear time series analysis. Secondly, the reliability of the results based on power spectrum analysis and nonlinear time series analysis of EMG signals for subjects with and without LBP needs to be investigated. Thirdly, it is necessary to determine the sensitivity of the analyses and the distribution of the values of the entropy for a group of subjects with and without LBP.

2. Clinical assessment of LBP

A clinical assessment of LBP is important as a diagnostic tool since we cannot distinguish subjects with genuine pain from those who fraudulently claim to suffer from pain (Chaffin, 1969). The potential cost to society from malingerers could be quite high. Additionally, the effectiveness of various rehabilitation interventions is difficult to assess without a clinical diagnosis of LBP. The interpretation of surface EMG data is not as reliable as that from needle EMG, for example. A clinical diagnosis based on surface EMG is desirable since it is widely accepted by the general population.

A clinical diagnosis of LBP using EMG should be based on properties of the signal that change drastically in the presence of pain/dysfunction. If this is the case, the observed quantities from subjects with LBP are expected to be different than those from subjects without LBP. Because a shift in the MF of the spectrum is explained by the change in the velocity of the action potential, it reflects a quantitative change of the signal during a fatiguing exercise. On the other hand, a change in the entropy of the signal reflects a qualitative change in the physiologic system.

Subjects with LBP often have reduced muscle strength and endurance, which compromises the functional capacity of the spine and increases the likelihood of re-injury (Cholewicki & VanVliet, 2002; Wilder *et al.*, 1996). In most cases, a compression of the power spectrum of the EMG signal to lower frequencies is observed during a fatiguing contraction. This compression is the result of slower muscle fiber action potential propagation and an alteration in shape due to changes in the excitability of the muscle cell membrane (Lindstrom *et al.*, 1974; Panjabi, 1992). These phenomena are referred to as "myoelectric manifestations of fatigue" and are typically seen during a prolonged muscle contraction. Individuals with better endurance are expected to exhibit a smaller shift of the MF (Mannion *et al.*, 1997b; Mannion *et al.*, 2001). It has been reported that subjects with LBP exhibit a larger shift of the MF than subjects without LBP (Mayer *et al.*, 1989; Roy *et al.*, 1989).

2.1 Noise in biological systems

The characterization of the power spectrum with a single frequency indicates that the time dependence of the signal is approximated by a simple oscillatory behavior. In contrast, the EMG signal looks irregular to the naked eye, and thus cannot be approximated by a periodic behavior. Seemingly irregular time series have been observed in many biological systems such as the electrocardiography signal of the human heartbeat, the electroencephalogram signal in instances of epilepsy and human gait, and others (Costa *et al.*, 2003; Costa, 2002; Goldberger *et al.*, 2002a).

It has recently been suggested that physiological time series contain "hidden information" (Goldberger *et al.*, 2002a). A biomechanical model of the human body emerges in which individual "units" interact in a nonlinear fashion such that feedback loops operate over long temporal and spatial ranges. This self-regulation leads to reduced variability which is important for maintaining physiological control of biological systems. For example, the prediction of homeostasis reveals that the output of a wide variety of systems, such as the normal human heartbeat, fluctuates in a complex manner even under resting conditions.

It is generally believed that the irregularity of the signal allows biological systems to respond to external disturbances that vary over a wide range of time scales. The velocity of the action potential determines the short-time behavior of the surface EMG signal. In contrast, the physiologic origin of its long-time behavior is unknown. It is not even clear whether observed fluctuations ("noise") in the signal are external or are intrinsic to the physiologic system. Intrinsic noise can be explained by the combined action of inhibitory and excitatory "units" or components of the system (Koppell, 2000). The presence of external fluctuations can have important consequences for complex systems. It has been shown, for example, that a system of oscillators can become synchronized, which may then explain the combined action of the entire system (Costa *et al.*, 2003).

It is not known which model of skeletal muscles explains the presence of intrinsic noise in the EMG signal. This is a common situation encountered in many studies of complex systems. Nonlinear time series analysis has developed numerous tools to distinguish nonlinear or chaotic behaviors within the system from external noise. For chaotic systems, the number of dynamic degrees of freedom can be determined from the signal that is (roughly) equal to the number of inhibitory and excitatory units in the system.

In nonlinear time series analysis, the characteristic behavior of a system is extracted from a mathematical analysis of the signal. The behavior of the signal is quantified using concepts and ideas borrowed primarily from statistical physics and signal processing. In particular, the information entropy has been proposed as a measure of the irregularity of the signal (Costa *et al.*, 2003; Costa, 2002; Goldberger *et al.*, 2002b; Pincus, 2001). A periodic signal and a complete irregular signal (or "white noise") have zero entropy. A random (or stochastic) signal with long-time correlations is characterized by a finite entropy, $S>0$. For a large variety of physiologic systems, it has been shown that dysfunction is associated with a decrease in the entropy of the time series. This suggests that physiological dysfunction leads to either complete order or excessive disorder.

2.2 Entropy of electromyography

In a mathematical description, the signal at (discrete) "time" n, x_n, is treated as a random, or stochastic, variable (Kantz, 2003; Sprott, 2003). It is assumed that the signal is "stationary," i.e., the quantity $\Sigma_{i=1}^{t} x_{n-1+i}$ does not depend on the initial time n. The mean-square displacement is then defined by $\Delta(t)=\langle[\Sigma_{i=1}^{t} x_{n-1+i}]^2\rangle$, where the average is taken with respect to the n. If the signal at time n is uncorrelated with the signal at a different time m, $\langle x_n x_m\rangle=0$, the mean-square displacement increases diffusively, $\Delta(t) \sim t$. This case is generally referred to as "white noise." In the presence of long-time correlations, $\langle x_n x_m\rangle \sim 1/|n-m|^{\nu}$ for some exponent $\nu>0$, fractional Brownian walk follows $\Delta(t) \sim t^{2H}$ (Mandelbrot, 1983). Here, the Hurst exponent is $H=2\nu+1$ with $0<H<0.5$ for sub-diffusive and $0.5<H<1$ for super-diffusive "behavior". The presence of long-time correlations implies that the signal has no characteristic time scales and looks the same on all time scales. In a certain mathematical limit, the mean-square displacement and the entropy are related to each other $S \sim \ln \Delta$.

The entropy reflects properties of the signal on many different time scales and, therefore, does not have a simple relationship with the velocity of the action potential. It follows that properties of the surface EMG signal obtained via nonlinear time series analysis are complementary to the analysis of the power spectrum. Entropy has many interdisciplinary applications as in aging psychology or macromolecular engineering (Allen *et al.*, 1998; Allen *et al.*, 2004). Regarding time series applications, biological time series are complex data that need to be distilled to useful information such as assessing an illness. Nonlinear analysis using fractal geometry and random walks theory proved to be useful in the analysis of a variety of time series such as correlations between global temperatures and solar activity (Scafetta & West, 2003), earthquake statistics (Scafetta & West, 2004), human heartbeat (Ivanov *et al.*, 1999), and shapes of red cells under flow stress (Korol & Rasia, 2003). Recently, nonlinear time series generated by the back muscles' electrical activity was investigated between subjects with and without LBP motivated by the need to develop an evaluation tool for LBP (Lee *et al.*, 2010; Sung *et al.*, 2005; Sung *et al.*, 2007a; Sung *et al.*, 2010).

Using random walk concepts, Collins and De Luca have studied the erratic motion of the center of pressure of a standing human body (Collins & De Luca, 1994; Collins & De Luca, 1995). They found a crossover from superdiffusive random walks for short times to subdiffusive random walks for longer times. In our entropic analysis of EMG time series from back muscles, we observed a crossover from subdiffusive, Hurst exponent $H \leq 0.5$, to self-organization, Hurst exponent $H \approx 0$. The Renyi entropy associated with diffusive processes grows linearly with the logarithm of time, and the rate of growth is independent of the Renyi parameter (Kaufman, 1985; Kaufman, 2007). The entropy is the rigorous measure of lack of information. The information, or Shannon, entropy for a particular experimental condition with a set of M possible outcomes is (Gage, 1992; S. Shannon, 1997):

$$S_{information} = -\sum_{j=1}^{M} p_j \ln(p_j) \tag{1}$$

where pj is the relative frequency of outcome #j. It is uniquely determined from the Khinchin axioms: (I) it depends on the probabilities p only; (II) the lowest entropy (S = 0) corresponds to one of the p's being 1 and the rest being zero (i.e., total information); (III) the largest value for the entropy is lnM and is achieved when all p's are equal to each other (i.e., the absence of any information); and (IV) S is additive over partitions of the outcomes. If the last axiom is relaxed to consider only statistically independent partitions, Renyi found that the information entropy is replaced by a one-variable function (Cybulski *et al.*, 2004):

$$S(\beta) = \frac{1}{1-\beta} \ln(\sum_{j=1}^{M} p_j^{\beta}) \,. \tag{2}$$

For β = 1, the Renyi entropy equals the Shannon entropy. The Renyi entropy is related to the Tsallis entropy which is central to the current massive research effort in nonextensive statistical mechanics (Vinga & Almeida, 2004).

In the continuum limit: $p_j \approx \rho(x,t)\Delta x$, where x is the random variable, e.g. displacement for random walker, and ρ is the probability distribution function. The actual experiment was conducted for measuring the electrical signal from back muscles (Sung *et al.*, 2005). Consider a time series x_t. Following Scafetta and Grigolini (Scafetta & Grigolini, 2002), the signal x_n was interpreted as a jump at time n. It was generated at all walks of time length t: $X_{m,t} = \sum_{j=0}^{t-1} x_{j+m}$. For a given time t, the ensemble of all the walks of time length t was considered and distinguished from one another by the initial time m. The range of X was divided in M equal bins, and the probability of finding a walker at that location was estimated by using the fraction of all X that fall in the bin. The results were obtained for M = 500 bins. The entropies were computed using Eqs. (1) and (2). The numerical time series were analyzed searching for a logarithmic dependence of the entropy.

Figure 1 indicates the EMG time series from the right thoracic muscle of the healthy individual and the entropy associated with walks generated from the healthy right thoracic muscle EMG time series as a function of the logarithm of time. At short times, $t < 0.01$ s, the slope is 0.26, 0.32, 0.34 for the Renyi parameter $\beta = 0, 1, 5$ respectively. Since the fit was done on only ten data points, there is a large uncertainty for those values. Similar slope values were extracted from the EMG data from all the muscles (both sides of the thoracic and lumbar erector spinae) for both individuals (HEALTHY and LBP subjects). At longer times, for 0.01 s < t < 1 s, the entropies exhibit a plateau. The plateau occurs at an entropy value well below the maximum possible entropy value lnM. Hence, it is not an artifact of the way we estimate the entropy; but it is an intrinsic property of the time series.

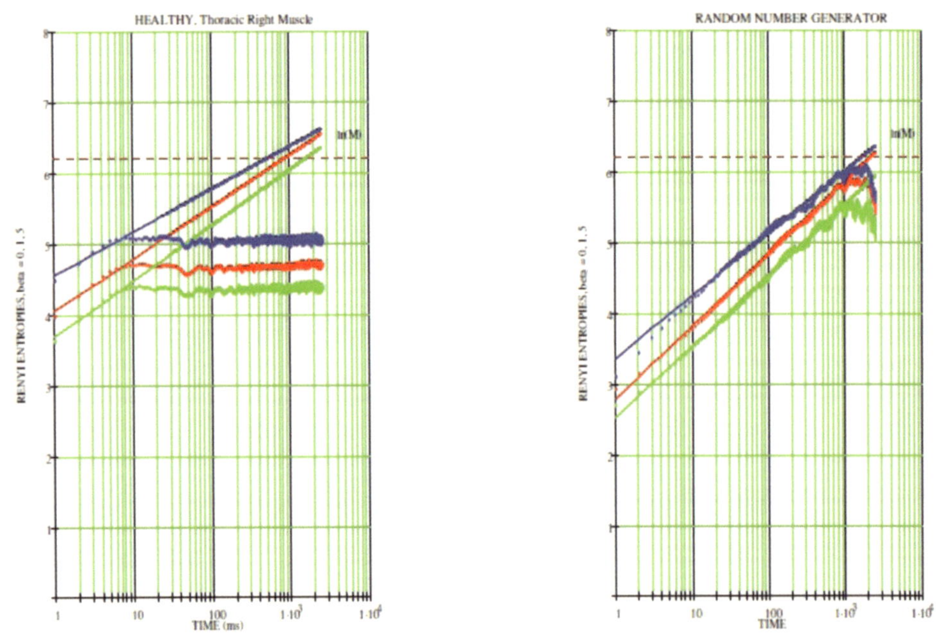

a. b.

Fig. 1. Entropy vs. ln$t$. Top curve $\beta = 0$, middle curve $\beta = 1$, bottom curve $\beta = 5$. a. Subject without LBP for the right thoracic erector spinae muscle; b. Random number generator.

The entropy plateau corresponds to the Hurst exponent $H \approx 0$. The power spectrum $P(f) \sim f^{\alpha}$ with an exponent $\alpha = 2H + 1 \approx 1$ follows $P(f) \sim 1/f$. Self-organization is generally associated

with $1/f$ noise, and this is the reason why the entropy plateau can be interpreted as a manifestation of self-organization (Buldyrev *et al.*, 2006). Qualitatively similar dependences were observed in the analysis of the erratic motion of the center of pressure of the human body (Collins & De Luca, 1994; Collins & De Luca, 1995). Though the details are not identical (e.g crossover time and slopes are different), we suspect that this type of crossover from large Hurst exponent random walks at short times to small Hurst exponent random walks at long times characterizes organized complex systems. In Figure 1b, the qualitatively different dependence of entropy on time exhibited by time series was generated with a commercial random number generator. The slopes of S versus ln$t$ for the random number generator data are 0.38, 0.45, 0.44 for $\beta = 0, 1, 5$ respectively. These values are quite close to the Brownian diffusion value $H = ½$. There is no plateau in the random number time series.
This comparison between the EMG data on one hand and random data on the other hand supports the idea that the system responsible for the back muscle signal is complex as opposed to noisy. The time evolution of entropy for EMG data also differs qualitatively from the time dependence of the entropy of chaotically advected tracers: the latter does not exhibit a crossover in time to self-organization, but it does exhibit a substantial dependence of the logarithmic amplitude on the Renyi parameter.
The entropy dependence on time constitutes a potential tool for differentiating between subjects with and without LBP. We show in Figure 2 below, side by side, graphs of the relative entropy $S/\ln(M)$ versus ln$t$ from four erector spinae (right and left thoracic and right and left lumbar) muscles of a healthy male and a LBP male of the same age. In each case, we computed the entropy using $M = 500$ bins.

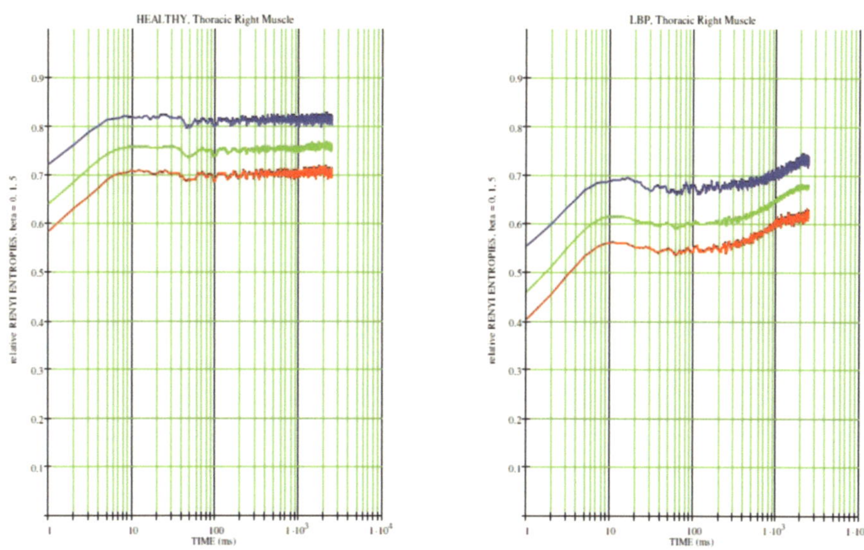

a b

Fig. 2. Relative Entropy on lumbar right muscle vs. ln$t$. Top $\beta = 0$, middle $\beta = 1$, bottom $\beta = 5$; a. Subject without LBP; b. Subject with LBP.

The plateau entropy is consistently higher for the healthy individual than for the LBP individual. A previous pilot study in our lab also demonstrated similar results involving ten healthy and ten LBP individuals, who were matched by gender, but not by age (Sung *et al.*, 2007b). The question of whether the plateau entropy constitutes a useful diagnostic tool for LBP needs further investigation with large groups of individuals matched by age, gender, body mass index, etc. It is worth emphasizing that Costa et al. and Chialvo argued based on heart time series that pathology is associated with less variability (lower entropy) as indicated in our study (Chialvo, 2002; Costa *et al.*, 2002).

To better understand the entropy time evolution, we show in Figure 3 the histograms used to determine the entropy for the left thoracic muscle of LBP subjects. In Figure 3a, we see the widening of the probability distribution with time corresponding to the entropy increase at short times $t < 10$ ms. In Figure 3b, the probability distribution is practically stationary corresponding to the entropy plateau at longer times 10 ms $< t <$ 500 ms. In Figure 3c, we show the probability distribution at $t = 1000$ ms, attempting to understand the increase in entropy apparent for $t > 500$ ms. We observe the occurrence of two peaks which may correspond to some sort of phase transition. In order to check this hypothesis, we computed the histogram using 66,000 data points rather than the 6,000 points window used in all other computations.

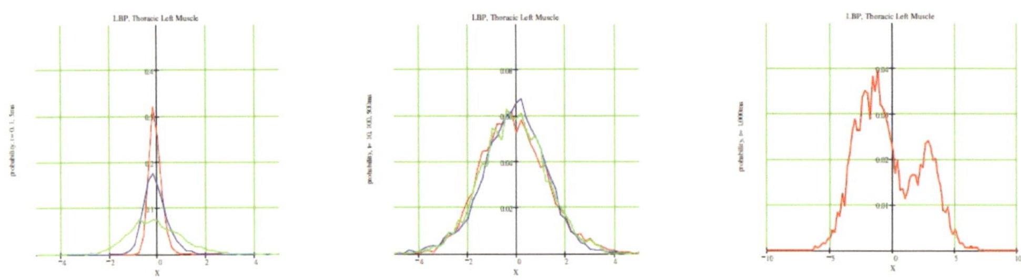

a. b. c.

Fig. 3. Probability distributions at short time, intermediate time, and long time for the thoracic left muscle in subjects with LBP at: (a) t = 0, 1, 5ms; (b) t = 10, 100, 500ms; (c) t =1000ms.

We reduced the original time series to 6,000 entries by averaging over 10 consecutive entries of the original time series. We labeled the resulting time series as *xn*, where the index *n* ('time') runs from 1 to 6,000. Nonlinear time series analysis assumes that the signal is stationary. To test this assumption, we calculated the mean and variance of 100 data points. The results for the subjects with and without LBP are shown in Figures 4A and 4B, respectively. Clearly, the EMG signal is stationary in both cases. Note that the average of the mean (μ) is nonzero, which reflects an offset in the calibration. For the numerical analysis below, we correct the offset by replacing *xn* with *xn* - μ. For nonlinear systems, signals at different times are correlated as shown in a phase portrait where the signal *xn*+1 at time *n*+1 is plotted vs the signal xn at time *n*.

For the subject without LBP (Figure 5A), the phase portrait has a circular shape. This portrait shows that the signals at consecutive times *n* and *n*+1 are statistically independent of each other. On the other hand, the phase portrait for the subject with LBP has the shape of an ellipse with the long axis directed along the diagonal (Figure 5B). The elliptical shape along the diagonal indicates the presence of correlations. Physicists have developed several

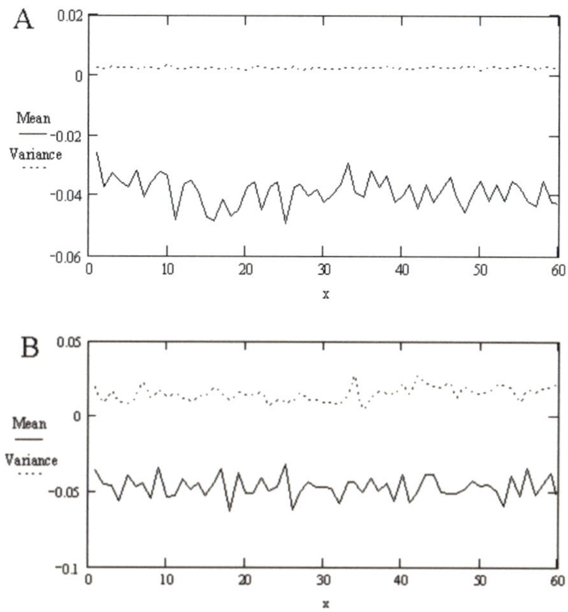

Fig. 4. Mean (solid line) and standard deviation (dashed line) for (A) subjects without and (B) subjects with LBP.

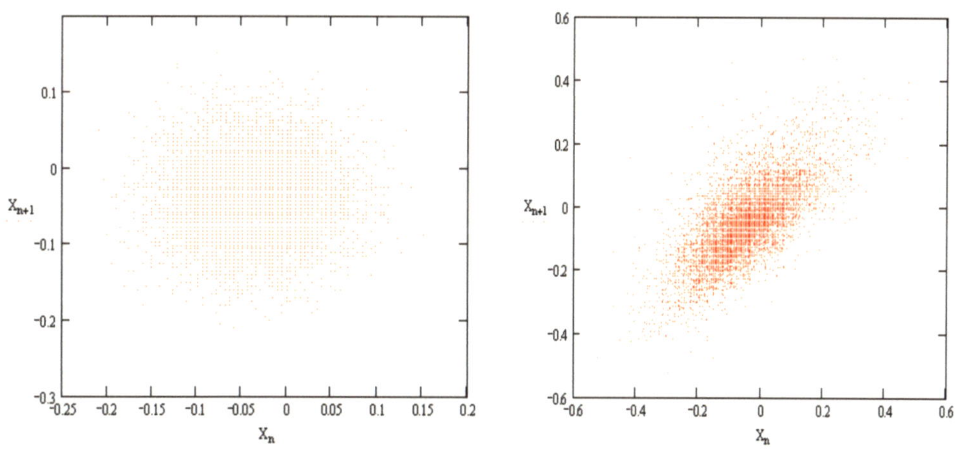

(A) (B)

Fig. 5. Phase portrait of (A) subjects without and (B) subjects with LBP.

methods to quantify the complexity of time series. One method explores the connection with random walks, or Brownian motion (Denny & Gaines, 2000). To this end, we interpret the signal xn as a jump at time n. It follows that the sum $X(t)=xn+xn+1+\ldots+xn+t$ is the displacement between times n and $n+t$. The average is zero $\langle X(t)\rangle=0$. The mean-square displacement is obtained by taking the square and then calculating the average with respect to the initial time n, $\Delta(t) = \langle X2(t)\rangle$. For deterministic motion, $\Delta(t) \sim t2$, while $\Delta(t) \sim t$ is for diffusion. In the general case, we write $\Delta(t) \sim t2h$ so that $0< h < 0.5$ and $0.5 < h< 1$ correspond to sub-

diffusive (negative correlations) and super-diffusive (positive correlations) behavior, respectively. In Figures 6A and 6B, we show the dependence of $\Delta(t)$ vs t in double-logarithmic plots.
A straight line corresponds to power-law behavior, and the Hurst exponent H (Mandelbrot, 1977) is determined by the slope. For the subject without LBP, we find H=0.5, corresponding to diffusive behavior. For the subject with LBP, we have H=0.2, which indicates the presence of long-time correlations in the EMG signal, in agreement with the results from the phase portrait. The mean-square follows (fractional) Brownian motion only for short-times. For long-times, $\Delta(t)$ appears to plateau. The determination of the Hurst Exponent is affected by large statistical fluctuations. In order to get a more reliable estimate of the Hurst exponent, an analysis of the entropy of the time series was undertaken.

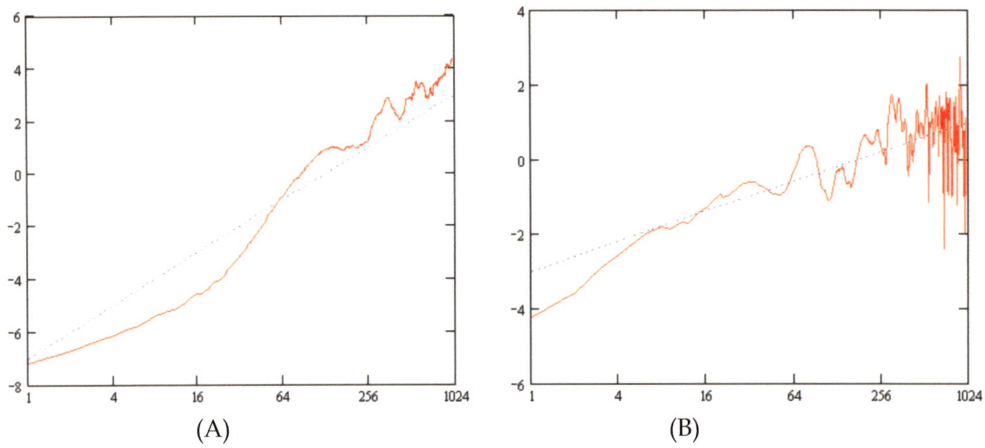

Fig. 6. Log-log plot Δ *vs.* t for (A) subjects without and (B) subjects with LBP.

One can characterize the complexity of time series by using the information (Shannon) entropy $S=-\Sigma pj \log pj$, where pj is the probability for outcome number 'j' of a given experiment (Allen *et al.*, 2004; Bezerianos *et al.*, 1995; Bezerianos *et al.*, 2003; Costa *et al.*, 2003). The above equation is the standard formulation of uncertainty as it has the following features: (i) the lowest entropy (S = 0) corresponds to one of the outcomes being certain [i.e. probability one] and the others never occurring [i.e. probability zero]; (ii) the largest value for the entropy, $S=\ln(M)$, is achieved when all outcomes are equally likely [all probabilities are equal to each other, $pj = 1/M$]; and (iii) S is additive over partitions of the outcomes. The results reported here were obtained for M = 1000 bins. The variation of S with t is expected to be logarithmic: $S(t) \sim H \ln t$, where H is the Hurst exponent introduced before. The entropic analysis of the time series from the subject without LBP and from the subject with LBP shows significant differences in how fast the entropy saturates.
In addition, there is a difference between the slopes of entropy and time function for subjects without and with LBP (Figure 7). The slopes represent estimates for the Hurst exponent H. In agreement with the variance of displacement analysis presented, there was a difference of the Hurst exponent between the subjects without LBP (H=0.5; Figure 6, A) and subject with LBP (H=0.4; Figure 6, B) were indicated. Note that the value of the exponent H for the LBP subject refers to short-times, while the behavior for long-times is characterized by the value 0.2 quoted before. The difference in the entropy vs time dependence exhibited

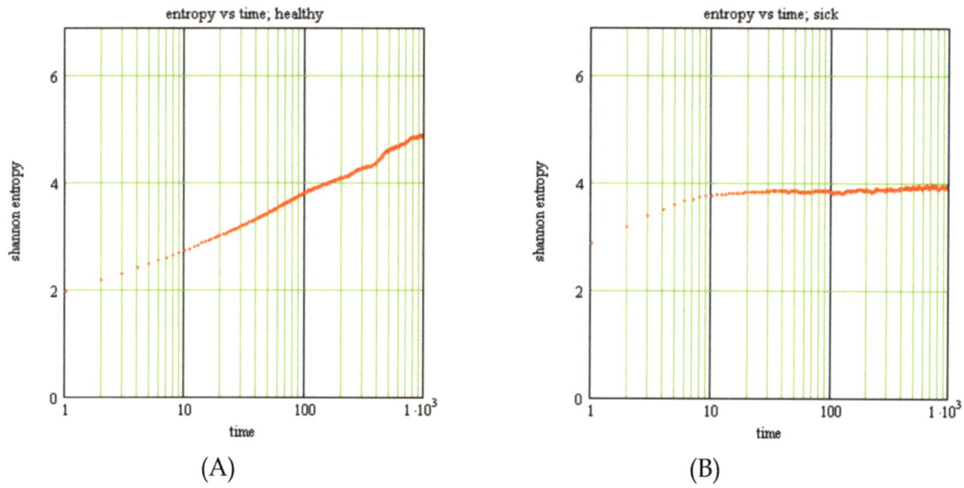

Fig. 7. Shannon entropy versus ln(t) for (A) subjects without and (B) subjects with LBP.

by the healthy and LBP subjects goes beyond the issue of the value of the Hurst exponent. The entropy associated with the LBP subject saturates at very short-times; two orders of magnitude shorter than for the healthy subject. Furthermore, the long time entropy of LBP is lower than for the healthy subject, a result consistent with non-linear analysis of other medical time series (Bezerianos *et al.*, 1995). It is generally observed that injuries result in a decrease in the complexity of biological systems.

In conculsion, nonlinear analysis of time series based on entropy can differentiate between complex biological sources and random sources of the data. While the EMG signal from an erector spinae muscle exhibits an entropy time dependence with a crossover from subdiffusive regime at short times to a self-organization regime (plateau) at longer time scales, time series generated with random number generators do not exhibit the plateau. The Renyi entropy time evolution also differentiates between this complex biological system and deterministic processes (e.g. tracers advection in polymer flows). The presence of the plateau points to the existence of anti-correlations of EMG signals separated in time by at least 0.01 s. Therefore, it is a manifestation of a complex self-organizing system in which individual units interact in a nonlinear fashion such that feedback loops operate over long temporal ranges (Goldberger *et al.*, 2002a).

2.3 Reliability of surface electromyography analysis

The reliability of surface EMG could be different between nonlinear analysis of time series and power spectrum analysis. Our previous study results indicated that the measurement of back muscle fatigability, especially the erector spinae muscle, indicated that the entropy analysis was a more reliable measure than the power spectral analysis (Sung *et al.*, 2008b).

It is well known that the observed EMG signal depends on anatomical factors, such as muscle geometry, subcutaneous fat, gender, and other confounding factors (Lindstrom *et al.*, 1974; Mannion *et al.*, 1997c; Pullman *et al.*, 2000; Roy *et al.*, 1997; Solomonow *et al.*, 1990). As a result, observed quantities from EMG signals show considerable variations even among a group of healthy subjects. A clinical diagnosis of musculoskeletal dysfunction using surface EMG is based on the assumption that dysfunction changes the values of the observed quantities. This underlying assumption is difficult to prove, however, because the EMG signal prior to an injury is generally not available.

One reliable indicator is MF, which is defined by dividing the area under the spectrum into two equal parts. However, use of the MF has led to contradictory results in muscle fatiguing experiments. It still remains to be seen whether a shift in the MF differentiates the various stages of non-acute LBP. The fatigability of back muscles might predispose individuals to LBP. A number of investigators have attempted to classify LBP via changes in the EMG signal during prolonged contraction of the paraspinal muscles (Lariviere *et al.*, 2002a; Lariviere *et al.*, 2002b; Mayer *et al.*, 1989; Peach & McGill, 1998; Roy *et al.*, 1997; Roy *et al.*, 1990). The MF of the back muscles is typically of the order of 100 Hz and is determined by the propagation of the action potential across the electrodes. That is, the MF reflects the behavior of the EMG signal on short-time scales.

Several studies have suggested that surface EMG power spectrum analysis could be used to evaluate patients undergoing rehabilitation in a non-invasive fashion (De Luca, 1984; Mannion *et al.*, 1998; Merletti *et al.*, 1999). The connection between fatigue and EMG spectral parameters is the basis for the use of EMG as an objective and noninvasive method of assessment of back muscle endurance (De Luca, 1984; Mannion *et al.*, 1997a). The original study linking LBP with fatigue was presented by De Luca (De Luca, 1984) who found that subjects with LBP have less endurance, and thus smaller MF slopes, during sustained muscle contractions (Merletti *et al.*, 1999; Roy *et al.*, 1989). However, contradictory results have subsequently been reported and have shown that MF slope is not better than chance in predicting LBP (Humphrey *et al.*, 2005; Lee *et al.*, 2010; Mannion *et al.*, 2001). Thus, a connection between spectral quantities and musculoskeletal pain/dysfunction remains elusive despite considerable efforts.

In recent studies, we applied methods from nonlinear analysis of time series and found that the time-dependent entropy calculated from the EMG signal shows a distinct plateau-like behavior for intermediate times (Kaufman, 2007; Sung *et al.*, 2005; Sung *et al.*, 2007b). The signal from EMG is the instantaneous algebraic summations of action potentials from muscle fibers, and its power spectrum is obtained from a fast Fourier transform of the signal. Recently, several studies in entropy measurements based on nonlinear time series analysis were published without reporting reliability and validity concerns (Goldberger *et al.*, 2002b; Kaufman, 2007; Sung *et al.*, 2007b). Therefore, it would be valuable to confirm the reliability of measurements for characterizing neuromuscular alterations by investigating differences between the power spectrum analysis and nonlinear time series analysis of entropy measures.

It has been found that the degree of randomness is a characteristic property of time series. Entropy is generally used to quantify the complexity. In particular, entropy is used to characterize non-periodic, random phenomena and indicates the rate of information production as it relates to dynamic systems (Richman & Moorman, 2000). Several research groups have compared entropy values for subjects with and without illness/dysfunction (Chialvo, 2002; Costa, 2002; Goldberger *et al.*, 2002a; Stanley *et al.*, 1992; West, 1990). This concept has been used to differentiate healthy subjects from those with heart disease using electrocardiogram time series as well; it is generally found that disease is associated with a lowering of the entropy. In several papers, we applied these ideas to EMG time series for the low back muscles. We found that subjects with LBP have lower entropies than healthy subjects, which is in agreement with the general finding. The traditional approach of EMG is based within the framework of linear systems for which a given input leads to a well-defined periodicity. This connection led to the notion of homeostasis, namely that the normal function of physiologic systems operates in a steady state and that fluctuations are suppressed. However, contradictory results have subsequently been reported without clear understanding of the reliability of entropy measures (Humphrey *et al.*, 2005; Sung *et al.*, 2008b).

Our previous studies indicated that the plateau entropy value was consistently higher for the healthy individual than for the LBP individual. However, the question of whether the plateau entropy constitutes a reliable assessment tool for LBP needs further investigation with large groups of individuals matched by age, gender, body mass index, etc. It is important to understand that Costa et al. and Chialvo argued that pathology/dysfunction is associated with less variability (lower entropy), which was consistent with our findings (Kaufman, 2007; Sung *et al.*, 2005; Sung *et al.*, 2007b).

Nonlinear analysis has proved to be useful in the analysis of a variety of physiologic time series such as human heartbeats (Ivanov *et al.*, 1999) and the shapes of red blood cells under flow stress (Korol & Rasia, 2003). Based on these empirical studies, it has been found that the time series from healthy subjects have higher entropy values than the time series from those with pathology/dysfunction. There are also several other studies indicating that traditional approaches to measuring the complexity of biological signals fail to account for the multiple time scales inherent in such time series. Generally, biological time series are complex data that need to be distilled to useful application to assess a pathology/dysfunction. However, no study has investigated the reliability of entropy measures to assess pathology/ dysfunction. In addition, despite much effort, the MF and the MF slope have not shown consistent measurements (De Luca, 1984; Mannion *et al.*, 1998; Merletti *et al.*, 1999; Sung, 2003).

In previous studies, we explored the use of entropy derived from time series as an alternative quantitative measure of EMG signals that can be used in a clinical assessment. We compared the values of the entropy between subjects with LBP and healthy subjects and found that healthy subjects have significantly higher entropies than subjects with LBP (Sung *et al.*, 2007b). However, it is important to examine the between-day variability of entropy, the MF, and the MF slope within the same sample group. In our current study, we compared the values of MF, MF slope, and entropy for two different measurements; and the results indicated the highest correlation for entropy, while the MF slope and MF demonstrated relatively weak correlations.

The results for the right back muscle are illustrated in Figures 8-13 in order to compare values with different measures. The consistent responses of the non-dominant side of the back could be less affected by hand dominance. The histogram of the entropy (Figure 8) demonstrated consistent distributions between pre- and post- measurement entropy values, which are plotted in Figure 9. The points representing the 32 subjects were plotted closely along the diagonal line, indicating that the two measurements reveal a relatively high correlation (R=0.75).

The mean and the standard deviations of the MF slope values for two measurements were analyzed, and the correlations ranged from 0.15-0.18, which does not indicate a significant difference between the MF slopes at two different observations. The intra class correlation coefficients (ICCs) ranged from 0.26-0.30, and the standard error of means (SEM) varied between 0.03 and 0.04, which were not significantly different for the distributions for two different times. Figure 10 compared two measurements of the MF slope for the right back muscle, and the number of subjects repeatedly demonstrated less similar results between the two measurements. The Pearson correlation coefficients ranged from 0.15-0.18 and were not statistically different. This result confirms the values of the MF slope of the right back muscle for post-measurement, which was plotted versus the values of pre-measurement in Figure 10 and shows no obvious difference. The points representing the subjects were distributed rather broadly, which was reflected in the low correlation coefficient (R=0.18).

The distribution of MF values from post-measurement shifted towards larger values. The correlations ranged from 0.38-0.47 and were statistically significant. Thus, there was a significant correlation between the distributions of the MF values from the measurements at two different times. The ICCs ranged from 0.54-0.64, and the SEM ranged from 3.10-3.60. The Pearson correlation coefficients ranged from 0.38-0.47 and were statistically significant. In Figure 12, two measurements of the MF for the right back muscle are compared, and the number of subjects repeatedly demonstrated less similar results between two measurements. Figure 12 depicts the histograms of the MF values. The two histograms indicated little difference except for two outliers for post-measurement values. Figure 13 depicts the MF values of the right back muscle, and the linear regression analysis yielded R=0.15. The values of MF for the two measurements were more highly correlated than those for the MF slope, although the correlation (R=0.38) was much lower than that for the entropy (Sung *et al.*, 2005).

Overall, the ICC values of entropy for between-day measurements were higher, and the SEM for entropy was lower than the MF and its slope. Therefore, the results of this study indicated that the entropy analysis could provide reliable measurements for muscle fatigability.

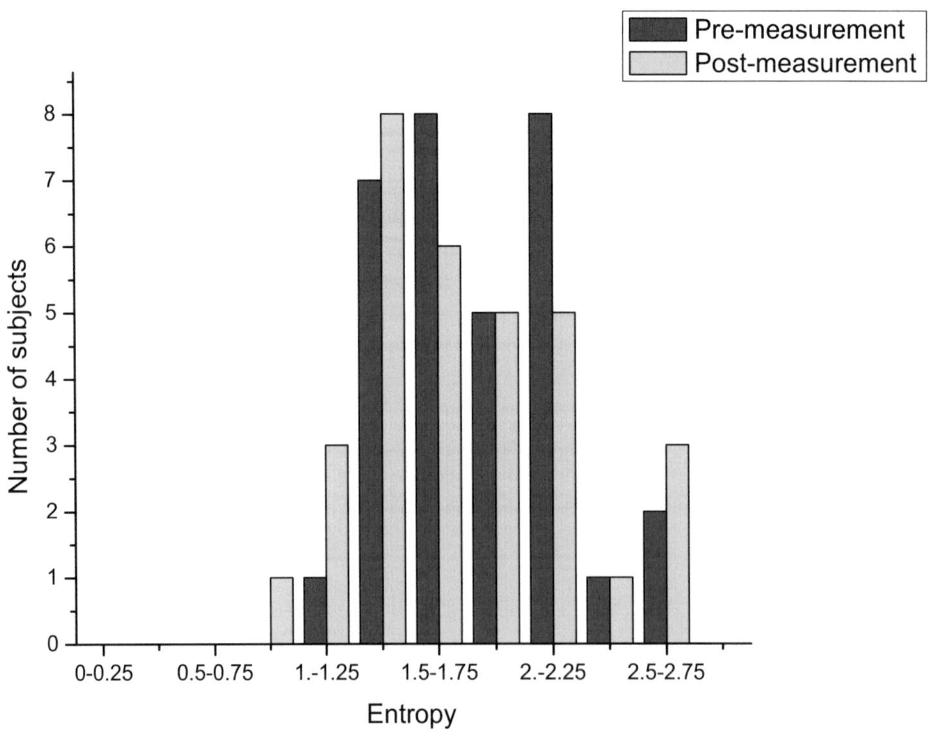

Fig. 8. Histogram of entropy measurements for the right back muscle.

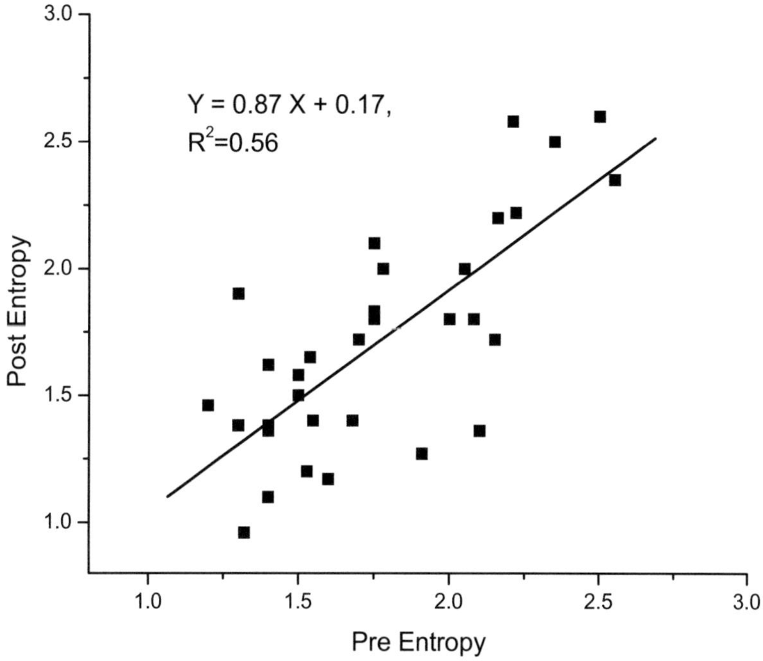

Fig. 9. The entropy values taken at two different measurements for the right erector spinae muscle. The correlation coefficient is R=0.75.

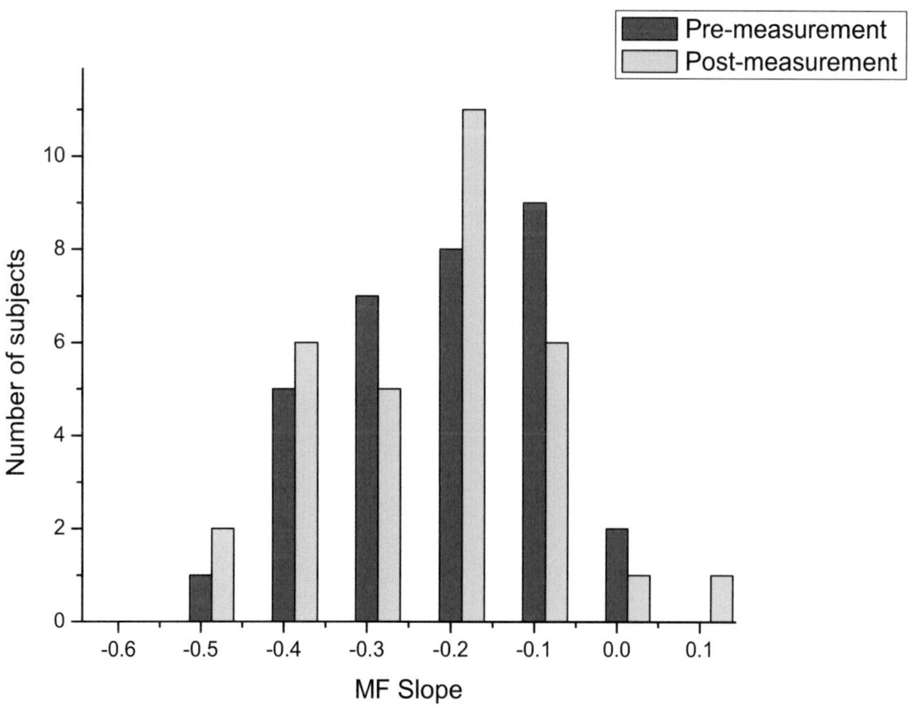

Fig. 10. Histogram of median frequency slope measurements for the right back muscle.

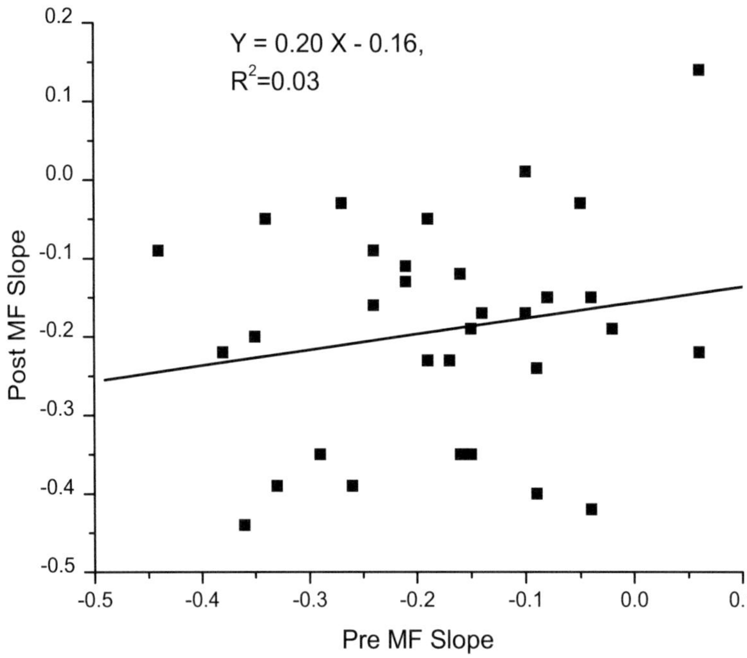

Fig. 11. The median frequency slope taken at two different measurements for the right back muscle. The correlation coefficient is R=0.18.

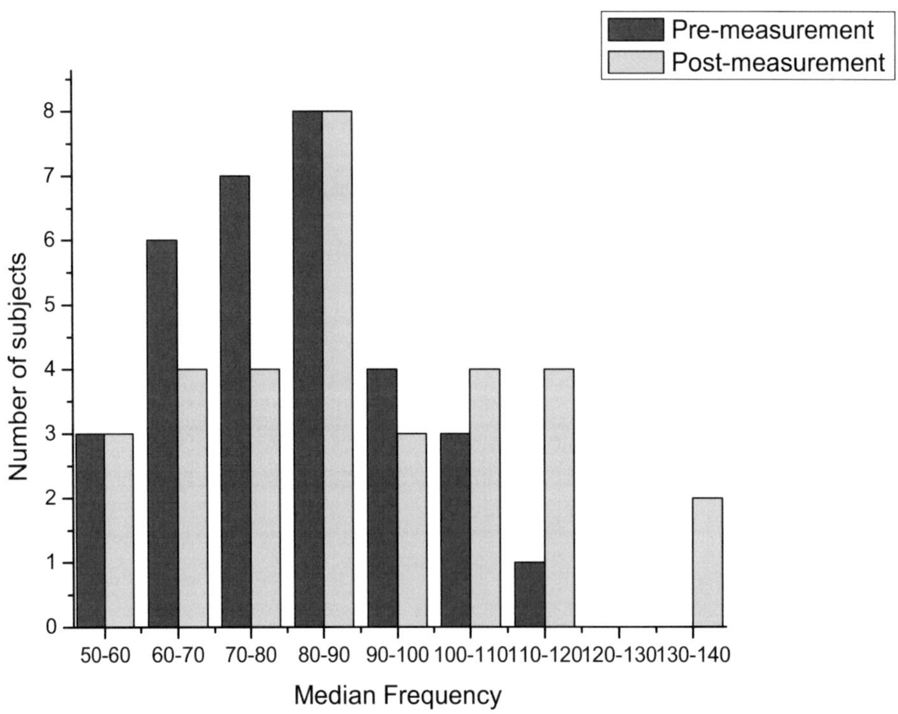

Fig. 12. Histogram of median frequency measurements for the right back muscle.

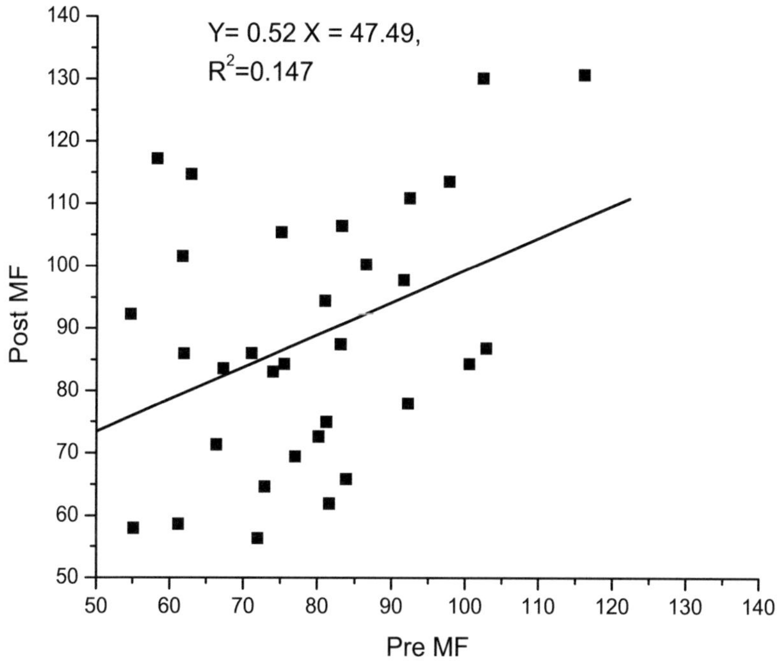

Fig. 13. The median frequency for the right back muscle at two different measurements. The correlation coefficient is R=0.38.

Overall, the entropy measurements for back muscles were more reliable than the power spectrum measures based on between-day reliability. Although there were no significant differences for between-day reliability for both entropy and MF slope, the test-retest reliability based on ICC values was higher for the entropy measure. The results of this study indicated that the complexity of time series analysis is a more reliable measure for the adaptability of biological systems than power spectral analysis.

A clinical assessment of LBP is important to objectively identify subjects with genuine pain and to assess the efficacy of therapeutic interventions. The entropy values from two measurements had the highest correlation, and we concluded that entropy is the most reliable measure from the low back muscles. The correlation of the MF slope and MF also demonstrated weak correlations and were statistically insignificant. Although there is a positive correlation between pain level and MF slope in back muscles, it is possible that the statistical use of correlation coefficients based on several validation studies was poor for reliability studies (Meyer, 1994).

In conclusion, it is important to compare the difference between nonlinear time series and power spectrum analysis regarding the irregularity of signals in biological systems. The quantities derived from nonlinear time series analysis of EMG signals will be compared with power spectrum analysis between subjects with and without musculoskeletal dysfunction/pain.

2.4 Sensitivity of surface electromyography analysis

As reported in our previous studies, the complexity of physiologic time series is a sensitive measure for muscle fatigability (Lee *et al.*, 2010). However, it is necessary to determine whether the observed Shannon (information) entropy, as compared with MF, was able to differentiate fatigability of the thoracic and lumbar parts of the erector spinae muscle following the intervention. Previously, our lab investigated tools for evaluating back muscle fatigability after spinal stabilization exercises in participants with chronic LBP (Lee *et al.*, 2010; Sung *et al.*, 2005; Sung *et al.*, 2008a; Sung *et al.*, 2010). The results of our previous study indicated that Shannon entropy might be a valuable tool to measure the differences of outcomes following the exercise intervention. The results indicated that the participants' pain levels decreased significantly after 4 weeks of spinal stabilization exercises. The entropy of the EMG signals also decreased and significantly interacted with pain level. The slope of the MF based on power spectrum analysis also decreased but did not demonstrate any interaction with pain level. Therefore, the entropy of the EMG signals might be a useful tool for measuring LBP.

In addition, the results indicated that the entropy clearly differentiated the two groups. However, the results of power spectrum analysis based on complexity of the EMG signal could be calculated with the entropy of the time series. The results indicated that healthy subjects revealed significantly larger entropy values than the subjects with LBP. These findings consistently demonstrated a connection between physiologic "health" and complexity (Costa *et al.*, 2003; Costa *et al.*, 2005; Li & Huston, 2002). Another important finding indicated that the entropy levels of the EMG signals demonstrated significant interactions between muscles and groups following treatment for muscle endurance. However, the MF did not demonstrate this interaction. The significant interaction effect of the entropy between muscles and groups following treatment during the one-minute back extension test supports the characteristics of the recorded signals that occurs with fatigue (Roy *et al.*, 1989). Exercises for graded activity programs can be used to increase trunk muscle endurance and to decrease pain (Jorgensen & Nicolaisen, 1986; Jorgensen & Nicolaisen, 1987). Undoubtedly, other muscles participated in the load sharing during the testing as well as when subjects performed the intervention exercises. The attachment of the lumbar muscles, rather than the thoracic back muscles, results in an effective lever arm for lumbar stabilization. Therefore, the lumbar muscle is more effective in creating a stabilizing moment over the lumbar vertebral segments during the test (Flicker *et al.*, 1993; MacIntosh & Bogduk, 1986).

Research in biology and medicine has shown that fluctuations in physiological systems may play a significant role (Costa, 2002; Goldberger *et al.*, 2002a; Liu *et al.*, 2002). In fractal physiology, the apparent random, or chaotic, signal is observed on different (time) scales. It is found that the signal looks similar, or self-similar. This means that a single time scale (e.g., the period of oscillation) is replaced by a family of time scales. It follows that the single state of the system is replaced by multiple non-equilibrium states that are correlated with each other. If the signal is completely random with no characteristic time scale, it would be modeled by "white noise" and the power spectrum would be flat with $P(f) \sim f0$. In general, the frequency spectrum is fitted to a power law $P(f) \sim 1/f\alpha$, with $0 < \alpha < 2$. In this case, the power spectrum does not define a MF. Other studies reported that for physiologic systems, a constant "output" requires other variables to fluctuate so that the system can adapt to sudden changes in demand or stimulus (Costa *et al.*, 2005). This extent of fluctuations in physiologic signals can be quantified by entropy calculated from their time series.

Nonlinear analysis is used to characterize "hidden" properties of physiologic time series. Following this approach, we interpreted the EMG signal in terms of a one-dimensional random walk in discrete time. We found that the mean-square displacement increased linearly for short times $t < 20$ ms and is nearly flat for intermediate times 20 ms $< t <$ 400 ms. This plateau behavior has been found for other biological systems and implies the existence of correlations in the signal (Costa *et al.*, 2005; Goldberger *et al.*, 2002a). However, these correlations cannot be explained within a linear model, and thus support the use of nonlinear analysis for EMG time series. This may also explain why the MF fluctuates during a sustained contraction, and why the connection between MF slope and LBP has proven elusive despite considerable efforts.

In conclusion, the nonlinear analysis to EMG time series was reviewed for low back muscles. The Shannon entropy is a standard measure of complexity and has been applied in cognitive science research, aging studies, heart failure research, and other fields (Allen *et al.*, 2004; Costa *et al.*, 2003; Costa *et al.*, 2005; Goldberger *et al.*, 2002a; Liu *et al.*, 2002). The time-dependent entropy of the EMG signal exhibits a plateau-like behavior which indicates the presence of long-time correlations in the signal. The plateau value of the entropy was lower for subjects with LBP than for individuals in the control group. This connection might prove to be useful in a clinical assessment of LBP. The existence of long-time correlations in the signal explains the large variability in the MF obtained from the power spectrum. The entropy clearly differentiated the two groups, whereas the MF exhibited significant overlaps between the groups.

3. Conclusion

This chapter covered comprehensive articles comparing the difference between nonlinear time series and power spectrum analysis regarding the irregularity of signals in biological systems. A clinical assessment of pain/dysfunction using EMG should be considered on properties of the signal that change drastically in the presence of pain/dysfunction. A shift in the MF of the spectrum is explained by the change in the velocity of the action potential, and it reflects a quantitative change of the signals. A change in the entropy of the signal also reflects a qualitative change in the physiologic system.

In this chapter, the quantities derived from nonlinear time series analysis of EMG signals was compared with power spectrum analysis between subjects with and without musculoskeletal dysfunction/pain. The fluctuations in physiologic signals can be quantified by entropy calculated from the nonlinear time series. The value of the entropy reflects the adaptability of biological systems; healthy systems are thus expected to have higher values than unhealthy systems. Finally, the distribution of the values of the entropy and power spectrum for a group of subjects with LBP and a group of healthy subjects was discussed.

4. Acknowledgment

This work was supported by Korea University and the Basic Science Research Program through the National Research Foundation of Korea funded by the Ministry of Education, Science and Technology (2010-0003015). This material is also the result of work supported in part by Drs. Miron Kaufman and Ulrich Zurcher of Cleveland State University, Cleveland, Ohio, for their critical analyses of the important intellectual content and interpretation of data. The author declares that no competing interests exist.

5. References

Allen, P. A., Kaufman, M., Smith, A. F. & Propper, R. E. (1998). A molar entropy model of age differences in spatial memory. *Psychol Aging*, Vol. *13*, No. 3, Sep, pp. 501-518

Allen, P. A., Murphy, M. D., Kaufman, M., Groth, K. E. & Begovic, A. (2004). Age differences in central (semantic) and peripheral processing: the importance of considering both response times and errors. *J Gerontol B Psychol Sci Soc Sci*, Vol. *59*, No. 5, Sep, pp. P210-219

Belair, J., Glass, L., An Der Heiden, U. & Milton, J. (1995a). Dynamical disease: Identification, temporal aspects and treatment strategies of human illness. *Chaos*, Vol. *5*, No. 1, Mar, pp. 1-7

Belair, J., Glass, L., Heiden, U. & Milton, J. (1995b). Dynamical Disease: Mathematical Analysis of Human Illness.

Bezerianos, A., Bountis, T., Papaioannou, G. & Polydoropoulos, P. (1995). Nonlinear time series analysis of electrocardiograms. *Chaos*, Vol. *5*, No. 1, Mar, pp. 95-101

Bezerianos, A., Tong, S. & Thakor, N. (2003). Time-dependent entropy estimation of EEG rhythm changes following brain ischemia. *Ann Biomed Eng*, Vol. *31*, No. 2, Feb, pp. 221-232

Buldyrev, S. V., Ferrante, J. & Zypman, F. R. (2006). Dry friction avalanches: experiment and theory. *Phys Rev E Stat Nonlin Soft Matter Phys*, Vol. *74*, No. 6 Pt 2, Dec, pp. 066110, ISSN 1539-3755 (Print) 1539-3755 (Linking)

Chaffin, D. B. (1969). Surface electromyography frequency analysis as a diagnostic tool. *J Occup Med*, Vol. *11*, No. 3, Mar, pp. 109-115, ISSN 0096-1736 (Print) 0096-1736 (Linking)

Chialvo, D. R. (2002). Physiology: unhealthy surprises. *Nature*, Vol. *419*, No. 6904, Sep 19, pp. 263

Cholewicki, J. & VanVliet, J. J. T. (2002). Relative contribution of trunk muscles to the stability of the lumbar spine during isometric exertions. *Clin Biomech (Bristol, Avon)*, Vol. *17*, No. 2, Feb, pp. 99-105

Collins, J. J. & De Luca, C. J. (1994). Random walking during quiet standing. *Physical Review Letters*, Vol. *73*, No. 5, Aug 1, pp. 764-767

Collins, J. J. & De Luca, C. J. (1995). Upright, correlated random walks: A statistical-biomechanics approach to the human postural control system. *Chaos*, Vol. *5*, No. 1, Mar, pp. 57-63

Costa, M., Goldberger, A. L. & Peng, C. K. (2002). Multiscale entropy to distinguish physiologic and synthetic RR time series. *Comput Cardiol*, Vol. *29*, pp. 137-140

Costa, M., Goldberger, A. L. & Peng, C. K. (2003). Multiscale entropy analysis: A new measure of complexity loss in heart failure. *J Electrocardiol*, Vol. *36 Suppl*, pp. 39-40

Costa, M., Goldberger, A. L. & Peng, C. K. (2005). Multiscale entropy analysis of biological signals. *Phys Rev E Stat Nonlin Soft Matter Phys*, Vol. *71*, No. 2 Pt 1, Feb, pp. 021906

Costa, M. G., A.J. Peng, C.K. (2002). Multiscale entropy analysis of complex physiologic time series. *Phys Rev Lett*, Vol. *89*, No. (6)

Cybulski, O., Babin, V. & Holyst, R. (2004). Minimization of the Renyi entropy production in the stationary states of the Brownian process with matched death and birth rates. *Phys Rev E Stat Nonlin Soft Matter Phys*, Vol. *69*, No. 1 Pt 2, Jan, pp. 016110, ISSN 1539-3755 (Print) 1539-3755 (Linking)

De Luca, C. J. (1984). Myoelectrical manifestations of localized muscular fatigue in humans. *Crit Rev Biomed Eng*, Vol. *11*, No. 4, pp. 251-279

Denny, M. & Gaines, S. (2000). Chance in Biology- Using Probability to Explore Nature.

Flicker, P. L., Fleckenstein, J. L., Ferry, K., Payne, J., Ward, C., Mayer, T., Parkey, R. W. & Peshock, R. M. (1993). Lumbar muscle usage in chronic low back pain. Magnetic resonance image evaluation. *Spine*, Vol. *18*, No. 5, pp. 582-586.

Furey, C. A. (1963). Clinical Indications for Electromyography. *J Med Soc N J*, Vol. *60*, Nov, pp. 514-517, ISSN 0025-7524 (Print) 0025-7524 (Linking)

Gage, J. S. (1992). The concept of meaning and the mathematical theory of communication. *MD Comput*, Vol. *9*, No. 3, May-Jun, pp. 146-148, ISSN 0724-6811 (Print) 0724-6811 (Linking)

Glass, L. (2001). Synchronization and rhythmic processes in physiology. *Nature*, Vol. *410*, No. 6825, Mar 8, pp. 277-284

Goldberger, A. L., Amaral, L. A., Hausdorff, J. M., Ivanov, P., Peng, C. K. & Stanley, H. E. (2002a). Fractal dynamics in physiology: alterations with disease and aging. *Proc Natl Acad Sci U S A*, Vol. *99 Suppl 1*, Feb 19, pp. 2466-2472

Goldberger, A. L., Peng, C. K. & Lipsitz, L. A. (2002b). What is physiologic complexity and how does it change with aging and disease? *Neurobiol Aging*, Vol. *23*, No. 1, Jan-Feb, pp. 23-26

Herzog, W., Nigg, B. M., Robinson, R. O. & Read, L. J. (1987). Quantifying the effects of spinal manipulations on gait, using patients with low back pain: a pilot study. *J Manipulative Physiol Ther*, Vol. *10*, No. 6, Dec, pp. 295-299, ISSN 0161-4754 (Print) 0161-4754 (Linking)

Hobbie, R. K. (1997). Intermediate Physics for Medicine and Biology.

Hoffmann, W. (1968). [Significance of clinical electromyography in childhood. 3. Electromyographic findings in movement disorders of central nervous origin]. *Padiatr Grenzgeb*, Vol. *7*, No. 1, pp. 13-25, ISSN 0030-932X (Print) 0030-932X (Linking)

Humphrey, A. R., Nargol, A. V., Jones, A. P., Ratcliffe, A. A. & Greenough, C. G. (2005). The value of electromyography of the lumbar paraspinal muscles in discriminating between chronic-low-back-pain sufferers and normal subjects. *Eur Spine J*, Vol. *14*, No. 2, Mar, pp. 175-184

Ivanov, P. C., Amaral, L. A., Goldberger, A. L., Havlin, S., Rosenblum, M. G., Struzik, Z. R. & Stanley, H. E. (1999). Multifractality in human heartbeat dynamics. *Nature*, Vol. *399*, No. 6735, Jun 3, pp. 461-465

Jorgensen, K. & Nicolaisen, T. (1986). Two methods for determining trunk extensor endurance. A comparative study. *Eur J Appl Physiol Occup Physiol*, Vol. *55*, No. 6, pp. 639-644

Jorgensen, K. & Nicolaisen, T. (1987). Trunk extensor endurance: determination and relation to low-back trouble. *Ergonomics*, Vol. *30*, No. 2, pp. 259-267.

Kantz, H. S., T. (2003). Nonlinear Time Series Analysis. Vol. *2nd Ed., Cambridge UP, Cambridge,*

Kaufman, A. (1985). Nonlinear Dynamics: Statistical Physics and Chaos in Fusion Plasmas. *Science*, Vol. *228*, No. 4698, Apr 26, pp. 485-486

Kaufman, M., Zurcher, U., Sung P. (2007). Entropy of Electromyography Time Series. *Physica A Statistical Mechanics and its Applications*, Vol. *386*, No. 2, 2007, pp. 698-707

Knowlton, G. C., Bennett, R. L. & Mc, C. R. (1951). Electromyography of fatigue. *Arch Phys Med Rehabil*, Vol. *32*, No. 10, Oct, pp. 648-652, ISSN 0003-9993 (Print) 0003-9993 (Linking)

Koppell, N. (2000). We Got Rhythm: Dynamical Systems of the Nervous System. Vol. *47*, pp. 6-16

Korol, A. M. & Rasia, R. (2003). Signatures of deterministic chaos in dyslipidemic erythrocytes under shear stress. *Chaos*, Vol. *13*, No. 1, Mar, pp. 87-93

Lariviere, C., Arsenault, A. B., Gravel, D., Gagnon, D. & Loisel, P. (2002a). Evaluation of measurement strategies to increase the reliability of EMG indices to assess back muscle fatigue and recovery. *J Electromyogr Kinesiol*, Vol. *12*, No. 2, Apr, pp. 91-102

Lariviere, C., Arsenault, A. B., Gravel, D., Gagnon, D., Loisel, P. & Vadeboncoeur, R. (2002b). Electromyographic assessment of back muscle weakness and muscle composition: reliability and validity issues. *Arch Phys Med Rehabil*, Vol. *83*, No. 9, Sep, pp. 1206-1214

Lee, T. R., Kim, Y. H. & Sung, P. S. (2010). Spectral and entropy changes for back muscle fatigability following spinal stabilization exercises. *Journal of Rehabilitation Research & Development*, Vol. *47*, No. 2, pp. 133-142, ISSN 1938-1352 (Electronic) 0748-7711 (Linking)

Li, J. S. & Huston, J. P. (2002). Non-linear dynamics of operant behavior: a new approach via the extended return map. *Rev Neurosci*, Vol. *13*, No. 1, pp. 31-57

Lindstrom, L., Magnusson, R. & Petersen, I. (1974). Muscle load influence on myo-electric signal characteristics. *Scand J Rehabil Med*, Vol. *0*, No. Suppl, pp. 127-148.

Liu, J. Z., Dai, T. H., Sahgal, V., Brown, R. W. & Yue, G. H. (2002). Nonlinear cortical modulation of muscle fatigue: a functional MRI study. *Brain Res*, Vol. *957*, No. 2, Dec 13, pp. 320-329

MacIntosh, J. E. & Bogduk, N. (1986). The biomechanics of the lumbar multifidus. *Clinical Biomechanics*, Vol. *1*, pp. 205-213

Mandelbrot, B. (1977). The Fractale Geometry of Nature.

Mandelbrot, B. (1983). Fractal Geometry of Nature.

Mannion, A. F., Connolly, B., Wood, K. & Dolan, P. (1997a). The use of surface EMG power spectral analysis in the evaluation of back muscle function. *J Rehabil Res Dev*, Vol. *34*, No. 4, Oct, pp. 427-439

Mannion, A. F., Connolly, B., Wood, K. & Dolan, P. (1997b). The use of surface EMG power spectral analysis in the evaluation of back muscle function. *Journal of Rehabilitation Research & Development*, Vol. *34*, No. 4, pp. 427-439

Mannion, A. F. & Dolan, P. (1994). Electromyographic median frequency changes during isometric contraction of the back extensors to fatigue. *Spine*, Vol. *19*, No. 11, Jun 1, pp. 1223-1229

Mannion, A. F., Dumas, G. A., Cooper, R. G., Espinosa, F. J., Faris, M. W. & Stevenson, J. M. (1997c). Muscle fibre size and type distribution in thoracic and lumbar regions of erector spinae in healthy subjects without low back pain: normal values and sex differences. *J Anat*, Vol. *190 (Pt 4)*, May, pp. 505-513

Mannion, A. F., Dumas, G. A., Stevenson, J. M. & Cooper, R. G. (1998). The influence of muscle fiber size and type distribution on electromyographic measures of back muscle fatigability. *Spine*, Vol. *23*, No. 5, Mar 1, pp. 576-584

Mannion, A. F., Muntener, M., Taimela, S. & Dvorak, J. (2001). Comparison of three active therapies for chronic low back pain: results of a randomized clinical trial with one-year follow-up. *Rheumatology (Oxford)*, Vol. *40*, No. 7, Jul, pp. 772-778

Mayer, T. G., Kondraske, G., Mooney, V., Carmichael, T. W. & Butsch, R. (1989). Lumbar myoelectric spectral analysis for endurance assessment. A comparison of normals with deconditioned patients. *Spine*, Vol. *14*, No. 9, pp. 986-991.

Merletti, R., Roy, S. H., Kupa, E., Roatta, S. & Granata, A. (1999). Modeling of surface myoelectric signals--Part II: Model-based signal interpretation. *IEEE Trans Biomed Eng*, Vol. *46*, No. 7, Jul, pp. 821-829

Meyer, J. J. (1994). The validity of thoracolumbar paraspinal scanning EMG as a diagnostic test: an examination of the current literature. *J Manipulative Physiol Ther*, Vol. *17*, No. 8, Oct, pp. 539-551

Nigg, B. M., Herzog, W. & Read, L. J. (1988). Effect of viscoelastic shoe insoles on vertical impact forces in heel-toe running. *Am J Sports Med*, Vol. *16*, No. 1, Jan-Feb, pp. 70-76, ISSN 0363-5465 (Print) 0363-5465 (Linking)

Panjabi, M. M. (1992). The stabilizing system of the spine. Part II. Neutral zone and instability hypothesis. *Journal of Spinal Disorders*, Vol. *5*, No. 4, pp. 390-396; discussion 397

Peach, J. P. & McGill, S. M. (1998). Classification of low back pain with the use of spectral electromyogram parameters. *Spine*, Vol. *23*, No. 10, May 15, pp. 1117-1123

Pincus, S. M. (2001). Assessing serial irregularity and its implications for health. *Ann N Y Acad Sci*, Vol. *954*, Dec, pp. 245-267

Pullman, S. L., Goodin, D. S., Marquinez, A. I., Tabbal, S. & Rubin, M. (2000). Clinical utility of surface EMG: report of the therapeutics and technology assessment subcommittee of the American Academy of Neurology. *Neurology*, Vol. *55*, No. 2, Jul 25, pp. 171-177

Rack, M. H. & Ross, H. F. (1975). Electromyography of human biceps during imposed sinusoidal movement of the elbow joint. *J Physiol*, Vol. *244*, No. 1, Jan, pp. 44P-45P, ISSN 0022-3751 (Print) 0022-3751 (Linking)

Richman, J. S. & Moorman, J. R. (2000). Physiological time-series analysis using approximate entropy and sample entropy. *Am J Physiol Heart Circ Physiol*, Vol. *278*, No. 6, Jun, pp. H2039-2049

Roy, S. H., De Luca, C. J. & Casavant, D. A. (1989). Lumbar muscle fatigue and chronic lower back pain. *Spine*, Vol. *14*, No. 9, pp. 992-1001

Roy, S. H., De Luca, C. J., Emley, M., Oddsson, L. I., Buijs, R. J., Levins, J. A., Newcombe, D. S. & Jabre, J. F. (1997). Classification of back muscle impairment based on the surface electromyographic signal. *Journal of Rehabilitation Research & Development*, Vol. *34*, No. 4, pp. 405-414

Roy, S. H., De Luca, C. J., Snyder-Mackler, L., Emley, M. S., Crenshaw, R. L. & Lyons, J. P. (1990). Fatigue, recovery, and low back pain in varsity rowers. *Med Sci Sports Exerc*, Vol. *22*, No. 4, Aug, pp. 463-469

Scafetta, N. & Grigolini, P. (2002). Scaling detection in time series: diffusion entropy analysis. *Phys Rev E Stat Nonlin Soft Matter Phys*, Vol. *66*, No. 3 Pt 2A, Sep, pp. 036130, ISSN 1539-3755 (Print) 1539-3755 (Linking)

Scafetta, N. & West, B. J. (2003). Solar flare intermittency and the earth's temperature anomalies. *Phys Rev Lett*, Vol. *90*, No. 24, Jun 20, pp. 248701

Scafetta, N. & West, B. J. (2004). Multiscaling comparative analysis of time series and a discussion on "earthquake conversations" in California. *Phys Rev Lett*, Vol. *92*, No. 13, Apr 2, pp. 138501

Shannon, C. E. (1997). The mathematical theory of communication. 1963. *MD Comput*, Vol. *14*, No. 4, Jul-Aug, pp. 306-317, ISSN 0724-6811 (Print) 0724-6811 (Linking)

Solomonow, M., Baten, C., Smit, J., Baratta, R., Hermens, H., D'Ambrosia, R. & Shoji, H. (1990). Electromyogram power spectra frequencies associated with motor unit recruitment strategies. *J Appl Physiol*, Vol. *68*, No. 3, Mar, pp. 1177-1185

Sprott, J. (2003). Chaos and Time-Series Analysis.

Stanley, H. E., Buldyrev, S. V., Goldberger, A. L., Hausdorff, J. M., Havlin, S., Mietus, J., Peng, C. K., Sciortino, F. & Simons, M. (1992). Fractal landscapes in biological systems: long-range correlations in DNA and interbeat heart intervals. *Physica A*, Vol. *191*, No. 1-4, Dec 15, pp. 1-12

Strogatz, S. H. (2001). Exploring complex networks. *Nature*, Vol. *410*, No. 6825, Mar 8, pp. 268-276

Sung, P. S. (2003). Multifidi muscles median frequency before and after spinal stabilization exercises. *Arch Phys Med Rehabil*, Vol. *84*, No. 9, Sep, pp. 1313-1318

Sung, P. S., Zurcher, U. & Kaufman, M. (2005). Nonlinear analysis of electromyography time series as a diagnostic tool for low back pain. *Med Sci Monit*, Vol. *11*, No. 1, Jan, pp. CS1-5, ISSN 1234-1010 (Print) 1234-1010 (Linking)

Sung, P. S., Zurcher, U. & Kaufman, M. (2007a). Comparison of spectral and entropic measures for surface electromyography time series: a pilot study. *Journal of Rehabilitation Research & Development*, Vol. *44*, No. 4, pp. 599-609, ISSN 1938-1352 (Electronic) 0748-7711 (Linking)

Sung, P. S., Zurcher, U. & Kaufman, M. (2007b). Comparison of spectral and entropic measures for surface electromyography time series: A pilot study. *J Rehabil Res Dev*, Vol. *44*, No. 4, pp. 599-610

Sung, P. S., Zurcher, U. & Kaufman, M. (2008a). Gender differences in spectral and entropic measures of erector spinae muscle fatigue. *Journal of Rehabilitation Research & Development*, Vol. *45*, No. 9, pp. 1431-1439, ISSN 1938-1352 (Electronic) 1938-1352 (Linking)

Sung, P. S., Zurcher, U. & Kaufman, M. (2008b). Reliability difference between spectral and entropic measures of erector spinae muscle fatigability. *J Electromyogr Kinesiol*, Dec 31

Sung, P. S., Zurcher, U. & Kaufman, M. (2010). Reliability difference between spectral and entropic measures of erector spinae muscle fatigability. *J Electromyogr Kinesiol*, Vol. *20*, No. 1, Feb, pp. 25-30, ISSN 1873-5711 (Electronic) 1050-6411 (Linking)

Vinga, S. & Almeida, J. S. (2004). Renyi continuous entropy of DNA sequences. *J Theor Biol*, Vol. *231*, No. 3, Dec 7, pp. 377-388, ISSN 0022-5193 (Print) 0022-5193 (Linking)

West, B. (1990). Fractal Physiology & Chaos in Medicine.

Wilder, D. G., Aleksiev, A. R., Magnusson, M. L., Pope, M. H., Spratt, K. F. & Goel, V. K. (1996). Muscular response to sudden load. A tool to evaluate fatigue and rehabilitation. *Spine*, Vol. *21*, No. 22, pp. 2628-2639.

9

sEMG Techniques to Detect and Predict Localised Muscle Fatigue

M. R. Al-Mulla[1], F. Sepulveda[2] and M. Colley[2]
[1]*Kuwait University*
[2]*Essex University*
[1]*Kuwait*
[2]*UK*

1. Introduction

Recent advances in physiological studies have demonstrated the importance of muscle fatigue detection and prediction in various aspects of our lives, including sports, rehabilitation and ergonomics. Automating muscle fatigue detection/prediction in wearable technology has the potential to aid in many applications. However, current research has made little progress towards automating muscle fatigue detection/prediction in computational models. The work presented in this chapter supports the idea that an automated muscle fatigue detection/prediction system can be used to aid sporting performance and to avoid injury. In support of this view, a wearable system that operates based on the detection and classification of three different stages of muscle fatigue (Non-Fatigue, Transition-to-Fatigue and Fatigue) has been developed. Current research focuses on only two muscle fatigue stages (Non-Fatigue and Fatigue); with this limitation in mind, data was analysed with the aim to develop features that best extract muscle fatigue content, using both statistical models and evolutionary computations tools to help find the number of muscle fatigue stages. This enabled the development of an automated muscle fatigue detection system, which provides true prediction capabilities. In doing so, a third stage of fatigue was identified, the so-called Transition-to-Fatigue stage, which occurs before the onset of fatigue. By identifying this transitional fatigue stage, it is possible to predict when fatigue will occur, which provides the foundation of the automated system. To demonstrate the applicability of the Transition-to-Fatigue class, the classification performance of the two class (Non-Fatigue and Fatigue) and three class approaches (Non-Fatigue, Transition-to-Fatigue and Fatigue) were compared. This chapter will include various studies that identify the most suitable methods to apply in the real-time autonomous system. The first section of studies developed various statistical features that best distinguished between the different classes of fatigue, resulting in new combined feature extraction methods called 1D spectro and 1D spectro_std. The second section used evolutionary computation, evolving features and creating pseudo-wavelets improving current state of the art. The various features evolved in this work all produced high classification accuracy from surface electromyography (sEMG) signals emanating from the biceps brachii during both isometric and non-isometric contractions. In the third section, a method to predict the time to fatigue was established using artificial neural network classification based on the three classes of fatigue. This technique was also implemented in the final study that developed a working prototype of the wearable autonomous system. One of the developed feature extraction methods, 1D spectro, was selected for implementation into the wearable autonomous system. This chapter presents preliminary empirical evidence demonstrating that the developed features and methods for fatigue detection/prediction improve the current state of the art. In this chapter, a definition of muscle fatigue is set, then, an overview of the detection of muscle fatigue will be given, followed by a discussion of specific approaches for extracting sEMG features which are related to muscle fatigue. The chapter then concludes with a summary of challenges for the future of this new and exciting technology.

1.1 Muscle fatigue definition

The term 'muscle fatigue' was first introduced by Bills (1943), who categorised it into three groups: subjective fatigue, which is influenced by psychological factors such as a lack of motivation; objective fatigue, which indicates a decline in productivity; and finally, physiological fatigue, which manifests itself by changes in physiological processes. Chaffin (1973) introduced the term 'localised muscle fatigue' as an example of physiological fatigue, which refers to the inability of a given muscle to maintain a desired force and is associated with localised pain.

Studies on localised muscle fatigue have focused mainly on the decline in the force of a muscle contraction during a sustained activity (Barry & Enoka, 2007), which results in a definition of fatigue as the inability of a muscle to continue exerting force or power. Barry & Enoka argue that this definition indicates that fatigue occurs quickly after the onset of a sustained period of exercise, although the subject may be able to sustain the activity. However, the muscle impairment will eventually lead to total fatigue, where it is impossible for the subject to continue performing the task (Bigland-Ritchie & Woods, 1984).

Muscle fatigue is a physiological phenomenon that can only be measured precisely by invasive means, which is clearly unsuitable for most applications, such as in sport science, human-computer interaction, ergonomics and occupational therapy. Therefore, non-invasive techniques have been developed to detect signals that are related to muscle fatigue. Generally, non-invasive clinical studies of muscle fatigue acquire such signals using two main techniques: mechanomyography (MMG) and/or electromyography (EMG). Historically, EMG has been chosen as the most suitable clinical research tool. MMG, on the other hand, is considered to be a mechanical equivalent of surface electromyography (sEMG), that works by recording the low-frequency oscillations that are produced by the muscle fibres when the muscle contracts and expands (Gordon & Holbourn, 1948). Nevertheless, there are other established techniques that are used to detect localised muscle fatigue, such as near infrared spectroscopy (NIRS) and ultrasound, and methods for assessing muscle fatigue, such as the Moore-Garg strain index and the CR Borg scale (Borg, 1970).

It has been known for at least 40 years that the sEMG signal carries information related to muscle fatigue (Edwards, 1981; Lindstrom et al., 1977), making it a suitable method for non-invasive muscle fatigue detection. Furthermore, the sEMG signal provides useful information when measuring and analysing localised muscle fatigue (Hagberg, 1981; Jorgensen et al., 1988; Petrofsky et al., 1982). Myoelectric manifestations of muscle fatigue can be seen in changes in signal frequency and amplitude and in the muscle conduction velocity (CV), while the mechanical factors related to muscle fatigue are manifested in a loss in the force exerted by the muscle (Asghari Oskœi et al., 2008). The myoelectric manifestations are perceived as an objective means by which to analyse muscle fatigue, since they disregard subjective motivators and, compared to mechanical factors, they provide early indicators of fatigue. In addition, sEMG is a very portable, easy to use and fairly inexpensive method.

1.2 How can muscle fatigue be detected ?

There are several techniques for signal detection which are often used in conjunction with each other for the study of muscle fatigue and it may be difficult to determine which to use in a particular application. Most modern research uses one or more of the methods described here in conjunction, such as an accelerometer with sEMG electrodes. Usually, the aim of combining sensors with sEMG or other sensors is validation, labelling or improving the signal to noise ratio.

To date, no consensus has been reached upon the ideal sensor technology to use for MMG recordings (Courteville et al., 1998; Gregori et al., 2003; Watakabe et al., 1998). The literature suggests that accelerometers are more appropriate than condenser microphones due to the effects of background noise. Also, accelerometers are inexpensive and reliable devices whereas condenser microphones are more expensive and have a much larger frequency range (20-2000 Hz) than that needed for accurately recording muscle vibrations (13-35 Hz) (Armstrong, 2010).

Compared to sEMG data collection, accelerometers are physically bulkier, more susceptible to noise from sudden movement and are significantly more expensive than sEMG electrodes. Limitations of NIRS are related to inconsistencies regarding muscle oxygenation during isometric exercise, making it a less reliable method. NIRS sensors are also very sensitive to movement, which makes NIRS an unsuitable candidate technique in sports and other movement-rich scenarios. It is possible to use the goniometer sensor to measure the development of fatigue in a realistic scenario. However, currently available goniometer sensors are expensive, have a short lifetime and must be handled with care. Electronic force gauges are also applicable in measuring fatigue but suffer from fragile construction, high cost and subject encumbrance in most scenarios. The Moore-Garg strain index and the modified Borg Scale can be used for fatigue detection in terms of translating facial/body cues using video processing, but these techniques suffer from privacy issues and can be highly subjective. In addition the Moore-Garg and Borg methods require a second person to measure the subjects' fatigue stages.

1.3 EMG signal pre-processing

Signal filtering is an important process that attenuates unwanted or erroneous electrical signals picked up by sensors and thus allows the experimenter to focus on a narrow energy band of interest. In general, filters attenuate signals within certain frequency ranges (the so-called stopband), thus limiting the frequency spectrum of the recorded signal to that of the so-called passband (De Luca, 1997). Filters can be categorised into four main types: low-pass, high-pass, bandpass and bandstop. Modern technologies have enabled the measurement of EMG signals of low noise and high signal fidelity (i.e., high signal to noise ratio). Filters can also be characterised by the width of their transition zone (De Luca, 1997), with more complex filter designs needed to produce tighter transition ranges. In general, the more complex the filter, the higher is its so-called 'order', i.e., a first order filter is a very simple order filter. The full effective bandwidth of the EMG signal can be measured using differential amplification. Bandpass refers to the range of frequencies from the low frequency to the high frequency limit of a signal. Typical bandpass frequency ranges are from between 10 and 20 Hz (high pass filtering) to between 500 and 1000 Hz (low-pass filtering). Movement artifacts, which are normally comprised of low frequency components (typically < 10 Hz), are removed by high-pass filtering, and signal aliasing is avoided by removing high frequency signal components through the use of low-pass filtering (Gerdle et al., 1999). Merletti (1999) states that the sEMG signals should be between the range of 5-500 Hz due to negligible contribution of the signals power density function outside of this range. Invasive EMG, on the other hand, should have a low-pass cut-off at no less than 1.5 kHz.

EMG signals are filtered by several classical filter types, including the Butterworth filter, Fourier series, the Chebyshev filter, the Elliptic filter and the Thompson or Bessel Filter, and filter equations are frequently recursive, such as in the Butterworth filter (De Luca, 1997). The purpose of the Butterworth filter is to produce a flat as possible frequency response in the passband, resulting in steep rolloffs in higher order filters, making it an ideal filter for conditioning the EMG signal (De Luca, 1997). Additionally its maximum passband gain, the cutoff frequency and the filter order are all clearly specified. In the past, sharp notch filtering was commonly used to remove power-line (A/C) noise components (i.e., either 50 or 60 Hz). However, since there are large signal contributions at these frequencies in EMG experiments, notch filtering results in a loss of information in this setting, and is thus usually avoided (Day, 2010).

Prior to the use of computers in signal processing, signals were mostly filtered by analogue means. Analogue filters usually employ electronic circuits, making use of three fundamental components: resistors, capacitors and inductors, which are arranged in circuits designed to meet particular needs (De Luca, 1997). The performance of an analogue filter is heavily dependent on the quality of the circuit design and the physical components that are used in building the circuit.Hence, digital filtering is often considered to be superior to analogue filtering (Hong & Bartlett, 2008). In the context of this thesis, the versatility of digital filtering makes it particularly suitable for the filtering of sEMG signals, where they are mostly used to remove noise, i.e., a band-pass filter, which combines low and high-pass filters, is used to cut off frequencies from 10-500 Hz. Signals can also be filtered through the application of a low-pass filter, so that slow changes in the signal amplitude are displayed and the signal is thus smoothed. According to Basmajian & De Luca (1985), the RMS signal voltage is the most suited approach to quantify the EMG signal, which is the mathematical equivalent to the standard deviation of the EMG signal.

1.4 Application of EMG in muscle fatigue research

EMG is an easy to use technique and has therefore been used in a vast range of research on muscle physiology. Generally, localised muscle fatigue occurs after a prolonged, relatively strong muscle activity, when a muscle or a group of muscles are fatigued. Due to the variability of inter-person muscle characteristics, there is no simple function of muscle load and timing that defines a precise muscle fatigue threshold. Changes in the EMG signals caused by fatigue are either measured in the time or frequency domain. Integrated EMG (IEMG) usually uses the time domain, and an increase in the signal period, amplitude and power reflect a higher muscle fibre recruitment for a fixed external force. The changes in EMG signal in the frequency domain relate to mean power frequency and median power frequency, which varies due to a shift towards lower frequencies, a small increase in low-frequency signal power, a relative decrease in high-frequency signal power, a decrease in low-frequency spectrum slope and an increase in high-frequency spectrum slope (Eberstein & Beattie, 1985; Gross et al., 1980; Petrofsky et al., 1982; Sato, 1982; Viitasalo & Komi, 1977). There are several reasons for these changes in the EMG signal, such as signal synchronisation, modulation of the recruitment firing rate, grouping and slowing of the CV (De Luca, 1979; Hermens et al., 1986; Viitasalo & Komi, 1977).

Although sEMG has been applied in many studies of localised muscle fatigue, it is not without its limitations, in particular, in studies of dynamic muscle contractions. The use of sEMG requires proper knowledge of the mechanisms of signal generation and propagation. Although signal acquisition *per se* is easy, inaccurate conclusions are easily drawn when inappropriate experimental methods are used (Merletti et al., 2003).

Most research concentrates on isometric contractions to establish typical sEMG readings when conducted in controlled settings. Changes in sEMG amplitude and centre frequency have been studied by Petrofsky et al. (1982), who found a decrease in the centre frequency of the spectrogram for all muscle groups. Research has also shown that a development in muscle fatigue correlates with changes in sEMG signal amplitude and MDF (Hagberg, 1981). Muscle fatigue causes MU recruitment, and the MU firing rate increases as a function of the elapsed time. These changes are not reflected in the EMG changes which occur during fatiguing isometric contraction of the arm flexors at 20-30% MVC (Maton & Gamet, 1989). However, it was recently found that the changes due to fatigue in the sEMG signal (increased amplitude and decreased frequency) suggest that the recruitment of MU firing rates correlates with sEMG amplitude (Calder et al., 2008).

Although CV strongly influences the power spectrum density (PSD) and has the highest inter-person repeatability, it has been argued that fatigue also compresses the frequency content of the sEMG signal in a proportional manner (Linssen et al., 1993). The PSD time-dependency can also be analysed, and is usually estimated from the instantaneous sEMG parameters, although there are shortcomings in the identification of changes in the short-period sEMG signals. A time-varying autoregressive (AR) model was proposed by Zhang et al. (2010), which produced a more stable and accurate instantaneous parameter estimation. Minning et al. (2007) studied differences in the rate of fatigue in the shoulder muscles during voluntary isometric contractions. They discovered day-to-day inconsistencies in the rate of fatigue in the middle deltoid muscle, which also fatigued more rapidly than other muscle groups. However, for the other muscles they found a consistent relationship between trial, day and muscle type. In a study on the relationship between short-time Fourier transform (STFT) and continuous wavelet transforms to analyse EMG signals from the back and hip muscles during fatiguing isometric contractions, it was found that the two methods reveal similar information regarding EMG spectral variables (Coorevits et al., 2008).

Although the success of sEMG is likely to be more prevalent in isometric muscle contractions, more recently EMG has been applied to the study of dynamic contractions (Singh et al., 2007). The analysis of the sEMG spectrum during cycling activities reveals a strong correlation between the onset of fatigue and the reduction of the MDF in dynamic contractions (Singh et al., 2007), and sEMG has been validated using biochemical analysis, indicating that the low-frequency band is a reliable indicator of muscle fatigue in dynamic contractions (Soo et al., 2009). By analysing the quantitative and qualitative changes in EMG patterns, such as IEMG and the frequency of the mean power, it has been argued that in dynamic contractions fatigue is related to qualitative changes in the pattern of MU recruitment, which occurs at a faster rate when the muscle has a higher degree of fast twitch muscles fibres. For the quantitative changes, only a small reduction in the amplitude of the IEMG signal was related to a high percentage of slow twitch muscle fibres (Komi & Tesch, 1979). Masuda et al. (1999) studied changes in sEMG patterns during static and dynamic fatiguing contractions by looking at the muscle fibre CV, MDF and mean amplitude in the vastus lateralis muscle. The muscle fibre CV appeared to be influenced by the metabolic state in the muscle, as it decreased significantly in isometric contractions, while it remained constant during dynamic contractions. This suggests that changes in the MDF cannot be explained wholly by shifts in the muscle fibre CV. Farina (2006) proposed a technique for detection and processing of muscle CV during dynamic contractions, and showed that a decline in CV reflects muscle fatigue. Another method for estimating muscle fatigue during dynamic contraction is to use a source separation technique related to independent component analysis to test whether the firing of MUs becomes more synchronised at the onset of localised muscle fatigue. As argued by Naik et al. (2009), it is widely accepted that lower-frequency sEMG signals indicate muscle fatigue due to MU synchronisation; however, there is little experimental evidence of this theory. Naik et al. concluded that during cycling movements, a global matrix is an applicable measurement for estimating localised muscle fatigue.

Several studies have identified the state of peripheral fatigue (Dimitrov et al., 2006; Gonzalez-Izal, Malanda, Navarro-Amezqueta, Gorostiaga, Mallor, Ibanez & Izquierdo, 2010). In a recent study, Gonzalez-Izal, Malanda, Navarro-Amezqueta, Gorostiaga, Mallor, Ibanez & Izquierdo (2010) compared several EMG parameters to assess peripheral fatigue during dynamic contractions. In that study, new spectral indices (FInsmX) developed by Dimitrov et al. (2006) were based on discrete wavelet transforms (DWT) and were compared to spectral parameters, such as mean average voltage, median spectral frequency and ratios between different scales obtained by DWT. Results showed the newly proposed spectral indices to be the best for assessing peripheral fatigue, both in correlation with the power output changes and in their regression. These new spectral indices have also been shown to be a useful tool in detecting changes in muscle power output in fatiguing dynamic contractions, and they can be used as predictors of changes in muscle power output (Gonzalez-Izal, Rodriguez-Carreno, Malanda, Mallor-Gimenez, Navarro-Amezqueta, Gorostiaga & Izquierdo, 2010).

Detecting muscle fatigue in an automated system requires a real-time measurement of changes in localised muscle fatigue. Stulen & De Luca (1982) developed a muscle fatigue monitor, which was a non-invasive device measuring localised muscle fatigue by spectral compression calculating median frequencies and two other parameters of the spectrum. This study used the MDF, which the author states is a more reliable analysis feature than other traditional parameters, e.g. mean or mode frequencies. Kramer et al. (1987) proposed a robust and relatively reliable parameter of fatigue that could be calculated off-line from computed, real-time sEMG data obtained from a simple analogue device. Wavelet coefficients can be used in non-stationary and time-varying signal processing, hence they have been applied in the assessment of localised muscle fatigue for both static and dynamic contractions using sEMG signals. The amplitude of approximation coefficients coincide with muscle fatigue development. Moshou et al. (2005) proposed a method for automating the detection of muscle fatigue by using NNs, where a two-dimensional self-organising map visualises the approximation of wavelet coefficients, enabling the visualisation of the onset of fatigue over time, and thus separating the EMG signal from fresh and fatigued muscles. Tepavac & Schwirtlich (1997) developed a technique which utilises the processed sEMG signal as an activation signal that changes the pattern to control a functional electrical stimulation (FES) system. Their technique is able to notify the user that a rapid drop in the muscle force is approaching, providing the capability of a simple on-off fatigue detection in FES applications. In the development of this technique the authors used seven different sEMG parameters, however the best relationship was established between the MDF and force changes, which were the parameters used to determine the prediction of the onset of fatigue and detection of fatigue. This is an interesting technique although it is not performed in autonomous, real-time system.

1.5 sEMG signal analysis and feature characterisation

Feature extraction is used in pattern recognition, being a form of dimensionality reduction (Samet, 2006). This method is used for transforming input data to a certain set of features which will extract the relevant information from that data. sEMG signals can be analysed to detect muscle fatigue by examining the changes in EMG measurements. Studies on sEMG show that an increase in EMG signal amplitude or shifts in the spectrogram are indicators of muscle fatigue in static contractions (Chaffin, 1973; De Luca, 1997; Duchene & Goubel, 1993; Kadefors et al., 1968; Lindstrom et al., 1977; Marras, 1990). Hagberg (1981) established that significant changes in the sEMG signal indicate muscle fatigue. Studies on muscle fatigue during isometric contraction have established typical sEMG readings when conducted in controlled settings. Changes in sEMG amplitude and centre frequency were studied by Petrofsky et al. (1982), who found a decrease in the centre frequency of the spectrogram for all muscle groups. It has also been shown that a development in muscle fatigue correlates with changes in amplitude and MDF (Hagberg, 1981). A variety of parameters have been used to investigate sEMG signals to determine muscle fatigue; however it is common to study the signal in terms of its frequency at a certain time, in both the time and time-frequency domains. Table 1 categorized the papers according to the feature extraction methods used by authors.

Feature extraction method	Refrence ID
RMS	(Basmajian & De Luca, 1985; Kumar & Mital, 1996)
STFT	(Merletti & Parker, 2004)
Total Band Power	(Welch, 1967)
New spectral parameter FI 1 to FI 5	(Dimitrov et al., 2006)
PSD	(Ortengren et al., 1975)
MDF	(Kumar & Mital, 1996)
IMDF	(Asghari Oskœi et al., 2008; Roy et al., 1998)
Cohen class transformations	(Cohen, 1995; Raez et al., 2006; Ricamato et al., 1992)
Gabor Transform	(Gabor, 1946)
Wavelet analysis	(Kumar et al., 2003; Laterza & Olmo, 1997)
Autogression analysis	(Graupe & Cline, 1975; Kim et al., 2005; Tohru, 1992)
Entropy	(Jaynes, 1957; Sung et al., 2008)
Recurrence Quantification Analysis	(Filligoi et al., 2010; Morana et al., 2009)
HOS	(Hussain et al., 2008; Kanosue et al., 1979)
Composite Features	(Boostani & Moradi, 2003; Hudgins et al., 1993; Phinyomark et al., 2009)

Table 1. Signal analysis and feature characteristics

1.5.1 Time domain and frequency domain analysis

A signal is acquired, and in some circumstances, analysed, in the time domain where the signal amplitude/voltage is represented as a function of time. However, for many analysis techniques, it is the frequency of the signal that is of greater value, and consequently the signal should be analysed in the frequency-domain, whereby the signal undergoes a Fourier transform so that it is represented as a function of frequency, rather than time.

Both the average rectified value, which measures the average of the absolute signal value, and the RMS, which is a measure of the signal power (Kumar & Mital, 1996), are used in the analysis of the raw EMG signal in the time domain. The RMS of the EMG signal calculates the square root of the average power of the raw EMG signal over a specific time period (Basmajian & De Luca, 1985). De Luca's group acknowledged both the average rectified value and RMS as appropriate analysis methods, however, several authors prefer the RMS (De Luca, 1997;

Merletti et al., 2003), since it can be used to obtain a moving average (Basmajian & De Luca, 1985). The moving average approach is used for processing raw EMG signals from dynamic contractions, as it identifies the rapid changes in the muscle activity during such contractions by using short duration sampling windows (Payton & Bartlett, 2008). Merletti et al. (2003) suggested that EMG analysis of dynamic contractions can make use of another processing method, the 'linear envelope', which uses a low pass filter to smooth the rectified EMG.

When a signal crosses the zero amplitude line, it is said to have made a 'zero-crossing'. When applied to sEMG data, the general idea is that an active muscle will produce more AP, and hence generate more zero crossings. However, at the onset of fatigue, the zero crossing rate drops dramatically due to the reduced conduction of electrical current in the muscle. Therefore zero-crossings are counted using geometric calculations to give an indication of the muscle status.

The total band power (TBP) of the sEMG signal can be estimated using the method by Welch (1967). This method has been used previously in several sEMG fatigue analyses (Cifrek et al., 2009; Helal et al., 1992) and has proved to be useful in quantifying the power of the EMG signals.

The frequency content of a signal can be determined by performing a Fourier transform to reveal its individual frequency components. The fast Fourier transform (FFT), a method for calculating the discrete Fourier transform, is suitable for use in stationary signals. EMG signals, which are non-stationary, should be represented in both the time and frequency domains. Therefore, the STFT, which analyses a small temporal section of the signal, can be used to determine the frequency and phase evolution of the EMG signal over time.

The time and frequency resolution depend upon the sampling rate and the temporal length of the signal section. Due to the inverse relationship between time and frequency in the Fourier transform, it follows that the higher the time resolution the lower the frequency resolution will be and *vice versa* (Merletti & Parker, 2004). The spectogram of the signal is the squared magnitude of the STFT.

Dimitrov et al. (2006) proposed a new spectral parameter with higher sensitivity than traditional indices for both dynamic and isometric contractions, which is a valid and reliable tool for the assessment of muscle fatigue. The parameter used the FFT to calculate ratios between different spectral moments measured over the power spectral density.

Following an FFT, this parameter represents the ratio between the low- and high-order spectral moments of the EMG power spectrum. Gonzalez-Izal, Malanda, Navarro-Amezqueta, Gorostiaga, Mallor, Ibanez & Izquierdo (2010) used this index to measure the changes in muscle power during a high-intensity dynamic protocol, and compared it to other frequency and amplitude parameters. It was found that the logarithm of this index detects the changes most accurately by assessing peripheral impairments.

EMG signals can be analysed in the time-domain using the PSD to describe how the power of a signal is distributed among its frequency components. Significant changes in the power spectrum indicate muscle fatigue (Ortengren et al., 1975), such that after fatigue onset the PSD is increased in the low frequency components and decreased in the higher frequency components.

Two of the most common frequency-dependent features in sEMG analysis are the MF and MDF. The MF is "the average frequency of the power spectrum and is defined as its first-order moment" (Asghari Oskœi et al., 2008), while the MDF is an index used in studies of spectral shifts and can be defined as "the frequency which divides the power spectrum in two parts with equal areas" (Kumar & Mital, 1996, p. 170). The power spectrum represents the MDF of the power, based on a continuous spectrum distribution. Hagberg (1981) stated that if the MDF decreases along with as the sEMG signal amplitude increases, which is a strong indication of fatigue.

The spectral frequency can be redefined to represent the non-stationary nature of the signal, or the instantaneous frequency, of the frequency content of the signal (Karlsson et al., 1999). The instantaneous median frequency (IMDF) was introduced by Roy et al. (1998). Studies by Asghari Oskœi et al. (2008) concluded that a significant decline in the IMDF of the signal is a significant manifestation of fatigue occurrence. In addition, Georgakis et al. (2003) demonstrated that the average instantaneous frequency is superior to the mean and median frequencies for the analysis of muscle fatigue during sustained contractions.

Some analysis methodologies use both the time and frequency domains to analyse the EMG signal. For example, the Cohen class transformation, a time-frequency representation applied in biomedical signal processing, is well-suited for analysis of signals from dynamic contractions. It is a distribution function introduced by Cohen (1995) using bilinear transformations, giving clearer results than the STFT. However, due to its use of bilinear transformations, the Cohen class is affected by cross-term contamination in its analysis of several functions, which can be avoided using window functions. The Wigner-Ville distribution function (WVD), proposed by Wigner in 1936 (Raez et al., 2006), was first used for corrections to classical statistical mechanics, however, it is also applicable as a transform in time-frequency analysis. This transform has higher clarity than the STFT and has more properties than most other time-frequency transforms, using all available information in the EMG signal. In 1948 Ville revised this function into a quadratic representation of the local time-frequency energy of a signal (Raez et al., 2006). It was discovered by Ricamato et al. (1992) that the WVD would detect the frequency ranges of the MUs, displaying recruitment patterns as muscles contract. However, Davies & Reisman (1994) found that the WVD joint density spectrum is noisy although its localisation properties are excellent and "generally concentrated around the instantaneous frequency of the signal". Another member of the Cohen's class functions is the Choi-Williams distribution (Davies & Reisman, 1994), which makes use of kernels to reduce the interference, something the Cohen's class distribution suffers from, although it is only possible for the kernel function to filter out the cross-term contamination.

The Gabor transform (named after Dennis Gabor) is a discrete Fourier transform utilising Gaussian windows, which is used in time-frequency analysis (Gabor, 1946). The transform determines the sinusoidal frequency and phase content of specific sections of a signal that changes over time, which is an advantage when representing local features. By using Gaussian windows, this function gives more weight to the signals near the time being analysed. Although this method is more precise than other methods, giving few errors, there are some major problems. The Gabor transform gives imaginary numbers with no physical meaning and it requires a lot of resources for full computation. Nevertheless, this transform guarantees energy conservation of the signal.

There are many time-frequency functions which can be used to analyse sEMG signals during localised muscle fatigue. Davies & Reisman (1994) showed that STFT can most precisely represent spectrum compression during muscle fatigue. Due to the cross-term contamination in the WVD, it is not possible to display the changes in the frequency components with muscle fatigue accurately. In a comparison between the STFT, the WVD, the continuous wavelet transform and the Choi-Williams distribution, Karlsson et al. (2000) found that the continuous wavelet transform resulted in a more precise estimation of EMG signals when applying various time-scale methods to analyse sEMG signals.

1.5.2 Wavelet analysis

By using a wavelet function (WF), the wavelet transform (WT) decomposes a signal into numerous multi-resolution components (Kleissen et al., 1998; Laterza & Olmo, 1997). It is used to detect and characterise the short time component within a non-stationary signal, providing information regarding the signal's time-frequency. The WF, being both dilated and translated in time and a linear function which does not suffer from cross-terms, undertakes a two-dimensional cross correlation with the time domain sEMG signal, making it an excellent alternative to other time-frequency parameters (Laterza & Olmo, 1997).

There are a number of so-called 'mother wavelets' that can be used for signal decomposition, including Symm-let, Coiflet, Haar, Morlet, Daubechies and Mexican Hat (Kumar et al., 2003). To select the most appropriate mother wavelet for a specific application and signal type, the properties of the WF and the characteristic of the signal should to be analysed and matched. Certain wavelets have somewhat established guidelines for their use, e.g., Db4 is said to be suited for signals using feature extractions and linear approximation with more than four samples, while Db6 is suited for signals that are approximated by a quadratic function over the support of six and finally coiflet6 is better suited for data compression results (Walker, 2000).

Guglielminotti & Merletti (1992) hypothesised that if the wavelet analysis is selected to fit with the shape of the MUAP, the WT would give the best energy location in a time-scale. Kumar et al. (2003) stated that the STFT does not give an optimal time or frequency resolution for the non-stationary signal, although the relatively short time windows may trace spectral variations with time. The WT, comprised of numerous WFs, can be used to decompose the sEMG signal. The output of the power transform domain is calculated and thus functions as a deciding parameter in selecting the most appropriate WF to give the highest contrast between sEMG cases. It has been shown that it is possible to detect muscle fatigue status by determining the Sym4 or Sym5 WFs and decomposing the signal at levels 8 and 9 (out of 10 levels). Kumar et al. (2003) discussed the effectiveness of decomposing the sEMG signal to measure its power in order to identify muscle fatigue as an automated process.

1.5.3 Autoregression analysis

Regression statistics is used to determine the relationship between an independent variable or variables and a dependent variable. An autoregressive (AR) model is a random process used in statistics and signal processing to model and predict natural phenomena. Graupe & Cline (1975) developed the AR moving average (ARMA) model to represent EMG signals, where the signals were split into short time intervals and the signal was considered to be stationary. However, Sherif (1980) replaced this model by a model using the AR integrated moving average (ARIMA) model, to be used on the non-stationary EMG signals. Hefftner et al. (1988) exploited the computational speed of the AR model for EMG feature discrimination.

Kim et al. (2005) measured fatigue in the trunk muscle using the first AR model, and concluded that the model was capable of assessing fatigue in static exercises, being sufficiently sensitive to detect fatigue at low force levels. Several authors have revised the AR parameters, adding a non-linear element (ARMA) (Bernatos et al., 1986) and a non-stationary identifier (Moser & Graupe, 1989). However, the ARIMA model is complex with a high computational cost and Tohru (1992) argued that more accurate models (ARMA and ARIMA) are not needed for studies on dynamic contractions.

1.5.4 Entropy

Entropy is a function that can be used in various fields, such as thermodynamics, communication and computer science. In physics, entropy is a statistical measure of disorder in a system, representing the probability that a certain outcome exists, while in information theory the basis of entropy relates to the randomness in a signal or in a random event (Jaynes, 1957). This is also applicable to a general probability distribution, rather than a discrete-valued event. Sung et al. (2008) argue that entropic measures reveal part of the sEMG signals that are not included in the power spectrum, and can be a useful tool in detecting muscle fatigue in gender differences.

1.5.5 Recurrence quantification analysis

Recurrence quantification analysis, a method of nonlinear data analysis which is used for the investigation of dynamical systems, is highly effective in detecting changes in the sEMG signal and is almost equivalent to the frequency domain analysis of the signal in non-isometric contractions (Filligoi et al., 2010). Morana et al. (2009) recently used recurrence quantification analysis in a study of muscle fatigue and stated that this method can be used to detect peripheral muscle fatigue.

1.5.6 Higher-order statistics

Higher-order statistics (HOS), a technique based on probability theory, characterises and analyses the nature of a random process, making it appropriate for use in the random time series produced by EMG signals. Due to the nature of the EMG signals, in particular when fatigue components are present in the signal, HOS will give more insight in terms of analysing the complexity of the EMG signal. In muscle fatigue HOS is used due to the increasing complexity of the EMG signal, the second order HOS (and higher orders) are used to detect non-gussian/non-linear properties of the signal. This is particularly useful method in muscle fatigue studies, which is an alternative of using the Gaussian/linear processes, such as the power spectrum of a signal giving the distribution of power among signal frequency. Moments and cumulants define the HOS of a signal. When analysing deterministic signals, moments are of great importance, while cumulants are useful for stochastic type signals (Gündoğdu et al., 2006). It has been used in sEMG studies to estimate the amplitude and the number of new MUAPs, as proposed by Kanosue et al. (1979). Several authors have studied HOS in sEMG signal processing, in particular testing it for Gaussianity and linearity, coherence and coupling of the signal. Their findings showed that during contractions at low- and high-force activity, HOS features are non Gaussian, while during the mid-level force the distribution is maximally Gaussian (Hussain et al., 2008; Raez et al., 2006; Shahid, 2007). HOS is also used to suppress Gaussian white noise in the sEMG signal (Hussain et al., 2008).

1.5.7 Composite features

The term 'composite features' relates to the use of a combination of common features to develop a new feature that aids in the analysis of sEMG signals. MacIsaac et al. (2006) presented a mapping function that maps segments of multiple myoelectrical signals for fatigue estimation of dynamic contractions, where the inputs are time domain features. This function is tuned by ANNs and is capable of use in real-time applications. Results show

that this function better maps the sEMG signals than either the MF or the IMDF for different conditions.
Although combining features is a fairly new approach in the field of localised muscle fatigue research, there has already been work on multiple features utilised for myoelectric control of prosthetics. The concept of multiple features was introduced to overcome the stochastic nature of the the EMG signal, which makes it difficult for only one parameter to reflect the uniqueness of the EMG signal to a motion command. Hence various features are used for extraction at different times of the signal. Hudgins et al. (1993) used this method first for time domain features, such as mean absolute value, mean absolute value slope, wavelength form, zero crossings and slope sign changes, which were then classified using an ANN. This new method of control increased the number of prosthetic functions which can be controlled by a single channel of myoelectric signal without the amputee having to increase his/her effort. Other researchers have also applied this multiple function technique. Phinyomark et al. (2009) calculated two novel features by modifying the mean and median frequencies. Instead of calculating the power spectrum, they calculated the mean and median of the amplitude spectrum (MMNF). Then they used a combination of the MMNF, a histogram of EMG and Willison amplitude as a feature vector in a classification task, giving a better classification recognition result of the EMG in noisy environment than other features. Boostani & Moradi (2003) aimed at selecting the best features which would give a high rate of motion classification for controlling an artificial hand. Nineteen EMG signal features were taken into account, including combining the WT with other signal processing techniques. The results of this study showed that the best features for motion classification were wavelet coefficients of EMG signals in nine scales, and the cepstrum coefficients. Although the above-mentioned studies do not investigate muscle fatigue *per se*, they all use a combination of features of the EMG signal to improve the classification outcome.

2. Feature selection

Feature selection is an important process that ensures that the selected features contain class related information, since most features do not hold such information. In machine learning and statistics, as well as pattern recognition and data mining, feature selection is a technique whereby a subset of relevant features is selected from the data, which is then applied in a learning algorithm (Sewell, 2010). Feature selection typically creates a model that facilitates the generalisation of the unseen dimensions and may substantially enhance the comprehension of the classifier model which is produced (Kim & Street, 2010). In supervised learning, which has been thoroughly investigated, the aim is to select a feature subset which produces high classification accuracy (Kim & Street, 2010). However, for unsupervised learning the goal is to identify an optimal subset that produces high quality clusters for a set number of clusters. There are two main types of feature selection: the wrapper approach and the filter approach.

2.1 The wrapper approach

The wrapper approach uses a classification method to evaluate the most optimal feature or feature sub-set. This model, often used in machine learning, is excellent for improving the performance of the classifier due to using the same bias for both the feature selection and the learning of the classifier (Kohavi & John, 1997). The wrapper method searches for the optimal feature subset or a near-optimal subset that will best suit a certain algorithm and a domain, and it differs from other approaches as the measure of relevance is defined as the accuracy obtained by nonlinear regression (Kohavi & John, 1997). The wrapper approach goes through two phases (Liu & Motoda, 1998). In the first phase, which is the feature sub-set selection, the best sub-set is selected based on the classifier's accuracy. It is only the optimal features with highest accuracy which is kept for use in the second phase. Learning and testing is the second phase, where a classifier learns and trains from the optimal sub-set and then tests it on the test data to obtain its predictive accuracy. Cross-validation is then used to estimate the accuracy as the accuracy of the training data may not ensure accuracy in the testing data. Although cross-validation may help in the difficult task of estimating the true accuracy, it will lengthen the process of feature selection. Other disadvantages of the wrapper approach is linked to being unable to handle great sizes of data and to the limitation in choice of classifiers (Liu & Motoda, 1998). As the classifier is rebuilt for each feature sub-set in the first phase it eliminates the use of classifiers which requires great computational resources.

2.2 The filter approach

The filtering approach has been linked to data mining, when a classifier cannot be directly linked with the data set and where the aim is data reduction (Liu & Motoda, 1998). In this model the relevance measure is defined independently from the learning algorithm. In the filtering approach the subset selection procedure is like a preprocessing step (Kojadinovic & Wottka, 2000). Even this model consists of two phases. Firstly, the feature selection uses separation index or other measures such as distance, dependency, consistency and information to get the best feature sub-set. Secondly, the classifiers learns from the training data set and tests it on the testing data set. This model can handle huge data sets due to the feature selection process in phase one, which is a less complex and time consuming method. The filter approach also tend to be much faster and cheaper than the wrapper approach, however, the disadvantage is that the best subset of variables may not be independent of the representational biases of the algorithm used in the learning phase (Kojadinovic & Wottka, 2000).

In research on localised muscle fatigue, feature selection is used to facilitate the pattern recognition and classification of the features analysing the sEMG signals (Tamil et al., 2008; Yan et al., 2008). Various methods have been applied in this process, however, the DBI for measuring clustering selection is commonly used for EMG pattern recognition (Huang & Chen, 1999; Petrofsky, 1981; Wang et al., 2004)

Clustering is generally considered as an unsupervised algorithm for grouping a heterogeneous population into a set of homogeneous classes. However, this strategy does not always ensure grouping similar classes together.

2.2.1 Davies-Bouldin index

Cluster validity is an important measurement of how well clusters are related to other clusters generated by clustering algorithms. In most applications the clustering result needs validation. The number of clusters is determined as a user parameter in the majority of clustering algorithms. There are many methods of finding the best number of clusters, however Davies & Bouldin (1979) developed the Davies-Bouldin index (DBI), which measures the ratio of the sum of within-cluster scatter to between-cluster separation, so that it uses both the clusters and their sample means. The DBI evaluates the cluster quality by utilising the average error of each class, serving as a measure of cluster quality by calculating the distance of the cluster members to the cluster centroids and the distances between the cluster centroids. In the DBI small values indicate that clusters are compact with their centres far apart. Hence, the optimal number of clusters is considered as the number that minimises the DBI. The formulation of the modified DBI proposed by Sepulveda et al. (2004) can be used to measure cluster quality. For data based on real numbers, the DBI always yields a real value ≥ 0. The DBI is a measure of the standard deviation of the signal. A small DBI indicates well separated and grouped clusters, which means that the lower the DBI the more separable are the classes. There are several methods to measure cluster quality, but the DBI has been applied in research on muscle fatigue (Boostani & Moradi, 2003). The DBI is related to the performance of the linear Fisher discriminant classifier to pairwise clusters.

3. Classification methods

Classification methods, used in statistics and computational problem solving, are supervised machine learning procedures where individuals are grouped according to their characteristics, which can also be called traits, variables, characters, etc. This method bases its training set on previously labelled individuals. There are many ways of classifying a signal. Signal classification methods can be in continuous time or discrete time, analog or digital, periodic or aperiodic, finite or infinite, and deterministic or random. Discrete/continuous classification is determined by whether the signal is countable (discrete) or continuous.

There are numerous ways to classify the sEMG signals, although the non-stationary nature of the signals make classification more complicated (Khezri & Jahed, 2007). A number of classification methods used for sEMG fatigue related signals are described below.

One common method for sEMG classification is to measure the Euclidean distance between the waveform of an MUAP; where a shimmer is generated in the representation of time-triggered and non-overlapping MUAPs (Raez et al., 2006). The shimmer is influenced by external factors, such as background noise and noise from offsets. In addition, the shimmer of the MUAP is affected by the variance within a class as well as the distance between the classes.

Christodoulou & Pattichis (1995) suggested using an ANN as a classification method, which can be implemented in three phases. The first phase is unsupervised learning, which is built on competitive learning and on a one-dimensional self-organising feature map. In the second phase the learning vector is quantified, which is a self-supervised learning method which aids classification performance. Finally, the third phase is that of classification. The fuzzy approach has been compared with the ANN method on four subjects, and very similar classification results were obtained. It is superior to the latter in at least three points: slightly higher recognition rate, insensitivity to over-training and consistent outputs demonstrating higher reliability (Chan et al., 2000). Table 2 categorized some papers according to the classification methods used by authors.

Classification method	Refrence ID
GP	(Holland, 1975; Koza, 1994; Poli et al., 2008)
GA	(Koza, 1994; Michalewicz, 1996; Raikova & Aladjov, 2002; Wang, Yan, Hu, Xie & Wang, 2006)
ANN	(Bishop, 1995; Xie et al., 2010; 2009)
Fuzzy systems	(Chan et al., 2000; Kiryu & Yamashita, 2007; Takagi & Sugeno, 1985)
LDA	(Balakrishnama & Ganapathiraju, 2010; Fisher, 1936)
Support Vector Machine	(Gunn, 1998; Hsu et al., 2003)
One Clause at a Time	(Torvik et al., 1999)
Cross validation	(Kohavi, 1995; McLachlan et al., 2004)
Confusion matrix	(Kohavi & Provost, 1998)

Table 2. Classification Methods

3.1 Evolutionary computation

Genetic programming (GP), which implements a learning engine based on Darwin's theory of the natural selection of the fittest, was founded by Koza (1994). GP is based on the concept of evolutionary algorithms introduced in 1954 by Nils Aall Barricelli, who applied it to evolutionary simulations. GP optimises a computer program in order to solve tasks and creates computer programs as part of the solution (Holland, 1975). The optimal program (fittest) is selected from three standard genetic operators (crossover, mutation and reproduction), which modify the GP's structure and create new (and often improved) offspring (generations) (Michalewicz, 1996). GP is closely related to genetic algorithms (GAs) (Holland, 1975), however, GP actually creates computer programs as part of the solution. GP uses a tree structure to represent the computer programs it produces and reproduces when a genetic program is run (Koza, 1994). The tree structures represent the population and the new generations which are created and is similar in construction (and appearance) to what is commonly known as a family tree. Setting a maximum tree depth avoids excessive growth of (tree-based) individuals during the evolutionary process (Koza, 1994). GAs and GPs also work according to the strategy of the survival of the fittest, this time searching the solution space of a function. GAs have proved to be a useful means to solve linear and nonlinear problems, where the areas of the state space are explored through mutation, crossover and selection operations applied to individuals in the population (Michalewicz, 1996). GAs and GP use the determination of six fundamental components: solution representation, selection function, genetic operators, initialisation, termination and a fitness function. This will be explained in the following sub-sections.

3.1.1 Solution representation

In order to describe each individual in the population of interest, GAs us a chromosome (or individual) representation in which each individual is made up of a sequence of genes. This scheme decides which genetic operators it should use, in addition to determining the structure of the problem (Houck et al., 1996). Each individual consists of a sequence of genes from a specific alphabet. Binary digits, floating point numbers, integers, symbols etc. can make up the alphabet. In this thesis, GAs are utilised that use an alphabet consisting of floating point numbers. Research shows that better solutions are produced with a more natural problem representation, and it is also more efficient (Michalewicz, 1996). Hence, bounded floating point numbers are a useful representation of individuals for function optimisation.

3.1.2 Selection function

In a GA, individuals are selected to produce successive generations. The selection is based upon the fitness of an individual, where the fittest individuals have an increased probability of being selected and any individual can be selected more than once (Nordin & Banzhaf, 1996).

3.1.3 Genetic operator

Genetic operators are the basis for the search mechanism of GAs. Based on present solutions in the population, the operators are utilised to establish new solutions. The two main operators are crossover and mutation. Crossover uses two of the existing individuals to reproduce two new individuals, while mutation randomly changes the genes in one individual to get a single new solution (Michalewicz, 1996). A reproduction operator selects a parent based on its fitness and creates identical copies of that parent in the next generation (Koza, 1994). There are several options for applying genetic operators to a multi-tree representation. It is possible to apply a particular operator that is selected to all trees within an individual. Another possibility is to iterate over the trees in an individual and select a potentially different operator for each. Finally it is possible to constrain crossover to occur only between trees at the same position in the two parents or it was possible to let evolution freely crossover different trees within the representation.

3.1.4 GA Initialisation and GA termination

An initial population must be provided for the GA and it is common for it to be randomly generated. Since GAs have the ability to produce exciting solutions, the initial population may sometimes be seeded with specifically chosen individuals amongst the otherwise randomly generated individuals. To obtain a termination the GA goes from generation to generation to select parents and reproduce offspring, which then go on to become the next generation of parents (Houck et al., 1996). One possible termination strategy is to use the population convergence criteria, where most of the whole population is forced to converge to a single solution. However, the most popular termination strategy is to decide on a specified maximum number of generations.

3.1.5 Fitness function

The fitness function is an important concept of GAs as this is the indicator for how well a generated solution solves a specific problem; it evaluates the quality of the individuals and guides the evolution to uncover progressively improved solutions during a system run, while the fitness measure specifies what needs to be done (Koza, 1994). In order to select the best suited individuals, a fitness measure is determined by the user and the program will measure the fitness based on a fitness function. The fitness function is objective and quantifies the optimality in solutions. There are two main classes of fitness functions: one where the fitness function can mutate and one where it cannot. In order to calculate the fitness the program may need to run several times with a variety of parameters so that the output can be evaluated (Garner, 2010); this is termed 'training'. One common way to represent the fitness is to measure the difference between the theoretical or ideal value and the actual value, which means that a low fitness value indicates less error.

3.2 Artificial neural networks

An artificial neural network (ANN), also called neural network (NN), is an information processing model inspired by how biological neural networks process information (Bishop, 1995). The key element of ANN is its structure, consisting of interconnected groups of artificial neurons that processes information by a connectionist approach to computation, solving a specific problem. It is called an artificial neural 'network' as the network describes the basis of the system with inter-connected neurons in various layers. ANNs are adaptable systems where the structure is changeable depending on internal and external information flowing through the network in the learning phase, and are capable of modelling complex relationships. ANNs are used in classification, in particular for pattern recognition, but also in data processing (e.g. filtering, clustering, blind source separation and compression) as well as for robotics, and regression analysis.

One of the advantages of ANNs is their ability to find meaning in complicated data (Bishop, 1995). In pattern recognition, where trends are complex and cannot be derived by humans or linear computer models, they act as an expert analysing the problem. In addition, ANNs have other capabilities such as creating their own organisation of information given in the training phase and learning tasks simply by training experience. ANNs are also a useful method in real-time operations, where computations are executed in parallel, hence special hardware devices can be used in order to take advantage of this capability.

3.3 Fuzzy systems

Fuzzy logic, a form of logic that is tolerant to contradictory data, is used in biomedical signal processing and classification to overcome problems where signals are stochastic and therefore may be contradictory in nature (Chan et al., 2000). Fuzzy systems can be trained to identify patterns which are not identifiable by other methods. Fuzzy systems determine fuzzy operators, which may be unknown, on fuzzy sets, requiring the use of 'IF-THEN' rules. Fuzzy systems are used to model or classify problems with variables and rules that can be analysed by a human user. A fuzzy classifier is an algorithm that labels objects by class, and it is argued that the classifier can predict the class label. Kucheva et al. (2000) argued that any classifier that uses fuzzy logic in its training set can be considered to be a fuzzy classifier. A fuzzy system has a vector that contains the values of the features for a specific task, and the system runs a training algorithm and a training data set. Once the system is trained it can be applied to unseen objects. There are several models of fuzzy classifiers, and the simplest method is a rule-based approach that works as an 'IF-THEN' rule system, where the class label is the consequent part of the rule. If the consequent part of the rule contains linguistic values the output will be a soft label with values from the discriminant function. Takagi & Sugeno (1985) identified a fuzzy classifier where the function is the consequent. This method also works according to the IF-THEN rule, however, the rule is a regressor over the feature data space.

3.4 Linear discriminant analysis

Linear discriminant analysis, (LDA), also related to Fisher's linear discriminant, is a technique applied in statistics, pattern recognition and machine learning which finds a linear combination of features for the characterisation or separation of two or more classes. The result can be used as a linear classifier or for dimensionality reduction in later classification. This model is closely related to other techniques, e.g. regression analysis, analysis of variance and principal component analysis, however, in LDA the variance is categorical. LDA can easily execute cases with unequal within-class frequencies, whose performance is examined on randomly produced test data (Balakrishnama & Ganapathiraju, 2010). In this method the ratio of between-class variance to the within-class variance is maximised in any data set, which ensures optimal separability.

There are two different approaches for the transformation of data sets and classification of test vectors in the transformed space: class-dependent transformation and class-independent transformation (Balakrishnama & Ganapathiraju, 2010; Fisher, 1936). The class-dependent transformation involves maximising the ratio of between-class variance to within-class variance. The main aim is high class separability, which is obtained by maximising this ratio. The data sets are transformed independently by the use of two optimising criteria. The class-independent transformation maximises the ratio of overall variance to within-class variance. In this method, only one optimising criterion is used to transform the data sets, which means that data points are transformed regardless of their class identity. In this approach, each class is considered as a separate class against all other classes. LDA is often used for the characterisation of two classes. Here the sample set is considered to be a training set which will find a good predictor for the second class. The following linear transformation describes the classification where the LDA maps the data (feature vector) x:

$$y = w^t x + w_0, \tag{1}$$

where w and w_0 are determined by maximising the ratio of between-class variance to within-class variance to guarantee maximal separability. The LDA uses two classes that are classified at one time:

$$X \in \begin{cases} Class\ 1, & \text{if } y > 0\,, \\ Class\ 2, & \text{if } y < 0\,. \end{cases} \tag{2}$$

3.5 Support vector machine

A support vector machine (SVM) is essentially a supervised learning method which can be used in classification and regression. By undergoing training, the SVM uses an algorithm to develop a model that will predict which category the examples in the training set belongs to. SVMs are a useful technique of data classification (Gunn, 1998; Hsu et al., 2003).

3.6 One clause at a time

One clause at a time (OCAT) is a classification function developed by Torvik et al. (1999), where the aim was to create a flexible, but simple prediction function. In their study on predicting if a muscle is fatigued or rested by investigating the peaks and characteristics fractile frequencies in the EMG signals, they found, in their comparison with other classification methods, that OCAT achieved the highest accuracy. Although ANNs also showed great accuracy they need subjective fine tuning and are complex in their interpretation. Nevertheless, they acknowledged that the more classical methods might be more powerful as long as valid assumptions are made, which is why they stated that more research is needed. This is an interesting but fairly dated approach that attempts to predict localised muscle fatigue.

3.7 Research on classification of EMG signals

There are several approaches to signal classification, but for EMG signal processing, NNs, described in section 3.2, have often been suggested. More specifically, the dynamic recurrent NN, which has two different adaptive parameters using fully interconnected neuron-like units and which maps the relationship between arm movement and EMG muscle activity, was proposed by Cheron et al. (1996). Del Boca & Park (1994) suggested ANNs as a suitable technique for real-time applications of EMG. Their method can precisely identify the features of the EMG signals, and the EMG features are extracted by Fourier analysis, using a fuzzy algorithm for clustering. The operations are undertaken in real-time by an FFT performed by the multipliers in a digital signal processor. The use of fuzzy systems, as described in section 3.3, is also a classification method that has been used in muscle fatigue research as a fatigue index, showing better results than conventional fatigue indices (Kiryu & Yamashita, 2007). Xie et al. used a fuzzy approximate entropy analysis of sEMG signals (Xie et al., 2009) and a cross-fuzzy entropy (Xie et al., 2010) as means by which to assess muscle fatigue.

As mentioned in section 3.1, GP, a specialisation within the field of GAs (Holland, 1975) and based on Darwin's theory of evolution, finds the best suited computer program to perform a set task. Whereas GAs search the space of a function to find an optimum solution, GP creates computer programs as part of the solution. Raikova & Aladjov (2002) used hierarchical

genetic algorithms (HGAs) to investigate the motor control for muscle forces during dynamic conditions. The HGA used genetic operators to find the moments of neural stimulation of all the MUs, which are the variables in genetic terms, so that the sum of MU twitches fulfills the set goals. Results showed that HGAs are a well suited method to examine motor control.
Wang, Yan, Hu, Xie & Wang (2006) have carried out several studies on classification of EMG signals using the wavelet packet method. One such study developed a classification method for sEMG signals based on discrete harmonic wavelet packet transform (DHWPT). Firstly, the relative energy of sEMG signals in each frequency band was extracted using DHWPT, and, secondly, a GA selected appropriate features that reduced the feature dimensionality. An NN would classify four types of prosthetic movement, utilising the selected features as the input vectors. This method produced high classification accuracy, in addition to saving computational time due to the fast algorithm in the DHWPT. In a similar study, Wang, Wang, Chen & Zhuang (2006) improved this sEMG signal classification method by using an optimal wavelet packet (OWP) method based on the DBI. Principle component analysis was applied for a reduction of the feature dimensionality of the outputs of the OWP decomposition. By using a neural network classifier to discriminate between the classes, the mean classification accuracy was 93.75%, outperforming the previous method developed by Wang, Yan, Hu, Xie & Wang (2006). Despite the fact that these two methods are based on EMG classification used for prosthetic movement, the classification methodologies are inventive and are of interest if they are applicable to sEMG signal classification of localised muscle fatigue.

3.8 Validation of classification

A statistical method for validation is cross validation, which evaluates how the classification results are applicable to an independent data set (Kohavi, 1995). Cross validation is based on an evaluation on the learning algorithm used for the applied classification technique. In cross validation the data is divided into two parts, out of which one is used for the training set and the other for the testing set (to validate the applied technique). There are several cross validation methods, such as repeated random sub-sampling validation, K-fold cross-validation, k x 2 cross-validation and leave-one-out cross-validation (Kohavi, 1995). Repeated random sub-sampling validation involves a random separation of the dataset into training and validation data. In every separation, the model fits the training set and predicts the outcomes for the data in the testing set (which is unseen). This strengths of this method are that it does not take long to compute compared to the other models and the proportion of the data set separation is not dependent upon the iterations (folds), however, some of the data may never be selected in the validation sub-sample while other data may be selected several times (Refaeilzadeh et al., 2008). K-fold cross validation partitions the original data set in for K sub-samples, out of which one subset is used for the validation process and the rest is used for the training set. This process is repeated K-times (iterations), ensuring that each of the K sub-samples are only used once in the validation and all of the observations are used for both training and validation (McLachlan et al., 2004). This is an advantage of this method, while the disadvantage is that the training algorithm needs to re-run several times, which means it requires a lot of time before it can make an evaluation. K $\times$ 2 cross validation is a variant of K-field validation, and this method is useful for large data sets, where the user randomly assign the data into two equal sets. Leave-one-out cross validation involves using a single observation from the original sample as the validation data, and the remaining observations as the training data. This is repeated such that each observation in the sample is used once as the validation data. This is the same as a K-fold cross-validation with K being equal to the number of observations in the original sample. Leave-one-out cross validation is also a method similar to K-fold classification, however, the number of iterations are equal to the number of data points in the sets, and each observation is used once as the validation data. This is an expensive method due to the number of times the training process is rerun.

4. Approaches in labeling the sEMG

In labelling the sEMG signal, only the kinematic data (the elbow angle and its standard deviation) were considered as they are reliable indicators in healthy individuals when assessing muscle fatigue onset (Barry, 1992; Guo et al., 2008; Herberts et al., 1980; James et al., 1995; Jarić et al., 1997; Taimela et al., 1999; Tho et al., 1997; Vedsted et al., 2006). The use of the kinematic variables defines the boundaries (Non-Fatigue, Transition-to-Fatigue and Fatigue) of the sEMG signal, providing the basis for training the sEMG classifier.

As the onset of muscle fatigue is diffuse, the use of fuzzy-logic classification is appropriate for setting the boundaries when labelling the sEMG. This study used both a fuzzy classifier to automate the labelling and human experts to verify the outcome of the fuzzy classifier. The two main criteria in labelling the sEMG signal are described below using fuzzy logic terms. The fuzzy classifier had two inputs (elbow angle and its standard deviation) and a single output. The labelling by the fuzzy classifier was verified by a human expert using Table 3 as a guide. The changes in the elbow angle and their indication of fatigue is based on a study by Van Roy et al. (2005). This study claims that changes in the elbow angle of 1.8 +/- 2.9 degrees in men indicates fatigue.

- Figure 1 indicates the fuzzy set input for the elbow angle provided by the goniometer (0 to 180°): Angles of 89° and above indicate Non-Fatigue, while angles below 86.5° indicate Fatigue. The figure also has a superimposed illustration of a single goniometer trial signal giving an example of how the fuzzy classifier identifies the boundaries to enable the labelling of the sEMG signal.
- Figure 2 indicates the fuzzy set input for the arm oscillations (Hristovski et al., 2010) (i.e., the standard deviation of the elbow angle), which was also provided by the goniometer: An increase in the standard deviation of the goniometer signals indicates either low angular oscillation or high angular oscillation. Calculation of the standard deviation was performed using a four-second non-overlapping window of the goniometer signal, then re-sampled to match the original signal size. Further examination of Figure 2, with the superimposed standard deviation signal, reveals that for this particular signal, at around 110 seconds, which resides at 0.6 standard deviations, the subject underwent the transition from the class of Non-Fatigue to that of Transition-to-Fatigue and at around 200 seconds indicates a Fatigue state at 1.0 standard deviations.

As with all fuzzy classifiers, only a single label was chosen as the final output (Slezak et al., 2005). Table 3 defines the rule base; the rule with the greatest firing strength was selected. The above fuzzy classifier inputs (elbow angle and amplitude of arm oscillation), when used in conjunction, were found to assist in finding the boundaries of the classes. Both inputs were used to define a 6 rule type-1 fuzzy classifier, using both triangular and trapezoidal antecedents and product inference.

Preliminary tests showed that the average sEMG signal in this data set was comprised of the muscle fatigue classes in the following estimated proportions: Non-Fatigue 54.5 %; Transition-to-Fatigue 43.18 % and Fatigue 2.32 %. These proportions varied between participants, with the only common feature being that the relative sizes and order of each

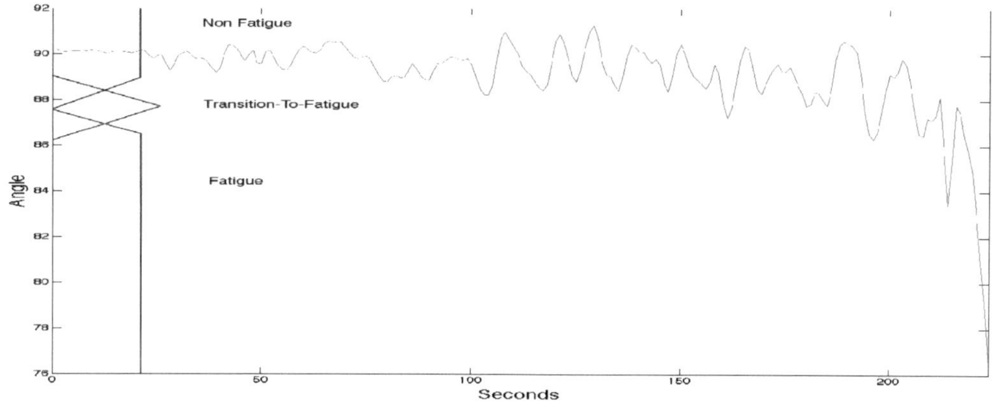

Fig. 1. The fuzzy set input for the angular position of the elbow.

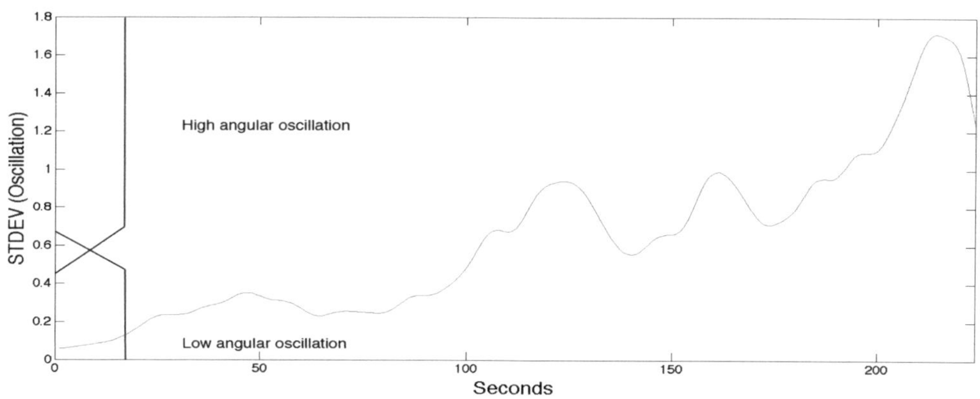

Fig. 2. The fuzzy set input for the angular oscillation (i.e., elbow angle standard deviation).

Rule	IF Input 1 (Elbow angle)	Input 2 (Oscillation)	THEN Output
1	Non-Fatigue	Low	Non-Fatigue
2	Non-Fatigue	High	Transition-to-Fatigue
3	Transition-to-Fatigue	Low	Transition-to-Fatigue
4	Transition-to-Fatigue	High	Transition-to-Fatigue
5	Fatigue	Low	Fatigue
6	Fatigue	High	Fatigue

Table 3. Rule base for signal labelling.

signal component were always the same: Non-Fatigue component > Fatigue component > Transition-to-Fatigue component. For illustration purposes, Figure 3 shows an outcome of the labelling process for a single trial.

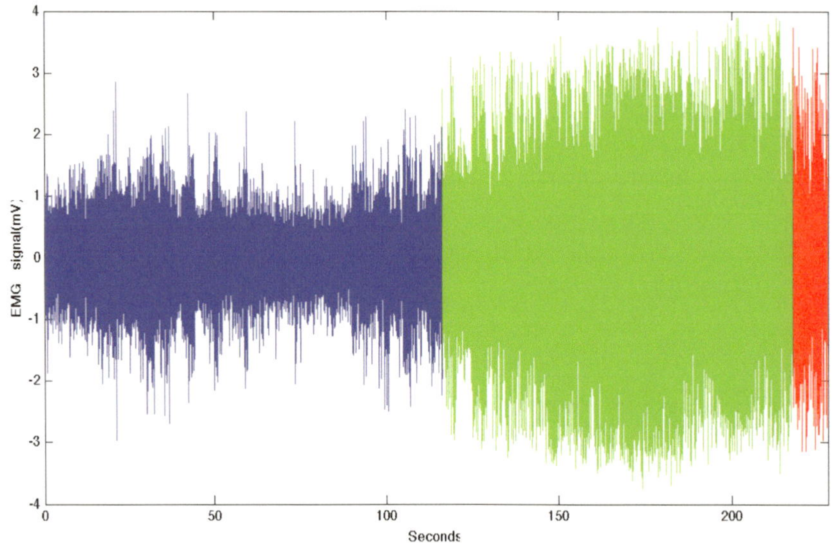

Fig. 3. An illustration of the sEMG signal after labelling (Blue=Non-Fatigue, Green=Transition-to-Fatigue and Red=Fatigue).

5. Conclusion

The defintion of localised muscle fatigue in the current litrutre has diffrent schools of thought, this chapter brought forward these definition to the reader. The chapter also looked at current state of the art in detecting, processing and calssification of sEMG for localized muscle fatigue. The novel concept of a three-phase approach to muscle fatigue(non-fatigue, transition-to-fatigue, and fatigue) was presented in this chapter.

6. References

Armstrong, W. J. (2010). Clinical applications of mechanomyography: technical brief, http://www.thefreelibrary.com/Clinical+applications+of+mechanomyography%3A+technical+brief-a0217771439.

Asghari Oskoei, M., Hu, H. & Gan, J. Q. (2008). Manifestation of fatigue in myoelectric signals of dynamic contractions produced during playing PC games, *Proceedings of the 30th annual international IEEE EMBS conference*, IEEE Engineering in Medicine and Biology Society, pp. 315–318.

Balakrishnama, S. & Ganapathiraju, A. (2010). Linear discriminant analysis -a brief tutorial, http://www.music.mcgill.ca/~ich/classes/mumt611_07/classifiers/lda_theory.pdf.

Barry, B. K. & Enoka, R. M. (2007). The neurobiology of muscle fatigue: 15 years later, *Integrative and Comparative Biology* 47(4): 465–473.

Barry, D. T. (1992). Vibrations and sounds from evoked muscle twitches, *Electromyography and clinical neurophysiology* 32: 35–40.

Basmajian, J. V. & De Luca, C. J. (1985). *Muscles alive: Their function revealed by electromyography*, Williams and Wilkins, Baltimore, MD, USA.

Bernatos, L., Crago, P. & Chizeck, H. (1986). A discrete-time model of electricity stimulated muscle, *IEEE Transactions on Systems, Man, and Cybernetics* pp. 829–838.
Bigland-Ritchie, B. & Woods, J. J. (1984). Changes in muscle contractile properties and neural control during human muscular fatigue, *Muscle Nerve* 7: 691–699.
Bills, A. G. (1943). *The psychology of efficiency*, Harper, New York, NY, USA.
Bishop, C. M. (1995). *Neural networks for pattern recognition*, Oxford University Press, New York, NY, USA.
Boostani, R. & Moradi, M. H. (2003). Evaluation of the forearm EMG signal features for the control of a prosthetic hand, *Physiological Measurement* 24: 309–319.
Borg, G. (1970). Perceived exertion as an indicator of somatic stress, *Scandinavian Journal of Rehabilitation Medicine* 2(2): 92–98.
Calder, K. M., Stashuk, D. W. & McLean, L. (2008). Physiological characteristics of motor units in the brachioradialis muscle across fatiguing low-level isometric contractions, *Journal of Electromyography and Kinesiology* 18: 2–15.
Chaffin, D. B. (1973). Localized muscle fatigue–definiton and measurement, *Journal of Occupational and Environmental Medicine* 15: 346–354.
Chan, F. H. Y., Yang, Y. S., Lam, F. K., Zhang, Y. T. & Parker, P. A. (2000). Fuzzy EMG classification for prosthesis control, *IEEE Transactions on Rehabilitation Engineering* 8(3): 305–311.
Cheron, G., Draye, J.-P. & Bourgeios, M. (1996). A dynamic neural network identification of electromyography and trajectory relationship during complex movements, *IEEE Transactions on Biomedical Engineering* 43(5): 552–558.
Christodoulou, C. I. & Pattichis, C. S. (1995). A new technique for the classification and decomposition of EMG signals, *IEEE international conference on neural networks (ICNN'95)*, Vol. 5, IEEE, Perth, Western Australia, pp. 2303–2308.
Cifrek, M., Medved, V., Tonkovi, S. & Ostoji, S. (2009). Surface EMG based muscle fatigue evaluation in biomechanics, *Clinical Biomechanics* 24: 327–340.
Cohen, L. (1995). *Time frequency analysis*, Prentice-Hall, Englewood Cliffs, NJ, USA.
Coorevits, P., Danneels, L., Cambier, D., Ramon, H., Druyts, H., Karlsson, S. J., Moor, G. D. & Vanderstraeten, G. (2008). Correlations between short-time Fourier- and continuous wavelet transforms in the analysis of localized back and hip muscle fatigue during isometric contractions, *Journal of Electromyography and Kinesiology* 18: 637–644.
Courteville, A., Gharbi, T. & Cornu, J. Y. (1998). MMG measurement: a high-sensitivity microphone-based sensor for clinical use, *IEEE Transactions on Biomedical Engineering* 45: 145–150.
Davies, D. L. & Bouldin, D. W. (1979). A cluster separation measure, *IEEE Transactions on Pattern Analysis and Machine Intelligence* 1(4): 224–227.
Davies, M. & Reisman, S. S. (1994). Time frequency analysis of the electromyogram during fatigue, *Proceedings of the 20th annual northeast bioengineering conference*, pp. 93–95.
Day, S. (2010). Important Factors in Surface EMG Measurement, `http://www.bortec.ca/Images/pdf/EMG20measurement20and20recording.pdf`.
De Luca, C. J. (1979). Physiology and mathematics of myoelectric signals, *IEEE Transactions on Biomedical Engineering* 26: 313–325.
De Luca, C. J. (1997). The use of surface electromyography in biomechanics, *Journal of Applied Biomechanics* 13: 135–163.
Del Boca, A. & Park, D. C. (1994). Myoelectric signal recognition using fuzzy clustering and artificial neural networks in real time, *IEEE international conference on neural networks (ICNN'94)*, IEEE, Orlando, FL, USA, pp. 3098–3103.

Dimitrov, G. V., Arabadzhiev, T. I., Mileva, K. N., Bowtell, J. L., Crichton, N. & Dimitrova, N. A. (2006). Muscle fatigue during dynamic contractions assessed by new spectral indices, *Medicine and Science in Sports and Exercise* 38: 1971–1979.

Duchene, J. & Goubel, F. (1993). Surface electromyogram during voluntary contraction: processing tools and relation to physiological events, *Critical Reviews in Biomedical Engineering* 21: 313–397.

Eberstein, A. & Beattie, B. (1985). Simultaneous measurement of muscle conduction velocity and EMG power spectrum changes during fatigue, *Muscle Nerve* 8: 768–773.

Edwards, R. (1981). Human muscle function and fatigue, *Ciba Foundation Symposium* 82.

Farina, D. (2006). Interpretation of the surface electromyogram in dynamic contractions, *Exercise and Sport Sciences Review* 34: 121–127.

Filligoi, G., Felici, F., Vicini, M. & Rosponi, A. (2010). Recurrence quantification analysis of surface electromyograms, `http://library.med.utah.edu/cyprus/proceedings/medicon98/medicon98.filligoi.giancarlo.pdf`.

Fisher, R. A. (1936). The use of multiple measurements in taxonomic problems, *Ann. Eugenics* 7: 179–188.

Gabor, D. (1946). Theory of communication, *Journal of the Institution of Electrical Engineers - Part III: Radio and Communication Engineering* 93: 422–457.

Garner, Z. (2010). An introduction to genetic programming, `http://www.generation5.org/content/2000/ga00.asp`.

Georgakis, A., Stergioulas, L. K. & Giakas, G. (2003). Fatigue analysis of the surface EMG signal in isometric constant force contractions using the averaged instantaneous frequency, *IEEE Transactions on Biomedical Engineering* 50: 262–265.

Gerdle, B., Karlsson, S., Day, S. & Djupsbacka, M. (1999). *Acquisition, processing and analysis of the surface electromyogram. Modern techniques in neuroscience*, Springer Verlag, Berlin, Germany.

Gonzalez-Izal, M., Malanda, A., Navarro-Amezqueta, I., Gorostiaga, E. M., Mallor, F., Ibanez, J. & Izquierdo, M. (2010). EMG spectral indices and muscle power fatigue during dynamic contractions, *Journal of Electromyography and Kinesiology* 20: 233–240.

Gonzalez-Izal, M., Rodriguez-Carreno, I., Malanda, A., Mallor-Gimenez, F., Navarro-Amezqueta, I., Gorostiaga, E. M. & Izquierdo, M. (2010). sEMG wavelet-based indices predicts muscle power loss during dynamic contractions, *Journal of Electromyography and Kinesiology* 20: 1097–1106.

Gordon, G. & Holbourn, A. H. (1948). The sounds from single motor units in a contracting muscle, *The Journal of Physiology* 107: 456–464.

Graupe, D. & Cline, W. K. (1975). Functional separation of EMG signals via ARMA identification, *IEEE Transactions on Systems, Man, and Cybernetics* 5: 252–259.

Gregori, B., Galie, E. & Accornero, N. (2003). Surface electromyography and mechanomyography recording: a new differential composite probe, *Medical and Biological Engineering and Computing* 41: 665–669.

Gross, D., Ladd, H. W., Riley, E. J., Macklem, P. T. & Grassino, A. (1980). The effect of training on strength and endurance of the diaphragm in quadriplegia, *American Journal of Medicine* 68: 27–35.

Guglielminotti, P. & Merletti, R. (1992). Effect of electrode location on surface myoelectric signal variables: a simulation study, *9th international congress of The International Society of Electrophysiological Kinesiology*, Florence, Italy.

Gündoğdu, U., Sayin, A., Akan, A., Arslan, Y., Orhan, E. & Baslo, M. (2006). Investigation of muscle fatigue using temporal and spectral moments, *Proceedings of the 5th WSEAS*

international conference on Signal processing, SIP'06, World Scientific and Engineering Academy and Society (WSEAS), Stevens Point, Wisconsin, USA, pp. 10–14.
URL: *http://portal.acm.org/citation.cfm?id=1983937.1983941*

Gunn, S. R. (1998). Support vector machines for classification and regression, *Technical report*, University of Southanpton, Southampton, UK.
URL: *http://eprints.ecs.soton.ac.uk/6459/*

Guo, J. Y., Zheng, Y. P., Huang, Q. H. & Chen, X. (2008). Dynamic monitoring of forearm muscles using one-dimensional sonomyography system, *Journal of Rehabilitation Research and Development* 45: 187–195.

Hagberg, M. (1981). Work load and fatigue in repetitive arm elevations, *Ergonomics* 24: 543–555.

Hefftner, G., Zucchini, W. & Jaros, G. G. (1988). The electromyogram (EMG) as a control signal for functional neuromuscular stimulation–Part I: autoregressive modeling as a means of EMG signature discrimination, *IEEE Transactions on Biomedical Engineering* 35: 230–237.

Helal, J.-N., Van Hoecke, J., Garapon-Bar, C. & Goubel, F. (1992). Surface myoelectric signals during ergocycle exrcises at various mechanical powers and pedalling rates, *Journal of Electromyography and Kinesiology* 2(4): 242–251.
URL: *http://www.sciencedirect.com/science/article/B6T89-4CDHXXY-5/2/e121acb16d3fc8c8480ee3e64fee8e18*

Herberts, P., Kadefors, R. & Broman, H. (1980). Arm positioning in manual tasks. An electromyographic study of localized muscle fatigue, *Ergonomics* 23: 655–665.

Hermens, H. J., Boon, K. L. & Zilvold, G. (1986). The clinical use of surface EMG, *Acta Belgica. Medica Physica* 9: 119–130.

Holland, J. H. (1975). *Adaptation in natural and artificial systems*, The University of Michigan Press, Ann Arbor, MI, USA.

Hong, Y. & Bartlett, R. (2008). *Routledge handbook of biomechanics and human movement science*, Routledge, New York, NY, USA.

Houck, C. R., A., J. J. & Kay, M. G. (1996). Comparison of genetic algorithms, random restart and two-opt switching for solving large location-allocation problems, *Computers and Operations Research* 23(6): 587–596.
URL: *http://dx.doi.org/10.1016/0305-0548(95)00063-1*

Hristovski, R., VenskaitytÆŠÃş, E., Vainoras, A., Balague, N. & Vazquez, P. (2010). Constraints-controlled metastable dynamics of exercise-induced psychobiological adaptation., *Medicina (Kaunas)* 46(7): 447–453.

Hsu, C. W., Chang, C. C. & Lin, C. J. (2003). A practical guide to support vector classification, *Technical report*, National Taiwan University, Taipei, Taiwan.
URL: *http://www.csie.ntu.edu.tw/ cjlin/papers/guide/guide.pdf*

Huang, H.-P. & Chen, C.-Y. (1999). Development of a myoelectric discrimination system for a multi-degree prosthetic hand, *IEEE International Conference on Robotics and Automation*, pp. 2392–2397.
URL: `http:{//dblp.uni-trier.de/db/conf/icra/icra1999-3.htmlHuangC99}`

Hudgins, B., Parker, P. & Scott, R. N. (1993). A new strategy for multifunction myoelectric control, *IEEE Transactions on Biomedical Engineering* 40: 82–94.

Hussain, M. S., Reaz, M. B. I. & Ibrahimy, M. I. (2008). SEMG signal processing and analysis using wavelet transform and higher order statistics to characterize muscle force, *ICS'08: Proceedings of the 12th WSEAS international conference on systems*, World

Scientific and Engineering Academy and Society WSEAS, Stevens Point, WI, USA, pp. 366–371.

James, C., Sacco, P. & Jones, D. A. (1995). Loss of power during fatigue of human leg muscles, *The Journal of Physiology* 484 (Pt 1): 237–246.

Jarić, S., Radovanović, S., Milanović, S., Ljubisavljević, M. & Anastasijević, R. (1997). A comparison of the effects of agonist and antagonist muscle fatigue on performance of rapid movements, *European Journal of Applied Physiology and Occupational Physiology* 76: 41–47.

Jaynes, E. T. (1957). Information theory and statistical mechanics, *Physical Review* 106(4): 620–630.

Jorgensen, K., Fallentin, N., Krogh-Lund, C. & Jensen, B. (1988). Electromyography and fatigue during prolonged, low-level static contractions, *European Journal of Applied Physiology and Occupational Physiology* 57: 316–321.

Kadefors, R., Kaiser, E. & Petersen, I. (1968). Dynamic spectrum analysis of myo-potentials and with special reference to muscle fatigue, *Electromyography* 8: 39–74.

Kanosue, K., Yoshida, M., Akazawa, K. & Fujii, K. (1979). The number of active motor units and their firing rates in voluntary contraction of human brachialis muscle, *The Japanese Journal of Physiology* 29: 427–443.

Karlsson, S., Yu, J. & Akay, M. (1999). Enhancement of spectral analysis of myoelectric signals during static contractions using wavelet methods, *IEEE Transactions on Biomedical Engineering* 46: 670–684.

Karlsson, S., Yu, J. & Akay, M. (2000). Time-frequency analysis of myoelectric signals during dynamic contractions: a comparative study, *IEEE Transactions on Biomedical Engineering* 47: 228–238.

Khezri, M. & Jahed, M. (2007). Real-time intelligent pattern recognition algorithm for surface EMG signals, *Biomedical Engineering Online* .

Kim, J.-Y., Jung, M.-C. & Haight, J. (2005). The sensitivity of autoregressive model coefficient in quantification of trunk muscle fatigue during a sustained isometric contraction, *International Journal of Industrial Ergonomics* 35: 321–330.

Kim, Y. & Street, W. N.and Filippo Menczer, F. (2010). Feature selection in data mining, `http://dollar.biz.uiowa.edu/~street/research/dmoc.pdf`.

Kiryu, T. & Yamashita, K. (2007). A ubiquitous wearable unit for controlling muscular fatigue during cycling exercise sessions, *Conference Proceedings - IEEE Engineering in Medicine and Biology Society*, pp. 4814–4817.

Kleissen, R. F., Buurke, J. H., Harlaar, J. & Zilvold, G. (1998). Electromyography in the biomechanical analysis of human movement and its clinical application, *Gait Posture* 8: 143–158.

Kohavi, R. (1995). A study of cross-validation and bootstrap for accuracy estimation and model selection, *Proceedings of the 14th international joint conference on artificial intelligence - Volume 2*, Morgan Kaufmann Publishers Inc., San Francisco, CA, USA, pp. 1137–1143.
URL: *http://portal.acm.org/citation.cfm?id=1643031.1643047*

Kohavi, R. & John, G. H. (1997). The wrapper approach.

Kohavi, R. & Provost, F. (1998). Editorial for the special issue on applications of machine learning and the knowledge discovery process, *Machine Learning* 30: 271–274.

Kojadinovic, I. & Wottka, T. (2000). Comparison between a filter and a wrapper approach to variable.

Komi, P. V. & Tesch, P. (1979). EMG frequency spectrum, muscle structure, and fatigue during dynamic contractions in man, *European Journal of Applied Physiology and Occupational Physiology* 42: 41–50.

Koza, J. R. (1994). *Genetic programming II: automatic discovery of reusable programs*, MIT Press, Cambridge, MA, USA.

Kramer, C. G., Hagg, T. & Kemp, B. (1987). Real-time measurement of muscle fatigue related changes in surface EMG, *Medical and Biological Engineering and Computing* 25: 627–630.

Kucheva, L. I., Whitaker, C. J., Shipp, C. A. & Duin, R. P. W. (2000). Is independence good for combining classifiers?, *Proc. of ICPR2000, 15th Int. Conference on Pattern Recognition, Barcelona, Spain*, Vol. 2, pp. 168–171.

Kumar, D. K., Pah, N. D. & Bradley, A. (2003). Wavelet analysis of surface electromyography to determine muscle fatigue, *IEEE Transactions on Neural Systems and Rehabilitation Engineering* 11: 400–406.

Kumar, S. & Mital, A. (1996). *Electromyography in ergonomics*, Taylor and Francis Ltd., London, UK.

Laterza, F. & Olmo, G. (1997). Analysis of EMG signals by means of the matched wavelet transform, *Electronic Letters* 33(5): 357–359.

Lindstrom, L., Kadefors, R. & Petersen, I. (1977). An electromyographic index for localized muscle fatigue, *Journal of Applied Physiology* 43: 750–754.

Linssen, W. H., Stegeman, D. F., Joosten, E. M., van't Hof, M. A., Binkhorst, R. A. & Notermans, S. L. (1993). Variability and interrelationships of surface EMG parameters during local muscle fatigue, *Muscle Nerve* 16: 849–856.

Liu, H. & Motoda, M. (1998). *Feature selection for knowledge discovery and data mining*, Kluwer Academic Publishers, Norwell, MA, USA.

MacIsaac, D. T., Parker, P. A., Englehart, K. B. & Rogers, D. R. (2006). Fatigue estimation with a multivariable myoelectric mapping function, *IEEE Transactions on Biomedical Engineering* 53: 694–700.

Marras, W. (1990). Industrial electromyography (EMG), *International Journal of Industrial Ergonomics* 6: 89–74.

Masuda, K., Masuda, T., Sadoyama, T., Inaki, M. & Katsuta, S. (1999). Changes in surface EMG parameters during static and dynamic fatiguing contractions, *Journal of Electromyography and Kinesiology* 9: 39–46.

Maton, B. & Gamet, D. (1989). The fatigability of two agonistic muscles in human isometric voluntary submaximal contraction: an EMG study. II. Motor unit firing rate and recruitment, *European Journal of Applied Physiology and Occupational Physiology* 58: 369–374.

McLachlan, G. J., Do, K. A. & Ambroise, C. (2004). *Analyzing microarray gene expression data*, Wiley, New York, NY, USA.

Merletti, R. (1999). Standards for Reporting EMG data., *Journal of Electromyography and Kinesiology* 9(1).

Merletti, R., Farina, D. & Gazzoni, M. (2003). The linear electrode array: a useful tool with many applications, *Journal of Electromyography and Kinesiology* 13: 37–47.

Merletti, R. & Parker, P. A. (2004). *Electromyography: physiology, engineering and non-invasive applications*, John Wiley and sons, Inc, New York.

Michalewicz, Z. (1996). *Genetic Algorithms + Data Structures = Evolution Programs*, Springer-Verlag, New York, NY, USA.

Minning, S., Eliot, C. A., Uhl, T. L. & Malone, T. R. (2007). EMG analysis of shoulder muscle fatigue during resisted isometric shoulder elevation, *Journal of Electromyography and Kinesiology* 17: 153–159.

Morana, C., Ramdani, S., Perrey, S. & Varray, A. (2009). Recurrence quantification analysis of surface electromyographic signal: sensitivity to potentiation and neuromuscular fatigue, *Journal of Neuroscience Methods* 177: 73–79.

Moser, A. T. & Graupe, D. (1989). Identification of nonstationary models with application to myoelectric signals for controlling electrical stimulation of paraplegics, *IEEE Trans Acoust Speech Sig Proc* ASSP-37(5): 713.

Moshou, D., Hostens, I., Papaioannou, G. & Ramon, H. (2005). Dynamic muscle fatigue detection using self-organizing maps, *Applied Soft Computing* 5: 391–398.

Naik, G. R., Kumar, D. K., Wheeler, K. & Arjunan, S. P. (2009). Estimation of muscle fatigue during cyclic contractions using source separation techniques, *Proceedings of the 2009 digital image computing: techniques and applications (DICTA 2009)*, IEEE Computer Society, pp. 217–222.

Nordin, P. & Banzhaf, W. (1996). Programmatic compression of images and sound, *in* J. R. Koza, D. E. Goldberg, D. B. Fogel & R. L. Riolo (eds), *Proceedings of the first annual conference on genetic programming*, MIT Press, Boston, MA, USA, pp. 345–350. URL: *ftp://lumpi.informatik.uni-dortmund.de/pub/biocomp/papers/gp96.ps.gz*

Ortengren, R., Andersson, G., Broman, H., Magnusson, R. & Petersen, I. (1975). Vocational electromyography: studies of localized muscle fatigue at the assembly line, *Ergonomics* 18: 157–174.

Payton, C. & Bartlett, R. (2008). *Biomechanical evaluation of movement in sport and exercise: The British Association of Sport and Science*, Routledge, New York, NY, USA.

Petrofsky, J. S. (1981). Quantification through the surface EMG of muscle fatigue and recovery during successive isometric contractions, *Aviation, Space, and Environmental Medicine* 52: 545–550.

Petrofsky, J. S., Glaser, R. M., Phillips, C. A., Lind, A. R. & Williams, C. (1982). Evaluation of amplitude and frequency components of the surface EMG as an index of muscle fatigue, *Ergonomics* 25: 213–223.

Phinyomark, A., Limsakul, C. & Phukpattaranont, P. (2009). A novel feature extraction for robust EMG pattern recognition, *Journal of Computing* 1(1).

Poli, R., Langdon, W. B. & McPhee, N. F. (2008). *A field guide to genetic programming*, Published via http://lulu.com. (With contributions by J. R. Koza). URL: *http://www.gp-field-guide.org.uk*

Raez, M. B., Hussain, M. S. & Mohd-Yasin, F. (2006). Techniques of EMG signal analysis: detection, processing, classification and applications, *Biological Proceedings Online* 8: 11–35.

Raikova, R. T. & Aladjov, H. T. S. (2002). Hierarchical genetic algorithm versus static optimization-investigation of elbow flexion and extension movements, *Journal of Biomechanics* 35: 1123–1135.

Refaeilzadeh, P., Tang, L. & Liu, H. (2008). Cross-validation, http://www.public.asu.edu/~ltang9/papers/ency-cross-validation.pdf.

Ricamato, A., Absher, R. G., M.T., M. & Tranowski, J. P. (1992). A time-frequency approach to evaluate electromyographic recordings, *Proceedings of the 5th annual IEEE symposium on computer-based medical system*, pp. 520–527.

Roy, S. H., Bonato, P. & Knaflitz, M. (1998). EMG assessment of back muscle function during cyclical lifting, *Journal of Electromyography and Kinesiology* 8: 233–245.

Samet, H. (2006). *Foundations of multidimensional and metric data structures*, Morgan Kaufmann, USA.

Sato, H. (1982). Functional characteristics of human skeletal muscle revealed by spectral analysis of the surface electromyogram, *Electromyography and Clinical Neurophysiology* 22: 459–516.

Sepulveda, F., Meckes, M. & Conway, B. (2004). Cluster separation index suggests usefulness of non-motor eeg channels in detecting wrist movement direction intention, *IEEE conference on cybernetics and intelligent systems*, pp. 943–947.

Sewell, M. (2010). Feature selection, `http://machine-learning.martinsewell.com/feature-selection/feature-selection.pdf`.

Shahid, S. (2007). *Higher order statistics techniques applied to EMG signal analysis and characterization of skeletal muscles*, PhD thesis, University of Limerick, Limerick, Ireland.

Sherif, M. F. (1980). *Stochastic model of myoelectric signals for movement pattern recognition in upper limb prostheses*, PhD thesis, School of Engineering and Applied Sciences, University of California at Los Angeles, Los Angeles, CA, USA.

Singh, V. P., Kumar, D. K., Polus, B. & Fraser, S. (2007). Strategies to identify changes in SEMG due to muscle fatigue during cycling, *Journal of Medical Engineering and Technology* 31: 144–151.

Slezak, D., Yao, J. T., Peters, J. F., Ziarko, W. & Xiaohua Hu, X. (2005). *Rough sets, fuzzy sets, data mining, and granular computing*, Springer, Berlin, Germany.

Soo, Y., Nishino, M., Sugi, M., Yokoi, H., Arai, T., Kato, R., Nakamura, T. & Ota, J. (2009). Evaluation of frequency band technique in estimating muscle fatigue during dynamic contraction task, *Proceedings of the 2009 IEEE International Conference on Robotics and Automation (ICRA'09)*, IEEE, pp. 933–938.
URL: *http:{//dx.doi.org/10.1109/ROBOT.2009.5152845}*

Stulen, F. B. & De Luca, C. J. (1982). Muscle fatigue monitor: a noninvasive device for observing localized muscular fatigue, *IEEE Transactions on Biomedical Engineering* 29: 760–768.

Sung, P. S., Zurcher, U. & Kaufman, M. (2008). Gender differences in spectral and entropic measures of erector spinae muscle fatigue, *Journal of Rehabilitation Research and Development* 45: 1431–1439.

Taimela, S., Kankaanpaa, M. & Luoto, S. (1999). The effect of lumbar fatigue on the ability to sense a change in lumbar position. A controlled study, *Spine* 24: 1322–1327.

Takagi, T. & Sugeno, M. (1985). Fuzzy identification of systems and its application to modeling and control, *IEEE Transactions on Systems, Man, and Cybernetics* 15(1): 116–132.

Tamil, E. M., Bashar, N. S., Idris, M. Y. I. & Tamil, A. M. (2008). Review on feature extraction and classification techniques for biosignal processing part III: electromyogram, *in* N. A. Abu Osman, F. Ibrahim, W. A. B. Wan Abas, H. S. Abdul Rahman & H.-N. Ting (eds), *4th Kuala Lumpur international conference on biomedical engineering*, Vol. 21 of *IFMBE Proceedings*, Springer Berlin Heidelberg, Germany, pp. 117–121.

Tepavac, D. & Schwirtlich, L. (1997). Detection and prediction of FES-induced fatigue, *Journal of Electromyography and Kinesiology* 7: 39–50.

Tho, K. S., Nemeth, G., Lamontagne, M. & Eriksson, E. (1997). Electromyographic analysis of muscle fatigue in anterior cruciate ligament deficient knees, *Clinical Orthopaedics and Related Research* pp. 142–151.

Tohru, K. (1992). Investigation of parametric analysis of dynamic EMG signals by a muscle-structured stimulation study, *IEEE Transactions on Biomedical Engineering* 39(3): 280–288.

Torvik, G. I., Triantaphyllou, E., Liao, T. & Waly, S. (1999). Predicting muscle fatigue via electromyography: A comparative study, `http://arrowsmith.psych.uic.edu/torvik/papers/iccie25_1999_torvik.pdf`.

Van Roy, P., Baeyens, J., Fauvart, D., Lanssiers, R. & Clarijs, J. (2005). Arthro-kinematics of the elbow: study of the carrying angle., *Ergonomics* 48(11): 1645–1656.

Vedsted, P., Blangsted, A. K., Søgaard, K., Orizio, C. & Sjøgaard, G. (2006). Muscle tissue oxygenation, pressure, electrical, and mechanical responses during dynamic and static voluntary contractions, *European Journal of Applied Physiology* 96: 165–177.

Viitasalo, J. H. & Komi, P. V. (1977). Signal characteristics of EMG during fatigue, *European Journal of Applied Physiology and Occupational Physiology* 37: 111–121.

Walker, J. S. (2000). *A primer on wavelets and their scientific applications*, Chapman and Hall/CRC, Boca Raton, FL, USA.
URL: *http://millenium.itesm.mx/record=i566853&searchscope=0*

Wang, G., Wang, Z., Chen, W. & Zhuang, J. (2006). Classification of surface emg signals using optimal wavelet packet method based on davies-bouldin criterion, *Medical and Biological Engineering and Computing* 44: 865–872. 10.1007/s11517-006-0100-y.
URL: *http://dx.doi.org/10.1007/s11517-006-0100-y*

Wang, G., Yan, Z., Hu, X., Xie, H. & Wang, Z. (2006). Classification of surface EMG signals using harmonic wavelet packet transform, *Physiological Measurement* 27: 1255–1267.

Wang, J., Yang, H. C. & Liu, J. H. (2004). Studies on the non-fatigue specificity of the fatigue-related sEMG signal parameters, *Space medicine and medical engineering Beijing* 17: 39–43.

Watakabe, M., Itoh, Y., Mita, K. & Akataki, K. (1998). Technical aspects of mechnomyography recording with piezoelectric contact sensor, *Medical and Biological Engineering and Computing* 36: 557–561.

Welch, P. D. (1967). The use of fast Fourier transform for the estimation of power spectra: a method based on time averaging over short, modified periodograms, *IEEE Transactions on Audio and Electroacoustics* 15: 70–73.

Xie, H.-B., Zheng, Y.-P., Guo, J.-Y. & Chen, X. (2010). Cross-fuzzy entropy: a new method to test pattern synchrony of bivariate time series, *Information Sciences* 180(9): 1715–1724.

Xie, H. B., Zheng, Y. P., Guo, J. Y., Chen, X. & Shi, J. (2009). Estimation of wrist angle from sonomyography using support vector machine and artificial neural network models, *Medical Engineering and Physics* 31: 384–391.

Yan, Z., Wang, Z. & Xie, H. (2008). The application of mutual information-based feature selection and fuzzy LS-SVM-based classifier in motion classification, *Computer Methods and Programs in Biomedicine* 90(3): 275–284.

Zhang, Z. G., Liu, H. T., Chan, S. C., Luk, K. D. & Hu, Y. (2010). Time-dependent power spectral density estimation of surface electromyography during isometric muscle contraction: methods and comparisons, *Journal of Electromyography and Kinesiology* 20: 89–101.

10

Clinical Application of Silent Period for the Evaluation of Neuro-Muscular Function in the Field of the Sports Medicine and Rehabilitation

Shinichi Daikuya[1], Atsuko Ono[1], Toshiaki Suzuki[2], Tetsuji Fujiwara[3] and Kyonosuke Yabe[4]
[1]*Kishiwada Eishinkai Hospital*
[2]*Kansai University of Health Sciences*
[3]*Kyoto University*
[4]*Nagoya University*
Japan

1. Introduction

A transient suppression of muscle activation was produced by electric stimulation to the innervating nerve during continued effort. This period of electrical inactivity, designated the mixed nerve silent period, results from several physiologic mechanisms (Kimura, 2001). On the other hand, the silent period during tonic muscle contraction demonstrated on electromyography is due to the rapid voluntary movement during tonic and mild muscle contraction (Ikai, 1955) and is elicited by cutaneous electrical stimulation of supplying nerve during muscle contraction (Higgins & Lieberman, 1968). In many previous studies about silent period, it was generally classified into three categories: (1) the quiet period of bursting wave activity on electromyography, recorded before the rapid motion in response to visual, auditory, light and/or sound stimulation (Yabe, 1976); (2) a transient suppression of muscle activation following electric stimulation of the mixed nerve innervating that muscle during continued effort (Kimura, 2001); (3) a pause of the muscle activity following the motor potential elicited by cortical magnetic stimulation during voluntary target muscle contraction (Calancie et al, 1987). In this study, we used the second category, according to which the silent period consists of several waves, including M wave, F wave and Long Latency Reflex (LLR).

The silent period in this article, which classified in the second category, is the duration of the inhibitory period of muscle contraction detected on surface electromyography, which is due to electrical stimulation at the innervating nerve during tonic muscle contraction (Figure 1). We have considered that the silent period of lower extremity is the total circuit time from the peripheral nerve stimulus point to the central nervous system (i.e., brainstem or motor cortex), because the M wave, F wave and LLR are included in the silent period on evoked electromyography. M wave is affected by the conductive condition of peripheral nerve and the muscle state (i.e. rest or contraction, length, volume and so on) (Fuglevand et al, 1993, Cupido et al, 1992, Behm & St-Pierre, 1997). F wave is influenced by the excitability of the spinal motor neuron function (Suzuki et al, 1993). LLR in the lower extremities is affected by the excitability of the spinal cord, brainstem or motor cortex (Roby-Brami & Bussel, 1987, Upton et al, 1971, Kuroiwa, 1986). Therefore, it has been thought that a variation of the silent period may be able to become an index of the degree of facilitation of the brainstem or motor cortex. So, the origin of silent period that we used in this study is thought to be influenced by muscle spindle function, afferent inhibited impulse from Golgi tendon organ or Ia fiber, recurrent inhibition in the spinal cord, inhibitive mechanism of cerebral cortex (Higgins & Lieberman, 1968, Upton et al, 1971, Anastasijevic & Vuco, 1980). And we have tried to apply the silent period to clarify the magnitude of facilitation of the brainstem or motor cortex in the field of physical therapy. In previous study, we had studied the neuromuscular function of healthy subjects in various conditions (i.e. control of degree of muscle contraction and alteration of postural condition) with a silent period using an electro-physiological method (Daikuya et al, 2003.). Though LLR may be included in silent period, LLR was usually distinguished under the supra-maximal stimulation, which was used to record the silent period. In addition, if the fluctuation of silent period was large, it was thought that it shown the possibility of having arrived in the level where electric stimulus differs every stimulus.

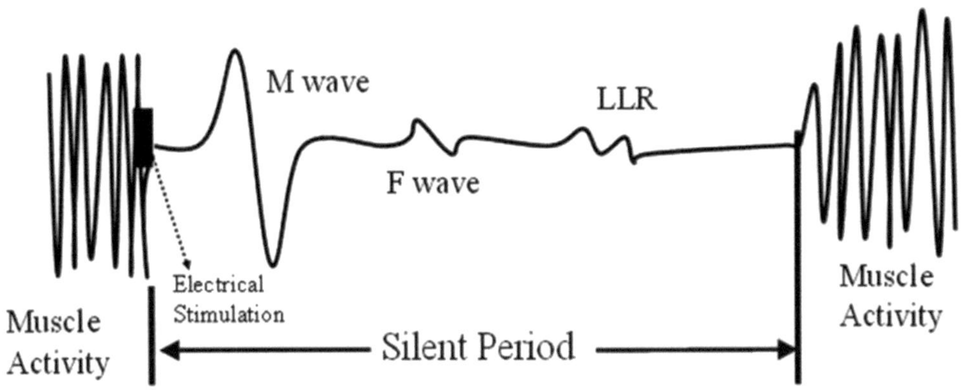

Fig. 1. Schematic Silent Period.

While, the state of improvement process after reconstruction of anterior cruciate ligament of the knee (ACL), following parameters were usually used as the index of recovery of physical function; muscle strength, range of motion (ROM), quality of sports performance, and so on. However, it is thought that results of their index and ability or disability of sports competition have little correlation, because we have experienced some cases with instability and/or a strange sensation of the knee during sports activity, although their muscle strength and ROM were good enough. Whereas, we have also experienced some cases without any problems, although their muscle strength and ROM were not enough. Therefore, we considered that as the index of recovery degree after reconstruction of ACL, only their parameters were not sufficient. And, we emphasized the necessity of evaluation of neuromuscular function after reconstruction of ACL. So, we had considered the neuromuscular function of healthy subjects in various conditions (i.e. control of degree of muscle contraction and alteration of postural condition.) with a mixed nerve silent period using an electro-physiological method (Daikuya et al, 2003.) and have attempted to apply the alteration of silent period aspects for the evaluation of the neuromuscular function of a lower extremity after reconstruction of ACL.

2. Silent period in healthy subjects; its aspects in relation to strength of tonic muscle contraction and postural alteration

Silent period aspects in healthy subjects were displayed as preliminary findings, which demonstrated the tendency of the change of the duration of silent period with an alteration of the strength of tonic muscle contraction, and the relationship between the duration of silent period and postural change in upper and lower extremity for application in the field of sports medicine.

2.1 Effect of electric stimulating condition on silent period recording

The effect of electric stimulation on silent period measurement was studied, in non-athlete, 9 healthy subjects with a mean age of 25.1 years (9 healthy subjects, 18 extremities, 8 males and 1 female). The experimental landscape was shown in Figure 2. The silent period was recorded from the opponens pollicis muscle under the following 3×3 electric stimulation conditions: 0.2Hz, 0.5Hz and 1.0Hz of frequency; 80%, 100% and 120% of intensity in maximal amplitude of M-wave. In this article, we defined the silent period as the duration from artifact produced by electrical stimulation of the muscle re-bursting on EMG, and the silent period was calculated the duration from the artifact due to electrical stimulation to reappearance or uninterrupted voluntary tonic muscle activity under the 200 or 500μV/div on a screen. The duration of silent period was expressed as the average of the latencies of all waves recorded.

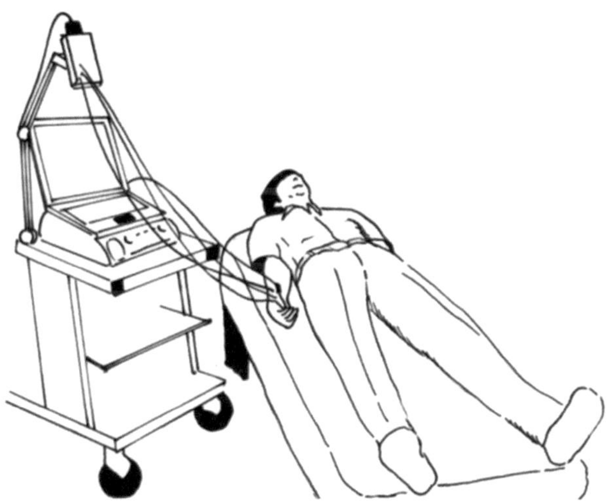

Fig. 2. Experimental landscape in upper extremity study.

The results were as follows; when the electric intensity was changed, the duration of silent period did not vary significantly. However, the silent period was become clearly with increase of intensity of the stimulation (Figure 3) and this mechanism was involved the "collision" effect. And more, with a faster frequency of stimulation, the duration of silent period became significantly shorter (Table 1). The present findings suggested that in silent period measurement, supra-maximal electric stimulation is most suitable. However, for frequency of electric stimulation, 1.0Hz stimulation is not suitable because there is the possibility that CNS is facilitated by the electric stimulation.

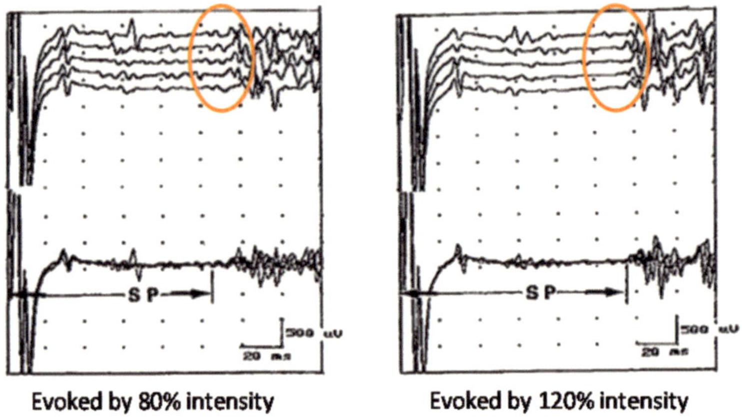

Fig. 3. Silent period due to 80% and 120% electric stimulus of intensity evoked the maximal amplitude of M-wave.
The upper shows typical 5 raw waves and the lower demonstrated the overlaid them.When the weak stimulus was provided, the starting point of muscle bursting was not clear (part of the circle on left figure) compared with providing the strong stimulus (part of the circle on right figure).

Frequency / intensity	80%	100%	120%
0.2Hz	105.3±5.3	107.2±6.5	106.4±6.4
0.5Hz	103.1±5.3	103.6±4.4	102.9±5.5
1.0Hz	102.2±4.6	101.9±4.3	101.8±5.5

(n=9, Average±SD ms)

Table 1. Effect of electric stimulating condition on silent period recording.
Silent period was shortened with increasing stimulation frequency (ANOVA and Tukey: $p<0.05$).

2.2 Silent period aspects in the strength change of background tonic muscle contraction

2.2.1 Upper extremity

We studied the silent period and its relation to isometric contraction in 15 healthy subjects, who were not athletes. Their mean age was 21.4 years. The silent period was recorded from opponens pollicis muscle by electrical stimulation followed by 25%, 50%, 75% and 100% of strength of tonic contraction with the maximal voluntary effort (MVE) under following conditions: subjects were in supine position at rest. The experimental landscape was also shown in Figure 2. Electrical stimulation (intensity: supra-maximal; duration: 0.2ms; frequency: 0.5Hz) was administered to median nerve at wrist. Recording electrode was placed on the opponens pollicis muscle and the reference electrode was put on the distal part of the first proximal phalanx, and samplings were repeated 20 times.
The acquired typical waveforms were demonstrated on Figure 4. Overall average, dominant side average and non-dominant side average in all subjects, the duration of silent period

showed significant differences in all combinations. In particular, the duration of silent period at 75%MVE was shortest (paired t-test; p<0.05, Table 2). This suggests that CNS may be more facilitated during 75%MVE of isometric contraction compared to other levels, and that the 75% level may be most suitable for preparing some types of movements.

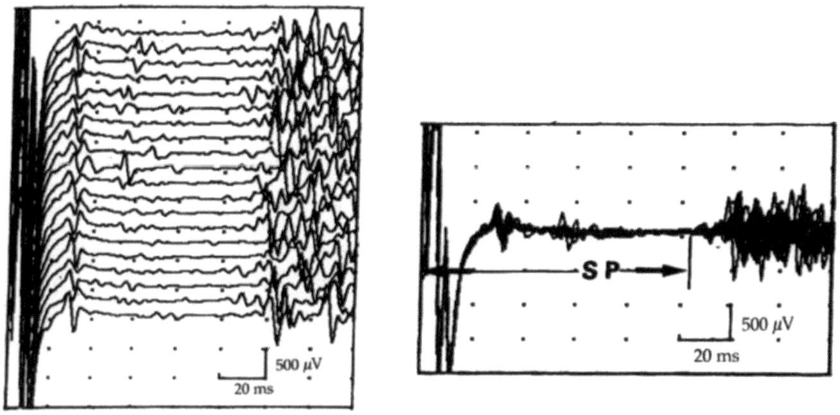

Fig. 4. Typical waveforms of silent period in upper extremity study.
The left figure shows typical 20 raw waves and the right figure demonstrates the overlaid them. Silent period on this figure was recorded at 25%MVE (Maximal Voluntary Effort).

Contraction level	25%MVE	50%MVE	75%MVE	100%MVE
Bilateral	108.8±6.4	106.9±7.2	105.8±6.6	107.6±8.0
Dominant	110.1±5.9	106.7±6.2	105.0±6.5	107.4±7.6
Non-dominant	107.5±6.6	107.1±8.1	106.7±6.6	107.8±8.4

Average±SD ms
MVE: Maximal Voluntary Effort

Table 2. The duration of silent period in the strength change of background tonic muscle contraction in upper extremity.

2.2.2 Lower extremity

The study was performed on the soleus muscles of 10 healthy non-athletes (20 lower extremities of healthy 8 males and 2 females, their mean age 25.2±2.7 years). The silent period was recorded from soleus muscle with same conditions of muscle contraction and sampling numbers as upper extremity. Subjects were in supine position with the hip and knee joints of the recorded side flexed at 45 degrees, and with the ankle joint kept 0 degree (Figure 5). Electrical stimulation was administered to tibial nerve at popliteal fossa with same condition as upper extremity. Recording electrode was placed on the soleus muscle and the reference electrode was put on the ipsilateral Achilles tendon.
The acquired typical waveforms were demonstrated on Figure 6. Similar to the results of upper extremity, the results indicated that the duration of silent period was the shortest during 75% of maximal effort (paired t-test; p<0.05, Table 3). It was considered that the

supra-spinal inhibition was remarkably released during sub-maximal effort level; in other words, CNS was most facilitated during sub-maximal effort.

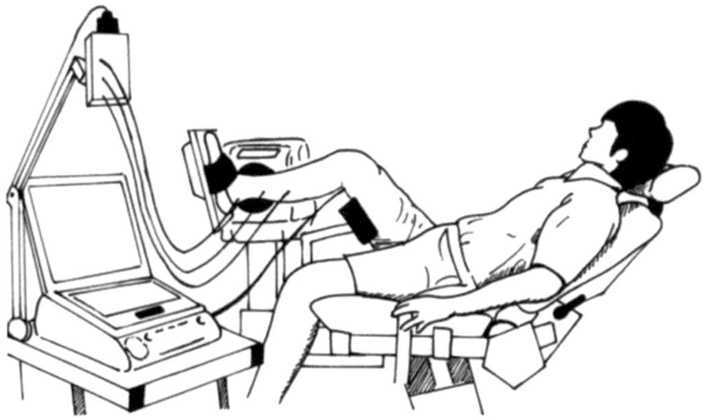

Fig. 5. Experimental landscape in lower extremity study.

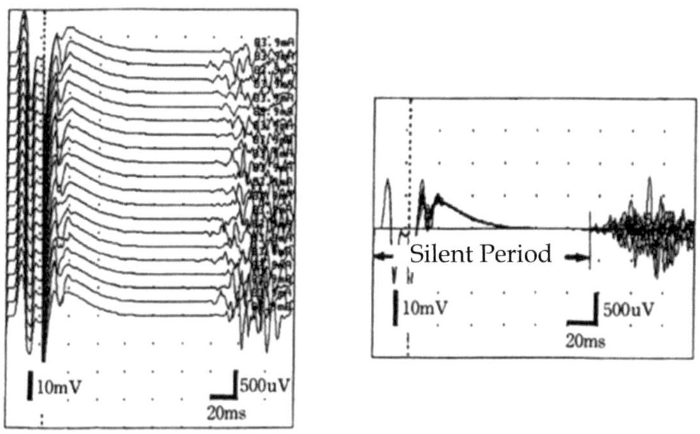

Fig. 6. Typical waveforms of silent period in lower extremity study.
The left figure shows typical 20 raw waves and the right figure demonstrates the overlaid them. Silent period on this figure was recorded at 25%MVE (Maximal Voluntary Effort).

Contraction level	25%MVE	50%MVE	75%MVE	100%MVE
Bilateral	153.0±15.4	142.3±14.2	127.6±14.5	144.3±13.7
Dominant	150.3±14.5	141.2±15.6	127.6±17.5	144.1±13.6
Non-dominant	155.7±16.5	143.4±13.5	127.6±11.7	144.5±14.6

Average±SD ms
MVE: Maximal Voluntary Effort

Table 3. The duration of silent period in the strength change of background tonic muscle contraction in lower extremity.

2.3 Silent period aspects in relation to postural change

2.3.1 Creeping posture

We measured the silent period in 10 healthy right-handed subjects (9 males and 1female), who were not athletes. Their mean age was 24.9±2.6 (range; 21-31) years and mean height was 169.7±7.8 (range; 152-182) cm. The silent period was recorded in the abductor pollicis brevis muscles (APB) of the dominant side. The subjects were asked to adapt 3 positions as follows in a shielded room. The 3 positions were all fours with bilateral elbows not bent (position 1), all fours with bilateral elbows bent at 45 degrees (position 2) and all fours with using the only dominant upper extremity (position 3).

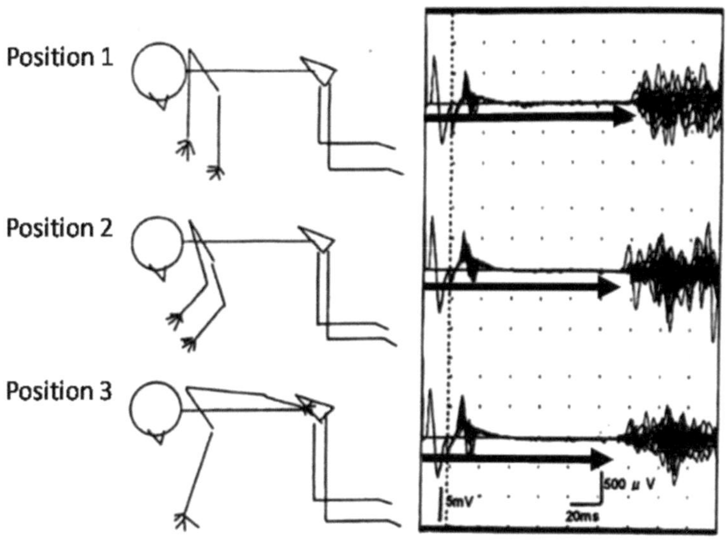

Fig. 7. Typical waveforms of silent period in relation to creeping posture.
The left figure shows the schematic three kinds of creeping postures and the right figures demonstrates the overlaid waveforms of the silent period on each posture.

And we confirmed that amplitudes of background EMG of APB were almost same in all positions. The silent period was recorded at APB with electrical stimulation of the median nerve in each position. The position sequence was randomized, and we let subjects take sufficient inter-test intervals to exclude the influence of contraction and electric stimulation of the previous test or muscle fatigue. Monopolar electrodes were used to measure surface EMG on median nerve stimulation at the wrist, and the sweep lime was 200ms. Electrodes were attached to the APB (recording), and the distal part of the proximal phalanx 1 (reference). The stimulus conditions were as follows; intensity: 1.2 times that which evoked maximum M wave, frequency: 0.5Hz, duration: 0.2ms, and number of recordings: 20 limes.
A representative pattern of the silent period is shown in Figure 7.
Table 4 summarizes the duration of silent period data in each position. The duration of silent period changed with alterations in posture. The duration of silent period in position 3 was the shortest. This finding indicates that the amount of weight bearing has an effect on the silent period and CNS function, because the amount of weight borne by the upper-extremity was the most in position 3.

	Position 1	Position 2	Position 3
Duration of silent period	124.3±15.2	119.6±13.7	112.0±13.9

(Average±SD ms)

Table 4. The duration of silent period from APB in the alteration of creeping postures. The duration of silent period in position 3 was the shortest. And the one in position 2 is shorter than in position 1 and longer than in position 3 (Paired t-test, $p<0.05$).

2.3.2 Standing posture

Subjects were 8 healthy males, with a mean age of 23.5±2.2 (21-27) years and a mean height of 170.8±2.4 (167-175) cm. Every subject's dominant leg was the right leg. The silent period by single stimulation to tibial nerve at the popliteal fossa was recorded from the dominant side soleus and gastrocnemius muscles during ten kinds of standing postures regulated by visual information, supporting or not by a finger and a width of base of support (Figure 8). And the silent period of each muscle was recorded during above ten kinds of standings under the following stimulus and recording conditions. The stimulating condition for

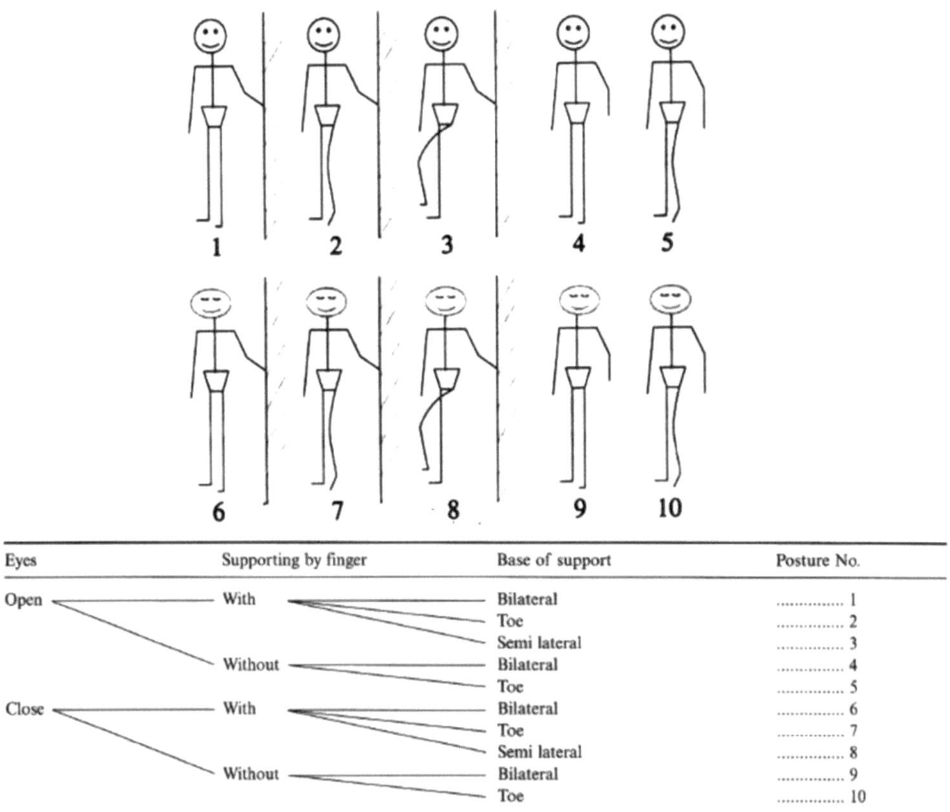

Fig. 8. Ten kinds of standing postures.

recording the silent period was as follows; intensity of supra-maximum, duration of 0.2ms, frequency of 0.5Hz and numbers of 30 times. As to the recording conditions of silent period, recording electrodes were placed on soleus and gastrocnemius (lateral head) muscles and reference electrode was put on the ipsilateral Achilles tendon. Sweep time on recording was 200ms. The raw data were amplified with a band pass between 20Hz and 2000Hz and averaged 30 times by a Nicolet Viking IIe. The silent period was calculated the duration from the artifact due to electrical stimulation to reappearance of uninterrupted voluntary tonic muscle activity under the 100μV or 200 μV/div on a screen. The difference of soleus and gastrocnemius silent periods was compared with the postural alteration as the ten kinds of standings. And a one-way analysis of variance (one-way ANOVA) was used as the statistical method to compare the data.

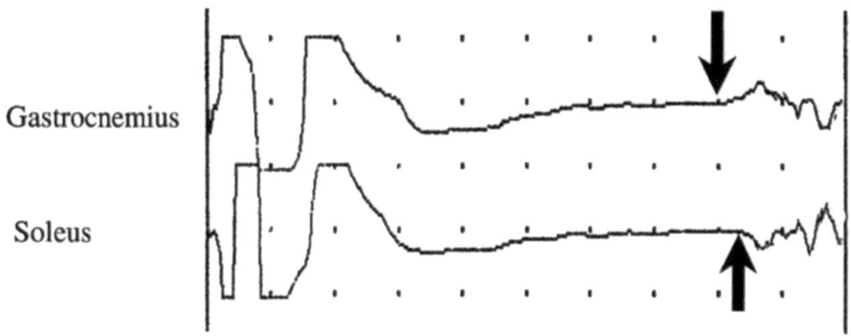

Fig. 9. Typical waveform of silent period on natural standing (posture 1).
Each arrow shows the re-bursting of the muscle activity. Each silent period was calculated the duration from starting of a waveform to a point demonstrated by arrow (22 y.o., male. Gain of amplitude: 100 μ V/div, Sweep: 200ms, Averaged: 30 times.).

Typical wave forms on natural standing of soleus and gastrocnemius silent periods were demonstrated on Figure 9. The duration of silent period on each standing was demonstrated on the Table 5. Both soleus and gastrocnemius silent periods did not change among 10 kinds of standing (One-way ANOVA, $F = 1.797$, $F = 1.786$). It is thought that a variation of the duration of silent period may reflect the magnitude of facilitation or disinhibition of the CNS including spinal, brainstem or motor cortex. As the result of this study in healthy persons, it was suggested that the degree of facilitation or disinhibition of CNS related to silent period from soleus and gastrocnemius was not different on ten kinds of standings regulated by visual information and a width of base of support.

3. Silent period application in the field of sports medicine - Silent period from soleus muscle as an index in a neuro-muscular function after reconstruction of anterior cruciate ligament

To clarify that silent period from soleus muscle may become an index expressed neuro-muscular function after reconstruction of anterior cruciate ligament (ACL), we studied the alteration of silent period from the soleus muscle in the patient with ACL reconstruction. Subjects of this study were three patients with anterior cruciate ligament (ACL) reconstruction, with two male athletes (case A and B) and one female sport instructor (case C). They have consented to be performed an electrophysiological study and to report their

	Gastrocnemius	Soleus
Position 1	160.5±27.3	165.9±26.7
2	135.5±28.9	144.0±28.3
3	129.3±18.9	143.8±18.8
4	146.5±21.3	157.8±17.8
5	130.1±20.4	135.6±20.9
6	157.0±22.2	164.9±19.5
7	136.7±21.8	148.5±24.5
8	121.3±15.9	129.7±14.3
9	147.1±25.1	157.7±21.7
10	137.1±23.3	147.1±23.9

(Average±SD ms)

Table 5. The duration of silent period on each standing.

own data in this study. Case A was a college soccer player for competition level. In rehabilitation process, he remarkably brought his nonl0Perative side lower extremity into the practice of running and cutting. Case B was a high school basketball player for competition level. Much instruction was need to alter his incorrect motion image related to sports activity on time, when his activity was growing in his rehabilitation process. Both case A and B was performed the left side ACL reconstruction immediately after the injury, and they reached to competition level in 6 months after operation. Case C was a sports instructor, and ACL reconstruction was provided to bilateral knee followed a conservative therapy for a few years after ACL tear. Rehabilitation after the operation was focused to acquired ability of her daily life, and she had no trouble when she returned to her occupation.

Rehabilitation protocol after ACL reconstruction was following (Figure 10). Hard type knee brace have been used for two weeks. Four weeks after, full weight bearing was permitted. Following the permission of full weight bearing, such various activities were trained as ambulation, jogging, running, cutting, splinting, jumping, and landing and so on with an adequate graded acquisition of sports activities. For the time of acquisition of sports activities, adequate grading was very important and was emphasized from the point of a dynamic energy and/or an Injury mechanism. Concretely, we have set the rehabilitation protocol as follows; stepping exercise for all direction and slow and fast stamping without sway for up and/or down and left or right were introduced at post eight weeks. From three to four months later, jogging and running without neither starting dash nor sudden stop, and side step cutting were started. At five months, exercises for jumping and landing were introduced. Post six months, which was final stage, following activities were acquired; a pursuit, a flight, a hopping and a contact under a therapist's control.

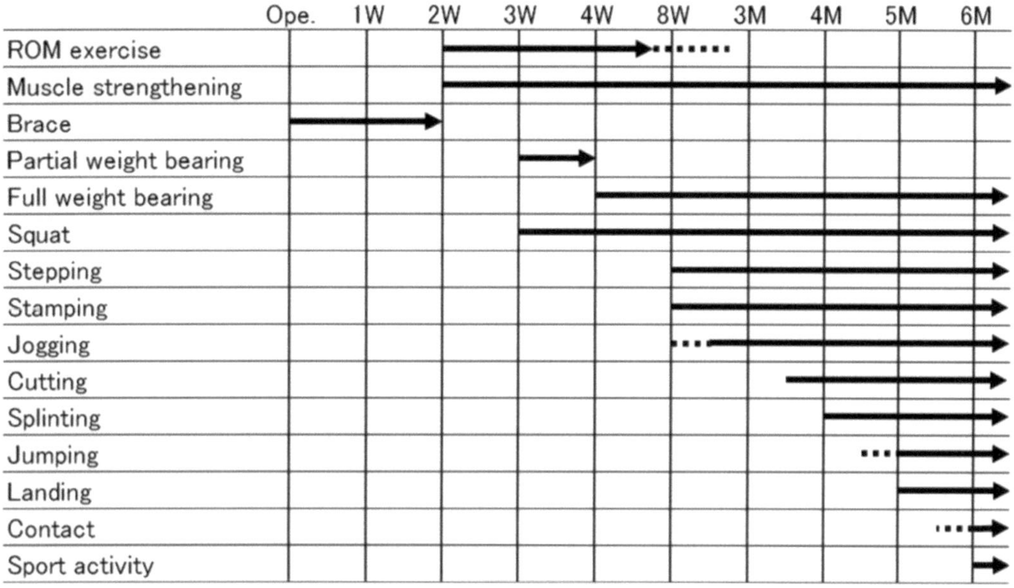

Fig. 10. Rehabilitation protocol after reconstruction of ACL.

Silent period from soleus muscle were recorded at every month after ACL reconstruction from post one month after operation (see Table 6). Silent period from soleus muscle were evoked by single stimulation to tibial nerve at the popliteal fossa on prone position with a tonic slight voluntary contraction of ankle plantar flexion. The stimulating conditions for recording the silent period were as follows; Intensity of supra-maximum, duration of 0.2 ms, frequency of 0.5 Hz and numbers of 16 times. As to the recording conditions of silent period, recording electrodes were placed on soleus muscle (leg medial and 4 or 5cm upper from ankle joint) and reference electrode was put on the ipsilateral attachment of Achilles tendon (calcaneus). Sweep time on recording was 200 ms. The raw data were amplified with a band pass between 20 Hz and 2000 Hz by a Nicolet Viking quest. And we determined a coefficient of variation of the duration of silent period in each recording.

	Post-surgery					
	1 m	2 m	3 m	4 m	5 m	6 m
Case A		Record	Record	Record	Record	
Case B	Record	Record	Record	Record	Record	Record
Case C	Record		Record	Record		Record

Table 6. Recording sessions of silent period in Case A, B and C.
Silent period was recorded for each subject at monthly intervals after ACL reconstruction as frequently as possible from one to six months post-surgery.
All subjects were able to return to sporting competition or her occupation at six months after their operations. (m: months)

Acquired raw waveforms, and the duration and the coefficient of variation of silent period in every subject were demonstrated in Figure 11-16. With case A, silent period of non-operative side shortened and a coefficient of variation of silent period increased in time of 2 months and 4months after the ACL reconstruction. In case B, bilateral silent period had no tendency in the mean value, however as for a coefficient of variation of silent period, it was little on non-operative side and it was large on operative side. Also, on operative side from one month to four months after ACL reconstruction, the fluctuation of silent period became large, and after four months it became the same as one of non-operative side. Furthermore, from one month after the operation, the long latency reflex (LLR) appeared in silent period

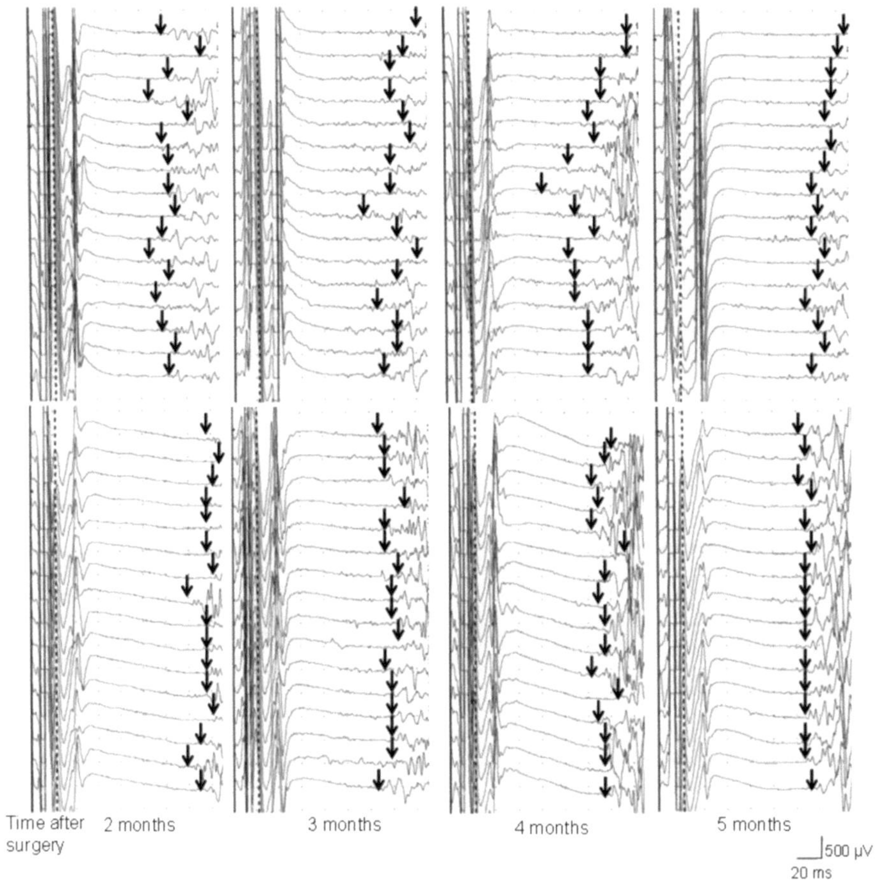

Fig. 11. Typical waveform of silent periods in Case A (Upper: non-operative side, Lower: operative side).
In non-operative side, a shortening of the duration and an increase in the coefficient of variation of the silent period were observed at 2 and 4 months post-surgery, when his overuse of the non-operative lower extremity was detected during sporting activity.
In operative side, no remarkable finding was observed and it was clarified that his neural functions related to soleus on the operative side did not change during the course of rehabilitation (Arrows show re-bursting points of voluntary muscle activation. The silent period was identified by the duration after the arrow).

recording, and it became most remarkable in four months and disappeared in six months after ACL reconstruction. With case C, remarkable and characteristic finding was not obtained in both duration and coefficient of variation of silent period.

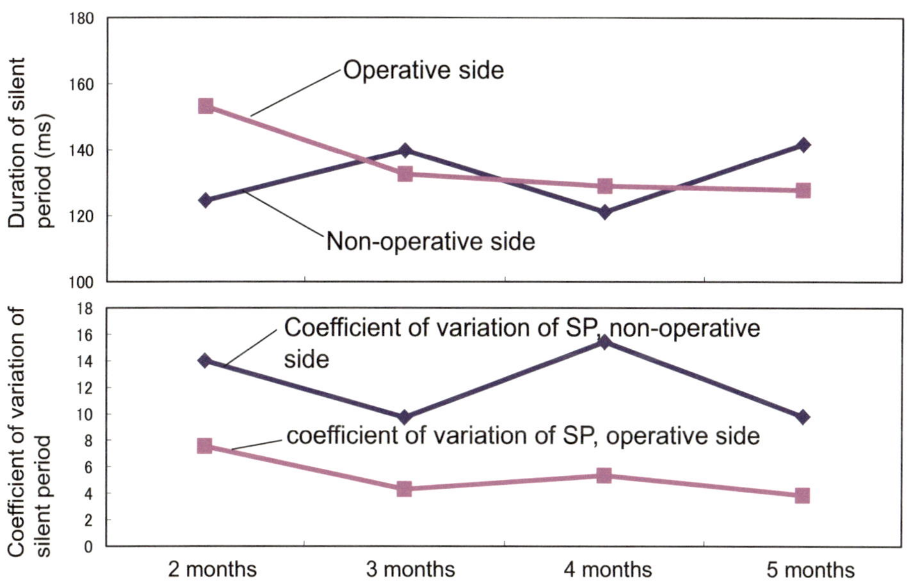

Fig. 12. The duration and coefficient of variation of silent period in Case A.
Coefficient of variation of the silent period increased at two and four months after ACL reconstruction.

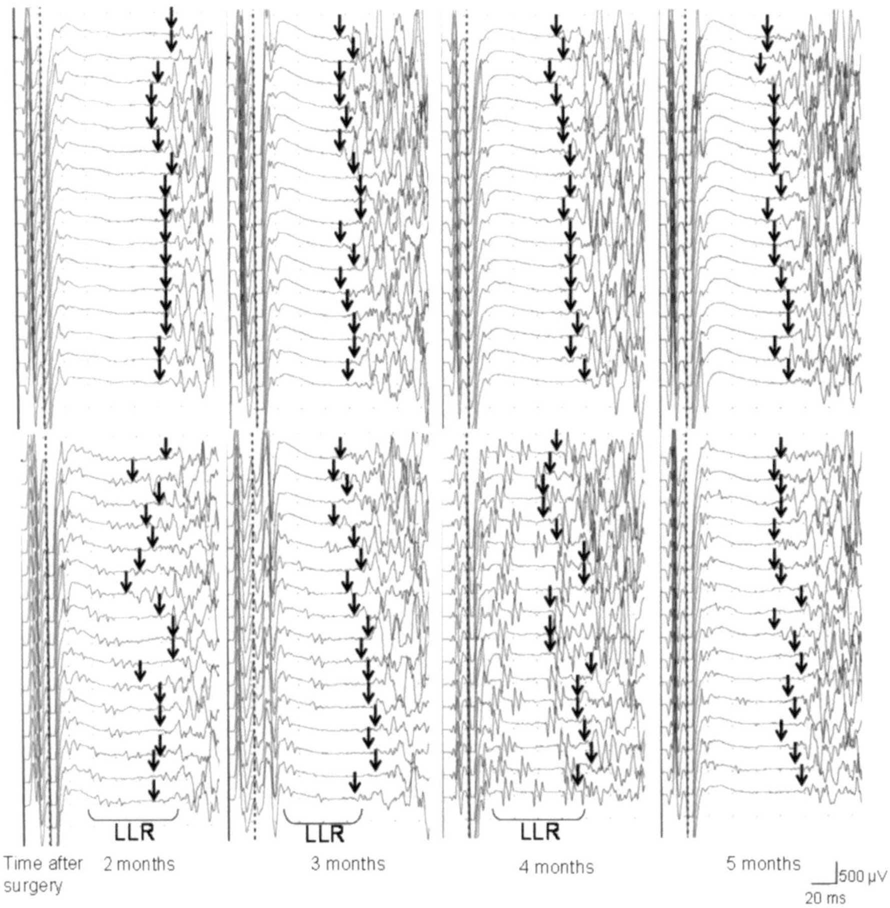

Fig. 13. Typical waveform of silent periods in Case B (Upper: non-operative side, Lower: operative side).
In non-operative side, no remarkable finding of the silent period was not observed.
In operative side, the appearance of LLR was the most clearest at 4 months post-surgery. After 4 months was the period when the patient had to re-acquire various activities at a higher rate and involved rapid step cutting in various directions. Large silent period variations indicated that this activated various neural functions (i.e., polysynaptic reflex on spinal and/or supra-spinal nervous system).
Arrows show re-bursting points of voluntary muscle activation. The silent period was identified by the duration after the arrow.

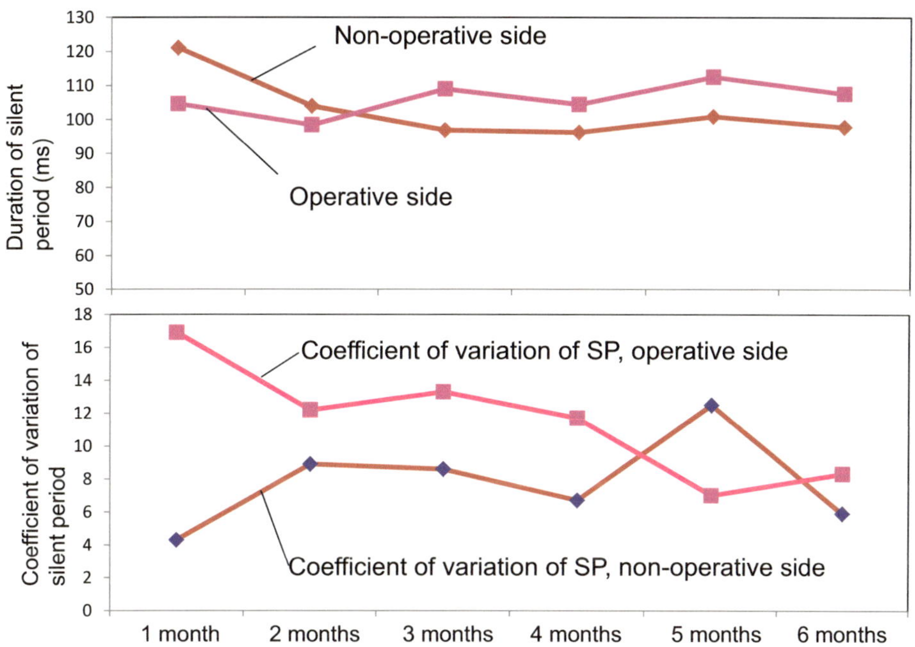

Fig. 14. The duration and coefficient of variation of silent period in Case B.
The large variation in the silent period from one to five months after operation needed to activate various neural functions (i.e., polysynaptic reflex on spinal and/or supra-spinal nervous system) for ankle plantar flexion in the prone position.

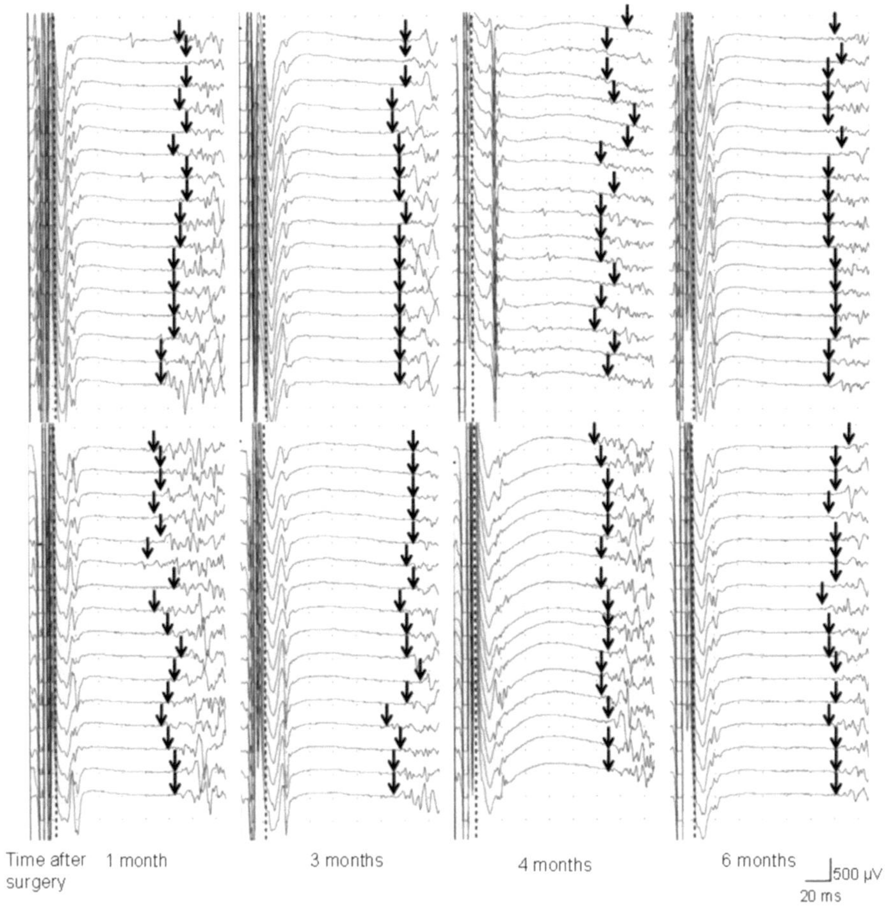

Fig. 15. Typical waveform of silent periods in Case C (bilateral reconstruction, Upper: right side, Lower: left side).
No remarkable findings of the silent period were observed on the non-operative side (Arrows show re-bursting points of voluntary muscle activation. The silent period was identified by the duration after the arrow.)

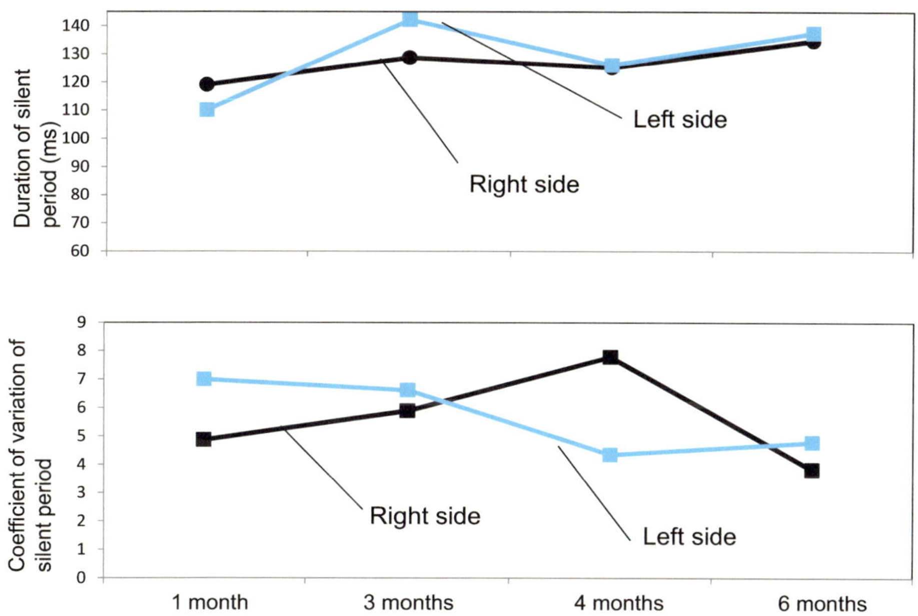

Fig. 16. The duration and coefficient of variation of the silent period in Case C. There was no typical finding.

From a result of this experiment, non-operative side silent period in case A presented a shortening of the duration and an increase of coefficient of variation of silent period when we could see his overusing activity of non-operative lower extremity in the sports activity. From the results of the shortening of the duration of silent period in case A, following speculation about neuro-muscular function of case A was acquired. When his overusing activity of non-operative side was observed, the excitability of spinal neural function has increased and supra-spinal neural function also has affected by his overuse. In operative side of case B, the appearance of LLR and the increase of coefficient of variation of silent period in simultaneous period were observed when much guidance was required in order to correct motion image in operative side. The appearance of LLR in operative side was most remarkably four months after the operation. As for the rehabilitation for the patient with ACL reconstruction, from operation to four months later, various activities has to be acquired; i.e., from no to full weight-bearing ambulation, squatting, jogging, and cutting. Therefore, they have to acquire the various activities rapidly within four months after the operation. With case B, his large silent period variation within four months after the operation indicated that it needed to activate various neural functions (i.e., polysynaptic reflex on spinal and/or supra-spinal nervous system) for ankle plantar flexion on prone position, which is easy and simple task. In case C, remarkable problem related to acquire the activity of daily life and to return her occupation did not appear, and she did not have any clinical findings in silent period. As for this, it was thought that neurological function related to silent period from soleus muscle did not affect with ACL reconstruction due to a long term conservative therapy and a sequential reconstruction in both side. Like above, it has been verified that silent period from soleus muscle has the possibility of reflecting the neural function according to recovery situation after the ACL reconstruction from three cases findings. Concretely, it has been cleared that silent period can become an index expressed neuro-muscular function during a process of acquisition the various activity, the motor learning and the adaptation after ACL reconstruction with a recovery state from injury and operation.

4. Conclusion

4.1 Clinical findings from healthy subject

From the examination in the healthy person, following findings were existed;

1. The duration of silent period was changed by strength of tonic muscle contraction.
2. The duration of silent period was also altered by intensity of muscle contraction of remote parts.
3. The duration of silent period was affected with amount of load of weight to extremity including recording muscle.
4. The duration of silent period was also affected with amount of load of weight to remote part.

4.2 Clinical application of silent period in the field of sports medicine

About the clinical application of silent period for the evaluation of neuro-muscular function in the field of the sports medicine and rehabilitation, we mention like below based on the experiment aimed at healthy subjects and its application to the patient with ACL reconstruction.

The silent period from soleus muscle has become an index expressed neuro-muscular function of lower extremity and supra-spinal function in the patient after reconstruction of ACL. From the examination in cases after the reconstruction of ACL, following findings were existed;

1. The duration and aspects of silent period have become the proof of observation view of case's sports activity and were able to become the index of the neuro-muscular function in the recovery phase after ACL reconstruction.
2. Silent period can apply to the evaluation of CNS function in the field of sports science, because the fluctuation of silent period was useful to search the adequate condition of readiness of sports activity and was able to clear the clinical and observational impression about athletes' sports activity.

5. References

Anastasijevic R & Vuco J (1980): Renshaw cell discharge at the beginning of muscular contraction and its relation to the silent period. *Experimental Neurology,* Vol.69, No.3, (Sep 1980), pp.589-598, ISSN 0014-4886.

Behm DG & St-Pierre DM (1997): Effects of fatigue duration and muscle type on voluntary and evoked contractive properties. *Journal of Applied Physiology,* Vol. 82, No.5, (May 1997), pp.1654-1661, ISSN 8750-7587.

Calancie B.; Nordin M, Wallin U & Hagbarth KE (1987): Motor-unit responses in human wrist flexor and extensor muscles to transcranial cortical stimuli. *Journal of Neurophysiology,* Vol.58, No.5, (Nov 1987), pp.1168-1185, ISSN 0022-3077.

Cupido CM.; Hicks AL & Martin J (1992): Neuromuscular fatigue during repetitive stimulation in elderly and young adults. *European Journal of Applied Physiology and Occupational Physiology* Vol.65, No.6, (1992), pp.567-572, ISSN 0301-5548.

Daikuya S.; Tanino Y, Nishimori T, Takasaki K & Suzuki T (2003): The silent period from soleus and gastrocnemius muscles in relation to conditions of standing. *Electromyography and Clinical Neurophysiology,* Vol.43, No.4, (June 2003), pp.217-222, ISSN 0301-150X

Fuglevand AJ.; Zackowski KM, Huey KA & Enoka RM (1993): Impairment of neuromuscular propagation during human fatiguing contraction at submaximal force. *Journal of Physiology,* Vol.460, (Jan 1993), pp.549-572, ISSN 0022-3751.

Higgins DC & Lieberman JS (1968): The muscle silent period and spindle function in man. *Electroencephalography and Clinical Neurophysiology,* Vol.25, No.3, (Sep 1968), pp.238-243, ISSN 1388-2457.

Ikai M (1955): Inhibition as an accompaniment of rapid voluntary act (Summary in English). *Nippon Seirigaku Zasshi (Journal of the Physiological Society of Japan),* Vol. 17, (1955), pp.292-298, ISSN 0031-9341.

Kimura J (2001): *Electrodiagnosis in diseases of nerve and muscle: principles and practice. Ed 3.,* Oxford university press, ISBN 0-19-512977-6, NY, USA.

Kuroiwa Y (1986): Long-loop reflex. *Rinsho Nouha (Clinical electroencephalography),* Vol.28, (1986), pp.353-362, ISSN 0485-1447. (Abstract in English)

Roby-Brami A & Bussel B (1987): Long-latency spinal reflex in man after flexor reflex afferent stimulation. *Brain,* Vol.110, No.Pt3, (Jun 1987), pp.707-725, ISSN 0006-8950.

Suzuki T.; Fujiwara T & Takeda I (1993): Excitability of the spinal motor neuron pool and F-waves during isometric ipsilateral and contralateral contraction. *Physiotherapy Theory and Practice,* Vol.9, (1993), pp.19-24, ISSN 0959-3985.

Upton AR.; McComas AJ & Sica RE (1971): Potentiation of 'late' responses evoked in muscles during effort. *Journal of Neurology, Neurosurgery & Psychiatry,* Vol.34, No.6, (Dec 1971), pp.699-711, ISSN 0022-3050.

Yabe K (1976): Premotion silent period in rapid voluntary movement. *Journal of Applied Physiology,* Vol.41, No.4, (Oct 1976), pp.470-473, ISSN 8750-7587.

Part 3

Diagnostics

11

Middle and Long Latency Auditory Evoked Potentials and Their Usage in Fibromyalgia and Schizophrenia

Hande Turker, Ayhan Bilgici[1] and Huseyin Alpaslan Sahin
Ondokuz Mayis University School of Medicine, Department of Neurology, Samsun
[1]Ondokuz Mayis University School of Medicine, Department of Physical Therapy and Rehabilitation, Samsun
Turkey

1. Introduction

1.1 Middle and long latency auditory evoked potentials and their usage in fibromyalgia

FM is a chronic syndrome that occurs predominantly in women and is marked by generalized pain, multiple defined tender points, fatigue, disturbed sleep, cognitive difficulty, and numerous other somatic complaints. The etiology and pathophysiology of FM remain unclear. Despite extensive research, no structural pathology has been identified in muscles or other tissues. The general and widespread nature of pain in FM strongly suggests the involvement of central mechanisms (Williams et al., 2006). Although psychological factors associated with chronic distress appear to be important for the development of FM in many patients, abundant evidence now indicates that pain in FM reflects abnormal pain processing in the central nervous system (ie. central sensitivity) (Herrero JF et al., 2000, Staud R. et al, 2001). Recent research suggested that FM patients might have deficiencies in central inhibitory mechanisms, such as diffuse noxious inhibitory control or the endogenous pain inhibitory system. Nevertheless, little is yet known about the brain mechanisms involved in the processing of nonpainful somatosensory information in FM (Monyoto P et al., 2006, Julien N. Et al., 2005).

Central mechanisms related to pathophysiology and hypervigilance have long been discussed for fibromyalgia. Nevertheless, research into this issue has been inconclusive so far. Our aim to design this study (Turker et al., 2008) was to determine whether central mechanisms played an important role in fibromyalgia via examining brain activity elicited by auditory evoked potentials in patients with FM and to assess relationship with clinical variables.

Middle latency evoked potentials (Middle Latency Auditory Evoked Potentials) are composed of several components that can be recorded from 10 to 50 msec after stimulus onset. The most stable components are Na and Pa, with latencies between 16-30 msec and 30-45 msec, respectively. Most of the MLAEP complex is thought to originate near the auditory cortex, although No, Po and Na may be generated by subcortical structures.

1.2 Patients and methods

33 female patients with a diagnosis of FM and 37 healthy women participated in the study. All patients met the American College of Rheumatology (ACR) criteria for FM (Wolfe et al., 1990).

Eighteen tender points accepted by the ACR for FM were evaluated. Each tender point was rated from 0 point (no pain) to 3 points (most severe pain). The sum of the 18 tender points was calculated as the total myalgic score (TMS). Other symptoms of FM were evaluated by using the Fibromyalgia Impact Questionaire (FIQ) and Health Assesment Questionary (HAQ) (Küçükdeveci et al.,2004,Bennett et al.,2005). The HAQ functional disability index was used to assess functional status. The instrument asks 24 questions regarding 8 activities of daily living areas.

The FIQ is a 20-item, self report instrument that measures multiple symptoms, functioning, and overall well-being. The first 10 items comprise a physical functioning scale; each item is rated on a 3-point Likert-type scale. On items 11 and 12, subjects indicate the days that they feel well or miss work because of fibromyalgia symptoms. Items 14 through 20 rate the difficulty in performing their job responsibilities, pain, fatigue, morning tiredness, stiffness, anxiety, and depression on a 10-cm visual analog scales (VAS). All subscores with the exception of the two work-related scores and physical function score were summed to yield the total score of fibromyalgia impact, which ranges from 0 (no impact) to 70 (maximum impact). Global disease severity was assessed with visual analogue scale (VAS) (0=very good, 10=very poor). The Hamilton Rating Scale for Depression and Hamilton Rating Scale for Anxiety were used to evaluate the affective condition of patients with FM (Hamilton et al., 1967).

Patients were excluded if they had evidende of traumatic injury, inflammatory rheumatic disease, a history of seizure, head trauma, or cerebrovascular disease; a lifetime history of pyschosis, or dementia; alcohol or substance dependence; if they received psychiatric treatment in the last 3 weeks or if there was a history of auditory impairment.

1.3 Evoked potentials recording procedure

All recordings of MLAEPs were performed at Dantec Keypoint. Electrode montage was adjusted as active electrode placed on ipsilateral mastoid and reference and ground electrodes at Cz and Fz, respectively. Silver surface electrodes were used for reference and ground electrodes. A scalp needle electrode was used as active electrode. Alternating clicks of 100 μsec duration were used and polarity was adjusted as vertex. The frequency of stimulation was 10/sec and the filtering was chosen as 10 Hz–200 Hz. Analysis time (sweep length) and sensitivity were 100msec and 0,2 μv/d, respectively. The intensity of the stimuli was chosen according to the auditory threshold. The ipsilateral ear was stimulated with an intensity of stimulus such as hearing threshold plus 60 DB, while the contralateral ear was masked with white noise. Averaging of 1000 signals was performed twice and overlapped for each ear. No, Po, Na, Pa, Nb, and Pb were sampled and latencies and amplitudes of each potential were determined and compared with age and gender matched controls. MLAEPs recordings were performed bilateraly i.e. 30 recordings were performed for patients and 30 recordings were performed for controls making a total of 60 recordings. No artifact rejection was employed. As hearing impairment can alter the MLAEPs, prior to beginning testing, the external ear canal was checked with an otoscope to assure that the canal was not blocked by cerumen. Patients with hearing problems assessed by otologic tests were excluded. MLAEPs

are known to be affected by medications, however all patients were under treatment and there was no other way to investigate them.
Recordings of MLAEPs and LLAEPs (Long latency auditory evoked potentials) were performed for both patients and controls, using an active electrode placed on ipsilateral mastoid and reference and ground electrodes at Cz and Fz, respectively. Binaural stimulation was performed for LLAEPs. No, Po, Na, Pa, Nb, and Pb were sampled for MLAEPs. N1, P1, N2 and P2 were sampled for LLAEPs. Latencies and amplitudes of each potential were compared with those of controls and correlation between clinical and electrophysiological parameters were investigated statistically. Our study was approved by the local committee of ethics.

1.4 Statistical methods

Statistical evaluation of data was performed via using descriptive statistical methods such as mean and standard deviations while student T test was used for quantitative data showing normal statistical distribution. Pearson and Spearman's correlation analysis methods were used to investigate the correlation between latencies of MLAEP and clinical parameters. The results were evaluated at a confidency interval of 95% and a statistical significancy of $p < 0.05$. Comparisons between groups were made using the chi-square test for categorical variables. No statistically significant differences were recognized in the comparison of demographical data (age, disease duration, education, occupation, education level and marital status) between the groups. Clinical measures of patients are shown in table 1.

Clincal parameter	Mean ± SD
HAQ (0-3)	0,87 ± 0,48
Number of tender points(11-18)	14,90 ± 4,14
Total myalgia score	35,09 ± 13,22
Anxiety score	23,06 ± 9,75
Depression score	19,15 ± 8,94
Global disease severity(0-10)	6,72 ± 1,89
	Mean ± SD
FIQ Total (0-70)	51,57 ± 15,08
Physical function score (0 – 30)	11,63 ± 5,49

HAQ: Health Assesment Questionary FIQ: Fibromyalgia Impact Questionaire

Table 1. Clinical measures of patients.

1.5 Results

The latencies of Na, Nb and Pb of MLAEPs in the patient group were statistically longer when compared with those of the healthy controls ($p<0.05$, $p<0.01$ and $p<0.01$ respectively). However No, Po and Pa did not show any statistical significant difference between the groups (Student t test). Latency of Na had statistically significant positive correlations with disease duration, FIQ total score, physical score and number of tender points ($p<0.05$). Latency of Pa had statistically significant positive correlations with age, disease duration, FIQ total score, physical score and FIQ 2, FIQ 3, FIQ 4 and FIQ 6 ($p<0.05$, $p<0.01$, $p<0.05$, $p<0.05$, $p<0.01$, and $p<0.05$ for the rest respectively) (Figure 1). Latency of Nb had statistically significant positive correlations with disease duration ($p<0.05$) (Figure 2), FIQ total score ($p<0.05$), FIQ 2 ($p<0.01$), FIQ 6 ($p<0.05$), global disease severity ($p<0.05$). Latency of Pb had statistically significant positive correlations with FIQ total score ($p<0.05$), FIQ 2 ($p<0.05$) and global disease severity ($p<0.05$) (Pearson and Spearman's correlation tests). Evaluation of groups regarding parameters of LLAEP showed that latencies of P1, N2 and P2 were statistically longer when compared with those of the healthy controls ($p<0.05$, $p<0.01$ and $p<0.01$ respectively) whereas N1 did not show any statistical significancy between the groups (Student t test).

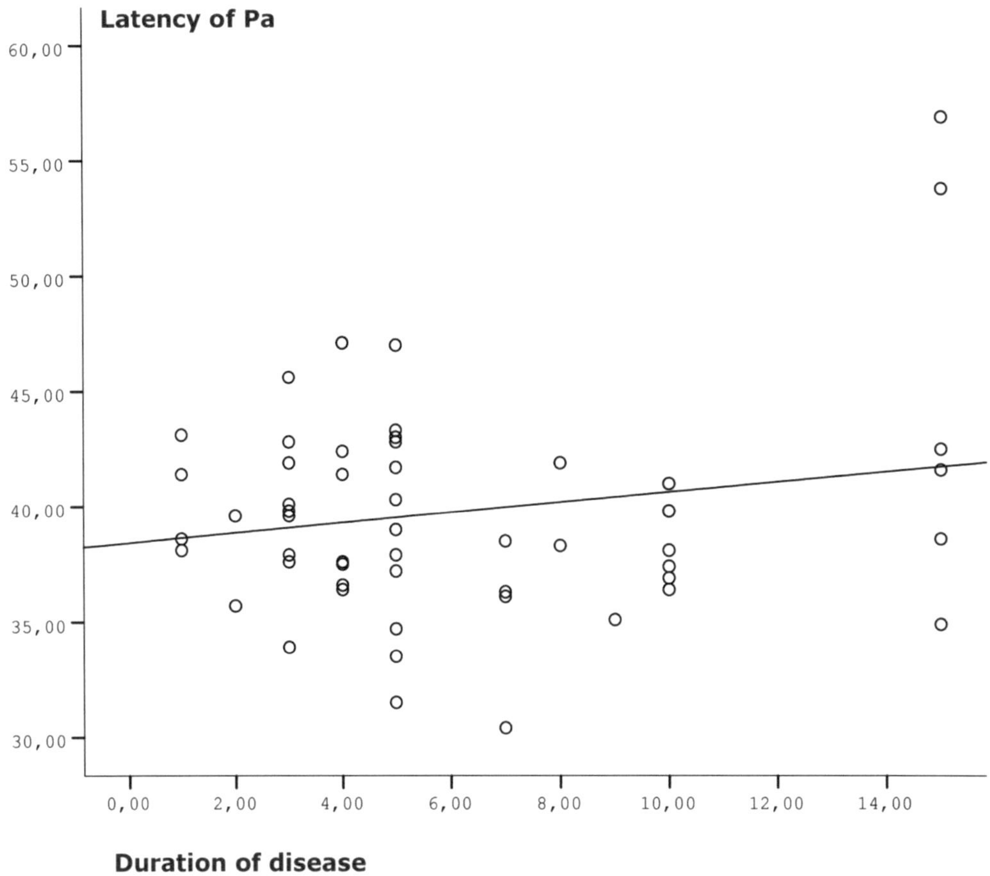

Fig. 1. Correlation analysis of Pa latency and disease duration.

Correlation studies of latencies of LLAEPs with clinical parameters showed that FIQ total score had a positive and statistically significant correlation with latency of N2 ($p<0.05$), while the same was valid for physical score and FIQ2 with latency of N1 ($p<0.05$). FIQ 5, 7 and 8 were positively correlated with latency of N2 ($p<0.05$, $p<0.01$ and $p<0.01$ respectively), while FIQ 9 and 10 were positively correlated with latency of N1 ($p<0.01$, $p<0.05$ respectively). HAQ and anxiety score had positive correlations with latency of N2 ($p<0.05$).

The amplitudes of Po, Pa and Nb of MLAEPs and P1, N1, P2 and N2 of LLAEPs in the patient group were statistically significantly very low when compared with those of the healthy controls ($p<0.01$) (Student t test). However, there were not any statistical significant differences of amplitudes of MLAEPs and LLAEPs between patients having different disease durations. Patients suffering from fibromyalgia for five or more than five years did not show statistically higher or lower amplitudes when compared with patients having the disease for less than five years. Patients having myalgia scores equal or more than 40 also did not show any statistical differences of amplitudes of MLAEPs and LLAEPs when compared with patients having myalgia scores less than 40. Patients having anxiety scores equal or more than 25 were also compared with the ones having scores less than 25 and no statistically significant differences of amplitudes were found. Same results were obtained when patients were compared regarding latencies of both MLAEPs and LLAEPs.

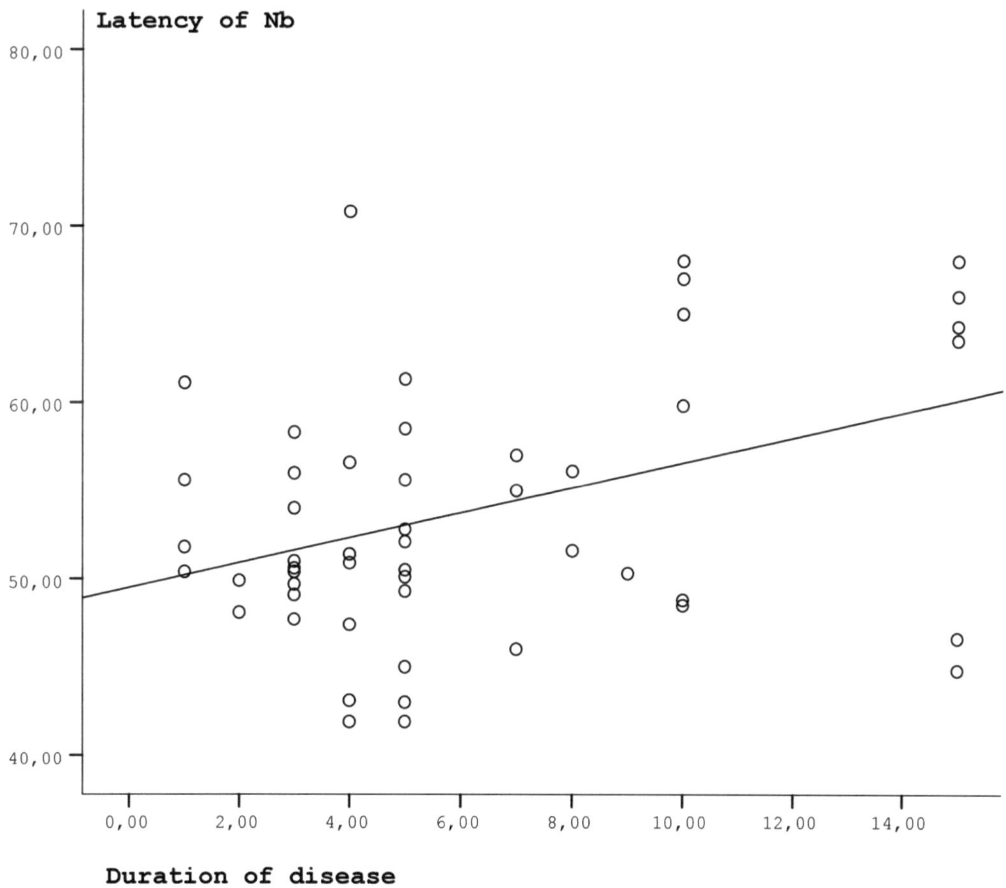

Fig. 2. Correlation analysis of Nb latency and disease duration.

A LLAEP trace of one of the patients with long latencies is shown in Fig. 3.

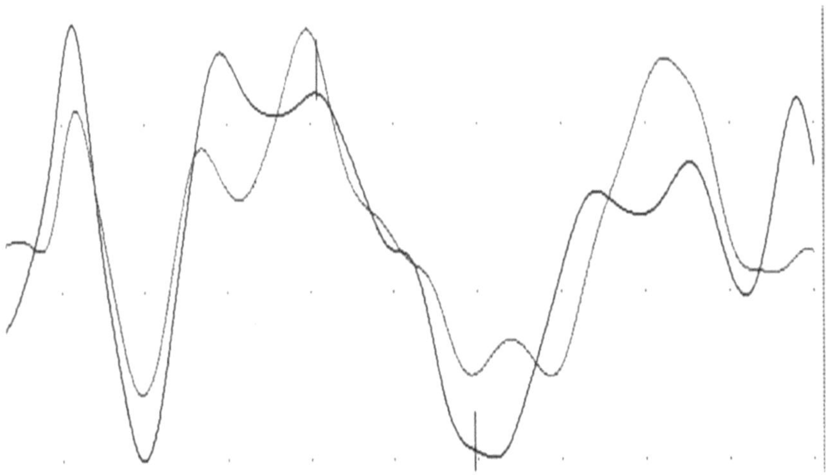

Fig. 3. A LLAEP trace of one of the patients with long latencies.

Correlation studies of amplitudes of LLAEPs with clinical parameters did not point out to any results of statistical significancy, whereas only one electrophysiological parameter in MLAEP amplitudes did. Amplitude of No showed a negative correlation with number of tender points ($p<0.05$) (Figure 4).

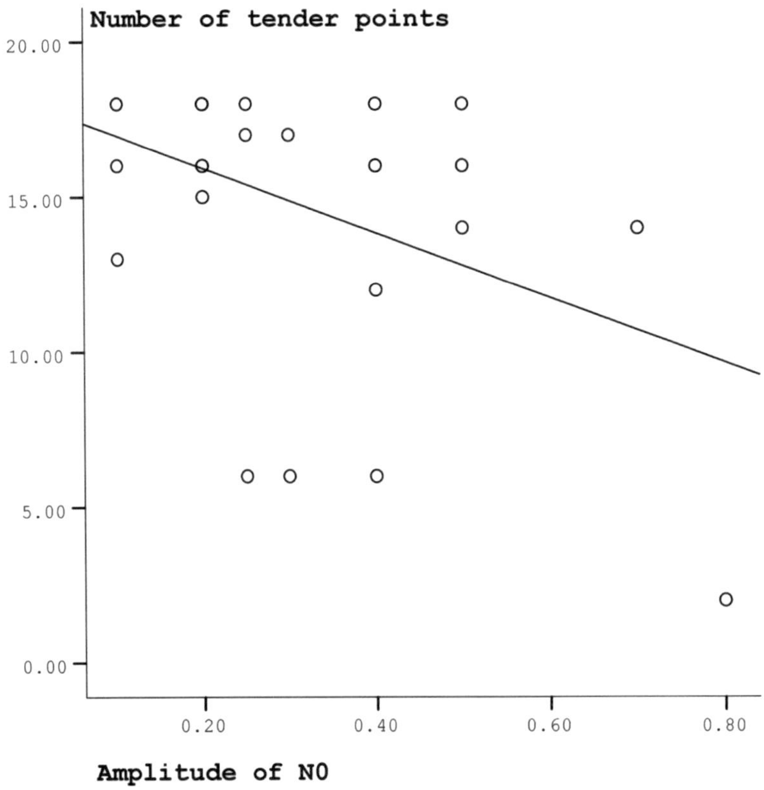

Fig. 4. Correlation analysis of number of tender points and amplitude of No.

Latencies of Na, Nb and Pb were statistically significantly longer in the patient group when compared with controls ($p<0.05$ and $p<0.01$ respectively).
The most important results for our study pointed out that Na, Pa and Nb latencies had positive correlations with disease duration which were statistically significant ($p<0.05$, $p<0.01$ and $p<0.05$ respectively) while the correlations between Na and HAQ and myalgia scores were positive although statistically insignificant ($p>0.05$). On the other hand, the number of tender points had a statistically significant positive correlation with Na ($p<0.05$). FIQ2 scores had negative and statistically very significant correlations with Pa and Nb ($p<0.01$ for both) while FIQ3 and FIQ scores had statistically positive correlations with Pa ($p<0.05$).

1.6 Discussion

Since 1990s, some possible explanations for the involvement of central pathways in fibromyalgia are discussed in various papers, though their number is still limited. To our knowledge, correlation of clinical parameters of fibromyalgia with MLAEPs has not been studied before.
In 1995, Johansson et al., reported significant focal flow decreases in dorsolateral frontal cortical areas of both hemispheres of fibromyalgic patients (Johansson et al., 1995). The AEPs also showed signs of dysfunction at least at the brainstem level. A large group of fibromyalgia patients were studied electrophysiologically by Rosenhall et al. in 1996 and significant differences were found in the study group regarding absolute and interpeak latencies in short latency AEPs, when compared with normals (Rosenhall et al, 1996). However sensorineural hearing loss was reported in 15% of patients. Bayazit et al., also studied short latency AEPs in fibromyalgia patients with and without cochleovestibular symptoms and reported no statistical difference of AEP abnormalities in these subgroups indicating that FM patients might complain of otologic symptoms without having a detectable ear disease and that a neural disintegration or some other events related to neural mediators might be the mechanism involved (Bayazit et al.,2002). Our group of patients did not have otological symptoms, however their MLAEPs showed statistically significant differences when compared with normal controls. This result of our study may be considered as being in agreement with the above study. Fann et al. studied MLAEPs in a similar patient group (chronic low back pain) and found a trend of increased latencies and lower amplitudes of P50 potential in the study group reporting also a decreased habituation of this very potential (Fann et al.,2005). Our study also indicated that Na, Nb and Pb (namely N16, N40 and P50 potentials) had longer latencies in the patient group when compared with normals. The origins of MLAEPs are still controversial. Most authors share the opinion that Pa potential (P30) is generated in the supratemporal auditory center of each hemisphere, but it is not clear that Pa represents the earliest cortical auditory response. Na and Pa are believed to be related with the activation of of the primary auditory cortex. Some authors imply that Pa is generated in the auditory cortex while Na is originated subcortically. No, Po and Na have origins of subcortical structures while most other MLAEP potentials have origins generated from sites near the auditory cortex. In 1991 Erwin RJ et al. reported that P50 (Pb) was generated in thalamus (Erwin RJ et al., 1991). In a review of functional MRI (Magnetic resonance imaging) findings in FM, decreased rCBF (regional cerebral blood flow) in the thalamus and in the caudate nucleus was reported as results of various studies, nevertheless indicating the fact that this finding was not unique to FM.

Latency, on the other hand, has been shown to reflect the efficiency and speed of information processing in cognitive function (Gracely et al., 2002).
Thus results of our study may well be interpreted that FM patients show a slower speed of information processing in areas which are responsible for complex auditory perceptions related highly to cognitive functions. In 2006 Montaya et al. found significant amplitude reductions in FM patients for the auditory but not the somatosensory modality and suggested also that there was abnormal information processing in FM patients characterized by a lack of inhibitory control to repetitive nonpainful somatosensory information during stimulus coding and cognitive evaluation (Montoya et al., 2006). Roth et al. also stated that women with chronic pain were particularly vulnerable to cognitive dysfunction in a study designed as a cross-sectional survey (Roth et al., 2005).

1.7 Conclusion

Our results may be interpreted that central mechanisms may be important in the evolution of fibromyalgia. CNS dysfunction may be both an etiological factor in the fibromyalgia syndrome and a pathophysiological mechanism explaining the clinical symptoms and signs.

2. The relationship between middle latency auditory evoked responses, and the neuropsychological profile in patients with schizophrenia

2.1 Introduction

Although variable time ranges are described for MLAEPs, recent reliable sources report that the middle latency auditory evoked responses (MLAEPs) are far-field potentials that appear between 10-50 ms following an auditory stimulus and are recorded on vertex. The upper range limit is also reported as 80-100 ms in some sources (Buchwald et al., 1989; Buchwald et al., 1991; Erwin et al., 1986; Erwin et al., 1987; Mauguire et al., 2007). Far field potentials are generated by movement of the charge, but the electrode sees the moving front of depolarization and repolarization rather than the direct charge flow between regions of depolarization and repolarization. Most evoked potentials are generated by charge movement in nerve tracts to and from the relay nuclei and are far-field potentials because of the depth of the neural generators. The near-synchronous volley of action potentials in the nerve tracts produces far-field potentials that are recorded at scalp electrodes (Mauguire et al., 2007).
In literature, it has been assumed that MLAEPs are composed of six waves; No, Po, Na, Pa, Nb, Pb. No and Po are the the earliest responses. Pa and Pb (P1, P50) are defined as positive waves occurring in the 29 msec and 45 msec after a stimulus, while Na and Nb are negative deflections in the 25 msec and 50 msec, respectively. The neural sources of these waves are still controversial (Misulis et al., 2001, Cacace et al., 1990). Most of the MLAEP complex is thought to originate near the auditory cortex, although No, Po and Na may be generated by subcortical structures.
Among components of MLAEPs, the most commonly studied wave is the Pb (synonyms: P1 or P50). The P1 potential is blocked by the muscarinic anticholinergic drugs. It is present during waking and rapid eye movement sleep and does not exist during deep slow wave sleep. It has also been reported that the P1 component may be associated with cognitive processes, especially attention and state. Abnormalities of MLAEPs have been reported in some neurodegenerative and psychiatric diseases such as Alzheimer's disease, Parkinson's

disease, schizophrenia, Huntington disease and autism (Buchwald et al.,1989, Woods et al., 1987, Green et al., 1995).

It has been assumed that latency in evoked potential studies reflect the efficiency and speed of information processing. Thus, the prolonged latency may reflect that the information processing speed slowed. Amplitude abnormalites, on the other hand, refer to axonal loss in related areas and show the overall efficiency of neural structures mediating a response.

Over thirty years, various MLAEP studies have been performed in patients with schizophrenia. In most of these studies, the sensory gating paradigm has been investigated and they demonstrated the P1 habituating phenomenon, recovery cycle abnormalities and P1 suppression deficiency (Aminoff et al., 1990; Buchwald et al., 1992; Dickerson et al., 1991). However the relationship between the P1 latencies, amplitudes and neurocognitive status stil remains unclear. In this study (Sahin et al, 2005; Turker et al., 2008) we investigated whether the MLAEPs correlated with the performances of neuropsychological tests in patients with schizophrenia and healthy controls.

2.2 Methods

2.2.1 Subjects

We examined 15 patients (8 female and 7 male) with schizophrenia, who met diagnostic criteria of DSM-IV for schizophrenia and compared them with control subjects (9 females and 6 males). Patients and control subjects were matched for age, gender, education levels and handedness.

Subjects who had other neurological or psychiatric disease, history of substance abuse and head trauma were not included in the study. All patients were psychiatrically stable (there were no psychotic symptoms and medication changes within at least two weeks prior to the assesment). Psychopathological symptoms severity in patiens was assessed by Positive and Negative Syndrome Scale (PANSS) (First, 1997). Informed consent was obtained from patients and control subjects before the study.

2.2.2 Evoked potentials recording procedure

All recordings of MLAEPs were performed at Dantec Keypoint. Electrode montage was adjusted as active electrode placed on ipsilateral mastoid and reference and ground electrodes at Cz and Fz, respectively. Silver surface electrodes were used for reference and ground electrode while a scalp needle electrode was used as active electrode. Alternating clicks of 100 μsec duration were used and polarity was adjusted as vertex. The frequency of stimulation was 10/sec and the filtering was chosen as 10 Hz-200 Hz. Analysis time (sweep length) and sensitivity were 100msec and 0,2 μv/d, respectively. The intensity of the stimuli was chosen according to the auditory threshold. The ipsilateral ear was stimulated with an intensity of stimulus such as hearing threshold plus 60 dB, while the contralateral ear was masked with white noise. Averaging of 1000 signals was performed twice and overlapped for each ear. No, Po, Na, Pa, Nb, and Pb were sampled and latencies and amplitudes of each potential were determined and compared with age and gender matched controls. MLAEPs recordings were performed bilateraly i.e. 30 recordings were performed for patients and 30 recordings were performed for controls making a total of 60 recordings. No artifact rejection was employed.

In MLAEP recording procedure, latency and amplitude measurements are usually done on the display, either manually or by an automatic peak detection algorithm that seeks the maximum value between preset time values. The amplitude can be expressed as a peak to peak value between adjacent positive and negative components or the peak value can be measured against some baseline, usually taken just before the stimulus is presented. Latency for MLAEPs can be described as the time till the peak of the negative or the positive potential has evolved and this may be labelled on the display after the click (Erwin et al., 1987)

As hearing impairment can alter the MLAEPs, the external ear canal was checked with an otoscope to assure that the canal was not blocked by cerumen before the test. Patients with hearing problems assesed by otologic tests were excluded. MLAEPs are known to be affected by medications, however all patients were under treatment and there was no other way to investigate them.

2.2.3 Neuropsychological evaluation

An extensive neuropsychological test battery was used to assess the cognitive functions; attention, language, visuospatial functions, verbal and visual memory, executive functions (Table 3).

2.2.4 Statistical methods

The age, gender, handedness, education, the latencies and amplitudes of MLAEPs the neuropsychological test parameters of the patients and controls groups were compared with student-t test. The pearson correlation coefficient was used to determine the correlation between PANNS scores, the neuropsychological test parameters, and disease duration.

2.3 Results

The demographic features of patient and control groups are presented in Table 2. There were no statistically significant difference between age, gender, handedness, and education levels of patient and control groups.

	Patients (n = 15)		Controls (n = 15)	p
Age	32.9 ± 10.6	29.8±2.3	NS	
Education	12.1 ± 3.7	12.6±2.6	NS	
MMSE	28.1 ± 2.7	29.6±0.8	S	
Gender	8M. 7F	9M. 6F		NS
Duration of disease (month)	135.3± 112.1	(-)		(-)

Table 2. Demographic Features.

2.3.1 Neuropsychological tests

Results are summarized in Table 4. Generally, in all the neuropsychological tests, performance of the patient group was poor when compared to control group. MMSE scores of the patient group were statistically significantly lower than those of the control groups.

There were statistically significant differences regarding the attention and the language tests. The scores of the tests assessing visuospatial functions, except BLO, were significantly different between patient and control groups. Also, patients got statistically significant lower scores on memory tests, and executive functions when compared with controls.

Mini mental state examination (MMSE)
Attention
WAIS-R Digit Span (DS)
Verbal Fluency (K-A-S Test)
Language
Boston Naming Test (30-items)
Visuo-spatial Functions
Benton's Line Orientation Test (BLO)
Benton's Facial Recognition Test (BFR)
WAIS-R BlocK Design (BD)
Hooper Visual Organization Test (HVOT)
Clock Drawing
Verbal Memory
California Verbal Learning Test (CVLT)
Visual Memory
WAIS-R subtest
Executive Functions
Wisconsin Card Sorting Test (WCST)
Stroop Test
Trail Making Test A and B (TMT A-B)

WAIS = Wechsler Adult Intelligence Scale.

Table 3. Neuropsychological Test Battery.

	Patients (n = 15)		Controls (n = 15)		
	Mean	SD	Mean	SD	p
MMSE	28.1	2.7	29.6	0.8	S
Attention					
WAIS-R DS-fwd	6	1.06	7.2	1.01	S
WAIS-R DS-bwd	3.6	1.29	5.2	1.08	S
Verbal Fluency (K-A-S Test)	35.07	13.96	48.47	12.18	S
K-A-S perseveration	0.67	0.81	0.07	0.25	S
Language					
Boston Naming Test (30-items)	27.60	2.79	29.27	1.28	S
Visuo-spatial Functions					
BLO	23.43	7.94	26.40	2.99	NS
BFR	18.07	3.38	21.93	2.63	S
BD	21.14	11.43	30.20	9.59	S
HVOT	17.79	4.04	21.00	1.89	S
Clock Drawing	9.26	0.79	9.93	0.25	S

	Patients (n = 15) Mean	SD	Controls (n = 15) Mean	SD	p
Verbal Memory					
CVLT					
Total of 5 trails	38.71	10.57	51.46	6.94	S
Long-delay free recall	7.92	2.97	12.53	2.06	S
Long-delay cued recall	8.21	2.96	13.20	1.65	S
Perseverations	5	4.11	3.40	3.08	NS
Free recall intrusions	2	2.21	1	1.81	NS
Cued recall intrusions	1.21	1.67	0.67	1.11	NS
Recognition	13.21	3.01	15.13	1.06	S
Discriminability (%)	88.09	9	96	3.5	S
False positive	1.5	1.6	0.46	1.06	S
Visual Memory					
WAIS-R subtest	8	3.2	11.67	1.1	S
Executive Functions					
WCST					
Total number of responses	117.50	18.25	95.6	15.37	S
Total categories completed	3.57	2.10	5.93	0.25	S
Number of perseverative responses	43.36	36.23	12.67	4.25	S
Total number of errors	51.64	25.42	22.67	8.30	S
Total number of correct responses	65.86	14.72	72.93	8.40	NS
Stroop 3	14.3	4	11.1	2.7	S
Stroop 5	27.9	9.6	25.1	8.2	NS
TMT A	69.72	25.7	35.35	13.18	S
TMT B	146.44	91.55	75.56	25.13	S

Table 4. Neuropsychological Test Results.

2.3.2 Evoked potentials

The results indicated that most of the MLAEPs data elicited from the patients showed statistically significant differences from controls. The pathological responses from both sides of the brains of patients did not differ significantly from each other as both right and left sides generated MLAEPs which were statistically significantly different from controls (Table 5-6). Apart from NoR and PaL, all latencies of other parameters of MLAEPs were prolonged in the patient group (Table 5). Apart from PbR, amplitudes of parameters of MLAEPs were statistically significantly lower in the patient group when compared with the control group, (Table 6).

We also found no correlations between PANSS scores, the scores of neuropsychological tests, the duration of disease, and the latencies and amplitudes of MLAEPs.

	Patients (n=15)		Control (n=15)		
	Mean	SD	Mean	SD	p
No_R	10.67	3.52	8.48	2.64	NS
No_L	11.18	3.26	8.04	2.25	S
Po_R	18.05	1.55	15.71	2.39	S
Po_L	19.14	3.87	15.36	2.38	S
Na_R	29.22	2.63	26.26	2.21	S
Na_L	29.98	3.55	26.65	2.79	S
Pa_R	40.16	3.32	37.70	2.64	S
Pa_L	43.01	6.35	39.77	3.31	NS
Nb_R	53.44	6.73	48.01	5.37	S
Nb_L	55.66	10.09	48.97	3.58	S
Pb_R	68.37	7.84	59.19	7.94	S
Pb_L	66.54	11.07	59.35	5.76	S

Table 5. Latencies of MLAEPs (Millisecond).

	Patients (n=15)		Control (n=15)		
	Mean	SD	Mean	SD	p
No_R	0.17	0.15	0.4	0.2	S
No_L	0.22	0.15	0.47	0.27	S
Po_R	0.22	0.13	0.49	0.25	S
Po_L	0.22	0.15	0.56	0.32	S
Na_R	0.39	0.35	0.86	0.50	S
Na_L	0.39	0.29	0.76	0.34	S
Pa_R	0.26	0.27	0.65	0.51	S
Pa_L	0.26	0.25	0.58	0.33	S
Nb_R	0.28	0.30	0.55	0.38	S
Nb_L	0.25	0.22	0.50	0.33	S
Pb_R	0.27	0.29	0.48	0.38	NS
Pb_L	0.19	0.10	0.50	0.31	S

Table 6. Amplitudes of MLAEP Potentials (Microvolt).

2.4 Discussion

In this study we found that the many parameters of MLAEPs except NoR and PaL for latency and PbR for amplidute, were significantly abnormal in the patient group. Also, the neuropsychological test performances of the patient group were poor when compared with normals.

According to our data, there were not any correlations between PANSS scores, the scores of neuropsychological test, the duration of disease, and the latencies and amplitudes of MLAEPs.

Although the neural sources of MLAEPs are still controversial, the studies suggest that Pa, Pb and Nb components of MLAEPs have a cortical generator (primary auditory cortex and adjacent areas) while No, Po, and Na have a brainstem-subcortical generator (medial geniculate body, polysensory thalamic nuclei) (Deiber et al., 1988; Diaz et al., 1990) It is well-known that human Pb (P1) potential is blocked by scopalamine, muscarinic cholinergic antagonists, and due to lesions including cholinergic pedunculopontine nucleus (Diaz et al., 1990)

In patients with schizophrenia, the abnormalities in auditory evoked potentials have been reported by other studies. Erwin et al. reported that the recovery cycle of the P1 component of auditory midlatency evoked potential is abnormal (Erwin et al.,1991). Boutros and coworkers suggested that there were morphological abnormalities of the MLAEPs in schizophrenia patients (Boutros et al.,2004). Clementz et al.showed that P50 suppression was deficient in these patients, indicating sensory gating abnormality (Clementz et al., 1997). All these findings were interpreted by authors as a deficiency of generators of MLAEPs, underlying neural structures and neurotransmitter systems in patients with schizophrenia.

We investigated the latency and amplitude features of MLAEPs recorded on dominant and non-dominant hemisphere in patients with schizophrenia but not the recovery cycle and sensory gating features. All patients and control subjects were strongly right-handed according to Edinburgh Inventory (Oldfield et al., 1971).

Our results revealed statistically significant differences both in latency and amplitudes of MLAEP components in the patient group when compared with the normal group.

Lateralization seems to be important in schizophrenic patients since some symptoms of the disease emerge when specific parts of the brain are involved. It was hypothesized that hypermetabolism of the left temporal lobe seemed to occur only if the patient was actively hallucinating for example (Mesulam et al., 1990).

In our study the pathological responses elicited from both sides of the brains of patients did not differ significantly from each other as both right and left sides generated MLAEPs which were statistically significantly different from controls. We believe this is an important finding since all our patients and controls were strongly right-handed. Thoma et al. concluded in one of their studies that converging evidence from EEG, MEG and neuropsychological measures pointed to left hemisphere dysfunction related to the well established sensory gating in schizophrenia (Thoma et al., 2003).

It has been assumed that latency in evoked potential studies reflect the efficiency and speed of information processing. Thus, the prolonged latency may reflect that the information processing speed slowed.

Amplitude abnormalites, on the other hand, refer to axonal loss in related areas and show the overall efficiency of neural structures mediating a response.

Amplitude abnormalities in evoked potentials of patients with schizophrenia have been reported with much more consistency than latency abnormalities. Munkundan and coworkers observed amplitude and recovery abnormalities but normal latencies of MLAEPs in schizophrenia patients (Munkundan et al., 1986). Williams and coworkers similarly found no latency abnormalities in a group of medicated schizophrenia patients (Williams et al, 2000). However, Boutros and coworkers demonstrated that schizophrenia patients had significantly longer latencies for the P50 and N100 components (Boutros et al., 2004). Our findings agree with results of the researchs in literature.

The many previous studies investigated the neuropsychological profile of the patients with schizophrenia. Almost all of these studies demonstrated the neuropsychological impairments in the multiple cognitive areas etc. memory, attention, language, executive functions (Bozikas et al., 2006; Brazo et al., 2005; Mohamed at al., 1999). However, it is still

unknown whether there is a relationship between the neuropsychological impairments and neuroanatomical changes. Also, it is unclear whether the negative and positive symptoms are associated with a spesific brain region and/or neuropsychological deficits. Andreasen et al. and Weinberg et al. have reported that the negative symptoms reflected primarily frontal lobe dysfunction (Andreasen, 1986; Weinberger, 1987). Berman et al. observed that negative symptoms associated with poor performances on cognitive tests reflected poor frontal lobe functions while positive symptoms were associated with poor attention representing widespread neural network (Berman et al., 1997). Liu et al. demonstrated that the negative schizophrenic patients had executive function deficits and lower rCBF perfusion in left prefrontal lobes (Liu et al, 2002). On the other hand, Morrison-Stewart et al. found no correlation between frontal lobe assessing neuropsychological tests and negative symptoms (Morrison et al., 2002). Addington et al. reported that there was no relationship between attention and negative and positive symptoms (Addington et al., 1997).
The results of our study showed that the cognitive functions assessing the comprehensive neuropsychological test battery were statistically significantly worse in the patient group when compared with the control group.
Schizophrenia is a heterogeneous mental disease which is characterized with thought disorder, hallucination, delusion and cognitive deficits.[45] Postmortem studies showed low neuron density, cortical volume reduction, pyramidal cell disarray, neurotransmitter disturbances such as glutamate, GABA, dopamine, and acetylcholine (Harrison et al.,1998; Sarter et al.,1998; Simpson at al, 1998). The longitudinal studies support that schizophrenia is largely a static disorder while others suggest a deteriorating course (Harrison et al.,1998; Gur et al., 1998; Vita et al., 1997).
The spectrum of disease duration of our patients was fairly widespread (min: 50 months max: 440 months). In our study there were no correlations between the disease duration, severity of the disease (by PANSS), EP measures, and neuropsychological profiles. This may perhaps support that schizophrenia is a static disorder rather than progressive.

3. Acknowledgements

This second work was partly supported by a research grant from Ondokuz Mayis University. The authors thanks to Prof. Dr. Yuksel Bek for statistical analysis.

4. References

Addington J, Addington D, Gasbarre L. Distractibility and symptoms in schizophrenia. J Psychiatry Neurosci 1997;22(3):180-4.

Andreasen NC, Nasrallan Z, Dunn VD, Olson SC, Grove WM, Ehrhardt JC, Coffman JA. Crossett JH. Structural abnormalities in frontal system in schizophrenia: a magnetic resonance imaging study. Arch Gen Psychiatry 1986;43:136-44.

Aminoff MJ, Goodin A, Goodin DS Electrophysiological features of the dementia of Parkinson's disease. Adv Neurol 1990;53:361-3.

Bayazit YA, Gursoy S, Ozer E, Karakurum G, Madenci E. Neurotologic manifestations of the fibromyalgia syndrome. J Neurol Sci. 2002 Apr 15;196(1-2):77-80.

Bennett R. The Fibromyalgia Impact Questionnaire(FIQ):a review of its development, current version, operating characteristics and uses. Clin Exp Rheumatol 2005;23(Suppl. 39):154-162.

Berman I, Viegner B, Merson A, Allan E, Pappas D, Green AL. Differential relationships between positive and negative symptoms and neuropsychological deficits in schizophrenia. Schizophr Res 1997;25(1):1-10.

Boutros NN, Korzyuko O, Oliwa G, Feingold A, Campbell D, Mcclain-Furmansk D, Struve F, Jansen BH. Morphological and latency abnormalities of the mid-latency auditory evoked responses in schizophrenia: a preliminary report. Schizophrenia Res 2004;70(2-3):303-13.

Bozikas Vp, Kosmidis MH, Kiosseoglou G, Karavatos A. Neuropsychological profile of cognitively impaired patients with schizophrenia. Compr Psychiatry 2006;47(2):136-43.

Brazo P, Delamillieure P, Morello R, Halbecq I, Marié RM, Dollfus S. Impairments of executive/attentional functions in schizophrenia with primary and secondary negative symptoms. Psychiatry Res 2005;133(1):45-55.

Buchwald JS, Erwın RJ, Read S, Lancker Dv, Guthrie D, Schawfel J, Tanhguay P. Midlatency auditory evoked responses: differential abnormality of P1 in Alzheimer disease. Electroencephalogr Clin Neurophysiol 1989;74(5):378-4.

Buchwald Js, Rubinstein EH, Schwafel J, Strandburg RJ. Midlatency auditory evoked responses. Electroencephalogr Clin Neurophysiol 1991;80(4):303-9.

Buchwald JS, Erwin RJ, Read S, Lancker DV, Cummings JL. Midlatency auditory evoked responses: P1 abnormalities in adult autistic subjects. Electroencephalogr Clin Neurophysiol 1992;84(2):164-71.

Cacace AT, Satya-Murti S, Wolpaw JR. Human middle latency auditory evoked potentials: vertex and temporal components. Electroencephalogr Clin Neurophysiol 1990;77(1):6-18.

Clementz BA, Geyer MA, Braff Dl. P50 suppression among schizophrenia and normal comparison subjects: a methodological analysis. Biol Psychiatry 1997;41(10):1035–44.

Deiber MP, Ibañez V, Fischer C, Perrin F, Mauguière F. Sequential mapping favours the hypothesis of distinct generators for Na and Pa middle latency auditory evoked potentials. Electroencephalogr Clin Neurophysiol 1988;71(3):187-97.

Diaz F, Cadaveria F, Grau C. Short- and middle-latency auditory evoked potentials in abstinent chronic alcoholics: preliminary findings. Electroencephalogr Clin Neurophysiol 1990;77(2):145-50.

Dickerson LW, Buchwald JS. Midlatency auditory evoked responses: Effects of scopolamine in cat and implication for brain stem cholinergic mechanisms. Exp Neurol 1991; 112(2):229-39.

Erwin RJ, Buchwald JS. Midlatency auditory evoked responses: differential recovery cycle characteristics. Electroencephalogr Clin Neurophysiol 1986;64(5):417-23.

Erwin RJ, Buchwald JS. Midlatency auditory evoked responses in the human and the cat model. Electroencephalogr Clin Neurophysiol Suppl 1987;40:461-7.

Erwin RJ, Mawhinney-Hee M, Gur RC, Gur RE. Midlatency auditory evoked responses in schizophrenia. Biol Psychiatry 1991;30(5):430-42.

Fann AV, Preston MA, Bray P, Mamiya N, Williams DK, Skinner RD, Garcia-Rill E. The P50 midlatency auditory evoked potential in patients with chronic low back pain (CLBP). Clin Neurophysiol. 2005 Mar;116(3):681-9. Epub 2004 Nov 23.

First MB, Spitzer RL, Gibbon M, Williams JBW. Structured Clinical Interview for DSM-IV Axis I disorders (SCID-I), clinical version. Washington, DC: American Psychiatric Press. 1997.

Gracely RH, Petzke F, Wolf JM, Clauw DJ. Functional magnetic resonance imaging evidence of augmented pain processing infibromyalgia. Arthritis Rheum. 2002 May;46(5):1333-43.

Green JB, Elder WW, Freed DM. The P1 component of tha middle latency auditory evoked potential predicts a practice effect during clinical trials in Alzheimer disease. Neurology 1995;45(5):962-6.

Gur RE, Cowell P, Turetsky BI, Gallacher F, Cannon T, Bilker W, Gur RC. A follow-up magnetic resonance imaging study of schizophrenia. Relationship of neuroanatomical changes to clinical and neurobehavioral measures. Arch Gen Psychiatry 1998;55(2):145-52.

Hamilton M. Development of a rating scale for primary depressive illness. Br J Soc Clin Psychol 1967;6:278-296.

Harrison PJ. The neuropathology of schizophrenia: a critical rewiew of the data and their interpretation. Brain 1999;122(4):593-624.

Herrero JF, Laird JM, Lopez-Garcia JA (2000) Wind-up of spinal cord neurones and pain sensation:much ado about something? Progress in Neurobiology 61(2);169-203.

Johansson G, Risberg J, Rosenhall U, Orndahl G, Svennerholm L, Nystrom S. Cerebral dysfunction in fibromyalgia:evidence from regional cerebral blood flow mesurements, otoneurological tests and cerebrospinal fluid analysis. Acta Psychiat Scand 1995;91:86-94.

Julien N, Goffaux P, Arsenault P, Marchand S. Widespread pain in fibromyalgia is related to a deficit of endogenous pain inhibition. Pain 2005;114:295-302.

Küçükdeveci AA, Sahin H, Ataman S, Griffiths B, Tennant A. Issues in cross-cultural validity: example from the adaptation, reliability, and validity testing of a Turkish version of the Stanford Health Asessment Questionnaire. Arthritis Rheum 2004;51:14-9.

Mauguire F, Butler SR, Ceranic B, Cooper R, Holder GE. Normal Findings by Modality in Clinical Neurophysiology Vol 1, eds. Binnie C, Cooper R, Mauguire F, 2007; 422.

Liu Z, Tam WC, Xie Y, Zhao J. The relationship between regional cerebral blood flow and the Wisconsin Card Sorting Test in negative schizophrenia. Psychiatry Clin Neurosci 2002;56(1):3-7.

Mesulam M. Schizophrenia and the brain. NEJM 1990; 322(12):789-94.

Mesulam M. From sensation to cognition. Brain 1998;121(6):1013-52.

Misulis KE, Fakhouri T. Spehlmann's Evoked Potential Primer, 3rd edition. Oxford Press, Butterworth Heinemann, Boston, 2001;6-7.

Mohamed S, Paulsen JS, O'leary D, Arndt S, Andreasen N. Generalized cognitive deficits in schizophrenia. Arch Gen Psychiatry 1999;56(8):749–54.

Montoya P, Sitges C, Garcia-Herrera M et al (2006) Reduced brain habituation to somatosensory stimulation in patients with fibromyalgia. Arthritis Rheum 2006;54(6);1995-2003.

Morrison-Stewart SI, Williamson PC, Corning WC, Kutcher SP, Snow WG, Merskey H. Frontal and non-frontal lobe neuropsychological test performance and clinical symptomatology in schizophrenia. Psychol Med 1992;22(2):353-9.

Munkundan CR. Middle latency components of evoked potential responses in schizophrenics. Biol Psychiatry 1986;21(11):1097-100.

Oldfield RC. The assessment and analysis of handedness: the Edinburgh Inventory. Neuropsychologia 1971;9(1):97-113.

Roth SR, Geisser ME, Theisen-Goodvich M, Dixon PJ. Cognitive complaints are associated with depression, fatigue, female sex, and pain catastrophizing in patients with chronic pain. Arch Phys Med Rehabil 2005;86:1147-54.

Rosenhall U, Johannsen G, Orndahi G. Otoneurologic and audiologic findings in fibromyalgia. Scand J Rehabil Med. 1996 Dec;28(4):225-32.

Şahin, HA., M. Sarıca, H. Türker, M. Baydın, Ö. Böke, B. Diren, "Şizofrenide semptom profili, kognitif durum ile beyin atrofisi arasındaki ilişki", 41. Ulusal Nöroloji Kongresi, Cilt 11, 70, İstanbul, 2005.

Sarter M, Bruno JP. Cortical acetylcholine, reality distortion, schizophrenia, and Lewy Body Dementia: too much or too little cortical acetylcholine? Brain Cogn 1998;38(3):297-316.

Simpson MD, Slater P, Deakin JF. Comparison of glutamate and gamma-aminobutyric acid uptake binding sites in frontal and temporal lobes in schizophrenia. Biol Psychiatry 1998;44(6):423-7.

Staud R, Domingo M(2001) Evidence for abnormal pain processing in fibromyalgia syndrome. Pain Med 2(3);208-215.

Turker, H., A. Bilgici, M.K. Onar, " The investigation of the correlation between middle and long latency auditory evoked potentials and clinical parameters in fibromyalgic patients," Proc. 13th European Congress of Clinical Neurophysiology, Istanbul, Clin Neurophysiol, Vol.119,104, Elsevier, Amsterdam, 2008.

Turker, H., H. Şahin, M. Sarica, O. Böke, " Middle latency auditory evoked responses in schizophrenia and correlation with hemishpere dominance," Proc. 13th European Congress of Clinical Neurophysiology, Istanbul, Clin Neurophysiol, Vol.119,103–104, Elsevier, Amsterdam, 2008.

Thoma RJ, Hanlon FM, Moses SN, Edgar JC, Huang M, Weisend, MP, Irwın J, Sherwood A, Paulson K, Bustillo J, Adler LE, Mıller GA, Cañive JM. Lateralization of auditory sensory gating and neuropsychological dysfunction in schizophrenia. Am J Psychiatry 2003;160(9):1595-605.

Vita A, Dieci M, Giobbio GM, Tenconi F, Invernizzi G. Time course of cerebral ventricular enlargement in schizophrenia supports the hypothesis of its neurodevelopmental nature. Schizophr Res 1997;23 (1):25-30.

Weinberger DR. Implications of normal brain development for the pathogenesis of schizophrenia. Arch Gen Psychiatry 1987;44(11):660-9.

Williams DA, Gracely RH. Biology and therapy of fibromyalgia. Functional magnetic resonance imaging findings in fibromyalgia. Arthritis Res Ther 2006;8(6):224

Williams LM, Gordon E, Wright J, Bahramali H. Late component ERPs are associated with three syndromes in schizophrenia. Int J Neurosci 2000;105(1-4):37-52.

Woods Dl, Clayworth CC, Knight RT, Simpson GV, Naeser MA. Generators of middle- and long-latency auditory evoked potentials: implications from studies of patients with bitemporal lesions. Electroenceph Clin Neurophysiol 1987;68(2):132-48.

Wolfe F, Smythe HA, Yunus MB et al. The American College of Rheumatology 1990 Criteria for the Classification of Fibromyalgia. Report of the Multicenter Criteria Committe. Arthritis Rheum 1990;33;160-172.

12

Non-Invasive Diagnosis of Neuromuscular Disorders by High-Spatial-Resolution-EMG

Catherine Disselhorst-Klug
Department of Rehabilitation & Prevention Engineering
Institute of Applied Medical Engineering, RWTH Aachen University
Germany

1. Introduction

Neuromuscular diseases are defined as pathological changes of the peripheral nerves (neuronal disorders), the neuromuscular junctions or the muscle fibres (muscular disorders). Since they are accompanied by weakness commonly, they have essential impact on the patient's movement performance. Especially in childhood, the consequences are serious and early diagnosis is essential for an adapted and task orientated therapy. The main aim in diagnostics of neuromuscular diagnosis is to distinguish between patients without any morbid changes in the MUs, patients with muscular disorders, and patients with neuronal disorders. Here, diagnostics avail on the fact that changes in the skeletal muscles, which take place during the progress of the disorder, are mostly on the level of single motor units (MUs). The MU is the smallest unit of the muscle, which can be activated independently by the central nervous system [Basmajian 1985]. Muscular disorders, for example, are characterised by a loss of single muscle fibres. This results in the fact that less muscle fibres contribute to an affected MU than to a healthy one. This is in contrast to neuronal disorders in which the motor neuron is destroyed. Consequently, complete MUs are affected. In this case the number of muscle fibres contributing to a MU is unchanged but the number of MUs available for force generation is reduced [Jerusalem 1979, Dubowitz 1991].
In human movement and locomotion the voluntary and active contraction of a muscle is initiated by the electrophysiological excitation of a pool of MUs. Since Electromyography (EMG) detects the electrophysiological signal generated by the muscle during excitation, it is a well established procedure utilised in studies of muscle function [Basmajian 1985]. During the last years surface electromyography (sEMG) has become more and more important. It offers a number of advantages when compared to invasive EMG procedures, like needle- or wire-EMG. For example, it causes no discomfort or risk of infection due to the insertion of the needle or the wire and it does not require the supervision by a physician. Compared to invasive measurements, the repeatability of surface EMG measurements is superior, and long term monitoring is possible, [Jonsson 1968]. In addition, the conventional needle-EMG is not suitable for investigations of the excitation spread. Compared to the needle EMG the wire EMG is less painful and allows the detection of the excitation spread. But after insertion the wire electrode tends to migrate within the muscle tissue even during isometric contraction [Jonsson 1968, Komi 1970]. Consequently, the reproducibility of the EMG signal detected with wire electrodes is limited.

The conventional sEMG has a limited spatial resolution and detects, therefore, a superposition of a large number of MUs. The separation of the activity of single MUs from simultaneously active adjacent ones is hard to achieve with surface electrodes. This task still needs highly specialised acquisition techniques, [Merletti 1989]. Consequently, sEMG is mainly used to obtain 'global' information about the muscle activation, like timing or intensity of the muscle activation. Therefore, for diagnostic purpose of neuromuscular disorders, the conventional sEMG techniques are not suitable, since information about the single MUs is needed to distinguish between patients without any morbid changes in the MUs, patients with muscular disorders, and patients with neuronal disorders. This is why in clinical practice still invasive Needle-EMG techniques are used, which gain the needed information about the single MU activity. The diagnostic selectivity of the commonly used Needle-EMG-procedures has been determined by comparing the Needle-EMG diagnosis and the result of a muscle biopsy [Hausmanova 1971, Black 1974, Buchtal 1982]. The most significant work is that of Buchtal and Kamieniekwa, which establishes a diagnostic selectivity of the Needle-EMG procedure of 77% in muscular disorders and 91% in neuronal disorders. However, in addition to the non-convincing diagnostic selectivity, the Needle-EMG methods are invasive and, consequently, painful for the patient.

2. High-spatial-resolution-EMG

In contrast to the conventional surface EMG techniques, the High-Spatial-Resolution EMG (HSR-EMG) allows the non-invasive detection of the single MU activity even during maximal voluntary contraction of the muscle. The methodology is based on the use of a multi-electrode array in combination with a spatial filter processing [Disselhorst-Klug 1998, Disselhorst-Klug 2000].

During a voluntary excitation of the muscle by the central nervous system, a time variable potential distribution is generated on the skin surface. Multi-electrode arrays can be beneficially used for the detection of the spatial potential distribution generated. From this information about the localisation of the source and its movement in time can be gained. Multi-electrode arrays are commonly used in electroencephalography and are recently becoming more popular in sEMG. In sEMG they have been described first by Rau [Rau1985], Masuda et al. [Masuda1985], De Luca et al. [de Luca 1987] and Reucher et al. [Reucher1987] and have been advantageously used in the fields of neurology, ergonomics, and biomechanics during the last years [Disselhorst-Klug 2000, Rau 2004]. Commonly used multi-electrode arrays consist of several (up to 240) pin-electrodes arranged either in a row or two-dimensionally with an inter-electrode distance of only a few millimetre. A multi-electrode array consisting of 16 gold-covered pin-electrodes (Figure 1) for example is used for the diagnostics of neuromuscular disorders. In this case the electrodes have a diameter of 0.5 mm and are springing-fitted to provide optimal contact with the skin surface. They are arranged two-dimensionally and have an inter-electrode distance between 2.5 mm and 5 mm depending on the muscle being investigated [Disselhorst-Klug 2000].

The potentials detected by the different electrodes of the array can be regarded as instantaneous spatial samples of the potential distribution generated on the skin surface by the excitation of the muscle fibres. To this potential distribution contribute different MUs in a different way. A small number of MUs, which are located very close to the skin surface, contribute to the resulting potential distribution with a spatially steep and high potential. On the contrary, MUs which are located more far away from the skin surface contribute

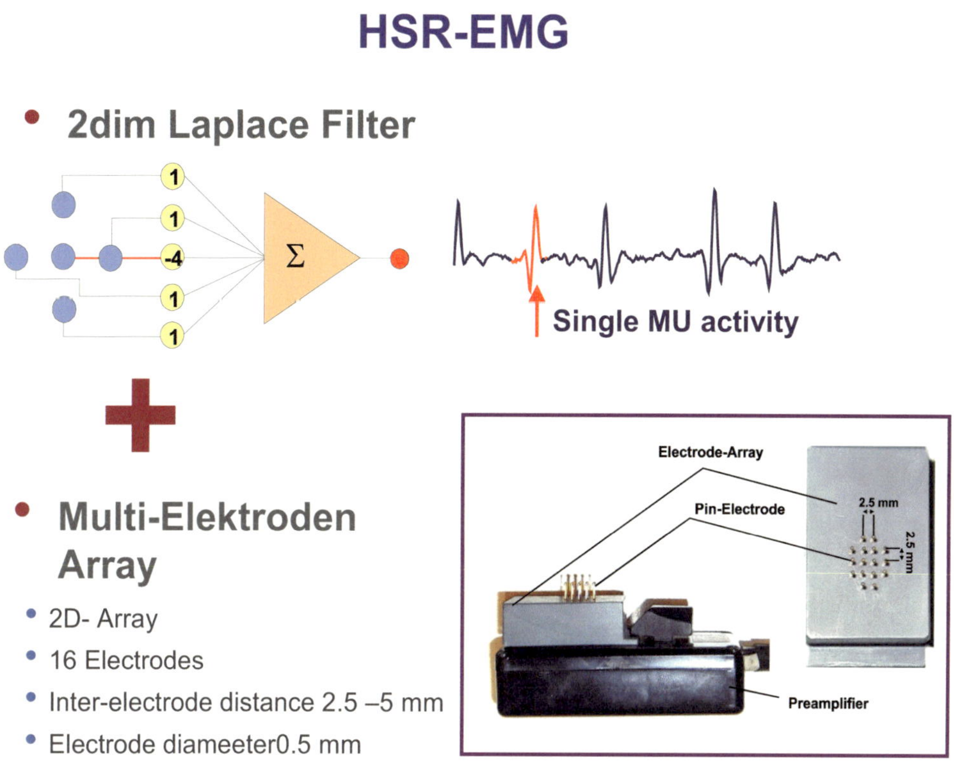

Fig. 1. HSR-EMG.
Multi-electrode array for the detection of the single motor unit activity during maximum voluntary contractions of the m. abductor pollicis brevis. By using an NDD-filter the single MU activity can be isolated in the signal. Adapted from [Disselhorst-Klug 2000].

lower and spatially more widened potential (Figure 2) [Disselhorst-Klug 1998]. This is due to the fact that caused by the electrical characteristic of the tissue between the source and the skin surface spatially high frequencies in the signal are more suppressed the deeper the source is located in the body [Lynn 1978]. Figure 2 shows an example of the potential distribution generated on the skin surface by two MUs located in different depth. If both MUs are excited at the same time. The potential distribution generated on the skin surface is equal to the superposition of the contributions of both MUs. Conventional sEMG applications are based on a bipolar lead with an inter-electrode distance of about 20 mm [Hermens 2000]. Due to this relatively large inter-electrode distance such an electrode arrangement detects the absolute value of the superimposed potential distribution, to which both MUs contribute in the same manner (Figure 2).
The volume conductor between the excited MU and the skin surface acts like a spatial low-pass filter. On the other hand, a spatial high-pass filter with an adequate cut-off frequency would transmit spatial frequencies higher than its cut-off frequency and would suppress spatially lower ones. Thus, by using a spatial high-pass filter the spatially high frequency contribution of MUs located close to the skin surface will be amplified and the contribution of MUs located more distantly will be reduced.

In a first approach, the simplest spatial high-pass filter - a bipolar lead with an inter-electrode distance in the mm-range and arranged in parallel to the muscle fibres - was used to improve the spatial selectivity of the non-invasive EMG-recording techniques (Figure 2) [Lynn 1978]. The bipolar lead differentiates the spatial potential distribution in the direction of the electrode arrangement. Due to this differentiation the bipolar lead enhances spatially steep components and reduces more flat ones (Figure 2). However, particularly at high force levels the bipolar lead with a small inter-electrode distance is not sufficient to discriminate the single MU activity in the signal course. Therefore, the principle of spatial filtering has been extended to more complex electrode arrangements.

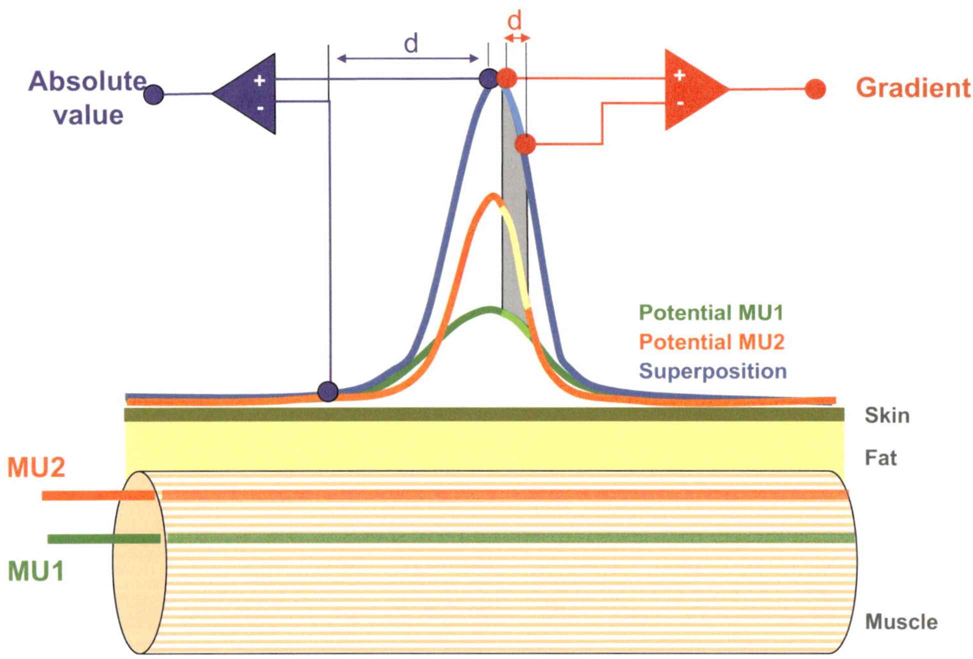

Fig. 2. Potential Distribution.
Potential distribution generated on the skin surface by two MUs located in differed distances from the skin surface. By using electrode distances d in the mm-range the contribution of the MU located close to the skin surface can be emphasised and the contribution of the more distantly located MU can be suppressed. Adapted from [Disselhorst-Klug 2000].

From image-processing it is known, that Laplace filters - which give the second spatial derivative - are well suited for the detection of edges perpendicular to the direction of differentiation. A one-dimensional Laplace filter can be realised with three electrodes arranged in a row. The central electrode has to be weighted with a factor of –2 and the two outer electrodes with a factor of 1. Such double differentiating filters have been first used in sEMG by Broman et al., [Broman 1985], and are now frequently used by different other groups. A higher spatial selectivity of the recording set-up can be achieved with two-dimensional Laplace filter arrangements [Reucher 1987, Disselhorst-Klug 1998]. It has been shown that a weighted summation of five cross-wisely arranged EMG leads forms the second spatial derivative of the potential distribution in two orthogonal directions (**N**ormal-**D**ouble-**D**ifferentiating-Filter). To perform a NDD-Filter the central electrode is weighted with a factor of –4 and the surrounding electrodes with a factor of +1. The NDD-Filter amplifies only the activity of MUs located directly below the centre electrode of the filter and reduces the signals of more distantly located sources. In this way, the activity of single MUs becomes clearly distinguishable in the signal course (Figure 1). Thus, the HSR-EMG allows the non-invasive detection of the single MU activity and seems, consequently, to be suitable for a non-invasive diagnosis of neuromuscular disorders [Disselhorst-Klug 1994, Farina 2003].

In initial clinical investigations the HSR-EMG has been validated in children suffering from Duchenne Muscle Dystrophy (Duchenne) or Spinal Muscle Atrophy (SMA) [Ramaekers 1993, Huppertz 1995, Rau 1997, Disselhorst-Klug 2000]. The investigations show that the HSR-EMG allows the detection of changes in the electrical activity of the muscle which are typical for each disorder and which might allow a reliable distinction between healthy volunteers and patients with neuromuscular disorders as well as between patients with muscular disorders and patients with neuronal disorders (Figure 3). In contrast to the HSR-EMG of healthy volunteers, the HSR-EMG pattern of patients with neuronal disorders shows high and isolated peaks within the signal course. However, the HSR-EMG pattern of patients with muscular disorders is characterised by low and wide MU action potentials, which are hard to distinguish within the signal course.

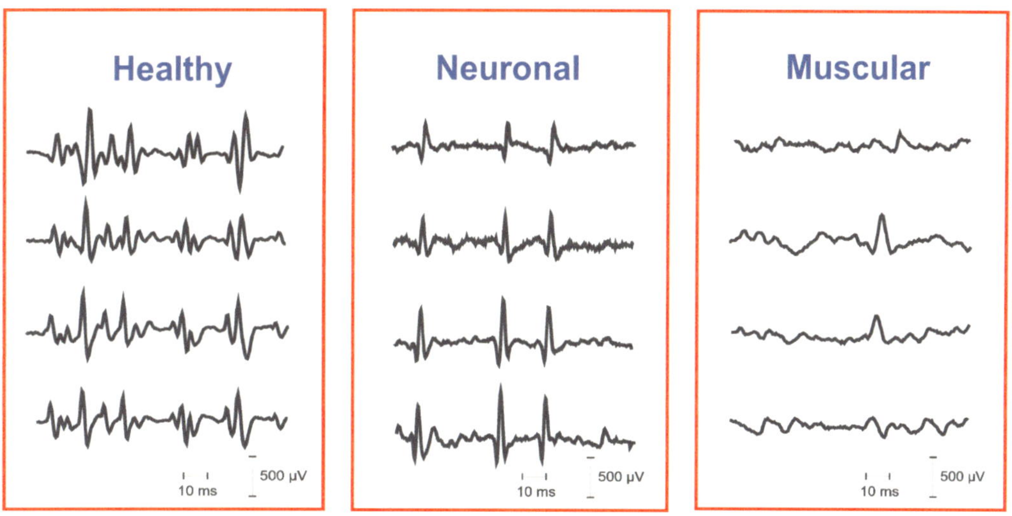

Fig. 3. Pathodological Changes.
Typical pathological changes in the HSR-EMG signal. Represented are four spatially filtered channels.

3. Quantitative evaluation of pathological changes in the HSR-EMG

Due to the first clinical experience with the HSR-EMG the question arises, whether the methodology allows a reliable distinction between healthy volunteers and patients with neuromuscular disorders as well as between patients with muscular disorders and patients with neuronal disorders. For that purpose a set of parameters has to be introduced, which allow a quantitative evaluation of the changes in the HSR-EMG pattern typical for each disorder. This can be understood as a classical feature extraction process. By an adapted classification procedure, which is based on extracted features, each patient can be assigned to one of the three disorder groups. In this way, the diagnostic selectivity of the non-invasive HSR-EMG can be determined.

Altogether seven parameters have been used for the validation of the typical differences in the HSR-EMG pattern of healthy volunteers, patients with muscular disorders and patients with neuronal disorders. The parameters can be divided into three groups regarding the excitation spread, the entire signal course in time as well as the shape of isolated peaks within the signal [Huppertz 1997]. Most of the parameters are well established in the field of signal processing and data analysis.

3.1 Parameters characterising the HSR-EMG signal in time

This group of parameters describes the entire signal course in time. In this way, the interaction of all MU located within the recording area of the spatial filter is regarded. The parameters belonging to this group are the signal **entropy (H)**, the **first zero crossing of the auto-correlation function (ACF_{zero})**, the **Chi-value (χ)** as well as the number of **values exceeding the RMS (T_{RMS})**.

The signal **entropy (H)** is a parameter well known in the field of signal processing. It describes the relation between the amplitude values of each sample within one measurement. Thus the entropy quantifies the predictability of the next measured amplitude value and characterises, in this way, the stochastic variability of the signal.

$$H = 1 - \sum_{i=\min}^{\max} \frac{p(x_i) \cdot \ln p(x_i)}{\ln(2)}$$

x_i = measured value
$p(x_i)$ = occurrence probability of x_i
min = smallest measured value
max = largest measured value

Comparable to the signal entropy the **first zero crossing of the auto-correlation function (ACF_{zero})** quantifies the stochastic variability of the signal too. The auto-correlation function (ACF) describes how similar different signal parts are. In the case of non-deterministic signals, like the HSR-EMG signal, the first zero crossing takes at higher values place, if the signal becomes more equal to itself.

$$ACF_{zero} = \frac{1}{2T} \sum_{t=-T}^{T} s(t) \cdot s(t+\tau)$$

s(t) = HSR-EMG signal
τ = time variable
T = smallest measuring duration
t = time

The **Chi-value (χ)** is based on the frequency distribution of the sample values. The frequency corresponds in this case to the probability that a sample with an amplitude within a given range is appears in the signal. The shape of the frequency distribution can be quantified by means of the χ^2-test which checks the probability that the frequency distribution is Gaussian. Here, as a quantifying parameter the Chi-value has been introduced. It corresponds not to the probability but to the absolute deviation to a Gaussian distribution.

$$\chi = \sum_{i=1}^{K} \frac{(X_i - N_i)^2}{N_i}$$

K = Number of different amplitude values
X_i = Frequency of a certain amplitude in the HSR-EMG signal
N_i = Frequency of a certain amplitude, when a Gaussian distribution is assumed
The parameter **values exceeding the RMS (T_{RMS})** has been defined as the number of samples with amplitude higher than the root mean square of the signal. To be independent from the recording time the parameter has been normalised to the total number of samples belonging to the signal.

$$T_{RMS} = \frac{1}{T}\sum_{i=1}^{n} t_i \quad \text{with} \quad \begin{array}{ll} t=1 & x_i > RMS \\ t=0 & x_i < RMS \end{array}$$

n = number of samples
T = measuring duration
t = time

3.2 Parameters regarding the isolated peaks

The excitation of a single MU can be identified in the signal by isolated peaks. Therefore, to the second group belong parameters describing the shape of isolated peaks. A signal part has been identified as a peak, if the following criteria are satisfied:

- The maximum amplitude must be higher than three times the RMS of the signal.
- Between the peak maximum and the adjacent minima the signal has to be continuous increasing respectively decreasing.
- The signal part identified as a peak is limited by the first crossing of the baseline before the minimum left to the peak maximum and by the first zero crossing of the baseline after the minimum right to the peak maximum

In initial investigations it has been shown that two parameters are sufficient to characterise the changes in the HSR-EMG pattern [Huppertz 1997]. These parameters are the **slope of the peak (S)** and the **peak amplitude frequency distribution (PAFD)**.
The parameter **slope of the peak** has been defined as the amplitude difference between the left minimum of the peak and its maximum divided by the time delay between both points. The parameter has been calculated for each peak detected within the HSR-EMG signal. The median value of all slops has been used standing in for all peaks which occur in the signal.

$$S = median\left[\left|\frac{x_{\min} - x_{\max}}{t_{\min} - t_{\max}}\right|\right]_P$$

P = number of peaks

The **peak amplitude frequency distribution (PAFD)** counts the number of peaks which have maximum peak amplitude within in a given interval. Similar to the frequency distribution of sample values the peak amplitude frequency distribution corresponds to the probability that a peak with maximum amplitude in a given interval can be found in the HSR-EMG signal. The PAFD of patients with muscular disorders shows high values for low amplitude peaks and low values for high amplitude peaks. This is in contrast to patients with neuronal disorders in which a typical biphasic shape of the PAFD can be found [Ramaekers 1993]. As a parameter describing the shape of the peak frequency distribution, the centroid of area has been calculated. The centroid of area is defined as the amplitude interval which divides the peak frequency distribution in two areas of the same size.

$$\sum_{i=1}^{a-1} N_i \Delta a < \frac{\sum_{i=1}^{A} N_i \Delta a}{2} < \sum_{i=a}^{N} N_i \Delta a$$

N_i = Frequency of maximum peak amplitudes within the interval i
A = Number of intervals
Δa = interval width
a = PAFD = bound which satisfies the inequality

3.3 Parameters regarding the excitation spread

The most significant parameter describing the excitation spread along the muscle fibres is **the conduction velocity in single MU (MUCV)**. The MUCV can be determined from the delay between the maximum amplitude of one peak in two adjacent and parallel to the muscle fibres orientated channels and their spatial distance (Figure 4). Since the conduction velocity depends on the temperature of the muscle, all MUCV values have been normalised to a temperature of 33°C [Rau 1997]. It has been shown earlier by Ramaekers et al. that the conduction velocity in single MUs is decreased in muscular disorders but unchanged in neuronal disorders [Ramaekers 1993].

3.4 Classification process

The parameter set can be used as a basis for the classification of the patients in healthy volunteers, patients with muscular disorders, and patients with neuronal disorders. Therefore, a classification procedure has been introduced based on a Fuzzy-approach [Kamel 1991].
Since the parameters have different diagnostic selectivity, the classification procedure has to be adapted to this specific classification task. This has been done by introducing weighting factors between 0 and 50 for each parameter. The weighting factors regard the contribution of each parameter to the classification result. They have been optimised by classifying a training data set generated with an especially developed muscle model [Disselhorst-Klug 1998]. This was to separate the training data set from the data set used for validation. The training data set consists of different simulated HSR-EMG signals regarding muscle structures with no pathological changes, muscle structures where a loss of muscle fibres takes place (muscular disorders), and muscle structures where a loss of entire MUs takes place (neuronal disorders) [Disselhorst-Klug 1998].
Performing the Fuzzy classification process, in a first step, all parameter values have been normalized to mean zero and variance 1. Starting the classification process, three clusters have been defined using a hierarchical cluster process like the nearest neighbourhood

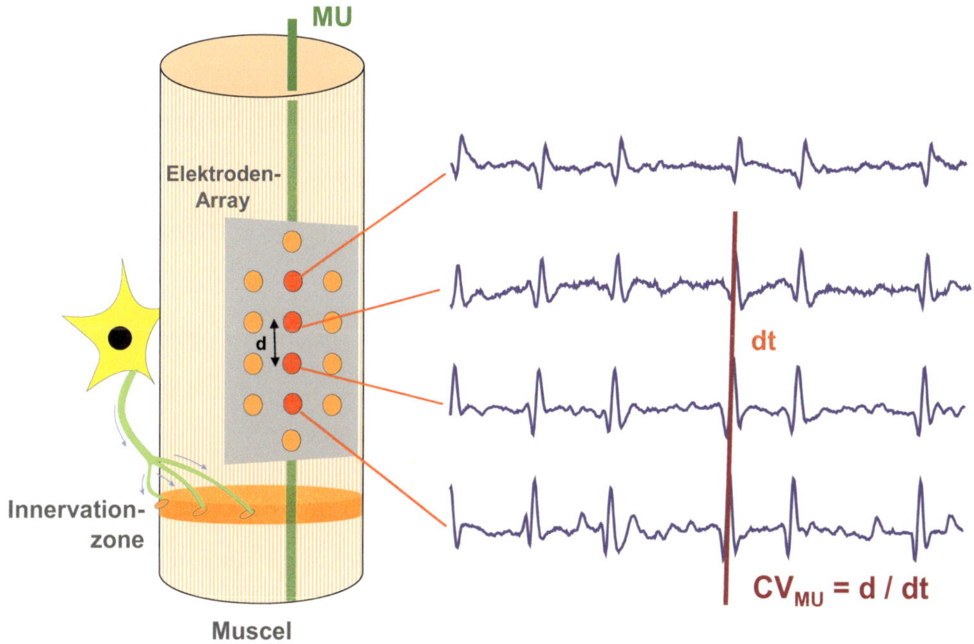

Fig. 4. Conduction velocity.
The conduction velocity of single motor units MUCV can be detected by several NDD-filtered channels arranged parallel to the muscle fibres.

algorithm. These three clusters represent the groups "neuronal disorder", "muscular disorder" and "healthy". The centroid of each cluster has been used to characterise its position in the feature space. After that, the Euclidian distances between the features of each HSR-EMG signal and the centroid of each cluster have been calculated. According to the Fuzzy classification process introduced by Kamel et al. [Kamel 1991], membership-values v_{ij} have been calculated:

$$v_{ij} = \frac{1}{\sum_{k=1}^{z} \left(\frac{d_{ij}}{d_{ik}} \right)^{\frac{1}{m-1}}}$$

v_{ij} = membership-values
m = 2: controlling the degree of fuzzyfication
d_{ij} = Euclidian distance between the $HSR\text{-}EMG_i$ and the centroid of the $cluster_j$
d_{ik} = Euclidian distance between the $HSR\text{-}EMG_i$ and the centroid of the $cluster_k$
z = 3: Number of clusters
Afterwards a new centroid for each cluster Z_j has been has been determined following:

$$\vec{Z}_j = \frac{\sum_{i=1}^{n} v_{ij} \vec{x}_i}{\sum_{i=1}^{n} v_{ij}}$$

n = 7: Number of parameters
x_i = set of parameter values calculated from the HSR-EMG$_i$
Due to the weighting of the set of parameter values calculated from the HSR-EMG signals with the membership-values, this iteration converges. The iteration process has been stopped when the following abort criterion is fulfilled:

$$\sum_{j=1}^{z}\sum_{k=0}^{n}\left|Z_{jk}^{(s)} - Z_{jk}^{(s-1)}\right| \;<\; \varepsilon$$

s = Number of iteration
ε = 0.9: defined value
Next the membership-ship values have to be normalised with:

$$\overline{v}_{ij} = \frac{v_{ij}}{\sum_{k=1}^{z} v_{ik}}$$

And finally, each HSR-EMG signal has been assigned to the cluster with the highest membership-value.
The training data set, consisting of simulated HSR-EMG signals and representing the different types of disorders, has been classified with all possible combinations of weighting factors. The optimal combination of weighting factors was found when a maximum number of simulated HSR-EMG signals were classified correctly. The weighting factor combination as a result of the optimisation process is shown in Table 1.

Parameter	Weighting-factor
Signal entropy	2
First zero crossing of ACF	1
Values exceeding the RMS	19
Chi-value	19
Slope of the peak	2
Peak frequency distribution	9
MUCV	40

Table 1. Weighting of the parameter.
Optimised weighting factors for each parameter. The weighting-factors take the diagnostic selectivity of each parameter into consideration. [Disselhorst-Klug 1998]

The same classification algorithm can be used to classify HSR-EMG signals recorded in patients suffering from neuromuscular disorders. Here, in a first step the parameter values have to be multiplied by the related weighting-factor. Afterwards the classification procedure has to be executed as described above.

4. Clinical validation

The HSR-EMG has been recorded at isometric, maximum voluntary contraction of the m. abductor pollicis brevis. The used electrode array consists of 16 gold covered pin electrodes

(0.5 mm diameter) in a two-dimensional arrangement. Due to the low distance between the m. abductor pollicis brevis and the recording side, the inter-electrode distance has been chosen to 2.5 mm. Directly at the electrode array, each of the 16 EMG-leads has been amplified and, later, transmitted to a recording unit. It consists of a band-pass filter (1 - 500 Hz) and a second amplifier. All 16 EMG-leads have been stored on a PC with a sampling frequency of 4000 HZ each. The spatial filtering of the EMG-data has been performed on the PC by specially developed software. From each spatially filtered channel, all evaluation parameters have been calculated. The value of each parameter has been averaged over all NDD-filtered channels. After determination of the parameter values, the HSR-EMG signal of each patient has been assigned to one of the three groups by the described Fuzzy classification process.
For the quantitative evaluation of the typical HSR-EMG patterns altogether 97 subjects, healthy volunteers (41) and patients with neuromuscular disorders (56), aged between the infancy and 25 years, have been investigated. The group of patients investigated consists of 35 patients with Duchenne Muscle Dystrophy (muscular disorder) and 21 patients with Spinal Muscle Atrophy (neuronal disorder). The diagnosis of the patients has been proofed by muscle biopsy. The parameters have been calculated in three different HSR-EMG recordings of each child. Afterwards, the median value of each parameter has been used, accounting for the typical HSR-EMG pattern. Some of the parameters, such as the conduction velocity in single MUs depend significantly on the age of the investigated child [Huppertz 1997]. Those parameters have been normalised to an age of eight.

Diagnostic selectivity of the HSR-EMG: 97%			
	Duchenne	Healthy	SMA
classified as muscular disorder	35	0	0
classified as healthy	0	41	3
classified as neuronal disorder	0	0	18
sensitivity	100%	100%	90%
specificity	100%	95,1%	100%
positive prediction	100%	93,2%	100%

Table 2. Diagnostic selectivity of the non-invasive HSR-EMG in children with Duchenne muscle dystrophy and spinal muscle atrophy. Shown, are the numbers of patients which have been classified in each group. Adapted from [Disselhorst-Klug 2000]

The result of the classification which was based on the weighted evaluation parameters is summarised in Table 2. With the classification, 100% of all investigated healthy children, 100% of all investigated patients with muscular disorders, and 87% of all investigated patients with neuronal disorders have been correctly identified. That mean, that on the average, in 97% of all investigated children the diagnosis by means of the non-invasive HSR-EMG was correct.

5. Conclusions

The High-Spatial-Resolution EMG provides information about the single MU activity in a non-invasive way even during maximum voluntary contraction of the muscle. Therefore, the methodology could be suitable for a non-invasive diagnosis of neuromuscular disorders. Earlier investigations of healthy children and children with Duchenne Muscle Dystrophy or Spinal Muscle Atrophy have shown, that there is a typical change in the HSR-EMG signal course in each patient group. These typical changes in the HSR-EMG pattern can be evaluated by seven parameters regarding the signal course in time, the shape of isolated peaks, and the excitation spread in single MUs. Based on these evaluation parameters and an especially developed classification procedure, it is possible to classify correctly 97% of all investigated children. That means, in this patient group, the diagnostic selectivity of the HSR-EMG is in the same range or even better than the commonly used needle-EMG techniques. This result could be reached, though the HSR-EMG methodology is limited to superficial muscles and MUs. Therefore, the HSR-EMG promises to be a suitable tool for a non-invasive diagnosis of neuromuscular disorders in clinical application.

6. References

Basmajian J.V. and De Luca C.J. (1985) Muscle Alive; Their Functions Revealed by Electromyography, *William & Wilkins 5th edition*

Black J.T:, Bhatt G.P., Dejesus P.V., Scotland D.L., Rowland L.P., (1974) Diagnostic accuracy of clinical data, quantitative electromyography and histochemistry in neuromuscular disease. *J. Neurol Science*, 21, 59-70.

Broman H., Bilotto G., and De Luca C. (1985) A note on non-invasive estimation of muscle fibre conduction velocity. *IEEE Tras. Biomed. Eng.*, 32, 311-319

Buchtal F., Kamieniecka Z. (1982) The diagnostic yield of quantitative electromyography and quantitative muscle biopsy in neuromuscular disorders. *Muscle Nerve*, 5, 265 - 280.

De Luca C., and Merletti R. (1987) Surface myoelectric signal cross-talk among muscles of the leg. *Electroencephalography. and Clin. Neurophysiol.* 69, 568-575

Disselhorst-Klug C., Bahm J., Ramaekers V., Trachterna A., Rau G. (2000): Non-invasive approach of motor unit recording during muscle contractions in humans. *European Journal of Applied Physiology*, 83: 144 - 150.

Disselhorst-Klug C., Silny J., Rau G. (1997): Improvement of spatial resolution in surface EMG: A theoretical and experimental comparison of different spatial filters. *IEEE Trans. Biomed. Eng.*, 44,7,567-574.

Disselhorst-Klug C., Silny J., Rau G. (1998): Estimation of the Relationship between the non-invasively Detected Activity of Single Motor Units and their Characteristic Pathological Changes by Modelling. *J. of Electromyography and Kinesiology*, Vol. 8/5, 323 - 335.

Dubowitz V. (1991) Atlas der Muskelerkrankungen im Kindesalter. *Hippokrates Verlag*.

Farina D, Schulte E, Merletti R, Rau G, Disselhorst-Klug C. (2003): Single motor unit analysis from spatially filtered surface electromyogram signals. PartI: spatial selectivity. *Med Biol Eng Comput.*, 41(3):330-7. IF 0,744

Hausmanova-Petusewicz I., Jedrezejowska H. (1971) Correlation between electromyographic findings and muscle biopsy in cases of neuromuscular disease. *J. Neurol. Science*, 13, 85-106.

Hermens H., Freriks B., Disselhorst-Klug C., Rau G. (2000): Development of recommendations for sensors and sensor placement procedures. *Journal of Electromyography and Kinesiology*, Vol. 10, 5, 361 - 374.

Huppertz H.-J. Disselhorst-Klug C., Silny J., Rau G., Heimann G. (1997) Diagnostic yield of non-invasive High-Spatial-Resolution-EMG in Neuromuscular Disease. *Muscle and Nerve*, in press.

Jerusalem F. (1979) Muskelerkrankungen, Klinik - Therapie - Pathologie. *Thieme Verlag Stuttgart.*

Jonsson B., Bagge U.E. (1968) Displacement, deformation and fracture of wire electrodes for electromyography. *Electromyography. 8. 328 - 347.*

Kamel M.S. (1991) A threshold Fuzzy c.means algorithm for semi-fuzzy clustering. *Pattern Recognition*, 27,9,

Komi P.V., Buskirk E.R. (1970) Reproducibility of electromyographic measurements with inserted wire electrodes and surface electrodes. *Electromyography*, 10, 357 - 367

Lynn P.A., Bettkes N.D., Hugh A.D. and Johnson S,W. (1978) Influence of electrode geometry on bipolar recordings of the surface electromyogram. *Med. Biol. Eng. Comput.*, 16, 651-660.

Masuda T., Miyano H., Sadoyama T. (1985) A surface electrode array for detecting action potential trains of single motor units. *Electroenceph. Clin. Neurophysiol.* 60, 435-443.

Merletti R. and De Luca C.J. (1989) New Techniques in surface electromyography. *In Desmedt J.E, (ed): Computer-Aided electromyography and expert systems., Elsevier, Amsterdam, 115-124.*

Papoulis A. (1965) Probability, random variables, and stochastic processes. *McGraw Hill, New York.*

Ramaekers V., Disselhorst-Klug C., Schneider J., Silny J., Forst J., Forst R., Kotlarek F., Rau G. (1993) Clinical Application of a non-invasive multi-electrode array EMG for the recording of single motor unit activity. *Neuropaediatrics*, 24, 134-138.

Rau G., Disselhorst-Klug C. (1997): Principles of high spatial resolution EMG (HSR-EMG): Single motor unit detection and the application in the diagnosis of neuromuscular disorders. *J. of Electromyography and Kinesiology*, Vol.7, No.4, 233-239.

Rau G., Disselhorst-Klug C., Silny J. (1997a) Non-invasive approach to motor unit characterization: muscle structure, membrane dynamics and neuronal control. *J. of Biomechanics*, Vol. 30, No. 5, 441 - 446.

Rau G., Reucher H. (1985) Muscular activity and surface EMG. In Perren S.M. and Schneider E. (ed.): Biomechanics: Current Interdisciplinary research, 27 - 35.

Rau G., Schulte E., Disselhorst-Klug C. (2004): From cell to movement: To what answers does EMG really contribute? *J. of Electromyography and Kinesiology*, 14, 611-617.

Reucher H., Rau G. and Silny J. (1987a) Spatial filtering of non-invasive multi-electrode EMG: Part I - Introduction to Measuring Technique and Applications. *IEEE trans. Bio-Med. Eng.*, BME-34,2, 98-105.

Reucher H., Silny J. and Rau G. (1987b) Spatial filtering of non-invasive multi-electrode EMG: Part II - Filter performance in theory and modelling. *IEEE Trans. Bio-Med. Eng.*, BME-34,2, 106-113.

13

EMG vs. Thermography in Severe Carpal Tunnel Syndrome

Breda Jesenšek Papež and Miroslav Palfy
University Clinical Centre Maribor, Slovenia

1. Introduction

Carpal tunnel syndrome (CTS) is one of the most common compressive neuropathies in the upper extremities (Bland, 2007) and a frequent cause of pain, paresthesias and impaired hand function. A syndrome is, by definition, a collection of signs and symptoms. Its clinical symptoms depend on duration and degree of the compression of the median nerve (MN). At first the sensory nerve fibres are affected, but as the compression persists, large calibre myelinated nerve fibres (sensory and motor) undergo damage as well. Clinical symptoms and signs alone are not sufficient to confirm the diagnosis and surgical release, electrodiagnostic methods are needed for this purpose (Rosenbaum & Ochoa, 2002).

Within the last decades, CTS reached epidemic proportions in many occupations and industries. It represents a large expense because of absence from work and wage compensation due to temporary incapacity for work. For this reason numerous researches, not only in the field of medicine, are looking for a non-invasive diagnostic method for determining those loads in workplaces that facilitate the development of CTS (Ammer, 1999, 2003; R.T. Herrick & S.K. Herrick, 1987; Schartelmüller & Ammer, 1996; Tchou et al., 1992).

Intelligent systems have turned out to be useful and successful aids in medicine for determining, classifying, sample searching, data analysis, and new knowledge discovery (Haas & Burnham, 2008). But thermography, on the contrary, did not receive due attention (American Academy of Neurology, 1990) in the area of determining entrapment neuropathies, despite its advantages (completely safe, passive investigation, without contact, painless and can be easily repeated with low costs of use) (Hackett, 1976).

1.1 Thermography

Thermography is a procedure for remote determination of temperature of objects, based on the detection of infrared radiation that the observed objects emit. As the name itself implies, thermographic or infrared cameras detect electromagnetic radiation below the frequency of red light. The range of wave lengths of infrared radiation includes lengths ranging from 700 nm to 1 mm, while thermographic cameras operate within an even narrower spectre, ranging from approx. 900 nm and 14 µm. As all objects emit infrared radiation, thermographic camera can determine an object's temperature on the basis of object's energy flux density. In this manner it can create a thermal image of observed objects (Fig. 1), where warmer objects usually appear in a warmer and lighter colour (light red to white) and colder objects appear in a colder and darker colour (blue to black) (Gaussorgues, 1994).

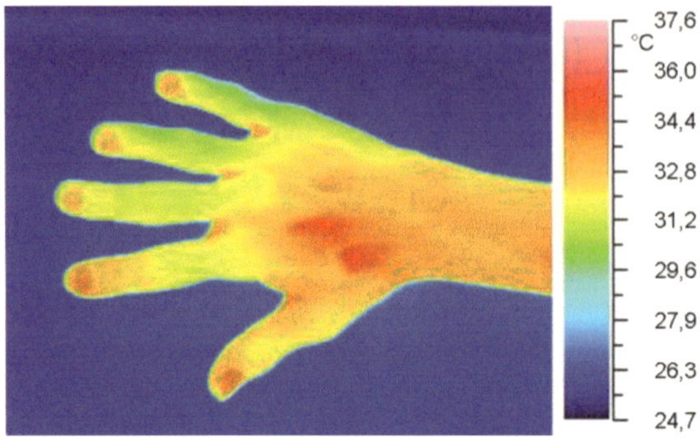

Fig. 1. Thermographic image of a patient's hand.

The possibility of detection of warmer objects on a colder background resulted in the development of thermography primarily for military and surveillance purposes, but with the decrease in prices of (initially very expensive) cameras, thermography established its position in numerous other areas too, such as industry, medicine, meteorology, and archaeology (Ring, 1995b).

Thermography, as we know it today, started to develop as late as the second half of the 20th century. Before this, remote temperature measurement was not possible, so surface measurements performed with various thermometers were used. The invention of the first thermometer is ascribed to the Venetian scientist Santorio Santorio, who improved Galileo's thermoscope in the beginning of the 17th century and equipped it with a scale, whereby enabling reading of ambient temperature. The precision of this thermometer was poor, because it was filled with air, and the effect of air pressure on the thermometer was not taken into account. The following improvement occurred in the mid 17th century - the use of alcohol in a closed bottle somewhat improved precision. The first mercury thermometer was made in 1714 by Gabriel Fahrenheit, who also takes credit for the first standardized temperature scale. He used the recently discovered freezing point and boiling point as reference values, and divided the intermediate interval to 180 degrees. He also added additional 32 degrees for values below the freezing point and set the lowest temperature 0, because this was the lowest temperature, which he achieved in his laboratory with a mixture of ice, water, and salt. In 1742, a Swedish scientist Anders Celsius developed his own scale by dividing the interval between the boiling point and the freezing point to 100 degrees. Interestingly enough, 0° was used to mark the boiling point, and 100° for the freezing point. The following year, Jean Pierre Cristin reversed the Celsius's scale and called it the hundred-degree scale. This name was in use until 1948, when it was renamed into the Celsius scale by international agreement. In 1848, a Scot William Thomson, later known as Lord Kelvin, proposed an absolute temperature scale with absolute zero at the lowest theoretical temperature the body can have -273.15°C. The standard unit for temperature is named after him - Kelvin (K).

At the end of the 16th century, a Neapolitan Giambattista della Porta was the first to notice the consequences of thermal radiation. In working on experiments with the concave glass he established that warmth or coldness can also reflect from glass, after placing candle flame and snowball in front of the glass. Almost two decades later, in 1790, a Swiss physicist, Pierre Prevost, introduced a theory, according to which all bodies, both warm and cold, thermally radiate, and that the quantity of radiation depends on body temperature. Only a few years later, a British astronomer of German descent, William Herschel, while diverting sunrays by means of prism discovered radiation beyond a still visible, red part of the light spectrum (Ring, 1987). With the thermometer he detected higher temperature beyond the red part of the spectrum and predicted that there is invisible light.

Herschel published his results in 1800, and named the invisible radiation "heat rays". The name infrared radiation was established as late as the second half of the 19th century. This was followed by the period of new developments in the area of thermodynamics. Firstly, in 1859, Gustav Kirchhoff introduced his law of thermal radiation, followed by Stefan (1879, by means of experiments) and Boltzmann (1884, with theoretical derivation) with the black body radiation law. In 1893, Wilhelm Wien introduced his relation between the wave length of the strongest radiation of black body and its temperature, which lead to Planck's black-body radiation law published in 1901. These laws represent physical background, which serves as the basis for the functioning of thermographic cameras.

One of the first steps in the development of the measurement of thermal radiation was the discovery of thermoelectric effect or the Seebeck's effect, named after his inventor, Thomas Johann Seebeck, Estonian physicist of German origin. In 1821 he discovered that voltage exists between two ends of metal rods, when these ends are at different temperatures. This resulted in the discovery of thermocouple. For measuring the created voltage he had to connect a metal rod to a conductor, which resulted in voltage opposite to the initial one. By using a different metal he was able to take advantage of the difference in both voltages, since it depends on the material used. He measured the created voltage and with it, indirectly, the temperature difference. Increase in temperature difference also increased the measured voltage, and this enabled him to calibrate the thermocouple and use it as a thermometer. Italian physicists Leopoldo Nobili and Macedonio Melloni increased the precision of temperature measurement by connecting several thermocouples. But in 1878, Samuel Pierpont Langley, an American astronomer, took a step further, as he invented a bolometer.

Langley used two platinum strips, covered with soot, as the ends of the Wheatstone bridge or the electrical resistance meter, equipped with a sensitive galvanometer and battery. One of the strips was exposed to infrared radiation, which caused the strip to warm up. This altered its resistance, which he was able to measure with his circuit. Thus he created the first temperature sensor, which exploits predictable variations of platinum resistance as the result of temperature variations. In the 20th century, the discovery of new combinations of materials lead to increasingly more precise and smaller bolometers, which in the mid 1980s resulted in the invention of the microbolometer - fields of temperature sensors made of silicon or vanadium oxide or amorphous silicon (Fig. 2). It was invented by the American corporation Honeywell for the US Department of Defense. After 1992 the technology became available to the wider public and is now used as the detection field in thermographic cameras of numerous producers (Cuthbertson, 1995).

Thermographic camera is an infrared camera, which generates a thermal image on the basis of measured values of infrared radiation of observed objects. Unlike a thermovision camera, which is used for watching in dark or under poor visibility conditions, a thermographic camera also determines actual values of surface temperatures of observed objects. The activity of thermographic camera can basically be compared to the activity of an ordinary digital videocamera, whereby the role of CCD sensors is assumed by the field of thermal IR sensors (microbolometers or semi-conductors with a narrow passage). By taking into account emissivity, distance, ambient temperature, and other factors, the camera calculates temperatures, which are detected by individual sensors, and generates thermal image on the basis of these temperatures. For the display of individual temperatures it uses a non-linear palette of so-called "non-primary colours", ranging from white for the highest temperature through red and yellow shades for higher temperatures to blue for lower, and black for the lowest temperatures (Fig. 1). The resolution of a thermal image rarely exceeds 320x240 pixels and is determined by the number of IR sensors (Fig. 2).

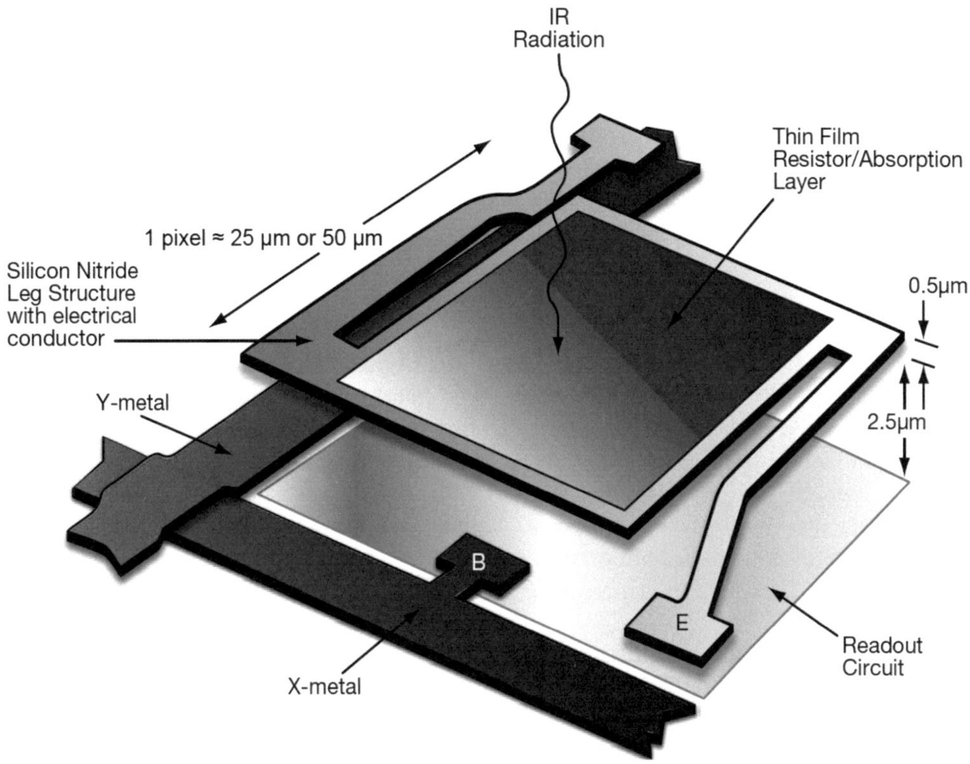

Fig. 2. The basis structure of a microbolometer (uncooled IR camera pixel).

Despite the initial development solely for military purposes, today thermographic cameras are used in different areas. Thermography is an excellent method of examination, also useful in the field of medicine for its safety (passive, no touch examination), lack of pain and invasiveness, easy reproducibility and low running costs (Hackett, 1976). Despite its advantages TG is not useful for routine diagnosis of CTS, since unmyelinated fibres remain intact until late in the severe nerve entrapment (American Academy of Neurology, 1990). Many patients with EMG diagnosed CTS have normal thermographic studies; however TG may show abnormalities in median nerve distribution in severe cases of CTS (Rosenbaum & Ochoa, 2002). To ensure reliability of TG pattern recognition we introduced a novel approach to thermal image analysis by using an artificial neural network (ANN).

1.2 Artificial neural networks

Data mining techniques provide a variety of different approaches for data analysis. ANNs are one of them (Larose, 2005). They are increasingly used in problem domains involving classification and are capable of finding shared features in a set of seemingly unrelated data.

An ANN is an abstract computational model of the human brain. Similar to the brain, an ANN is composed of artificial neurons and interconnections. When we view such a network as a graph, neurons can be represented as nodes and interconnections as edges (Fig. 3). There are many known variations of ANNs, differing in their topology, orientation of connections and approaches to learning (Kasabov, 1996). Probably the most established are "feed-forward backpropagation" neural networks (a.k.a. multilayer perceptrons). Due to its efficiency and relatively simple training process this type of ANN was chosen for our classification (diagnosis of CTS, based on collected data).

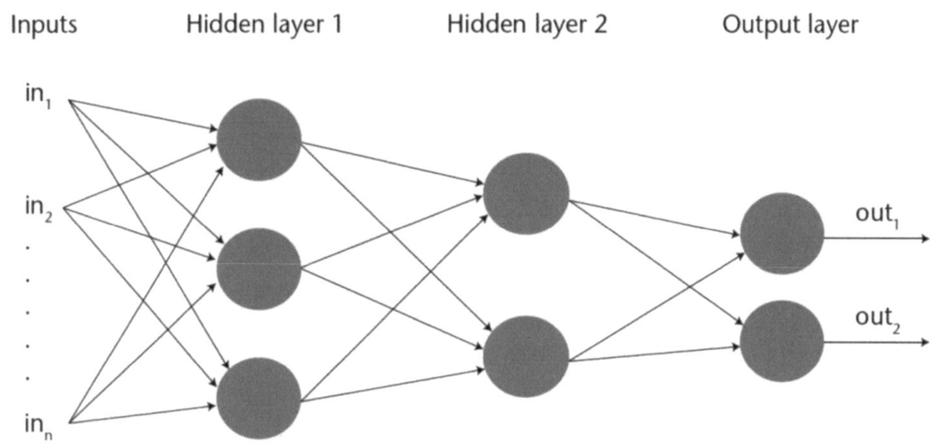

Fig. 3. Example of an ANN (multilayer perceptron).

A multilayer perceptron consists of layers of neurons, more specifically an input layer, an output layer and at least one hidden middle layer. Neurons on the same layer are not connected; all interconnections are directed from the input layer towards the output layer. The input layer is represented by normalized numerical values or inputs, passed on to the neurons on the 1st hidden layer. These neurons generate their own numerical outputs and pass them on to the next layer. This process continues until the last (output) layer and resembles the transmission of impulses inside the brain. Each connection in a network is weighted. The weights are internal parameters of an ANN and simulate the biological synaptic strengths in a natural neuron (McCulloch & Pitts, 1943).

An artificial neuron generates its output through an activation function (Fig. 4) which accepts as its input the sum of weighted outputs from neurons on the previous layer and an externally applied bias, denoted by b_k (1). The bias has the effect of increasing or lowering the net input of the activation function, depending on whether it is positive or negative. Weights and biases directly affect the importance of individual connections.

$$net_k = x_1 w_{k1} + x_2 w_{k2} + \cdots + x_m w_{km} + b_k \tag{1}$$

Different activation functions are commonly used. We chose the log-sigmoid function (2).

$$f(net_k) = \frac{1}{1+e^{-net}} \tag{2}$$

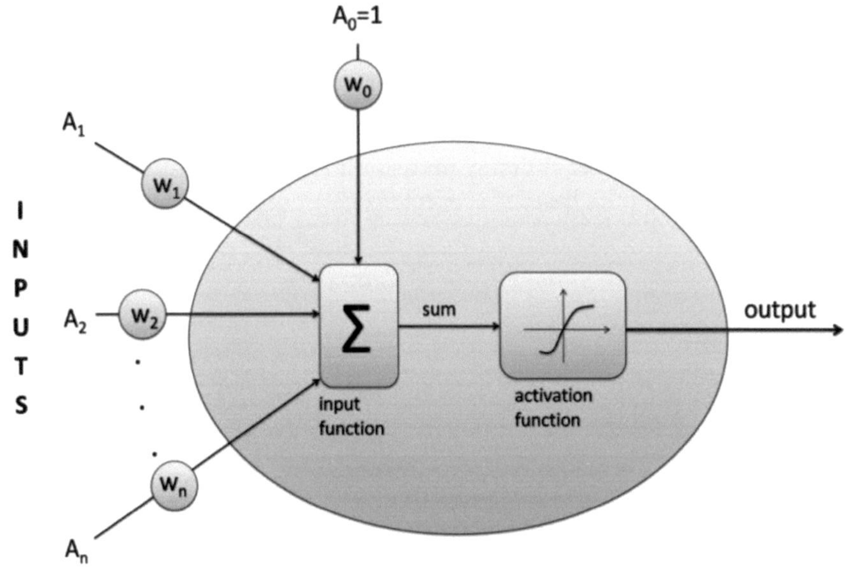

Fig. 4. Model of an artificial neuron.

The output of a multilayer perceptron consists of numerical values, generated by the last (output) layer. It is usually mapped into a binary value, identifying the class of the object, represented by its numerical descriptors at the input level. In order to successfully classify input objects an ANN must go through a thorough process of supervised learning. It consists of applying a large number of training examples to the inputs of an ANN and adjusting the parameters (weights) according to a highly popular algorithm known as the "error back-propagation algorithm".

First, numerical descriptors of an object from the training set are applied to the inputs of the ANN. The network classifies the object by calculating the output values. The output is compared to the desired (correct) result and an error value is calculated. If this error exceeds the defined threshold value, the sequence of corrective adjustments to the weights is started. Adjustments are done from the output towards the input layer as the error signal travels backwards. After the corrections are done, the network generates a smaller error when classifying the same object, thus improves itself through learning. A more detailed description of the error back-propagation algorithm is beyond the scope of this chapter and is well documented in literature (Rojas, 1996). More knowledgeable readers might find it interesting that weight adjustments were done under *generalized delta rule* which included a *momentum* constant, increasing the rate of learning while avoiding the danger of instability (Kantardzic, 2003).

In theory, if the training set is large and diverse enough, an ANN can accumulate enough knowledge to reliably classify unknown objects.

To test the reliability of an ANN the data to be classified is usually divided into two sets. The first set consists of cases used for the learning process through which an ANN adapts itself and the second set consists of cases, previously unknown to trained ANN. These cases are then classified and the results are compared to actual class values.

2. Background

There have been several studies published that have used thermography as a diagnostic tool for determining various entrapment neuropathies (Ammer, 1999, 2003; R.T. Herrick & S.K. Herrick, 1987; Schartelmüller & Ammer, 1996; Tchou et al., 1992). There is a generally accepted opinion that thermography is not appropriate for routine diagnostics of CTS and other entrapment neuropathies, as they predominantly affect thick myelinated fibres, while thermography (indirectly through the arrangement of temperature changes) enables only an assessment of the functional status of thin, mostly unmyelinated, nociceptor and sympathetic, vasomotor nerve fibres (Rosenbaum & Ochoa, 2002). However, since MN contains motor, sensory and sympathetic fibres, we can justifiably expect involvement of the autonomous nervous system and consequently thermoregulation of hand, when entrapment occurs. A quick, precise, dynamic, very sensitive, and non-invasive surface detection of temperature changes of the skin is within the domain of thermography (Jones & Plassmann, 2002).

3. Methods

Monitoring the dynamics of thermographic changes in CTS aided by artificial intelligence, represented the basic research challenge. We asked ourselves if the artificial intelligence system can identify the typical CTS pattern from the thermogram of a hand, and, if so, at what stage of entrapment. Much like in other entrapment neuropathies, the myelinated fibres are the ones that are primarily affected, but chronic or extremely severe acute entrapment also captures thin sympathetic (autonomous) nerve fibres (Benaroch, 2007). However, it is necessary to point out that the latter have the capacity of improving much faster (Marotte, 1974).

In 1976, for the purposes of thermographic diagnostics in the area of entrapment neuropathies, researchers developed the provocative cold stress test (Ring, 1995a). In this test the patient's hands wrapped in thin plastic gloves are submerged in cold water (in different researchers temperature varies from 1°C to no more than 20°C) for 1 minute. After a 10 to 15-minute adaptation to the room temperature the temperature changes of the hand are determined using an IR camera. Thermographic images are taken before and after the stress test, in specific time intervals. During this process the patient should not touch anything.

According to a theory, provocation excites sympathetic autonomous nerve fibres of the hand and induces vasoconstriction. Quantitative thermography (measurement of hand temperature after a specific time interval) is used for estimating the response of the autonomous nervous system. It is expressed as vasodilation or reactive hyperthermia, which consequently normalizes hand temperature. A healthy person develops reactive hyperthermia relatively early (within 10 minutes) and equally on all fingers. But in CTS, by using thermography, we discovered different temperature changes. Neurophysiologic basis of the procedure is the measurement of the response of the sympathetic nervous system. Autonomous nerve fibres, which innervate the skin, run together with sensory fibres of peripheral nerves and also have the same arrangement within an individual nerve (Kline & Hudson, 1990). The autonomous, vegetative, nervous system of the hand controls sweat secretion and vasomotorics. The latter is responsible for the control of skin circulation required for maintaining body temperature. In vasodilation body temperature is diverted from the body and, vice versa, in vasoconstriction the temperature is retained. The initial response of the body to the provocation cold stress test is vasoconstriction.

We believe that the provocation stress test is more useful for research purposes. In our previous clinical practice the method did not stand the test. We often tried with different water temperatures. We have used ice cold water, in line with the published standard and protocol for clinical thermography (International Academy of Clinical Thermology, 2002), as well as warmer water, up to 20°C, which is recommended by Ring (Ring, 1995a). The latter claims that in the case of cold water the regeneration period is (too) long, while the Guidelines advise against water that is warmer than ice cold, as otherwise sympaticus stimulation would not be sufficient. The basic deficiencies of the test we have come across in clinical use are: it is too time consuming, unpractical (requires putting on and taking off thin plastic gloves with as little contact as possible), "old-fashioned" (the majority of patients thought it was too banal holding hands in a vessel with usually cold water, and for this reason they were not very cooperative), and unpleasant (people with impaired autonomous nervous system experience holding hands in cold water as pain). Numerous volunteers have declared that they would rather undergo EMG investigation again than the provocation cold stress test. Clear and simple instructions not to touch the wall or bottom of the vessel have frequently been breached. Constant supervision was required for a very simple test. Obviously, other clinicians have also come across similar problems, because we found no literature sources on published clinical (just research) studies using the provocation stress test on a sufficiently large population, which would provide enough data for a reliable statistical analysis. For the reasons described above our attention has been directed to finding a method that would enable us to abandon the stress test.

In currently published studies, thermographic images were analysed by means of commercial computer programmes and manual definition of fields of interest (Ammer, 1999, 2003; R.T. Herrick & S.K. Herrick, 1987; Schartelmüller & Ammer, 1996; Medical Imaging Research Group, University of Glamorgan, 2004). The analysis of thermographic images is a demanding and time-consuming task, because the precision in determining the fields of interest of images is the decisive factor for a proper diagnosis. We often require measurements with a precision of 0.1°K.

For this purpose we have developed software tool, which provided us with an exact analysis of thermographic images and automated the CTS diagnosis procedure, while eliminating the need for the preliminary provocation cold stress test (Fig. 5).

We have used the well-known advantages of machine learning by using data mining (Kantardzic, 2002). We have developed a neural network, which is capable of diagnosing CTS on the basis of very discrete temperature differences that are invisible to the eye on a thermographic image.

Patients were selected from a pool of clinically suspect CTS patients referred by general practitioners and various specialists to our department. The exclusion criteria for participation was: previous operation for CTS, negative electrodiagnostic test for CTS, abnormal hand anatomy (amputations, injuries, other anomalies) preventing the acquisition of standard images of hands. Volunteers who did not exhibit symptoms of CTS and were subsequently diagnosed by electromyography as not having the syndrome were used to acquire images of healthy hands (dorsal and palmar views).

For our pilot study 112 images were examined: 23 patients (15 females, eight males; mean age 51.4 years, range 26-71 years) were used to acquire 60 images depicting 30 hands (dorsal and palmar views) at different stages of CTS; 13 volunteers (eight females, five males; mean age: 48.3 years, range 28-66 years) who did not exhibit symptoms of CTS and who were subsequently diagnosed by EMG as not suffering from the syndrome were used to acquire 52 images of healthy hands (dorsal and palmar views of 26 hands).

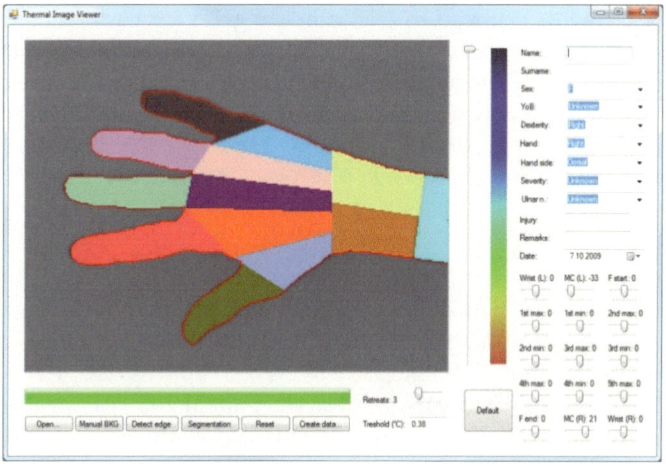

Fig. 5. Computer software for identification of mean temperatures of individual hand segments.

The results of a pilot study were very promising. In the majority of performed measurements classification exceeded the 77% effectiveness (Table 1).

The most important segments turned out to be fingers, especially the index finger and the little finger (which also coincides with the anatomic distal innervation area for the median or ulnar nerve (ulnaris). The results also coincided with a similar study carried out by Schartelmüller and Amer in relation to the thoracic syndrome pathology by means of manual analysis of thermograms (Schartelmüller & Ammer, 1996). Successful classification of our neural network was supported by the fact that whenever we excluded the majority of fields of interest of MN (thumb, index finger, and middle finger), the efficiency was not better, only accidental.

Included segments	**Success rate (%)**
All dorsal segments (reference case)	80.6
All segments	74.3
All palmar segments	65.6
All dorsal but thumb	81.8
All dorsal but index finger	77.3
All dorsal but middle finger	81.8
All dorsal but ring finger	79.2
All dorsal but little finger	75.2
All dorsal but index and little finger	70.8
All dorsal but thumb, index and middle finger	64.5
All dorsal without wrist segments	82.5
All dorsal without metacarpal segments	78.4

Table 1. Pilot study CTS classification success rates (each success rate percentage is the mean of five repeat runs on 22 randomly selected hands).

The findings of our pilot study spoke in favour of the applicability of the intelligent system for discerning CTS from thermovision images. In a smaller number of study and test cases (n = 112) the efficiency of classification exceeded our expectations. We were aware of the fact that a small set of elements can lead to misleadingly good (or bad) results. Therefore, for a realistic evaluation of efficiency of classification we have collected a significantly larger data base. In total we acquired 502 images of 251 hands (dorsal and palmar side of each hand). 71 patients (52 females and 19 males with mean age 56.8 years, range 23 - 90 years) contributed 274 images of 137 hands (in 5 patients only one hand met the inclusion criteria) and 57 volunteers (35 females, 22 males; mean age 47.6 years, range 25 - 74 years) contributed 228 images of 114 healthy hands.

3.1 Statistical analysis

All statistical analyses were performed using the R Project for Statistical Computing, a software language and environment for statistical computing, available as free software under the terms of GNU General Public License. Where appropriate, data are presented as mean ± SD or as percentages. Comparisons between patient and volunteer groups regarding segment temperatures were analysed by non-parametric Mann-Whitney-Wilcoxon test since it is used to compare two independent groups of sampled data and unlike the parametric t-test, makes no assumptions about the distribution of the data (e.g., normality). A p-value < 0.05 was considered to be statistically significant.

4. Study results

The prevailing opinion in literature states that for determining CTS by using thermography dorsal segments of the hand are more important than the palmar ones (R.T. Herrick & S.K. Herrick, 1987). Even more so, we have confirmed that palmar segments are not useful for detecting CTS by means of IR thermography (Fig. 6).

The finding was a surprise to us, because we have initially expected palmar changes, considering the distal innervation sample of MN. Our explanation is that obvious temperature differences on the dorsal or palmar side are the result of hand complexity. They originate both from anatomical and physiological and functional features of the hand. In anatomical terms, the skin on the hand is thinner and contains essentially more sweat glands (>450/cm^2) than on the dorsal side (Tortora & Derrickson, 2008). In physiological terms, the emotional stress is initially reflected by palm sweating (next to feet and armpits). In the majority of basic hand functions (grasping, leaning, carrying) the palmar side of palms and fingers is burdened. Everything we have described above has an important influence on local temperature changes even in a healthy person, which is in our opinion a sufficient reason why the palmar side of hands is not the most appropriate for a credible analysis of thermograms in CTS cases.

One of our further objectives, after having expanded our data base, was the attempt of classifying CTS with thermography, while considering neurophysiological levels of MN entrapment. For this purpose we have developed a neural network, which is capable of classifying data into four classes (no entrapment, mild, moderate, severe). However, the results of this classification were even weaker. We have also tried using other methods of machine learning (Podgorelec et al., 2002), but they did not produce favourable results either, so we abandoned the idea. On the basis of statistical data processing (Table 2), which has shown significant difference among healthy patients and the severe level of CTS entrapment, we have decided to use only the latter for classification.

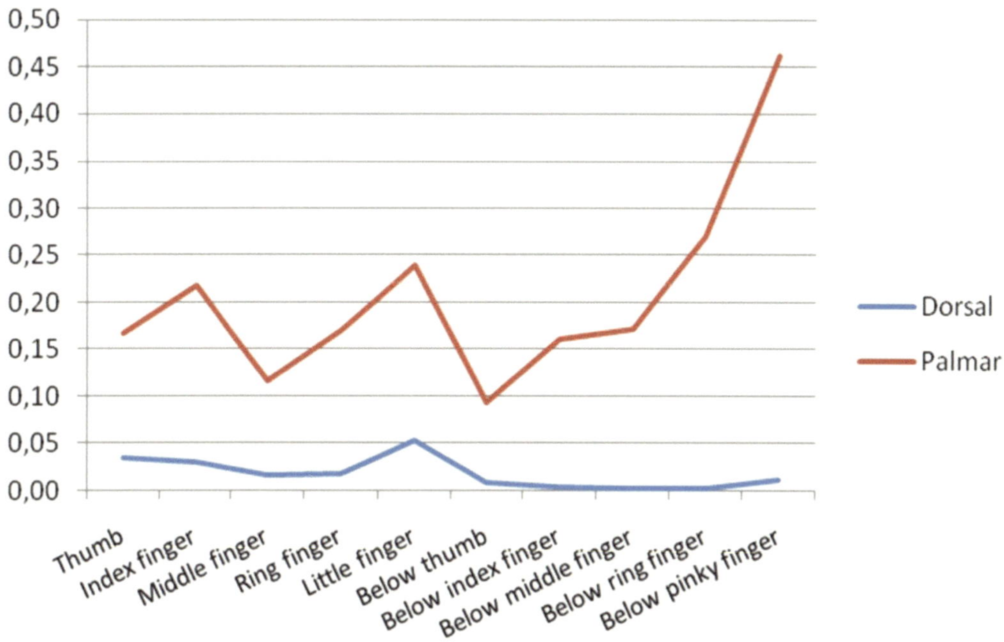

Fig. 6. Statistical significances of differences between segment temperatures in patients' and volunteers' hands (Mann-Whitney-Wilcoxon test, p=0.05), for dorsal and palmar side.

Segment	Mild-Normal	Moderate-Normal	Severe-Normal	All CTS-Normal
Whole hand	0,237400	0,285800	1,79E-006	0,007162
Thumb	0,244800	0,509300	5,07E-005	0,034990
Index finger	0,295100	0,449800	6,19E-005	0,029850
Middle finger	0,470900	0,397900	4,90E-005	0,017270
Ring finger	0,550600	0,557500	3,49E-005	0,017840
Little finger	0,473400	0,619200	4,03E-004	0,053060
Below thumb	0,111200	0,165400	2,32E-006	0,008782
Below index finger	0,166000	0,218600	3,36E-007	0,004250
Below middle finger	0,175600	0,228700	1,42E-007	0,003147
Below ring finger	0,176200	0,279400	1,24E-007	0,003551
Below pinky finger	0,132300	0,318200	1,69E-006	0,011470

Table 2. Statistical significances of differences between dorsal segment temperatures in different NCS severity levels (Mann-Whitney-Wilcoxon test, p=0.05).

After repeated learning and testing of the neural network on the basis of these reduced results (dorsal images of the severe CTS and healthy hands; n = 185), we have achieved our best results. The efficiency of classification has exceeded 83% (Table 3).

Classification run	Incorrectly classified	Correctly classified	Success rate (%)
1	6	31	83,78
2	5	32	86,49
3	8	29	78,38
4	5	32	86,49
5	7	30	81,08
Mean	6.2 ± 1.30	30.8 ± 1.30	**83.24 ± 3.52**

Table 3. CTS diagnosis success rate when only dorsal segments of severe cases and healthy hands were used (n=37, 20% of all hands, each success rate percentage is the mean of five repeat runs).

5. Discussion

On the basis of such results, we can claim that thermography is a useful method for assessing severe CTS levels, even without using a preliminary stress test. Our attention has to be directed to the interpretation of thermograms in relation to the clinical picture, because pathological thermographic samples can be a result of neuropathic changes, local inflammation, or vascular diseases.

In terms of pathophysiology, we differentiate between four basic thermographic patterns of neuropathic origin (Rosenbaum & Ochoa, 2002):

1. Warm pattern I: sympathoparalytic vasodilatation;
   It occurs due to the loss of vasoconstrictor activity of sympaticus, (such as blockade of sympaticus or local blockade of somatic nerve). The skin is warm. Mechanism of action: the result of reduced vasomotor tonus of arteriolesis vasodilation, which is expressed as increased blood flow to the skin.
2. Cold pattern I: Denervation supersensitive vasoconstriction;
   The result of chronic interruption of postganglionic sympathetic neuron, which supplies the skin, leads to hypothermia of denervated area (sympathetic denervation supersensitivity). The skin is cold. Postsynaptic abnormality in the smooth muscles. Mechanism of action: the result of increased vasomotor tonus of arterioles is vasoconstriction, which is expressed as reduced blood flow to the skin.
3. Cold pattern II: Somatosympathetic reflex vasoconstriction;
   It is the result of the excitation of sensory receptors from the skin or irritation of sensory nerve, which is reflected as sudden cooling of skin on the area, where afferent impulses originate from. It is a reflex action, and afferent sensory fibres in this case are sympathetic.
4. Warm pattern II: Antidromic vasodilatation;
   Hyperthermia occurs due to vasodilatation, which does not depend on sympathetic activity, but on neurosecretion of vasodilatatory substances. Every stimulus, which reaches sufficient intensity to stimulate noniceptive nerve endings, can induce neurosecretory functions and consequently antidromic vasodilatation. The skin, which is cold due to symptomatic vasodilatation, retains the capacity for reflex sympathetic vasoconstriction.

In CTS, including rare cases of painful MN entrapment, we can come across any of the pathological samples mentioned above. However, further attention is required for the interpretation of results, because changes in vasomotor tonus are not exclusively the result of stimulation of sympathetic nerve fibres (Aminoff, 1979; Ochoa & Verdugo, 1995; Ochoa, 2002). And namely:

1. Reflex sympathetic activity can merely be physiological response to pain;
2. Vasoconstriction is often the result of denervation supersensitivity rather than of sympathetic hyperactivity;
3. Antidromic vasodilatation can also be caused by stimulation of sensory nociceptors;
4. Vasomotor disorders can simply be a result of the non-use of hand (Ochoa & Yarnitsky, 1994).

Giordano and others (Giordano et al., 1992) examined 40 patients with idiopathic CTS by applying electroneurography and thermography, and compared them to 30 healthy volunteers. Abnormal hypothermia and hyperthermia were attributed to changes in vasoconstrictor tonus caused by the compression of thin non-myelinated sympathetic fibres. With regard to complex thermoregulation mechanisms, autonomous activity of vegetative nervous system and individual reaction of individuals, the interpretation of thermograms is not uniform and must be done in conjunction with anamnesis, clinical picture and/or electrodiagnostics. It is commonly known that clinical signs for CTS are highly specific, but also not sensitive (Gunnarsson et al., 1997; Kuhlman & Hennessey, 1997; Kuntzer, 1994; Seror, 1993; Uncini et al., 1993). D`Arcy and Mc Gee have published work in which they present an overview of literature covering the period from April 1966 to December 2000, which discuss symptoms and signs for CTS diagnostics, in comparison to electrodiagnostic testing. They have established that sensitivity and specificity of clinical investigation vary considerably (D'Arcy & McGee, 2000). As part of our research we decided to compare thermograms with electrodiagnostics, since the latter is considered the most specific, sensitive (over 90%), and objective test for CTS diagnostics (Cassvan et al., 1988; Hennessey & Johnson, 1996; Hilburn, 1996; Jackson & Clifford, 1989; Johnson, 1993; Lew et al., 2005; Seror, 1987).

Rosenbaum and Ochoa warn that thermography cannot simply be equated with the CTS diagnostics, because it does not say much about the patophysiological basis of thermographic changes and entrapment, other than presenting changes in body temperature in a very precise and spectacular manner (Rosenbaum & Ochoa, 2002). In currently published clinical studies on CTS it has been reported that many patients with the clinically and electrodiagnostically confirmed CTS had normal thermographic samples (So et al., 1989; Myers et al., 1988). Thermograms were manually read. Y.T. So and others registered pathological samples in no more than 55% (So et al., 1989. In 1992 Tchou and others compared thermograms of 61 patients with CTS and 40 volunteers. Thermograms were considered abnormal, if at least 25% of distal median area was affected by temperature increase by more than 1°C. They have noted 93% sensitivity and 98% specificity of the thermographic method in impaired MN in the carpal tunnel, but only in the case of unilateral CTS (Tchou et al., 1992).

Our study also includes use of artificial intelligence, because we wanted to avoid the provocation cold stress test and manual interpretation of thermograms. By using neural networks of the multi-level perceptron type, we have, after preliminary supervised training, automated the analysis of thermograms and the CTS diagnosis procedure. As it turned out, by using a new software tool we were able to register very discrete temperature changes, which are not perceived macroscopically on the thermogram, and which the neural network successfully classified into the pathological sample. By using artificial intelligence we were able to abandon the need for contralateral comparison with the "healthy" side, which represented reference values in currently manually analysed thermograms. With regard to

the findings of our research we can claim that the use of thermography in detecting CTS is useful even in the case of bilateral impairment. Considering this, the method achieved wider indication area, as by its definition CTS is more frequently bilateral (Rosenbaum & Ochoa, 2002). Our neural network was used on a group of patients with predominantly bilateral impairment, and the threshold for successful classification was set at 80%.
The assessment of the autonomous nervous system, in MN entrapment, was evidenced only by few authors (Aminoff, 1979; Verdugo et al., 2004; Verghesse et al., 2000). As a matter of fact, the incidence of these symptoms is not completely clear both in healthy people and in people with some other hand pathology. Burke and other discuss that more than a half of all patients with electrodiagnostically confirmed CTS, and also approximately two thirds of those without CTS, mentioned hand sweating. The entrapment of autonomous median fibres in the carpal tunnel was assessed with the sympathetic skin response, which was pathological in one third of all those patients with CTS, who stated symptoms, consistent with vegetative symptomatics (Burke et al., 1999). Yarnitsky and Ochoa claim that symptoms, which potentially belong to the autonomous nervous system disorder (finger sweating, dry palms, Raynaud's phenomenon, and finger pallor), can only be noticed in 17% to 32% of patients with CTS, and don't have high diagnostic value (Yarnitsky & Ochoa, 1991). But on the contrary, Verghese and others point out that the involvement of autonomous nervous system in CTS is frequent (55%), especially in the group of people with severe neurophysiological level of entrapment (Verghesse et al., 2000).
The results of our research are in line with the latter; as a matter of fact, the classification was by far the most successful in the group with the most severe level of entrapment in terms of electrodiagnostics (Table 3). In this group, even pathophysiologically, we can already expect impairment of thin, non-myelinated, autonomous, nerve fibres.

6. Conclusion

After an in-depth deliberation we believe that a pathophysiologically-substantiated doubt, with regard to the mechanism of the incidence of temperature changes in CTS, doesn't diminish the applicability of thermography in diagnosing MN entrapment by using artificial intelligence. As is often the case in medicine, temperature is a symptom and reflects a certain condition. By using artificial intelligence, considering reliable electrodiagnostic criteria, we have succeeded in classifying the discussed condition on hands as the result of severe level of MN entrapment in the carpal tunnel. Doctrinally, even though this is the best and the most frequently researched entrapment neuropathy on hands, there is currently no consensus reached with regard to treatment (Gerritsen et al., 2002; Gunnarsson et al, 1997; Hui et al., 2005; Kanaan & Sawaya, 2001; O'Gradaigh & Merry, 2000; Padua et al., 2001). Usually, mildly expressed CTS symptomatics in clinical terms is initially treated conservatively. With regard to the decision when and which type of operative relaxation of MN is the most appropriate, there are no uniform scientifically-supported evidences (Chang et al., 2008; Finsen & Russwurm, 2001; Iida et al., 2008; Mondelli et al., 2001). In patients, who refuse surgical procedures, neurophysiological investigation with a very clear clinical picture makes no sense, because it doesn't change their treatment in any way. Not taking into account results of neurophysiological measurements, it is conservative (disburden, braces), which means cheap, non-invasive, and completely reversible. Likewise, it also does not make sense to refer patients with CTS symptoms, which last less than six months, to neurophysiological measurements, because the probability of spontaneous healing is particularly high in the early period (Padua et al., 2001). Considering the described doctrine, recommendation, and clinical practice, we can diagnose CTS in cases of severe entrapment with a high level of reliability by using thermography and appropriate software tool. Simultaneously, critical interpretation of thermograms, considering anamnesis and clinical picture, is also sufficient for the beginning of CTS treatment. Patients with severe level of entrapment (where typical thermogram is registered), if they consent to the operative procedure, are referred to EMG investigation and then to decompression; all others are treated conservatively for the next six months.

On the basis of the conducted study, IR thermography cannot be recommended as an equal diagnostic method to the already established EMG investigation. However, we are determining that it can be used as a successful, non-invasive method for detecting severe CTS cases. It could also be useful in preventive examinations of a wider population, such as in different industries, where ergonomic conditions of work represent a major risk for the development of CTS (repeating hand and wrist movements, work with vibration machines, work in extreme wrist positions along with simultaneous pressure on palms, work in cold atmosphere, professional drivers, etc.), as well as in pregnant women and children and those symptomatic patients, who as a principle reject EMG and operative therapy.

Considering good results we have obtained by using neural networks in the group of severe entrapments we recommend thermography as a screening method for determining CTS. Indirectly, the method can also be useful in reducing long waiting periods for EMG investigation, which is the major deficiency of this generally established, standard diagnostics. By using non-invasive thermography we would focus on the group of patients most at risk, who would be given priority for EMG investigation.

The method we have developed with a clear indication for or restriction only to severe cases of entrapment is recommended as a screening method for determining CTS and as pre-level of EMG investigation, which otherwise still remains the most reliable standard in the area of diagnostics of entrapment neuropathies.

7. References

American Academy of Neurology [AAN]. (1990). Report of the American Academy of Neurology and Therapeutics and Technology Assessment Subcommittee. Assessment: Thermography in neurologic practice. *Neurology*, Vol. 40, No.3, pp. 523-525, ISSN 0028-3878

Aminoff, MJ. (1979). Involvement of peripheral vasomotor fibers in carpal tunnel syndrome. *J Neurol Neurosurg Psychiatry*, Vol.42, No.7, pp. 649-55, ISSN 0022-3050

Ammer, K. (1999). Diagnosis of nerve entrapment syndromes by thermal imaging, *Proceedings of the First Joint BMES/EMBS Conference*, Vol.2, p. 1117, ISBN 0-7803-5674-8, Atlanta, Georgia, USA, October 13-16, 1999

Ammer, K. (2003). Nerve entrapment and skin temperature of the human hand, In: *A case book of infrared imaging in clinical medicine*, A. Jung, J. Zuber, F. Ring, (Eds.), 94-96, Medpress, ISBN 83-916116-2-0, Warsaw, Poland

Benaroch, EE. (2007). The Autonomic nervous system: Basic anatomy and physiology. *Continuum Lifelong Learning Neurol*, Vol.13, No.6, pp. 13-32, ISSN 10802371

Bland, JDP. (2007). Carpal tunnel syndrome, BMJ, Vol.335, No.7615, pp. 343-346, ISSN 0959-8138

Burke, DT.; Burke, MA.; Bell, R.; Stewart, GW.; Mehdi, RS. & Kim, HJ. (1999). Subjective swelling: a new sign for carpal tunnel syndrome. *Am J Phys Med Rehabil*, Vol.78, No.6, pp. 401-405, ISSN 0894-9115

Cassvan, AA.; Ralescu, S.; Shapiro, E.; Moshkovski, FG. & Weiss, J. (1988). Median and radial sensory latencies to digit 1 as compared with other screening tests in carpal tunnel syndrome. *Am J Phys Med Rehabil*, Vol.67, No.5, pp. 221-224, ISSN 0894-9115

Chang, MH.; Wei, SJ. & Chen, LWA. (2008). Practical electrophysiological guide for non-surgical and surgical treatment of carpal tunnel syndrome. *J Hand Surg Eur Vol*, Vol.33, No.1, pp. 32-37, ISSN 1753-1934

Cuthbertson, GM (1995). The development of IR imaging in the United Kingdom, In: *The Thermal Image in Medicine and Biology*, Ammer, K. & Ring, EFJ. (Eds.), pp. 21-32, Uhlen-Verlag, ISBN 3-900466-57-2, Vienna, Austria

D'Arcy, CA. & McGee, S. (2000). The rational clinical examination. Does this patient have carpal tunnel syndrome?. *JAMA*, Vol.283, No.23, pp. 3110-3117, ISSN 0098-7484

Finsen, V. & Russwurm, H. (2001). Neurophysiology not required before surgery for typical carpal tunnel syndrome, *J Hand Surg Br*, Vol.26, No.1, pp. 61-64, ISSN 0266-7681

Gaussorgues, G. (1994). Infrared Thermography, Chapman & Hall, ISBN 0412479001, Cambridge, UK

Gerritsen, AA.; de Krom, MC.; Struijs, MA.; Scholten, RJ.; de Vet, HC. & Bouter, LM. (2002). Conservative treatment options for carpal tunnel syndrome: a systematic review of randomised controlled trials. *J Neurol*, Vol.249, No.3, pp. 272-280, ISSN 0340-5354

Giordano, N.; Batissti, E.; Franci, A.; Magaro, L.; Marcucci, P.; Cecconami, L. & Marcolongo, R. (1992). Telethermographic assesment of carpal tunnel syndrome. *Scand J Rheumatolo*, Vol.21, No.1, pp. 42-45, ISSN 0300-9742

Gunnarsson, LG.; Amilon, A.; Hellstrand, P.; Leissner, P. & Philipson, L. (1997). The diagnosis of carpal tunnel syndrome. Sensitivity and specificity of some clinical and electrophysiological tests. *J Hand Surg Br*, Vol.22, No.1, pp. 34-37, ISSN 0266-7681

Haas, OCL. & Burnham, KJ. (Eds.)(2008). Intelligent and Adaptive Systems in Medicine, Taylor & Francis, ISBN 978-0-7503-0994-3, London, UK

Hackett, MEJ. (1976). The place of thermography in medicine. *Acta thermographica*, Vol.1, pp. 176–180, ISSN 0391-9846

Hennessey, WJ. & Johnson, EW. (1996). Carpal tunnel syndrome, In: *Practical electromyography*, 3rd ed., Johnson EW., Pease WS. (Eds.), 195-216, Williams and Wilkins, ISBN 0683044575, Baltimore, USA

Herrick, RT. & Herrick, SK. (1987). Thermography in detection of carpal tunnel syndrome and other compressive neuropathies. *J. Hand Surg Am*, Vol.12, No.5, Pt.2, pp.943-949, ISSN 0363-5023

Hilburn, JW. (1996). General principles and use of electrodiagnostic studies in carpal and cubital tunnel syndromes. *Hand Clin*, Vol.12, No.2, pp. 205-221, ISSN 0749-0712

Hui, ACF.; Won, SG.; Leung, CH.; Tong, P.; Mok, V.; Poon, D.; Li-Tsang, CW.; Wong, LK. & Boet, R. (2005). A randomized controlled trial of surgery vs steroid injection for carpal tunnel syndrome. *Neurology*, Vol.64, No.12, pp. 2074-2078, ISSN 0028-3878

Iida, J.; Hirabayashi, H.; Nakase, H. & Sakaki, T. (2008). Carpal tunnel syndrome: electrophysiological grading and surgical results by minimum incision open carpal tunnel release. Neurol Med Chir (Tokyo), Vol.48, No.12, pp. 554-559, ISSN 0470-8105

International Academy of Clinical Thermology. (2002). *Thermography guidelines: Standards and protocols in clinical thermographic imaging*. June 2011, Available from: http//www.iact-org.org/professionals/thermog-guidelines.html#/imaging

Jackson, DA. & Clifford, JC. (1989). Electrodiagnosis of mild carpal tunnel syndrome. *Arch Phys Med Rehabil*, Vol.70, No.3, pp. 199-204, ISSN 0003-9993

Johnson, EW. (1993). Diagnosis of carpal tunnel syndrome. The gold standard. *Am J Phys Med Rehabil*, Vol.72, No.1, p. 1, ISSN 0894-9115

Jones, BF. & Plassmann, P. (2002). Digital Infrared thermal imaging of human skin. *IEEE Eng Med Biol Mag*, Vol.21, No.6, pp. 41-48, ISSN 0739-5175

Kanaan, N. & Sawaya, RA. (2001). Carpal tunnel syndrome: modern diagnostic and management techniques. *Br J Gen Pract*, Vol.51, No.465, pp. 311-314, ISSN 0960-1643

Kantardzic, M. (2002). *Data Mining: Concepts, Models, Methods, and Algorithms*. Wiley-Interscience, ISBN 0471228524, Hoboken, New Jersey, USA

Kasabov, NK. (1996). *Foundations of Neural Networks, Fuzzy Systems, and Knowledge Engineering*. MIT Press, ISBN 0262112124, Cambridge, Massachusetts, USA

Kline, DG. & Hudson, A. (1990). Acute injuries of peripheral nerves. In: *Neurological Surgery*, Youmans RJ., (Ed.), 2423-2510, WB Saunders Co, ISBN 0721620949, Philadelphia, USA

Kuhlman, KA. & Hennessey, WJ. (1997). Sensitivity and specificity of carpal tunnel syndrome signs. *Am J Phys Med Rehabil*, Vol.76, No.6, pp. 451-457, ISSN 0894-9115

Kuntzer, T. (1994). Carpal tunnel syndrome in 100 patients: sensitivity, specificity of multi-neurophysiological procedures and estimation of axonal loss of motor, sensory and sympathetic median nerve fibers. *J Neurol Sci*, Vol.127, No.2, pp. 221-229, ISSN 0022-510X

Larose, DT. (2005). *Discovering Knowledge in Data: An Introduction to Data Mining*. John Wiley, ISBN 978-0-471-66657-8, Hoboken, New Jersey, USA

Lew, HL.; Date, ES.; Pan, SS.; Wu, P.; Ware, PF. & Kingery, WS. (2005). Sensitivity, specificity, and variability of nerve conduction velocity measurements in carpal tunnel syndrome. *Arch Phys Med Rehabil*, Vol.86, No.1, pp. 12-16, ISSN 0003-9993

Marotte, LR. (1974). An electrone microscope study of chronic median nerve compression in guinea-pig. *Acta Neuropathol*, Vol.27, pp. 69-82, ISSN 0001-6322

McCulloch, WS. & Pitts, W. (1943). A Logical Calculus of the Ideas Immanent in Nervous Activity. *Bulletin of Mathematical Biophysics* , Vol.5, pp.115-133, ISSN 0007-4985

Medical Imaging Research Group, University of Glamorgan. (2004). CTHERM Demo, June 2011, Available from: http://www.comp.glam.ac.uk/pages/staff/pplassma/MedImaging/Resources/CTHERM_Demo/Intro.htm

Mondelli, M.; Reale, F.; Padua, R.; Aprile, I. & Padua, L. (2001). Clinical and neurophysiological outcome of surgery in extreme carpal tunnel syndrome. *Clin Neurophysiol*, Vol.112, No.7, pp. 1237-1242, ISSN 1388-2457

Myers, S.; Vermeire, P.; Sherry, B. & Cross, D. (1988). Liquid crystal thermography: quantitative studies of abnormalities in the carpal tunnel syndrome. *Neurology*, Vol.39, No.11, pp. 1465-1469, ISSN 0028-3878

Ochoa, JL. (2002). Pathophysiology of chronic neuropathic pains, In: *Surgical management of pain*, Burchiel KJ, (Ed.), 25-41, Thieme Medical, ISBN 0865779120, New York, USA

Ochoa, JL. & Verdugo, RJ. (1995). Reflex sympathetic dystrophy. A common clinical avenue for somatoform expression. *Neurol Clin*, Vol.13, No.2, pp. 351-63, ISSN 0733-8619

Ochoa, JL. & Yarnitsky, D. (1994). The triple cold syndrome: Cold hyperalgesia, cold hypoaesthesia and cold skin in peripheral nerve disease. *Brain*, Vol.117, No.1, pp. 185-197, ISSN 0006-8950

O'Gradaigh, D. & Merry, P. (2000). Corticosteroid injection for the treatment of carpal tunnel syndrome. *Ann Rheum Dis*, Vol.59, No.11, pp. 918-919, ISSN 0003-4967

Padua, L.; Padua, R.; Aprile, I.; Pasqualetti, P. & Tonali, P. (2001). Multiperspective follow-up of untreated carpal tunnel syndrome: a multicenter study. *Neurology*, Vol.56, No.11, pp. 1459-1466, ISSN 0028-3878

Podgorelec, V.; Kokol, P.; Stiglic, B. & Rozman, I. (2002). Decision trees: an overview and their use in medicine. *J Med Syst*, Vol.26, No.5, pp. 445-463, ISSN 0148-5598

Ring, EFJ. (1995a). Cold stress testing of the hand, In: *The Thermal Image in Medicine and Biology*, Ammer K., Ring EFJ., (Eds.), 237-240, Uhlen Verlag , ISBN 3-900-4666-572, Vienna, Austria

Ring, EFJ. (1995b). The history of thermal imaging, In: *The Thermal Image in Medicine and Biology*, Ammer, K. & Ring, EFJ. (Eds.), pp. 13-20, Uhlen-Verlag, ISBN 3-900466-57-2, Vienna, Austria

Rojas, R. (1996). *Neural Networks: A systematic introduction*, Springer-Verlag, ISBN 3540605053, Berlin, Germany

Rosenbaum, RB. & Ochoa, JL. (2002). *Carpal tunnel syndrome and other disorders of the median nerve: Anatomy of the Median Nerve* (2nd ed.), Butterworth - Heinemann, ISBN 0-7506-7314-1, Boston, Massachusetts, USA

Schartelmüller, T. & Ammer, K. (1996). Infrared Thermography for the Diagnosis of Thoracic Outlet Syndrome. *Thermologie Österreich*, Vol.6, pp.130-134, ISSN 1021-4356

Seror, P. (1987). Electroclinical correlations in the carpal tunnel syndrome. Apropos of 100 cases. *Rev Rhum Mal Osteoartic*, Vol.54, No.10, pp. 643-648, ISSN 0035-2659

Seror, P. (1993). Sensitivity of various electrophysical studies for the diagnosis of carpal tunnel syndrome. *Muscle & Nerve*, Vol.16, No.12, pp. 1418-1419, ISSN 0148-639X

So, YT.; Olney, RK. & Aminoff, MJ. (1989). Evaluation of thermography in the diagnosis of selected entrapment neuropathies. *Neurology*, Vol.39, No.1, pp. 1-5, ISSN 0028-3878

Tchou, S.; Costich, JF.; Burgess, RC. & Wexler, CE. (1992). Thermographic observation in unilateral carpal tunnel syndrome: report of 61 cases. *J Hand Surg Am*, Vol.17, No.4, pp.631-637, ISSN 0363-5023

Tortora, JG. & Derrickson, BH. (2008). The Integumentary system. In: *Principles of Anatomy and Physiology*, 12th ed., pp. 140-159, John Wiley & Sons, ISBN 0470279877, New York, USA

Uncini, AD.; Muzio, A.; Awad, J.; Kanente, G.; Tafuro, H. & Cambi, D. (1993). Sensitivity of three median-to-ulnar comparative tests in diagnosis of mild carpal tunnel syndrome. *Muscle & Nerve*, Vol.16, No.12, pp. 1366-1373, ISSN 0148-639X

Verdugo, RJ.;, Bell, LA.; Campero, M.; Salvat, F.; Triplett, B.; Sonnad, J. & Ochoa, JL. (2004). Spectrum of cutaneous hyperalgesias/allodynias in neuropathic pain patients. *Acta Neurol Scand*, Vol.110, No.6, pp. 368–376, ISSN 0001-6314

Verghesse, J.; Galanopoulou, AS. & Herskovitz, S. (2000). Autonomic dysfunction in idiopathic carpal tunnel syndrome. *Muscle Nerve* , Vol.23, No.8, pp. 1209-1213, ISSN 0148-639X

Yarnitsky, D. & Ochoa, JL. (1991). Differential effects of compression-ischaemia block on warm sensation and heat-induced pain. *Brain*, Vol.114, No.2, pp. 907-913, ISSN 0006-8950

14

Functional Significance of Facilitation Between the Pronator Teres and Extensor Carpi Radialis in Humans: Studies with Electromyography and Electrical Neuromuscular Stimulation

Akira Naito[1], Hiromi Fujii[2], Toshiaki Sato[2], Katsuhiko Suzuki[2] and Haruki Nakano[1]
[1]*Yamagata University*
[2]*Yamagata Prefectural University of Health Sciences*
Japan

1. Introduction

Excitatory (facilitation) or inhibitory spinal reflex arcs (inhibition) mediated by group I afferent fibers from the muscle spindles (group Ia afferents) and Golgi tendon organs (group Ib afferents) among muscles in the human upper limb have been studied (Fig. 1) (Aymard et al., 1995; Baldissea et al., 1983; Cavallari & Katz, 1989; Cavallari et al., 1992; Creange et al., 1992; Day et al., 1984; Fujii et al., 2001; Katz et al., 1991; Kobayashi et al., 2000; Lourenço et al., 2007; Marchand-Pauvert et al., 2000; Miyasaka et al., 1995, 1996, 1998, 2007; Naito et al., 1996, 1998a, 2001; Naito, 2003, 2004; Nakano et al., 2005, 2006; Ogawa et al., 2005; Pierrot-Deseilligny & Mazevet, 2000; Rossi et al., 1995; Sato et al., 2002; Shinozaki et al., 2001; Suzuki et al., 2005, 2007; Wargon et al., 2006). These reflex arcs modulate motoneuron excitabilities to coordinate smooth muscular movements (Naito, 2003, 2004; Pierrot-Deseilligny et al., 1981; Rothwell, 1994; Tanaka, 1989). The facilitation must function for co-contraction of muscles and the inhibition for alternating or reciprocal contraction among muscles (Naito, 2003, 2004).

Musculus (m.) pronator teres (PT) arises from the medial epicondyle of the humerus (humeral head) and the coronoid process of the ulna (ulnar head) and attaches on the lateral surface of the shaft of the radius (Basmajian, 1982; Jenkins, 2008; Standring et al., 2005). It is innervated by the median nerve. M. extensor carpi radialis longus (ECRL) arises mainly from the distal third of the supracondylar ridge of the humerus and attaches to the radial side of the dorsal aspect of the base of the second metacarpal. M. extensor carpi radialis brevis (ECRB) arises mainly from the lateral epicondyle of the humerus and attaches on the radial side of the base of the third metacarpal. Both muscles (ECR) are innervated by the radial nerve. Most textbooks of anatomy describe that PT acts as a forearm pronator and ECR as a wrist extensor and abductor. Our previous studies have demonstrated facilitation between PT and ECR (ECRL, ECRB) in humans (Fig. 1) (Nakano et al., 2005, 2006). The facilitation seems to be mediated by group Ia afferents through a monosynaptic path. It is known that monosynaptic facilitation mediated by group Ia afferents is usually observed

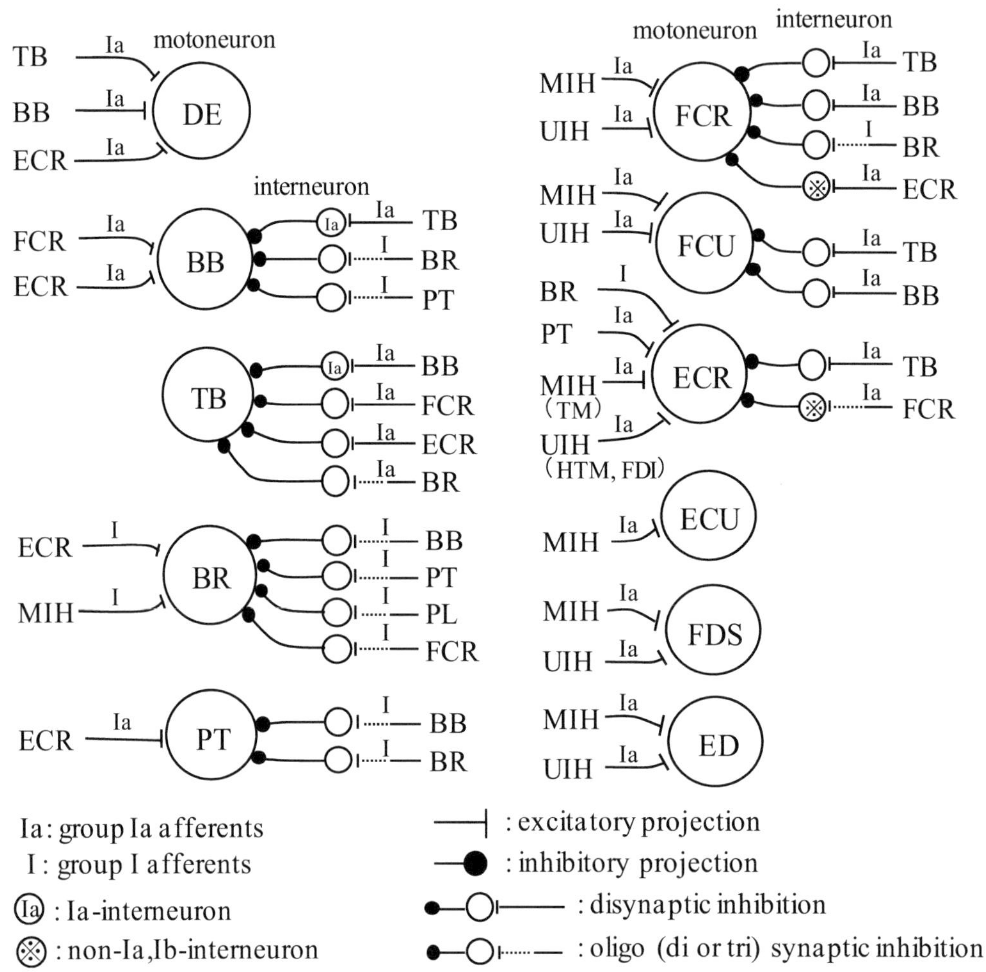

Fig. 1. Excitatory (facilitation) and inhibitory spinal reflex arcs (inhibition) studied among muscles in the human upper limb (homonymous facilitation mediated by group Ia afferents and homonymous inhibition mediated by group Ib afferents are omitted). The facilitation is illustrated on the motoneuron's left, the inhibition on the right. DE: musculus (m.) deltoideus (anterior fibers), BB: m. biceps brachii, TB: m. triceps brachii, BR: m. brachioradialis, PT: m. pronator teres, PL: m. palmaris longus, ECR: m. flexor carpi radialis, FCU: m. flexor carpi ulnaris, ECR: mm. extensor carpi radialis longus and brevis, ECU: m. extensor carpi ulnaris, FDS: m. flexor digitorum superficialis, ED: m. extensor digitorum, MIH: hand muscles innervated by the median nerve, UIH: hand muscles innervated by the ulnar nerve, TM: thenar muscles, HTM: hypothnar muscles, FDI: m. interosseus dorsalis prima, Abbreviations in this as well as Figs. 2-7.

among synergistic muscles (Naito, 2003, 2004; Pierrot-Deseilligny et al., 1981; Tanaka, 1989). However, since PT and ECR are not synergistic, the functional significance of the facilitation is still unclear. This chapter describes the significance elucidated by studies using an electromyography (EMG) and electrical neuromuscular stimulation (ENS).

2. EMG study

Observations of activities of two muscles during repetitive movements must reveal activation of facilitation or inhibition between them. The facilitation must be active during co-contraction of the muscles and the inhibition must be during alternating or reciprocal contraction between the muscles. Since PT belongs to forearm pronators and ECR (ECRL, ECRB) to wrist extensors, activities of the muscles during repetitive movements of dynamic forearm pronation/supination, and those of static (isometric) wrist extension and dynamic wrist extension/flexion were studied using EMG.

For EMG recording, bipolar intramuscular electrodes made of teflon-coated stainless steel wire (75 μm in diameter, SUS 316, AM system, Carlsborg WA, USA) with distance of about 4 mm were used (Basmajian & Deluca, 1985; Fujii et al., 2007; Naito et al., 1998b; Perotto, 1994). The electrodes were implanted percutaneously into the muscles with 25 gauge-injection needles (Naito et al., 1998b, Riek et al., 2000). A wet bandage was put round the shoulder and used as reference. EMGs were amplified, band pass filtered (10-1,000 Hz), and sampled at 2,048 Hz. Then they were integrated (rectified and averaged) with an EMG integration program (Multi-Computer System, Giga Tex Co., Osaki, Japan).

2.1 The repetitive movements of dynamic forearm pronation/supination

EMGs of m biceps brachii (BB), PT, ECRL, ECRB, m. extensor carpi ulnalis (ECU), and m. flexor carpi ulnaris (FCU) were recorded in five normal subjects (male, age range 23-46 years). Movements tested were repetitive movements of dynamic forearm pronation/supination between the maximum prone (90 degrees of pronatioon) and spine positions (90 degrees of supination) with maintenance of the wrist neutral position (0 degrees of flexion/extension, 0 degrees of adduction/abduction). The subject sat on a chair with the shoulder joint flexed to 0 degrees of flexion and the elbow joint flexed to 90 degrees of flexion (Fig. 2A). In order to obtain adequate EMGs of the muscles (Basmajian and Deluca, 1985; Naito et al., 1998b), a belt weighing 1.0-2.0 kg was wound around the hand (palm) as a load. The movements were pictured with three digital video cameras (NW-GS 100, Panasonic, Tokyo, Japan) (anterior, superior, and medial aspects). Trajectories of the styloid process of the radius during the movements were traced using a 3-D-position sensor (3DPS) system (Liberty, POLHEMUS, USA), which delivered coordinate (x, y, z). A terminal probe of the 3DPS system was put on the skin of the styloid process with adhesive tape. Lissajou's curves (trajectories in the coronary plane) was drawn with the data (x, y) using a 2-D Lissajou presentation program (RO299-4588G, Gigatex, Osaki, Japan). Video pictures and data of the 3DPS system were fed into a simultaneous recording system of digital video pictures and electric signals (The Teraview, Gigatex, Osaki, Japan) with EMGs (Sagae et al., 2010; Sato et al., 2007).

During the movements, BB showed activities increasing and decreasing and PT, ECRL, and ECRB parallel activities decreasing and increasing at the supination and pronation phases, respectively, in all the five subjects (Fig. 2B, C). These fluctuations resulted in peaks and troughs of BB activities, and troughs and peaks of PT, ECRL, and ECRB activities at the maximum supination and pronation, respectively (Table 1). ECU showed parallel activities to PT, ECRL, and ECRB activities in all the subjects and those to BB activities (Fig. 2C) in two subjects. Peaks of the parallel activities of the latter were much lower than those of the former. FCU showed parallel activities to BB activities in three subjects (Fig 2B). In one subject, large and regular activities of which peaks followed the peaks of BB activities and small irregular activities were observed (Fig. 2C). In the remaining one subject, FCU showed no activities during the movements.

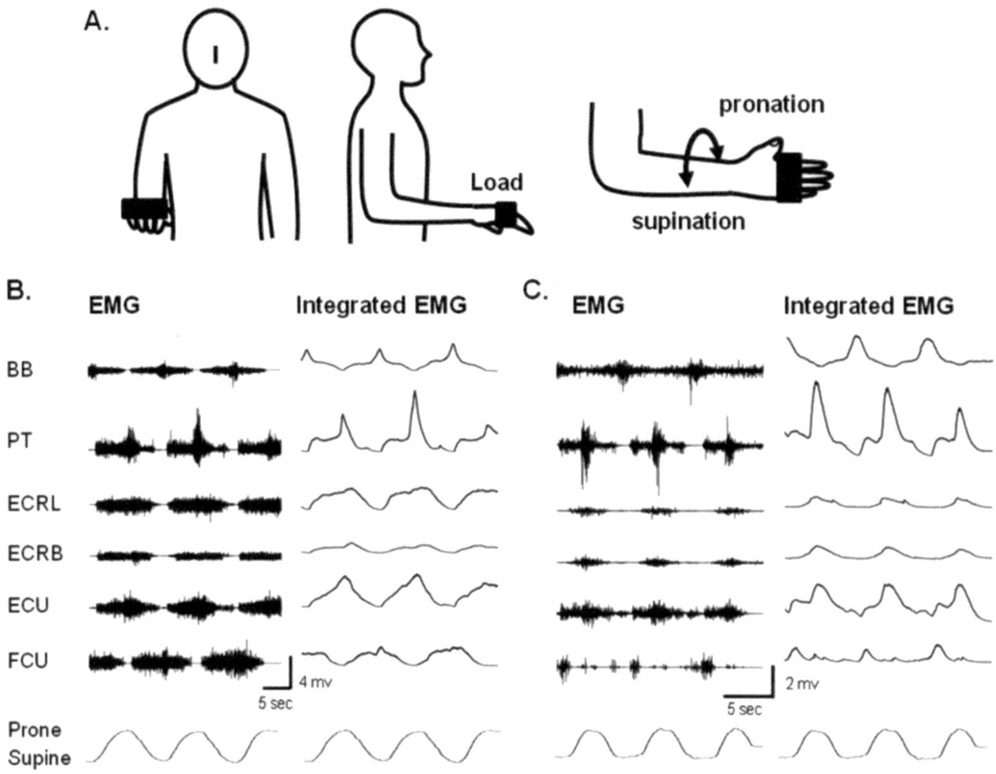

Fig. 2. An electromyographic (EMG) study of repetitive movements of dynamic forearm pronation/supination with maintenance of wrist neutral position in normal human subjects. **A**: The posture of the subject. During the experiment, the subject sits on a chair and keeps the shoulder joint at 0 degrees of flexion/extension, adduction/abduction, and external/internal rotation, the elbow joint at 90 degrees of flexion, and the wrist joint at 0 degrees of flexion/extension and adduction/abduction (neutral position). In order to evoke adequate EMG activities, a belt weighing 1.0-2.0 kg is surrounded around the hand. **B, C**: EMGs of BB, PT, ECRL, ECRB, ECU, and FCU during the movements in two subjects. The bottom solid lines indicate changes in the position of the forearm. Note that parallel activities of ECRL, ECRB, and PT increasing and decreasing at the pronation and supination phases, respectively, are observed in both the subjects.

Among BB, PT, ECR (ECRL, ECRB), ECU, and FCU in humans, facilitation between PT and ECR (Nakano et al., 2005, 2006), and from ECR to BB (Cavallari & Katz, 1989) and inhibition between BB and PT (Miyasaka et al., 1996; Naito et al., 1998a), and from BB to FCU (Cavallari et al., 1992) have been studied (Fig. 1). The EMG study showed that activities of BB increased and decreased and those of PT and ECR decreased and increased at the supination and pronation phases, respectively, in all the five subjects. This observation suggests that reciprocal contraction between BB and PT, and BB and ECR, and co-contraction of PT and ECR occur during the movements. The inhibition between BB and PT

	Peaks		Troughs	
	MaxS	MaxP	MaxS	MaxP
BB	5	0	0	5
PT	0	5	5	0
ECRL	0	5	5	0
ECRB	0	5	5	0
ECU	0	5	5	0
FCU	3	0	0	4

MaxS: the maximum supination, MaxP: the maximum pronation, BB: musculus (m.) biceps brachii, PT: m. pronator teres, ECRL: m. extensor carpi radialis longus, ECRB: m. extensor carpi radialis brevis, ECU: m. extensor carpi ulnaris, FCU: m. flexor carpi ulnaris, Abbreviations in this as well as Tables 2, 3.

Table 1. Peaks and troughs of activities of muscles during repetitive movements of dynamic forearm pronation/supination with maintenance of the wrist neutral position in five subjects.

(Miyasaka et al., 1996; Naito et al., 1998a) must be active during the reciprocal contraction and the facilitation between PT and ECR (Nakano et al., 2005, 2006) must be during the co-contraction. The facilitation must work effectively for the parallel activities increasing at the pronation phase. The facilitation from ECR to BB (Cavallari & Katz, 1989) seems to be inactive during the movement. In the EMG study, parallel activities of ECU to PT and ECR activities and BB activities were seen in all and two subjects, respectively. The parallel activities of the latter were much smaller than those of the former. These results suggest that co-contraction of PT, ECR, and ECU, and reciprocal contraction between BB and ECU occur during the movement. The EMG study also showed that parallel activities of FCU to BB activities were observed in three subjects and activities of FCU of which peaks followed the peaks of BB activities in one subject. This observation suggests that co-contraction of BB and FCU, and reciprocal contraction between FCU and PT, and FCU and ECR occur during the movements. The inhibition from BB to FCU (Cavallari et al., 1992) seems to be inactive during the movements. Observations of the co-contraction and reciprocal contraction suggest a possibility that facilitation between PT and ECU, and ECR and ECU, and inhibition between PT and FCU, ECR and FCU, and ECU and FCU exist in humans. Further studies are required to elucidate existences of the facilitation and inhibition.

2.2 The repetitive movements of static wrist extension and dynamic wrist extension/flexion

EMGs of PT, ECRL, ECRB, and FCR were recorded in twelve normal human subjects (male 9, female 3, age range 20-40 years) (Fujii et al., 2007). EMGs were fed into a data recorder (RECTI-HORIZ-8K, NEC, Tokyo, Japan) and pen recorder (RCD-928, Shinko, Tokyo, Japan). Movements tested were repetitive movements of static (isometric) wrist extension and dynamic wrist flexion/extension in the prone (about 80 degrees of pronation), semiprone (neutral), and supine positions (about 80 degrees of supination) of the forearm (Fig. 3A). The subject sat on a chair and put the forearm on an experimental table with the shoulder joint flexed to 0-20 degrees of flexion and the elbow joint flexed to 70-90 degrees of flexion (Fig. 3A). In the movements of the static wrist extension, the subject made an effort to extend the wrist in the position of 0-20 degrees of extension against resistance for about 5 sec. The resistance was produced by the experimenter's hand. The hand pressed the dorsum of the subject's hand to prevent the wrist from extending. The effort was performed 3-5 times at interval of about 5 sec. In the movements of the dynamic wrist flexion/extension, the subject performed a to-and-fro motion from the maximum flexion to the maximum extension of the wrist 5 times for about 25 sec. Angular changes of the wrist in flexion/extension direction were measured using an electrogoniometer (PH510, Denkikeisoku Hanbai, Tokyo, Japan). Data of the angular changes were fed into the data recorder and pen recorder with EMGs.

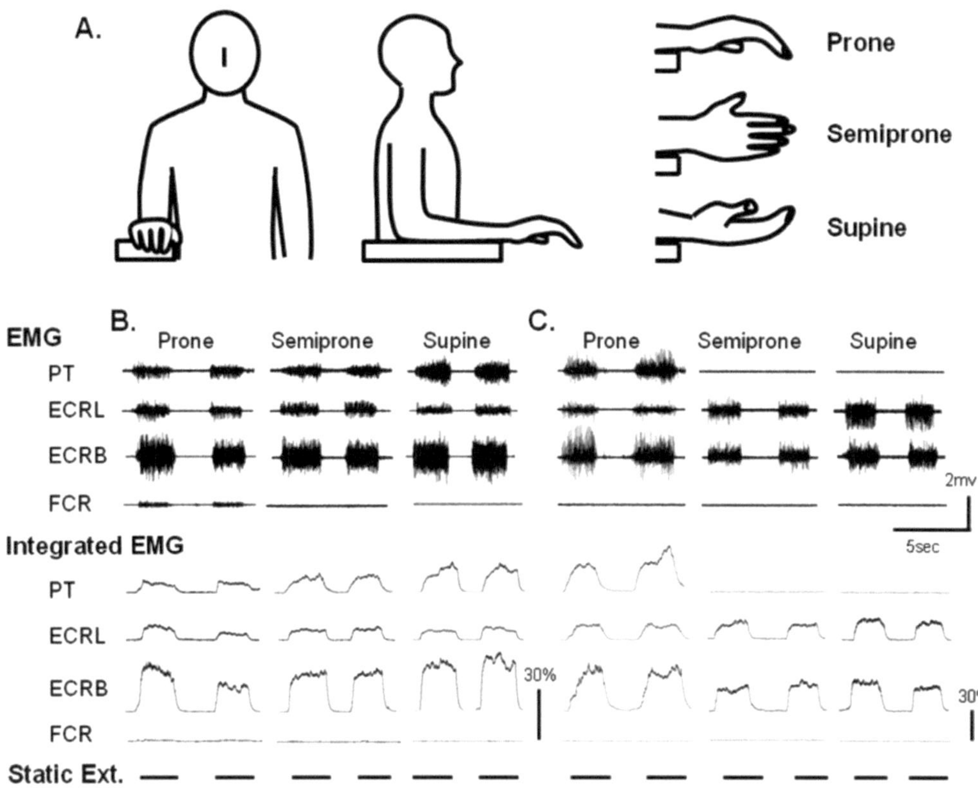

Fig. 3. An EMG study of repetitive movements of static (isometric) wrist extension with maintenance of the forearm in the prone, semiprone (neutral), and supine positions in normal human subjects. **A**: The posture of the subject. During the experiment, the subject sits on a chair and puts the pronated, semipronated, and supinated forearm on an experimental table with the shoulder joint at 0-20 degrees of flexion/extension, 0 degrees of adduction/abduction, and external/internal rotation, the elbow joint at 70-90 degrees of flexion. Static wrist extension is performed against the resistance produced by the experimaner's hand. **B, C**: EMGs of ECRL, ECRB, PT, and FCR during the movements in two subjects. The bottom thick lines indicate the period of the extension. Parallel activities of PT, ECRL, and ECRB are observed in the prone, semiprone, and supine positions in one subject (**B**) and in the prone position in another (**C**). Calibration bars for integrated EMGs: a percentage of the amplitude produced by the maximum contraction. Reproduced with permission from Fujii et al. (2007).

During the movements of the static wrist extension, ECRL and ECRB showed activities in the prone, semiprone, and supine positions of the forearm in all the twelve subjects (Table 2, Fig. 3B, C). Slight or no activities were seen in FCR. PT showed activities in the prone, semiprone, and supine positions in all, eight, and eight subjects, respectively. The activities were parallel with those of ECRL and ECRB. In the remainders, PT showed no activities during the movements.

During the movements of the dynamic wrist flexion/extension, activities of ECRL and ECRB increased at the extension phase and those of FCR at the flexion phase in all the twelve subjects (Fig. 4). Therefore peaks of the activities of ECRL and ECRB appeared at the extension phase and those of FCR at the flexion phase (Table 3). Activities of PT increased at the extension phase in all, eight and five subjects, respectively, and at the flexion phase in zero, four, and five subjects, respectively, in the prone, semiprone, and supine positions. In three subjects (YE, SY, SK in Table 3), the activities increased at both the extension and flexion phases in the semiprone and supine positions. The activities of PT at the extension and flexion phases were parallel with those of ECRL and ECRB, and FCR (Fig. 4A), respectively.

	Prone				Semiprone				Supine			
Subject	ECRL	ECRB	PT	FCR	ECRL	ECRB	PT	FCR	ECRL	ECRB	PT	FCR
K.S.	+	+	+	–	+	+	+	+	+	+	–	–
Y.E.	+	+	+	–	+	+	–	–	+	+	–	–
H.F.	+	+	+	–	+	+	–	–	+	+	–	–
M.S.	+	+	+	–	+	+	–	–	+	+	–	–
K.S.	+	+	+	–	+	+	+	–	+	+	+	–
S.Y.	+	+	+	+	+	+	+	–	+	+	+	–
H.T.	+	+	+	–	+	+	+	+	+	+	+	–
Y.K.	+	+	+	–	+	+	–	+	+	+	+	–
A.M.	+	+	+	–	+	+	+	–	+	+	+	+
Y.U.	+	+	+	–	+	+	+	–	+	+	+	–
S.K.	+	+	+	+	+	+	+	+	+	+	+	–
Y.W.	+	+	+	–	+	+	+	–	+	+	+	–

FCR: m. flexor carpi radialis. Abbreviations in this as well as Table 3.

Table 2. Activities of muscles during repetitive movements of static wrist extension in twelve subjects.

Among PT, ECR, and FCR in humans, inhibition between ECR and FCR (Aymard et al., 1995; Baldissera et al., 1983; Day et al., 1984), and facilitation between PT and ECR (Nakano et al., 2005, 2006) have been studied (Fig. 1). In the EMG study, during the repetitive movements of the dynamic wrist flexion/extension ECR (ECRL and ECRB) and FCR showed increments of activities at the extension and flexion phases, respectively, regardless of the positions of the forearm in all the subjects. Therefore alternating contraction between the muscles occurred during the movements. The inhibition between ECR and FCR (Aymard et al., 1995; Baldissera et al., 1983; Day et al., 1984) must be active during the alternating contraction. In the EMG study, in the prone, semiprone, and supine positions of the forearm, PT and ECR showed parallel activities during the movements of the static wrist extension in all, eight, and eight subjects and at the extension phase of the movements of the dynamic wrist extension/flexion in all, eight and five subjects, respectively. Therefore co-contraction of the muscles occurred during the wrist extension movements at least with the prone forearm. The facilitation between PT and ECR (Nakano et al., 2005, 2006) must be

Subject	Prone				Semiprone				Supine			
	ECRL	ECRB	PT	FCR	ECRL	ECRB	PT	FCR	ECRL	ECRB	PT	FCR
K.S.	E	E	E	F	E	E		F	E	E		F
Y.E.	E	E	E	F	E	E	E F	F	E	E	E F	F
H.F.	E	E	E	F	E	E		F	E	E		F
M.S.	E	E	E	F	E	E	E F	F	E	E	F	F
K.S.	E	E	E	F	E	E	E	F	E	E		F
S.Y.	E	E	E	F	E	E	E F	F	E	E	E F	F
H.T.	E	E	E	F	E	E		F	E	E	F	F
Y.K.	E	E	E	F	E	E	E	F	E	E	E	F
A.M.	E	E	E	F	E	E	E	F	E	E		F
Y.U.	E	E	E	F	E	E		F	E	E		F
S.K.	E	E	E	F	E	E	E F	F	E	E	E F	F
Y.W.	E	E	E	F	E	E	E	F	E	E	E	F

E: extension phase, F: flexion phase

Table 3. Peacks of activities of muscles during repetitive movements of dynamic wrist flexion/extension in twelve subjects.

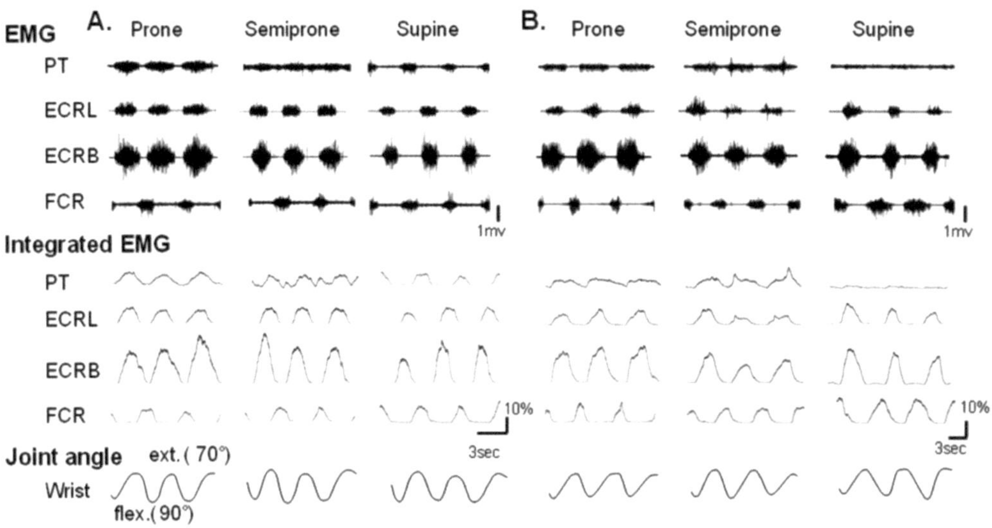

Fig. 4. An EMG study of repetitive movements of dynamic wrist flexion/extension with maintenance of the forearm in the prone, semiprone (neutral), and supine positions in normal human subjects. The subject performed the movements in the posture as well as Fig. 3A. **A, B**: EMGs of ECRL, ECRB, PT, and FCR during the movements in two subjects. The bottom trace represents the position of the wrist in flexion/extension direction. Parallel activities of PT, ECRL, and ECRB are seen at the extension phase in the prone and semiprone positions in both subjects (**A, B**). PT and FCR show parallel activities at the flexion phase in the supine and semiprone positions in one subject (**A**). Calibration bars for integrated EMGs: a percentage of the amplitude produced by the maximum contraction. Reproduced with permission from Fujii et al. (2007).

active during the co-contraction. In the EMG study, during the movements of the dynamic wrist flexion/extension parallel activities of PT and FCR were seen at the flexion phase in the semiprone and supine positions in four and five subjects, respectively. This observation of co-contraction seems to indicate existence of facilitation between PT and FCR. It therefore seems likely that the facilitation between PT and ECR is activated with pronating the forearm and that between PT and FCR is with supinating the forearm. Further studies are required to elucidate influence of the forearm position on the facilitation.

3. ENS study

Motions of the forearm and wrist produced by ENS to PT and ECRL were examined in the same twelve subjects of the EMG study in 2.2 (Fujii et al., 2007). The subject sat on a chair the shoulder joint flexed to 0-20 degrees of flexion and the elbow joint flexed to 70-90 degrees of flexion as well as in EMG study in 2.2 (Fig. 3A). The forearm was put on an experimental table in the prone, semiprone, and supine positions. For electrical stimulation, monopolar electrodes made of teflon-coated stainless steel wire (above-mentioned product) were implanted percutaneously into each motor point of ECRL and PT with 27 gauge injection-needles (Fujii et al., 2007; Naito et al., 1994, 2002; Sagae et al., 2010). A guide needle of a 25 gauge spinal-needle (length: 89 mm, Top Co., Tokyo, Japan) was percutaneously inserted into the subcutaneous tissue along to the lateral intermuscular septum of the arm and used as reference. Before the implantation, locations of the motor points were examined by electrical stimulation with surface electrodes. During the implantation, electrical rectangular pulses (duration: 0.2 ms, amplitude: -20-0 V, frequency: 1 or 20 Hz) were occasionally delivered to the muscles through the wire electrodes and contraction of individual muscles was confirmed by inspecting and palpating the tendon or belly of them (Albright & Linburg, 1978; Basmajian, 1982; Standring, 2005; Yoshida, 1994). Also it was carefully checked that no contraction of any other muscles was induced by the stimulation. For the ENS study, electrical rectangular pulses (duration: 0.2 ms, amplitude: -20 - 0 V, frequency: 20 Hz) were delivered using a computer-controlled multi-channel functional electrical stimulation (FES) system which we had developed to restore motor functions of paralyzed extremities with intramuscular wire electrodes (Handa et al., 1989; Hoshimiya et al., 1989). EMGs of ECRL and PT were recorded with two pairs of surface electrodes (Ag/AgCl Paste Applied with PVC Tape, Vitrode, NIHON KODEN, Tokyo, Japan), which were put on the central part of the contracted muscle belly longitudinally with the distance of about 1 cm. EMGs were amplified and band pass filtered (10-350 Hz). A wet bandage put round the shoulder was used as reference. Stimulation intensities (voltage) for the motor threshold (MT) and maximum contraction (MC) in individual muscles were determined by monitoring EMGs (motor wave) of the muscles and palpating the belly and tendon of them. In order to stimulate each of the muscles with the intensity between MT and MC, the voltage data for MT and MC were put into the FES system. Before ENS, the examined forearm was in the prone, semiprone, and supine positions. Then motions of the forearm and wrist induced by ENS were taken video with a digital video system (NV-MX2500, Panasonic, Tokyo). Angular changes of the motions of the wrist in flexion/extension direction and the forearm in pronation/supination direction were measured with the electrogoniometers mentioned above. A motion of the wrist in abduction/adduction direction was checked with video pictures. During ENS, EMGs of PT and ECRL were recorded with the pairs of the surface electrodes mentioned above. Data of the angular changes and EMGs were fed into the data recorder and pen recorder. ENS to ECRL was examined in all the twelve subjects. Since ENS to PT resulted in activation of PT and the other muscles innervated by the median nerve, i.e. FCR, m. palmaris longus, in one subject, it was examined in the remaining eleven subjects. The stimulus intensity was increased linearly from MT to MC for 4-5 sec.

ENS to PT induced a motion of forearm pronation from the prone, semiprone, and supine positions to the maximum pronation (90 degrees of pronation) in all the eleven subjects. ENS to ECRL induced motions of wrist extension to the maximum extention (70 degrees of extension) and abduction (radial flexion) to 5-20 degrees of abduction regardless of the positions of the forearm in all the twelve subjects. When the forearm was pronated before ENS, 30-80 degrees supination of the forearm from the prone position was induced in all the twelve subjects (Fig. 5).

Combined ENS to PT and ECRL was examined in the eleven subjects. An increase of the stimulus intensity of ENS to PT from MT to MC fixed the forearm in the maximum pronation (Fig. 6). Then an increase for ENS to ECRL from MT to MC resulted in motions of wrist extension to the maximum extension and abduction to 5-20 degrees of abduction without a motion of supination in all the eleven subjects. In this situation, a decrease of the intensity of ENS to PT from MC to MT resulted in a motion of 40–90 degrees supination from the maximum pronation while holding the wrist extension and abduction. Then the increase of the intensity of ENS to PT from MT to MC resulted in a motion of pronation to the maximum pronation while holding the extension and abduction (Fig. 6D).

4. Functional significance of the facilitation between PT and ECR

The ENS study showed that ENS to PT produced forearm pronation from the prone, semiprone, and supine positions to the maximum prone position and that to ECRL wrist extension to the maximum extension and abduction to 5-20 degrees of abduction in the forearm prone, semiprone, and supine positions in all subject. These results suggest that PT acts as a forearm pronator and ECRL as a wrist extensor and abductor independent of the forearm position. The EMG study of the repetitive movements of dynamic forearm pronation/supination with maintenance of the wrist neutral position showed parallel activities of PT, ECRL, and ECRB increasing and decreasing at the pronation and supination phases, respectively, in all subject. This result suggests that the facilitation between PT and ECR is active during the co-contraction and works effectively at the pronation phase of the movements. Since at the pronation phase pronating force of PT must be used to pronate the forearm and extending and abducting force of ECR must be to support the weight of the hand, the facilitation seems to be convenient for maintenance of the wrist position.

The ENS study showed that ENS to ECRL produced 30-80 degrees forearm supination from the prone position in all subject. This result suggests that ECRL act as not only a wrist extensor and abductor but also a forearm supinator when the forearm is in the prone position. Hence forearm supination from the prone position should be added to one of the actions of ECRL. The EMG study showed parallel activities of PT, ECRL, and ECRB during the movements of static wrist extension and at the extension phase of the movements of dynamic wrist extension/flexion in the prone position of the forearm in all subject. This result suggests that co-contraction of PT and ECR occurs during both static and dynamic wrist extension movements at least with the prone forearm. The facilitation must be active during the co-contraction. Since during the wrist extension movements extending and abducting force of ECRL must be used to extend the wrist and pronating force of PT must be to counteract supinating force of ECRL, the facilitation seems to be very convenient for maintenance of the forearm position. Actually the ENS study confirmed that combined ENS to PT and ECRL resulted in wrist extension and abduction with maintenance of the forearm prone position. The results of the EMG and ENS studies suggest that the facilitation is between antagonistic muscles. It is of no ordinary type.

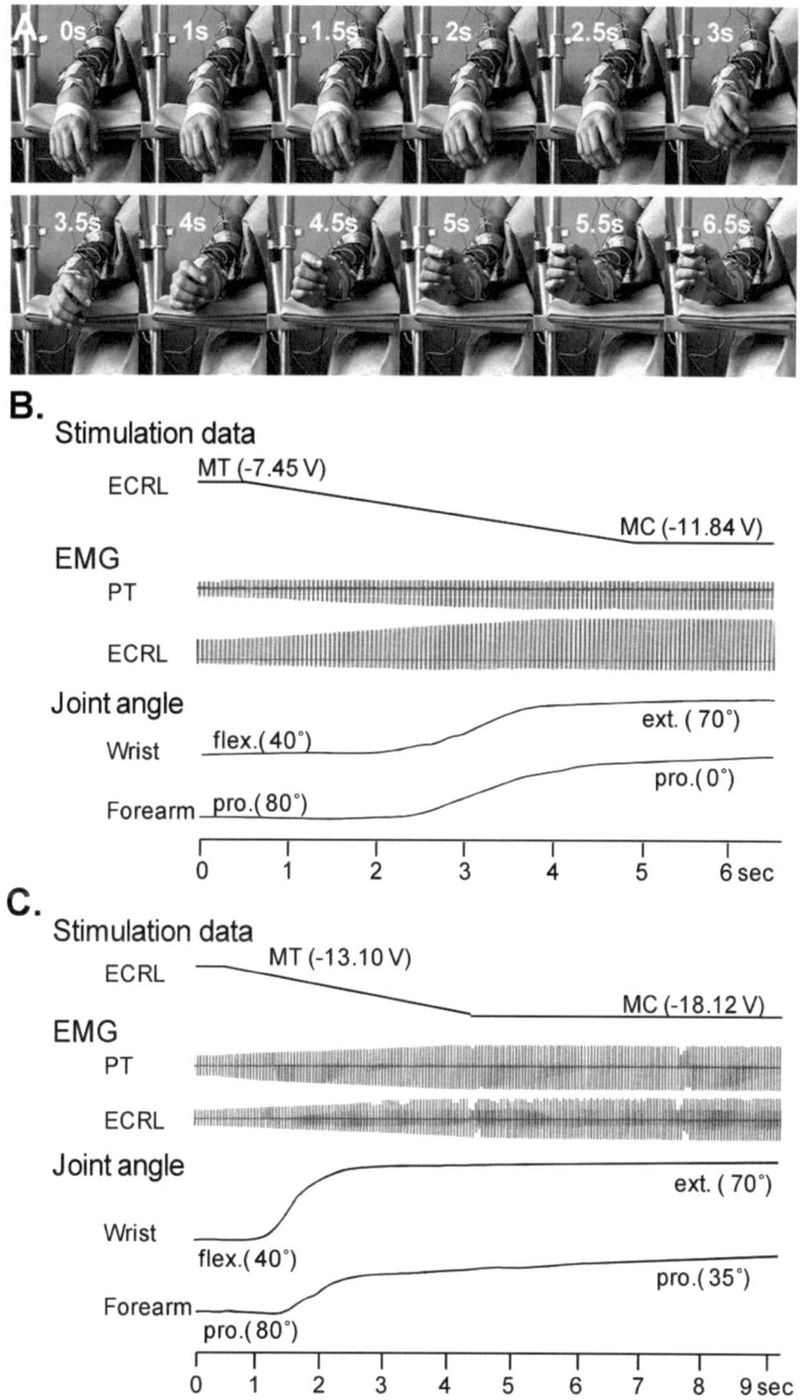

Fig. 5. An electrical neuromuscular stimulation (ENS) study: Motions produced by ENS to ECRL in normal human subjects. **A**: Pictures showing a sequence of the motions in a subject at 0.5-1 s interval. Before ENS (0 s), the forearm is in the prone position. Motions of wrist

extension and abduction (radial flexion), and forearm supination are induced (1-6.5 s). **B, C**: Results in two subjects, of which one (**B**) is of the subject in **A**. Prior to ENS, the forearm in the prone position. The stimulation intensities increased linearly from the motor threshold (MT) to the maximum contraction (MC) for 4.5 s in **B** and 4 s in **C**. Motions of wrist extension from 40 degrees of flexion to 70 degrees of extension and forearm supination from 80 to 0 degrees of pronation are induced in **B** and those of extension from 50 degrees of flexion to 70 degrees of extension and supination from 80 to 35 degrees of pronation are in **C**. No voluntary contraction of ECRL and PT are observed in EMG in both subjects (**B, C**). Abbreviations in this as well as Fig. 6. Reproduced with permission from Fujii et al. (2007).

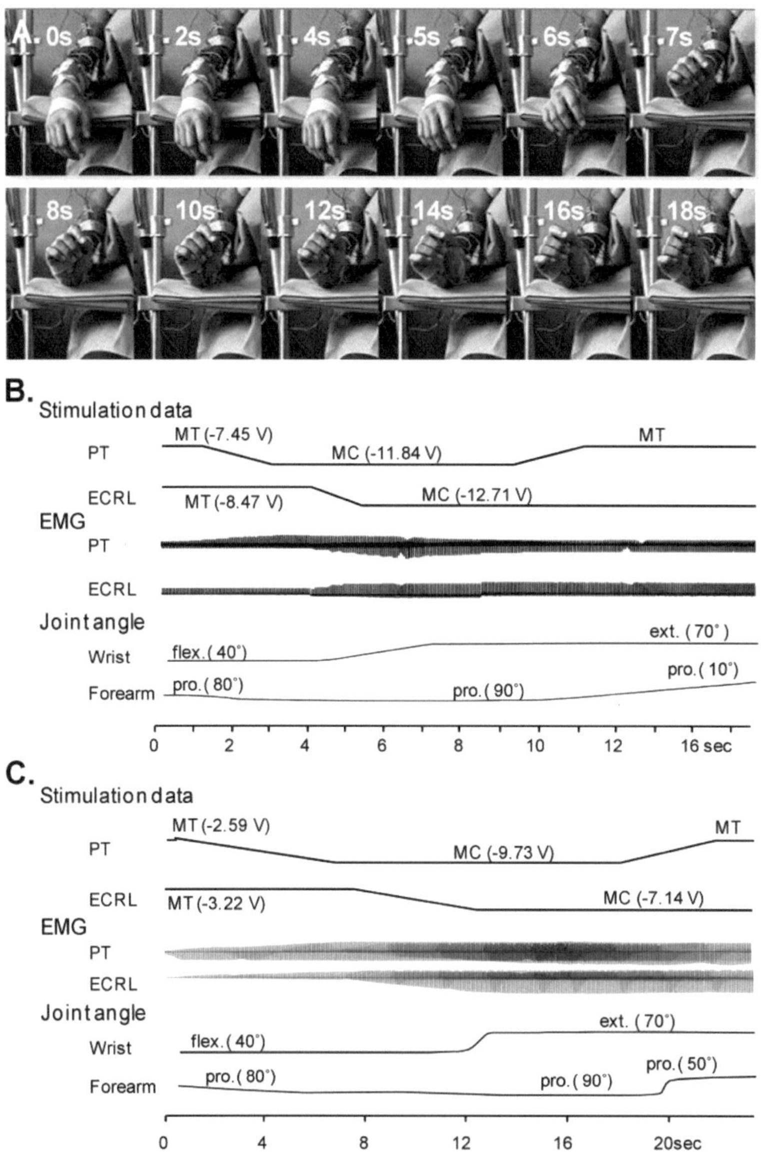

Fig. 6. (Continued)

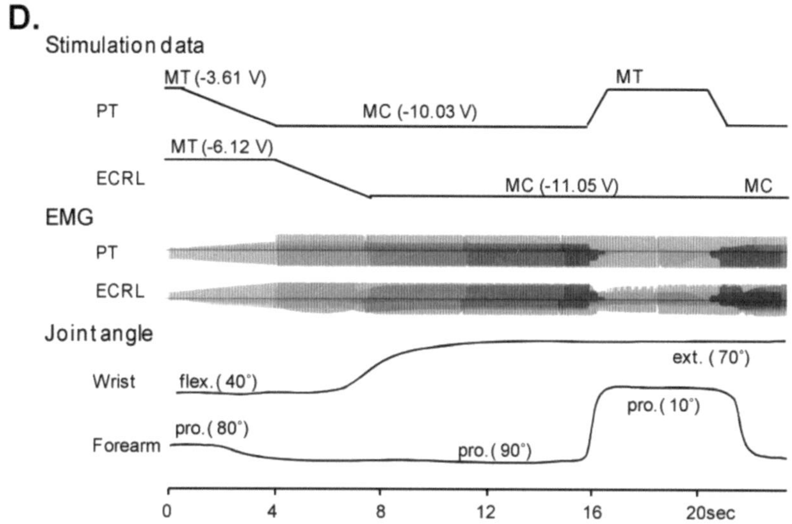

Fig. 6. An ENS study: Motions produced by a combined ENS to PT and ECRL in normal human subjects. **A**: Pictures showing a sequence of the motions in one subject at 1-2 s interval. Before ENS (0 s), the forearm is in the prone position. ENS to PT induces a motion of pronation to the mamimum pronation of the forearm (1-4 s). Then ENS to ECRL produces a motion of wrist extension and abduction with maintenance of the maximum pronation (4-8 s). Then a reduction of ENS to PT results in a motion of supination with maintenance of the extension and abduction (8-18 s). **B-D**: Results in three subjects, of which one (**B**) is of the subject in **A**. In all the three subjects (**B-D**), an increase of the stimulation intensity of ENS to PT from MT to MC induces a motion of pronation from 80 to 90 degrees of pronation (from the prone position to the maximum pronation). Then an increase of the intensity of ENS to ECRL from MT to MC induces a motion of wrist extension from 40 degrees of flexion to 70 degrees of extension (the maximum extension) with maintenance of the maximum pronation. Then a decrease of the intensity of ENS to PT from MC to MT results in a motion of supination from the maximum supination to 10 (**B**), 50 (**C**), and 10 degrees of pronation (**D**) with maintenance of the maximum extension. In one subject (**D**), then an increase of the intensity of ENS to PT induces a motion of pronation to the maximum pronation with maintenance of the maximum extension. No voluntary contraction is observed in EMG in all the subjects (**B-D**). Reproduced with permission from Fujii et al. (2007).

5. Effects of wrist extension and flexion on forearm supinating force

It is known that FCR acts as not only a wrist flexor and abductor but also a forearm pronator (American Society for Surgery of the Hand, 2011; Basmajian, 1982). The ENS study has shown that ECRL acts as a wrist extensor and abductor and a forearm supinator when the forearm is in the prone position (Fujii et al., 2007). It therefore is support an idea that forearm supinating force is increased and decreased by wrist extension and flexion, respectively.

Our previous study showed effects of wrist extension and flexion on forearm supinating force in humans (Otaki et al., 2009). In our study, the forces produced by maximal supination with the wrist relaxed (R-Sup), maximally flexed (F-Sup), and maximally extended (E-Sup) in the forearm 90° (prone), 60°, 30°, and 0° pronated (neutral) positions were measured in eight normal human subjects (male 7, female 1, age range 20-41 years). Also activities of BB, which acts as an elbow flexor and forearm supinator, FCR, and ECR (ECRL and ECRB) were recorded with EMG using surface electrodes. In the EMG study, FCR and ECR respectively showed activities during wrist flexion and extension (Fig. 7A, B). BB showed activities increasing concomitantly with increased the force. Usually, E-Sup produced larger BB activities than R-Sup and F-Sup; and F-Sup decreased FCR activities and increased ECR activities. In the force study, the respective force of R-, F-, and E-Sup decreased with changing position from prone to neutral. Assuming the force of R-Sup in each position as 100%, that of E-Sup was 163±20%(mean ±S.D.), 142±17%, 134±15%, and 118±23%, and those of F-Sup was 81±7%, 90±14%, 78±13%, and 80±10%, respectively, in the prone, P60°, P30°, and neutral positions (Fig. 7C). In every position, the force of E-Sup was larger and that of F-Sup was smaller than that of R-Sup. The increment of the force of E-Sup decreased with changing the position from prone to neutral.

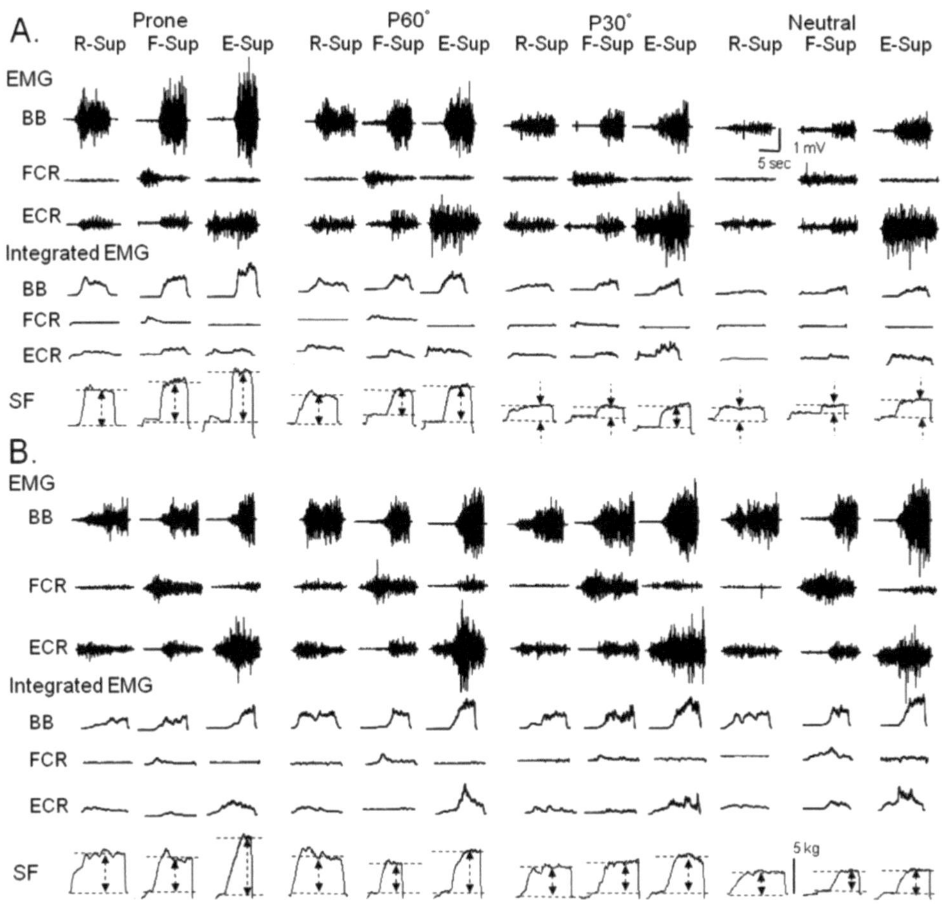

Fig. 7. (Continued)

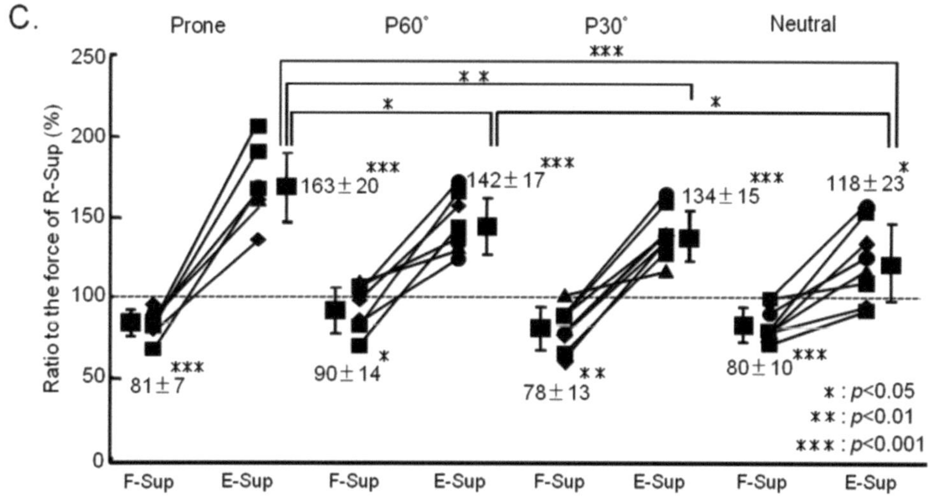

Fig. 7. Effects of wrist extension and flexion on forearm supinating force (SF) in normal human subjects. **A, B**: EMGs of BB, FCR, and ECR, and SF during maximal forearm supination with the wrist relaxed (R-Sup), maximally flexed (F-Sup), and maximally extended (E-Sup) in the forearm 90 degrees (Prone), 60 degrees (P60°), 30 degrees (P30°), and 0 degrees pronated (Neutral) positions in two normal human subjects. SF is indicated by the length of double broken arrow or the distance between two broken arrows. In every forearm position, E-Sup produces larger BB activities than R- and F-Sup. A decrease of FCR activities and an increase of ECR activities are observed during F-Sup. **C**: A graph showing ratio (%) of SF of F- and E-Sup to that of R-Sup in the forearm Prone, P60°, P30°, and Neutral positions in eight subjects. Individual data of the ratio of SF, and average and standard deviation are illustrated in the graph. In every position, SF of E-Sup is larger and that of F-Sup is smaller than that of R-Sup. Note that the increment of SF of E-Sup decreases with the forearm position from Prone to Neutral. Reproduced with permission from Otaki et al. (2009).

The results of the force study suggest that the supinating force is reinforced by the extension and weakened by the flexion and the reinforcement effect decreases with supination of the forearm. Since reflex arcs of facilitation from ECR to BB, inhibition between FCR and ECR, and from BB to FCR exist in humans (Fig. 1) (Aymard et al., 1995; Baldissera et al., 1983; Cavallari & Katz, 1989; Cavallari et al, 1992), the results of the EMG study suggest that the effects result not only from actions of the muscles but also from activations of the reflex arcs. Our recent study further showed an increase and decrease of forearm pronating force by wrist flexion and extension, respectively, in humans (Sato et al., 2011).

6. Summary

The functional significance of facilitatory spinal reflex arcs (facilitation) between musculus (m.) pronator teres (PT) and m. ectensor carpi radialis (ECR; ECR longus: ECRL, ECR brevis: ECRB) in humans was studied using an electromyography (EMG) and electrical neuromuscular stimulation (ENS). The EMG study of dynamic forearm pronation/ supination movements with maintenance of the wrist neutral position (PS-movements) showed parallel activities (co-contraction) of PT and ECR increasing and decreasing at the pronation and supination phases, respectively. The facilitation must be active during the co-contraction and work effectively at the pronation phase. The EMG study of static and dynamic wrist extension movements with the prone forearm (WE-movements) also showed co-contraction of the muscles. The facilitation must be active during the co-contraction. The ENS study showed that ENS to PT produced forearm pronation and that to ECRL wrist extension and abduction independent of the forearm position. Since at the pronation phase of the PS-movements pronating force of PT must be used to pronate the forearm and extending and abducting force of ECR must be to support the weight of the hand, the facilitation seems to be convenient for maintenance of the wrist position. The ENS study also showed that ENS to ECRL produced forearm supination from the prone position. This result suggests that ECRL acts as not only a wrist extensor and abductor but also a forearm supinator when the forearm is in the peone position. Since during the WE-movements extending force of ECR must be used to extend the wrist and pronating force of PT must be to counteract supinating force of ECR, the facilitation seems to be convenient for maintenance of the forearm position. The results of EMG and ENS studies suggest that the facilitation is between antagonistic muscles. Finally, an increase and decrease of forearm supinating force respectively by wrist extension and flexion were briefly described.

7. Acknowledgment

The authors thank Dr. Takuji Miyasaka, Dr. Shinji Kobayashi, Dr. Katuhiro Shinozaki, Dr. Masaaki Sagae, Dr. Aya Narita, Mr. Makoto Nagamuma, Mr. Hiroto Kobayashi, Mr. Wataru Hashizume, Ms. Saori Yoshida, Mr. Katsuhiko Kato, and Mr. Inazo Eguchi for their excellent assistance. Thanks are also tendered to students of Yamagata University School of Medicine and Yamagata Prefectural University of Health Sciences for their helpful cooperation. This study was supported, in part, by a Grant-in-Aid from Japanese Ministry of Education, Science, Sport and Culture (17590146) and by grants from the Yamagata Health Support Society Foundation.

8. References

Albright, J.A. & Linburg, R.M. (1978) Common variations of the radial extensors. *J Hand Surg*, Vol. 3, pp.134-138, ISSN 1531-6564

American Society for Surgery of the Hand (2011) *The electric textbook of hand surgery. Anatomy of the hand. Muscles.* E-HAND. COM, http://www.eatonhand.cpm/hom/hom033.htm

Aymard, C.; Chia, L.; Katz R.; Lafitte, C. & Penicaud, A. (1995) Reciprocal inhibition between wrist flexors and extensors in man: a new set of interneurones? *J Physiol (Lond)*, Vol. 487, pp.221-235, ISSN 0022-3751

Baldissera, F.; Campadelli, P. & Cavallari, P. (1983) Inhibition of H-reflex in wrist flexors by group I afferents in the radial nerve. *Electromyogr Clin Neurophysiol*, Vol.23, pp.187-193, ISSN 0301-150X

Basmajian, J.V. (1982) *Primary Anatomy* (8th Ed.), Williams and Wilkins, ISBN 0-683-00550-2, Baltimore, pp 150-164

Basmajian, J.V. & Deluca, C.J. (1985) *Muscle Alive: Their Functions Revealed by Electromyography* (5th Ed.), Williams and Wilkins, ISBN 0-683-00414-X, Baltimore, pp 265-289

Cavallari, P. & Katz, R. (1989) Pattern of projections of group I afferents from forearm muscles to motoneurones supplying biceps and triceps muscles in man. *Exp Brain Res*, Vol. 78, pp.465-478, ISSN 0014-4819

Cavallari, P.; Katz, R. & Penicaud, A. (1992) Patterns of projections of group I afferrents from elbow muscles to motoneurones supplying wrist muscles in man. *Exp Brain Res*, Vol. 91, pp. 311-319, ISSN 0014-4819

Creange, A.; Faist, M.; Katz, R. & Panicaud, A. (1992) Distributions of heteronymous Ia facilitation and recurrent inhibition in the human deltoid motor nucleus. *Exp. Brain Res*, Vol. 90, pp. 620-624, ISSN 0014-4819

Day, B.L.; Marsden, C.D.; Obeso, J.A. & Rorhwell, J.C. (1984) Reciprocal inhibition between the muscles of the human forearm. *J Physiol (Lond)*, Vol. 349, pp.519-534, ISSN 0022-3751

Fujii, H.; Kobayashi, S.; Shinozaki, K.; Naito, A.; Sato, T.; Miyasaka, T. & Shindo, M. (2001) Inhibitory projections of muscle afferents between the brachioradialis and flexor carpi radialis in humans. *Neurosci Res*, Suppl 25, S87, ISSN 0168-0102

Fujii, H.; Kobayashi, S.; Sato, T.; Shinozaki, K. & Naito, A. (2007) Co-contraction of the pronator teres and extensor carpi radialis during wrist extension movements in humans. *J Electromyogr Kinesiol*, Vol. 17, pp.80-89, ISSN 1050-6411

Handa, Y.; Hoshimiya, N.; Iguchi, Y. & Oda, T. (1989) Developments of percutaneous intramuscular electrode for multi-channel FES system. *IEEE Trans Biomed Eng*, Vol. 36; pp.705-710, ISSN0018-9294

Hoshimiya, N.; Naito, A.; Yajima, M. & Handa, Y. (1989) A multichannel FES system for the restoration of motor functions in high spinal cord injury patients: A respiration-controlled system for multijoint upper extremity, *IEEE Trans Biomed Eng*, Vol. 36; pp.754-760, ISSN0018-9294

Jenkins, D.B. (2008) *Hollinshead's Functional Anatomy of the Limbs and Back* (9th ed.), WB Saunders, ISBN 978-1-4160-4980-7, Philadelphia

Katz, R.; Penicaud, A. & Rossi, A. (1991) Reciprocal Ia inhibition between elbow flexors and extensors in the human. *J Physiol (Lond)*, Vol. 437; pp.269-286, ISSN 0022-3751

Kobayashi, S.; Naito, A.; Hayashi, M.; Ogino, T.; Fujii, H. & Tonosaki, A. (2000) Inhibitroy projections of muscle afferents from the brachioradialis to the flexor carpi radialis motoneurones in humans. *Acta Anat Nippon*, Vol. 76, p.130 (in Japanese), ISSN 0022-7722

Lourenço, G.; Iglesias, C. & Marchand-Pauvert, V. (2007) Effects produced in human arm and forearm motoneurones after electrical stimulation of ulnar and median nerves at wrist level. *Exp Brain Res*, Vol. 178, pp.267-284, ISSN 0014-4819

Marchand-Pauvert, V.; Nicolas, G. & Pierrot-Desilligny, E. (2000) Monosynaptic Ia projections from intrinsic hand muscles to forearm motoneurones in humans. *J Physiol (Lond)*, Vol. 525, pp.241-252, ISSN 0022-3751

Miyasaka, T.; Sun, Y.-J.; Naito, A.; Morita, H.; Shindo, M.; Shimizu, Y. & Yanagisawa, N. (1995) Reciprocal inhibition between biceps brachii and brachioradialis in the human. In abstract, *4th IBRO World Congress of Neuroscience*; Rapid Communications, Oxford New York, p.334

Miyasaka, T.; Sun, Y.-J.; Naito, A. & Shindo, M. (1996) Inhibition projections from the biceps brachii to the pronator teres motoneurones in the human. *Neurosci Res*, Suppl 20, S183, ISSN 0168-0102

Miyasaka, T.; Naito, A.; Morita, H.; Sun, Y.-J.; Chishima, M. & Shindo, M. (1998) Inhibitory neural connection from the brachioradialis to the pronator teres in human. *Neurosci Res*, Suppl 22, S159, ISSN 0168-0102

Miyasaka, T.; Naito, A.; Shindo, M.; Kobayashi, S.; Hayashi, M.; Shinozaki, K. & Chishima, M. (2007) Modulation of bracioradialis motoneuron excitabilities by group I fibers of the median nerve in humans. *Tohoku J Exp Med*, Vol. 212, pp.115-131, ISSN 0040-8727

Naito, A.; Handa, Y.; Handa, T.; Ichie, M.; Hoshimiya, N. & Shimizu, Y. (1994) Study on the elbow movement produced by functional electrical stimulation (FES). *Tohoku J Exp Med*, Vol. 174, pp.343-349, ISSN 0040-8727

Naito, A.; Shindo, M.; Miyasaka, T.; Sun, Y.-J. & Morita, H. (1996) Inhibitory projections from brachioradialis to biceps brachii in human. *Exp Brain Res*, Vol. 111, pp.483-486, ISSN 0014-4819

Naito, A.; Shindo, M.; Miyasaka, T.; Sun, Y.-J.; Momoi, H. & Chishima, M. (1998a) Inhibitory projections from pronator teres to biceps brachii motoneurones in human. *Exp Brain Res*, Vol. 121, pp.99-102, ISSN 0014-4819

Naito, A.; Sun, Y.-J.; Yajima, M.; Fukamachi, H. & Ushikoshi, K. (1998b) Electromyographic study of the elbow flexors and extensors in a motion of forearm pronation/supination while maintaining elbow flexion in humans. *Tohoku J Exp Med*, Vol. 186, pp.267-277, ISSN 0040-8727

Naito, A.; Shinozaki, K.; Kobayashi, S.; Fujii, H.; Sato, T.; Miyasaka, T. & Shindo, M. (2001) Excitatory projections of muscle afferents between the bracchioradialis and extensor carpi radialis in humans. *Neurosci Res*, Suppl 25, S87, ISSN 0168-0102

Naito, A.; Yajima, M.; Chishima, M. & Sun, Y.-J. (2002) A motion of forearm supination with maintenance of elbow flexion produced by electrical stimulation to two elbow flexors in humans. *J Electromyogr Kinesio*l, Vol. 12, pp.259-265, ISSN 1050-6411

Naito, A. (2003) Spinal mechanism for motor control: neural connections among muscles in the human upper limb. *Yamagata Med J*, Vol. 21, pp.155-169 (in Japanese) , ISSN 0288-030X

Naito, A. (2004) Electrophysiologircal studies of muscles in the human upper limb: the biceps brachii. *Anat Sci Int*, Vol. 79, pp.11-20, ISSN 1447-6959

Nakano, H.; Miyasaka, T.; Sagae, M.; Fujii, H.; Sato, T.; Suzuki, K.; Ogawa, K.; Shindo, M. & Naito, A. (2005) Facilitation from the pronator teres to extensor carpi radialis motoneurons in humans: Studies using a post-stimulus time-histogram technique. Acta Anat Nippon, 80 suppl, p.5, ISSN 0022-7722

Nakano, H.; Miyasaka, T.; Sagae, M.; Fujii, H.; Sato, T.; Suzuki, K.; Shindo, M.; Ogino, T. & Naito, A. (2006) Facilitation between pronator teres and extensor carpi radialis: Studies with a PSTH method. *Clin Neurophysiol*, Vol. 117, S160, ISSN 1388-2457

Ogawa, K.; Suzuk,i K.; Fujii, H.; Sato, T.; Nakano, H.; Sagae, M.; Miyasaka, T.; Naito, A. & Watanabe, H. (2005) Facilitation from thernar muscles to extensor carpi radialis in humans: A study using an electromyogram-averaging method with mechanical conditioning stimulation. *Yamagata Med J*, Vol. 23, pp.107-105 (in Japanese with English abstract and figure legends), ISSN 0288-030X

Otaki, R.; Sato, T.; Naganuma, M.; Suzuki, K.; Narita, A.; Sato, A.; Miyasaka, T.; Fujii, H. & Naito, A. (2009) Effects of wrist flexion and extension on forearm supination force.

Structure Function, Vol. 8, pp.13-18 (in Japanese with English abstract and figure legends), ISSN 1347-7145

Perotto, A.O. (1994) *Anatomical Guide for the Electromyographer: The Limb and Trunk* (3rd ed.), Charles C. Thomas, ISBN 0-398-05900-4, Springfield IL

Pierrot-Deseilligny, E.; Morin, C.; Bergego, C. & Tankov, N. (1981) Pattern of group I fiber projections from ankle flexor and extensor muscles in man. *Exp Brain Res*, Vol. 42:, pp.337-350, ISSN 0014-4819

Pierrot-Deseilligny, E. & Mazevet, D. (2000) The monosynaptic reflex: a tool to investigate motor control in humans. Interest and limits. *Neurophysiol Clin*, Vol. 30, pp.67-80, ISSN 0987-7053

Riek, S.; Carson, R.C. & Wright, A. (2000) A new technique for the selective recording of extensor carpi radialis longus and brevis EMG. *J Electromyogr Kinesiol*, Vol. 10, pp.249-253, ISSN 1050-6411

Rossi, A.; Decchi, B.; Zalaffi, A. & Mazzocchio, R. (1995) Group Ia non-reciprocal inhibition from wrist extensor to flexor motoneurones in humans. *Neurosci Lett*, Vol. 191, pp.205-207, ISSN 0304-3940

Rothwell, J. (1994) *Control of Human Voluntary Movement* (2nd ed.) Chapman & Hall, ISBN 0-412-47700-9, London, pp149–181

Sagae, M.; Suzuki, K.; Fujita, T.; Sotokawa, T.; Nakano, H.; Naganuma, M.; Narita, A.; Sato, T.; Fujii, H.; Ogino, T. & Naito, A. (2010) Strict actions of the human wrist extensors: A study with an electrical neuromuscular stimulation method. *J Electromyogr Kinesiol*, Vol. 20, pp.1178-1185, ISSN 1050-6411

Sato, T.; Fujii, H.; Naito, A.; Tonosaki, A.; Kobayashi, S.; Shinozaki, K.; Miyasaka, T. & Shindo, M. (2002) Inhibition of muscle afferents from the brachioradialis to triceps brachii motoneurones in humans: Central pathway. *Acta Anat Nippon*, Vol. 77 Suppl, H511, ISSN 0022-7722

Sato T, Suzuki K, Sotokawa T, Fujita T, Sagae M, Nakano H, Naganuma M, Fujii H, Kato K & Naito A (2007) Simultaneous recording system for digital video pictures and electric signals. *Structure Function*, Vol. 6, pp.3-8 (in Japanese with English abstract and figure legends), ISSN 1347-7145

Sato, T.; Sato, T.; Konishi, Y.; Naganuma, M.; Suzuki, K.; Narita, A.; Fujii, H.; Hashizume, W. & Naito, A. (2011) Effects of wrist flexion and extension on forearm pronation force. *Structure Function*, Vol. 9, pp.59-63 (in Japanese with English abstract and figure legends), ISSN 1347-7145

Shinozaki, K.; Naito, A.; Kobayashi, S.; Miyasaka, T.; Shindo, M. & Tonosaki, A. (2001) Pathways of facilitatory projections between the bracioradialis and extensor carpi radialis in humans. *Acta Anat Nippon*, Vol. 76, p.130 (in Japanese) , ISSN 0022-7722

Standring, S.; Ellis, H.; Healy, C.; Johnson, D. & Williams, A. (2005) *Gray's Anatomy* (39th ed.) Elsevier, Churchill Livingstone, ISBN 0-443-07168-3, Edinburgh, pp.879–880

Suzuki, K.; Nakano, H.; Sato, T.; Fujii, H.; Ogawa, K.; Watanabe, H. & Naito, A. (2005) Facilitation from the median nerve innervating hand muscles to extensor carpi radialis in humans: A study using an electromyogram-averaging method. *Yamagata Med J*, Vol. 23, pp.59-68 (in Japanese with English abstract and figure legends), ISSN 0288-030X

Suzuki, K.; Fujita, T.; Sotokawa, T.; Naganuma, M.; Sato, T.; Fujii, H.; Nakano, H.; Narita, A.; Miyasaka, T.; Shindo, M. & Naito, A. (2007) Facilitation from hand muscles innervated by the ulnar nerve to extensor carpi radialis in humans: A study using an electromyogram-averaging method. *Jpn J Clin Neurophysiol*, Vol. 35, p.449-450 (in Japanere), ISSN 1345-7101

Tanaka, R. (1989) Spinal mechanisms for human motor control. In: *Annual Review of Neuroscience,* edited by M. Ito & H. Narabayashi, Igaku-Shoin, IBSN4-260-17303-0, Tokyo, pp. 61-91 (in Japanese)

Wargon. I.; Lamy, J.C.; Baret, M.; Ghanim, Z.; Aymard, C.; Penicaud, A. & Katz, R. (2006) The disynaptic group I inhibition between wrist flexor and extensor muscle revisited in humans. *Exp Brain Res*, Vol. 168, pp.203-217, ISSN 0014-4819

Yoshida, Y. (1994) Anatomical studies on the extensor carpi radialis longus and brevis muscles in Japanese. *Okajima's Folia Anat Jpn*, Vol. 71, pp.123-136, ISSN 0030-154X

Part 4

Evoked Potential

15

Visual and Brainstem Auditory Evoked Potentials in Neurology

Ashraf Zaher
Department of Neurology, Faculty of Medicine, University of Mansoura, Mansoura, Egypt

1. Introduction

Historically, Richard Caton (1875) discovered evoked potentials and the electroencephalogram (EEG) at the same time. The evoked potentials provided a useful tool for neurophysiological research (Shagass, 1976).
Evoked potentials are the voltage changes generated in the brain, the sense organ and the pathway leading to the brain in response to an external stimulus. This stimulus has to be somewhat above its subjective detection threshold so as to be clearly discernible, as well as to be of abrupt onset and /or offset so, that discrete volley is set up in the afferent pathway, hence capable of eliciting distinct cortical potential changes (Kriss, 1980).
Chiappa et al., 1987 defined an evoked potential as the record of the electrical activity produced by groups of neurons within the spinal cord, brain stem, thalamus or cerebral hemispheres following stimulation of one or another specific system by means of visual, auditory, or somatosensory input.
EEG recording may be obtained in a relatively direct manner by amplifying and displaying the activity picked up by electrodes placed on the scalp (Shagass, 1976), but most evoked potential (EP) activity due to their low amplitude, 0.1-20 microvolts relative to the normal background activity of EEG, their activity can not be clearly displayed, however with the development of micro-computers in the seventies (special signal averaging process) helping the extraction of the evoked potential from the EEG activity which is of much greater amplitude leading to their widespread clinical use (Kimura, 1985).

2. Visual evoked potentials (VEPs)

2.1 Introduction

The visual evoked potentials (VEPs) result from change of brain activity following application of intermittent visual stimulus to the visual system. They provide a quantitative measure of the functional integrity of the visual pathways (Celesia, 1988). The function measured includes that of the optic nerve, through the optic chiasma and tract, to the lateral geniculate bodies and the geniculocalcarine projection to the visual cortex "area 17" (Yiannikas and Walsh, 1983).
Since the VEP measures the pathway from the retina to area 17, a normal P100 does not exclude lesions of the visual pathway beyond area 17. For this reason, the VEP may be normal in patients with the diagnosis of cortical blindness. The usefulness of VEP is limited in

malingering and hysterical visual loss (Bodis-Wollner et al., 1977). It is useful when a normal VEP is recorded, but abnormal responses are of limited diagnostic value in such cases.

The most important fact to consider is that, although the axons from the nasal half of the retina decussate at the optic chiasm, the temporal axons do not. Therefore, retrochiasmatic lesions may not be detected by full-field checkerboard stimulation. VEPs are most useful in testing optic nerve function and less useful in postchiasmatic disorders. In retrochiasmatic lesions, the MRI is a more useful test. Partial-field studies may be useful in retrochiasmatic lesions; however, they are not performed routinely in clinical settings (Chiappa, 1990).

Recordings of this evoked potential are recognized as a reliable diagnostic procedure in the investigation of lesions of the anterior visual pathway (Halliday et al., 1976). However, it is not specific with regard to etiology. A tumor compressing the optic nerve, an ischemic disturbance, or a demyelinating disease may cause delay in the P100; only additional clinical history and, often, MRI are needed to uncover the etiology (Leslie et al., 2002).

2.2 Normal components of pattern reversal visual evoked potential (PRVEP) (Figure 1)

The cerebral pattern reversal evoked potential to full field stimulation consists of three peaks in normal subjects. The peak polarities are negative, positive and negative (NPN) and the mean peak latencies are 70, 100 and 145 milliseconds (msec) respectively. The first negative wave (N1 or N70) may be difficult to identify in some normal subjects and many patients likewise, the second negative peak (N2 or N145) is too inconsistent in latency and amplitude to be of clinical value. Thus, waveform identification in the pattern shift visual evoked potential consists of the large positive peak (P1 or P100). Depending on the stimulating device in use, and the presence or absence of abnormalities, it may be found any where from 90 to 250 msec (chiappa, 1982).

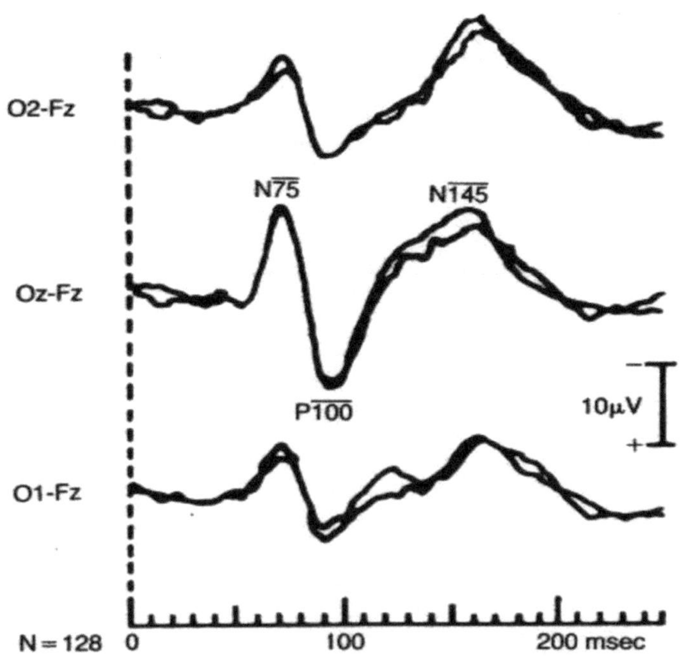

Fig. 1. Normal Visual Evoked Potential (VEP) (Poon's, 2003a).

	Latency (msec.)	R-L Difference	Amplitude (μV)	R-L Difference
N70	71.1 (<81.8)	9.4	3.8 (>0.1)	5.1
P100	95.8 (<112.0)	9.3	10.1 (>1.8)	7.0
Steady state P1	95.5 (<118.1)	21.0	8.3 (>6.1)	6.1

Table 1. Visual Evoked Potential Normative Data From Celesia (1985).

	Full field VEP			
	Mean	**Range**	**SD**	**Mean + 3 SD**
P100 latency	102.3 msec.	89-114	5.1	117.6
L-R difference	1.3 msec.	0-6	2.0	7.3
P100 amplitude	10.1 uV	3-21	4.2	22.7
P100 amp. Diff.	1.6 uV	0-5.5	1.4	5.8

Table 2. Visual Evoked Potential Normative Data From Chiappa (1990).

Check size	**VEP Check Size Effects**						
	Latency (msec.)				**Amplitude (uV)**		
	Latency Mean (SD) (Range)	**Latency ULN**	**L-R Diff Mean (SD) (Range)**	**L-R Diff ULN**	**Amplitude Mean (SD) (Range)**	**L-R Diff Mean (SD) (Range)**	**L-R Diff ULN**
17"	106.8 (6.4) (96.7-128.8)	126.0	2.73 (2.32) (0-8.80)	9.7	8.34 (3.71) (1.6-18.7)	1.48 (1.19) (0.2-5.2)	5.1
35"	102.9 (7.4) (88.6-121.4)	125.1	2.53 (2.91) (0-13.4)	11.3	7.13 (3.68) (1.0-19.8)	1.69 (2.00) (0-8.6)	7.7
70"	103.8 (6.9) (88.2-122.5)	124.5	2.18 (2.59) (0-12.7)	10.0	7.95 (3.64) (1.8-19.8)	1.29 (1.16) (0-4.8)	4.8
144"	107.3 (8.8) (91.1-130.6)	133.7	2.44 (2.55) (0-12)	10.1	7.72 (2.95) (1.5-16.1)	1.36 (1.22) (0-5.4)	5.0
288"	113.5 (11.8) (91.4 -142)	148.9	3.95 (4.03) (0 -15.2)	16.0	7.31 (2.74) (2.6 -14)	1.10 (1.05) (0 -3.9)	4.3

ULN = Upper Limit of Normal (Mean + 3 SD) *(Chiappa, 1990).*

Table 3. Check size 25.8" *(Chiappa, 1990).*

P100 is usually seen in all normal subjects and has a variability small enough to make it reliable in clinical practice, in addition to measuring the absolute latency of P100, determining the inter-ocular latency difference, amplitude, inter-ocular amplitude difference ratio and duration of P100 has increased the diagnostic yield of the test (chiappa, 1983).

The "W" morphology is most often an individual variation, although decreasing the stimulation frequency from 2 Hz to 1 Hz usually converts the W shape into a conventional P100 peak. Check size and alternation rate are factors in this; the responses can be manipulated to a "W" or a conventional P100 response by changing these parameters. Large checks tend to produce VEPs similar to those produced by flash stimulation (Leslie et al., 2002).

Blumhardt and Halliday, (1979) noted that the ipsilateral hemisphere evoked potential was actually a series of waves with negative components preceding and following P100 wave at latencies of approximately 75, 145 msec respectively. The contralateral hemisphere response consists of a triphasic complex occurring synchronously but of opposite polarity with a major negativity at about 100 msec and smaller positive deflections at 75 and 145 msec.
Maximum value for P100 is 115 msec in patients younger than 60 years; it rises to 120 msec thereafter in females and 125 msec in males. Even though published norms are available in the medical literature, each individual laboratory should have its own norms to control for lab-to-lab variability in technique **(Leslie et al., 2002).**

2.3 Generator source of pattern reversal visual evoked potential (PRVEP)

In relation to the generator sources of PRVEP Chiappa,(1983) claimed that P100 is generated in the striate and pre-striate occipital cortex as a result of both primary activation and subsequent thalamocortical volleys. However, the exact sources of P100 are not well defined. Positron tomographic mapping of human cerebral metabolism during reversal checkerboard stimulation revealed strong activation of both primary and association visual cortical areas (Phelps et at., 1981).
Ikeda et al., 1998 studied generators of VEP by dipole tracing in the human occipital cortex. Current source generators (dipoles) of human VEP to pattern-onset stimuli were investigated. A visual stimulus, a checkerboard pattern, was presented for 250 ms in each of the 8 quadrants. Central and peripheral parts of each of the 4 quadrant fields were evaluated. The results from these analyses of VEP indicated topographic localization of the dipoles around the calcarine fissure.

2.4 Principles of recording of VEP

2.4.1 Technical details (Leslie et al., 2002)

Dark room; Patient seated 70-100 cm from the screen; Corrective lenses used if necessary (acuity check prior to commencement of VEP); Pupil size and any abnormality should be noted(The pupils should not be dilated by mydriatics to prevent interference with accommodation); Sedation should not be used, and note should be taken of medications that the patient is taking regularly; Checkerboard pattern is used as stimulation; Check size of approximately 30 seconds of visual angle; Contrast between 50-80 percent; Stimulus rates of 1-2 Hz are recommended (producing a reversal every 500 msec); Filter setting should be 1 to 200 Hz bandwidth (outside limit is 0.2-300 Hz); The recommended recording time window (i.e. sweep length) is 250 ms; 50-200 responses are to be averaged; A minimum of 2 trials should be given.

2.4.2 Stimulation procedures

There are two general types of visual stimuli that are most often used to elicit visual evoked potential. These are the un-patterned flashing lights and the patterned stimuli which in clinical laboratories are usually checkerboards (Sokol, 1980).
Unpatterned flashing stimuli can be produced with a photo stimulator similar to that used in EEG recordings for photic driving. The intensity, color and rate of stimulation of the flash light can be varied. But, the variability in amplitude and latency of the evoked potential is much greater than in patterned stimuli (Halliday, 1982).
Patterned stimuli can be presented in three ways. These are the flashing patterned stimulus, the pattern onset, offset and the pattern reversal. A flashing patterned stimulus is produced

by placing a photo stimulator behind a large photographic transparency of black and white checks (Harter and White, 1968). In pattern onset, offset the checks appear for discrete amount of time (500 msec) and then disappear. While, in the pattern reversal stimulation, checks are visible all the time. In order to maintain a constant luminance level, one half of the checks increases in luminance, while the other half decreases. This can be accomplished electronically by using T.V. monitor to generate the checks (Arden et al., 1977b).
Checkerboard pattern reversal are the most frequently used stimuli in clinical investigations of the visual pathway as they evoke relatively large potentials (Halliday et al.,1987 and Chiappa, 1988) with variability in latency less than in flash stimuli and it is more sensitive to the presence of conduction defects in the visual pathway (Chiappa, 1982). The fovea is estimated to generate 65% of the pattern-reversal response; flash stimuli, in contrast, tend to generate response from the peripheral retina as well. The insensitivity of flash VEPs, particularly in retrochiasmatic lesions, has been based on diagnostic studies in which patient recordings must differ from normative population data by 2 standard deviations (SDs) to be considered abnormal (Berson, 1994).

Characteristics of pattern reversal stimulation

Erwin, 1980 outlined seven basic characteristics of pattern-reversal stimulation:
1-The rate of pattern-reversal is the number of times that the pattern changes within a second. The direction of pattern reversal is not considered since usually all the pattern reversal responses are averaged together. 2-The reversal time is the total time taken to change from one pattern to its opposite. 3-Stimulus luminance is an essential attribute for visual stimulus. 4-The type of the pattern is obviously important. The most commonly used stimulus is a checkerboard. 5-Vertical-horizontal orientation of the pattern evokes larger responses than oblique orientation. 6-The size of the pattern elements can be described in two ways. The visual angle subtended by each element can be measured. As well, the spatial frequency (the number of intensity cycles through light and dark per degree of visual field) can be used. Another aspect of the stimulus related to the spatial extent of the pattern elements is the spatial rate of luminance change. 7-Two of the most important aspects of the stimulus are its field size and relationship to fixation.

2.4.3 Electrode montage

Responses are collected over Oz, O1, and O2 and with hemifield studies at T5 and T6 electrodes using the standard EEG electrode placement. Scalp electrodes are positioned as follows:

a. Electrode number one: 5 cms above the inion posteriorly in the middle line (Oz).
b. Electrodes number two and three: 5 cms lateral on either side of electrode one (O1, O2).
c. Two additional electrodes: 10 cms away on each side from the middle electrode (T5, T6). Optional to be used in hemifield studies.
d. Reference electrode: is usually FZ. (e) Ground electrode: over the ear lobule (Halliday, 1982).

Both eyes are tested at first, then each eye is tested at a time, (while the other is covered with an eye patch) to avoid masking of a unilateral conduction abnormality. The subject is instructed to gaze at a dot in the center of the pattern during display. The pattern stimulator is operated at about two reversals per second. Patient having field defects or amblyopia may shift their center of gaze into the good visual field. So in order to offset this, a 1° to 2° blank strip may be inserted on either side of the fixation point during partial field stimulation (Chiappa, 1983).

2.4.4 Interpretation

Abnormalities of VEPs have been described in many disorders of the optic nerve, chiasma and retrochiasmatic visual pathways. The VEP is considered abnormal when the latency of P100 wave is outside the boundaries established for normals, or the P100 is absent. The most frequent abnormality is characterized by normal amplitude but prolonged latency of N70 and P100, but a prolonged latency may sometimes be associated with decreased amplitude. The most sever abnormality is an absent VEP (Celesia and Tobimatsu, 1990).

Monocular VEP abnormality

This abnormality suggests a conduction defect in the left/right visual pathway anterior to the optic chiasm. Although demyelinating disease is the most common aetiology for such a finding, various other possibilities cannot be excluded e.g. retinal disease and compressive lesions of the optic nerve (Poon's, 2003a).

In patients with small monocular delays in N70 and P100, it is useful to look at the intereye latency difference. A latency difference between the two eyes greater than 10 msec is clearly indicative of pathology on the side with the longer latency (Celesia and Tobimatsu, 1990).

Binocular VEP abnormality

These abnormalities suggest conduction defects in the visual pathways bilaterally. However, because of the binocular nature of the findings, the lesion location (retina, optic nerve, tracts or radiations) cannot be determined (Poon's, 2003a).

2.4.5 Pitfalls

Check size of 27 seconds of visual angle may result in normal P100 latency in a patient with cortical blindness; smaller checks (i.e. 20 seconds of visual angle or less) should be used to demonstrate the abnormality. If cortical blindness is suspected, large checks should not be used (Bodis-Wollner, 1977).

In conditions such as retinal disease or refractory errors, the amplitude may be smaller and, at very small check sizes, the latency may increase. For this reason proper refraction is of great importance (Chiappa, 1990).

2.5 Factors affecting VEP

Factors which affect VEP are either technical and / or subject factors.

2.5.1 Technical factors

2.5.1.1 Screen luminance

A decrease in brightness results in delaying P100 i.e. increase in its latency (Halliday et al., 1973). Stochard et al., 1979 showed that the pupillary diameter has an effect on retinal illumination and thus also on P100 latency.

2.5.1.2 Degree of contrast

Reduction in the degree of contrast between the black and white squares of checkerboard pattern increases P100 latency and reduces the amplitude (Mackay and Jeffreys, 1973).

2.5.1.3 Size of the stimulating pattern

A decrease of the size of the stimulating pattern (degree of visual angle) results in a reduction of the amplitude of the response (Asselman et al., 1975).

2.5.1.4 Check size

Smaller checks give the highest amplitude responses (Leserve and Romand, 1972).

2.5.1.5 Electrode placement

Ipata et al., 1997 assessed interhemispheric visual transfer of information in humans. Estimates of interhemispheric transfer time ranged between 5.77 and 12.54 msec, depending upon the type of component and the location of the electrode sites. More anterior locations yielded shorter values and overall transfer time tended to be 7 msec shorter for the N70 component than for the P100 component.

2.5.1.6 Stimulus rate

When the rate of pattern reversal is increased, changes in P100 latency is noticed. Increasing the rate beyond 8 per second transforms the evoked responses into a steady state evoked potential (a long train of repetitive wave with a sinusoidal appearance) (Stockord et al., 1979).

2.5.2 Subject factors

2.5.2.1 Age

There is an increase in the latency for subjects of ages starting from the end of the second decade onwards. This increase amounts to 2 msec per decade (Celesia and Daly, 1977). However, Stochard et al., 1979 found no change in P100 latency for subjects of age until the fifth decade. Then, the latency increases at a rate of 2 msec per decade.

2.5.2.2 Sex

Females have usually shorter P100 latency than males. This may be due to difference in the head size (Stockard et al., 1979). However, Shearer and Dustman, (1980) reported no such difference.

2.5.2.3 Visual acuity

Changes in visual acuity markedly affect P100 amplitude. In visual acuity lower than 6 / 18, no latency changes is observed but the amplitude is reduced (Fitzgerald et al., 1980). Diminution of visual acuity has a greater effect on latency using smaller checks (giving visual angle 12) than larger checks (giving visual angle 48). (Sokol et al., 1981).

2.5.2.4 Body temperature

No significant change in P100 latency results by raising body temperature in normals (Matthews et al., 1979). Also, little effect on P100 latency is noticed in patients having multiple sclerosis.

2.5.2.5 Physiological changes of serum glucose level

Sannita et al., 1995 evaluated the correlation between amplitude and latencies of the pattern-reversal VEP and serum glucose level in healthy volunteers. Pattern VEP and serum glucose levels were obtained at 2-hour intervals during an 8-hour experimental session. At serum glucose concentrations within the physiological range of variability (55-103 mg/dL), the P100 latency increased with increasing serum glucose level, with a 6.9% estimated latency difference between lower and higher glucose concentrations.

2.5.2.6 Medications

2.5.2.6.1 Carbamazepine

Certain drugs, such as carbamazepine, prolong VEPs. The effects of carbamazepine monotherapy on VEPs were studied in epileptic children by Yuksel et al., 1995. Pattern-reversal VEPs were determined before administration of the antiepileptic drugs and after 1 year of therapy. The VEP amplitude showed no consistent changes after 1 year of therapy, but VEP P100 latencies were significantly prolonged after 1 year of carbamazepine therapy. The conclusion was that carbamazepine slows down central impulse conduction.

2.5.2.6.2 Lithium

Previous reports in the literature have suggested that lithium medication does not affect the VEP to flash stimulation. It was predicted that this would not be true for pattern reversal stimulation. Seven patients had their pattern evoked potential measured using a 42' check to fractional pattern displacement of 1/4, 1/2, 3/4 and Full Square. The VEP was measured before, 1 week after and 5 weeks after the commencement of lithium medication. The results show that there is a significant increase in both the N70-P100 and P100-N145 amplitudes when the 'before lithium' sessions are compared to 'after lithium.' Seven normal subjects matched for the age and sex of the patient group were tested twice, once as a 'control' and a further 5 weeks after this. No significant differences were found in the 'control' sessions between patient and normal groups although a significant difference in both the N70-P100 and P100-N145 amplitude after the treatment of the patient group with lithium was found (Fenwick and Robertson, 1983).

2.5.2.6.3 Levodopa

Pattern visual evoked potentials (PVEPs) were recorded at three luminance levels and five different check sizes in a group of 16 control subjects before and after the oral administration of levodopa. At the lower luminance levels, significant decrease in PVEP latencies were found. For PVEPs the latency changes occurred only at small check sizes. No changes were observed in control experiments without levodopa administration. These results are in agreement with a VEP delay found in Parkinson's disease and with a VEP latency increase in rats after dopamine depletion (Gottlob et al., 1989).

2.6 Clinical applications of VEP

Clinical usefulness of VEPs includes the following

- More sensitive than MRI or physical examination in prechiasmatic lesions.
- Objective and reproducible test for optic nerve function.
- Abnormality persists over long periods of time.
- Inexpensive as compared with to MRI.
- Under certain circumstances, may be helpful to positively establish optic nerve function in patients with subjective complaint of visual loss; normal VEP excludes significant optic nerve or anterior chiasmatic lesion (Leslie et al., 2002).

With abnormal VEP, some of the differential diagnostic considerations are as follows

- Optic neuropathy.
- Optic neuritis.

- Toxic amblyopia.
- Glaucoma.
- Leber's hereditary optic neuropathy.
- Retrobulbar neuritis.
- Ischemic optic neuropathy.
- Multiple sclerosis.
- Tumors compressing the optic nerve e.g. Optic nerve gliomas, meningiomas, craniopharyngiomas, giant aneurysms and pituitary tumors (Andrew et al., 2002).

2.6.1 VEP in Optic neuritis

Prolongation of P100 latency is the most common abnormality and usually represents an optic nerve dysfunction. VEP is clearly more sensitive than physical examination in detecting optic neuritis. Elvin et al., 1998 used Doppler ultrasonography, MRI and VEP measurements to study abnormal optic nerve function. VEP assessments were performed in 16 patients. Patients with impairment of visual acuity and a prolonged VEP initially had a more swollen nerve and increased flow resistance in the affected optic nerve. Statistically significant side-to-side differences were found in the optic nerve diameter and in the resistance to flow in the central retinal artery between the affected and unaffected eyes.

2.6.2 VEP in Multiple Sclerosis

Visual evoked potentials have become widely accepted in diagnostic schemes for the assessment of multiple sclerosis. It has been shown that a deviation in latency is a better criterion than a deviation in amplitude, since amplitude varies widely among subjects, whereas evoked potential latency remains restricted rather to a narrow range (McDonald and Brans, 1992).

VEPs has the ability to reveal the presence of a clinically silent lesion in the visual pathway in a patient having signs of demyelination evident in other parts of the CNS, thus confirming the diagnosis of multiple sclerosis (Russel et al., 1991).

In multiple sclerosis, P100 absolute latency may be increased unilaterally or a significant interocular difference may occur (Cutler et al., 1985). Moreover, broad response of P100 latency and abnormal shape of NPN was found in majority of multiple sclerosis patients (Glaser, 1990).

In a review of 180 patients with multiple sclerosis 73 % had abnormal VEPs; more importantly, VEPs were abnormal in 54 % of patients without any symptoms or signs referable to the visual system. Such patients are often in the early stages of the disease, when diagnosis is difficult even with modern neuroimaging techniques (Halliday et al., 1977). MRI demonstrated high-signal lesions in 84-88 % of symptomatic patients, whereas VEPs were abnormal in 100% of cases (Kojima et al., 1990).

Brigell et al., 1994 described the pattern VEP using standardized techniques. They concluded that the peak latency of pattern-reversal VEP is a sensitive measure of conduction delay in the optic nerve caused by demyelination. Pattern-reversal VEPs were recorded from 64 healthy subjects and 15 patients with resolved optic neuritis. The results showed that the N70 and P100 peak latencies and N70-P100 interocular amplitude difference were sensitive measures of resolved optic neuritis.

2.6.3 Flash VEP in Cerebral stroke

Ipata et al., 1997 studied left-right asymmetry of flash VEPs in patients after stroke. The VEP amplitude was smaller over the ischemic hemisphere than over the intact hemisphere. This finding indicates that the left-right asymmetry in VEPs of patients after brain damage may be a result of changes in the conductivity of the volume conductor, due to the ischemic region between the source and the electrodes.

2.6.4 Pattern-reversal VEP in classic and common migraine

Shibata et al., 1997 recorded pattern-reversal VEP to transient checkerboard stimulus in 19 patients with migraine with visual aura (i.e. classic migraine), 14 patients with migraine without aura (i.e. common migraine) in the interictal period, and 43 healthy subjects. Latencies and amplitudes of pattern-reversal VEPs in each group were analyzed. In patients with classic migraine, P100 amplitude was significantly higher than in healthy subjects, whereas latencies of pattern-reversal VEPs did not differ significantly. No significant differences were noted in latency between the common migraine group and healthy subjects or in latencies and amplitudes of pattern-reversal VEP between the classic migraine and common migraine groups. These results suggest that patients with classic migraine may have hyperexcitability in the visual pathway during interictal periods and that the increased amplitude of pattern-reversal VEPs after attacks may be due to cortical spreading depression.

2.6.5 VEP in adrenoleukodystrophy

Adrenoleukodystrophy is an X-linked metabolic disorder with very long-chain fatty acid (VLCFA) accumulation and multifocal nervous system demyelination, often with early involvement of the visual pathways. Kaplan et al., 1993 found that pattern-reversal VEPs were abnormal in 17% of patients with adrenoleukodystrophy; no evidence indicated that reduction of VLCFA levels improved or retarded visual pathway demyelination.

2.6.6 functional disorders

In malingering and hysterical visual loss normal VEP usually suggests continuity of the visual pathways ruling out disease up until area 17 but does not exclude fully cortical blindness in such cases (Bodis-Wollner, 1977).

2.6.7 VEPs in retinopathies and maculopathies

Diseases of the retina, especially diseases affecting the macular region, are associated with abnormal VEPs. In maculopathies, simultaneous recording of pattern Electroretinogram (ERG) and VEPs may be diagnostically useful in differentiating between involvement of the macula and optic nerve. In maculopathies and retinopathies involving the macular region, pattern ERG are absent or have a prolonged b-wave latency. The retinocortical time remains within the normal boundaries, indicating that the P100 delay occurs at the retinal level. In optic nerve diseases VEPs may be absent or prolonged, but pattern ERG are normal; the retinocortical time is thus prolonged, indicating that the pathology is postretinal (Celesia and Kaufman, 1985).

In patients with retinopathies the latency of P100 was found to be prolonged by a mean of 19.6 msec with a range of 6 to 39 msec. Delays in latency that exceeded the limits of normality by more than 45 msec usually indicate optic nerve dysfunction especially in multiple sclerosis (Lennerstrand, 1982).

3. Brainstem Auditory Evoked Potentials (BAEPs)

3.1 Introduction

On applying auditory stimulus to one ear, activation of peripheral and central auditory pathways occurs. Brain stem auditory evoked potentials (BAEPs) are the electrical activities resulting from the activation of the eighth nerve, cochlear nucleus, tracts and nuclei of the lateral lemniscus and inferior colliculus (Chiappa, 1983).

Brain stem auditory evoked potential recording is a physiological technique which can be used to evaluate the auditory pathway. It has the advantage of not requiring a voluntary response by the patient and occurring during sleep (Stephen, 1983).

3.2 Description and origin of BAEPs (Figure 2,3)

Clinical stimuli delivered to one or both ears evoke seven submicrovolt vertex-positive waves that appear at the human scalp in the first 10 msec after each stimulus (Picton et al., 1974). They are named according to their sequence in roman letters (from I to VII) (Chiappa et al., 1978).

Wave (I)

This wave is generated from the auditory portion of the eighth cranial nerve, probably from the proximal portion of that nerve just lateral to the brain stem in contact with the spiral ganglia. It is a prominent initial upgoing peak in the ipsilateral ear recording channel. It is important as a reference point for interwave latency measurement (Rowe III, 1978). Patients who have only central nervous system problems should have a preserved wave I. Conversely, patients who have a significant peripheral hearing impairment may have a very poor formed or absent wave I, but may have relatively normal waves II-V (Nuwer et al., 1994).

Wave I can sometimes be seen to have two separate components. The first, earlier component is present and higher in amplitude especially during high intensity, high pitched stimulation. This component should be used for scoring whenever it is present. The second, slightly later lower amplitude component of wave I, is present at a more wide range of stimulus intensities and pitch (Matsuoka et al., 1994).

Waves (II)

This wave may be generated near or at the cochlear nucleus (Row III, 1978). A portion of it can come from the eighth nerve fibers around the cochlear nucleus, and this part of II can be preserved despite brain stem death. Wave II is poorly defined in some adults and most neonates. It sometimes appears as a small peak along the downgoing slope of the wave I. At other times, it merges into the upgoing slope of wave III. It is more often prominent on the contralateral channel recording, where it has a slightly prolonged latency compared to the ipsilateral channel, sometimes fusing with wave III into an M-shaped II-III complex (Aminoff et al., 1994).

Wave (III)

This wave is probably generated from the lower pons as the pathway travels through the superior olive and trapezoidal body (Row III, 1978). The nuclei or fiber tracts that are most responsible for generating this potential are unknown and may be multiple.

Wave III is usually a prominent peak and is followed by a prominent III trough. In the contralateral channel wave III often appears smaller and earlier than on the ipsilateral channel, because its amplitude is similar at the vertex and contralateral ear (Goodin et al., 1994).

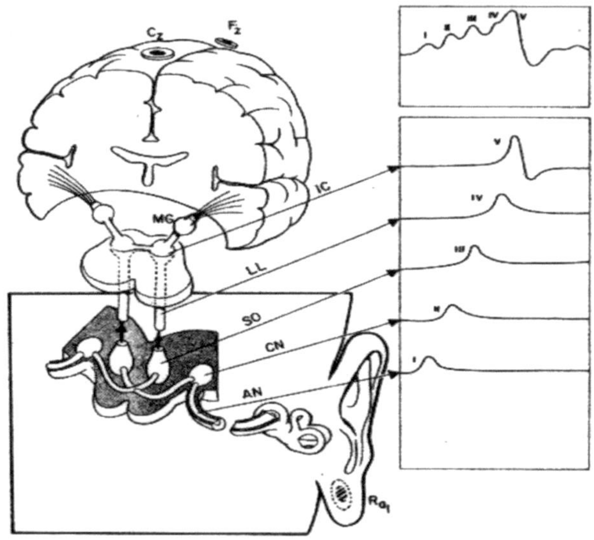

Figure 93. **Auditory evoked response studies. AN = auditory nerves; CN = cochlear nuclei; SO = superior olives; LI = lateral lemnisci; IC = inferior colliculi; MG = medial geniculates.**

Fig. 2. Anatomical-electrophysiological correlation of BAEP *(Poon's, 2003b).*

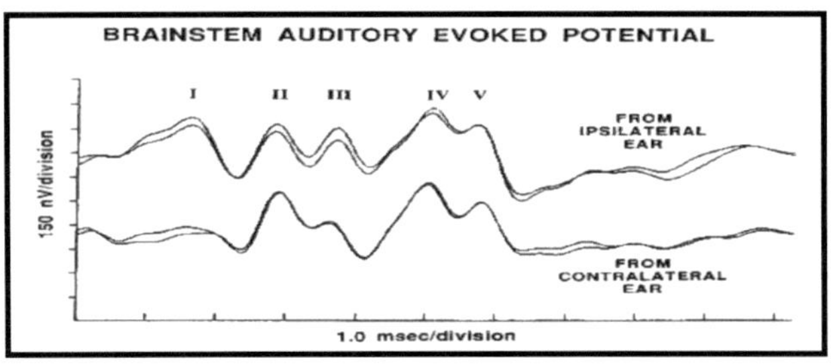

Fig. 3. Normal components of BAEP *(Nuwer et al., 1994).*

Waves (IV) and (V)

Contribution to these two potentials probably includes generators in the upper pons or lower midbrain, in the lateral lemniscus and the inferior colliculus. There are conflicting reports about whether these peaks are generated in the ipsilateral or contralateral brain stem, but the preponderance of evidence favors a contralateral brain stem generator site for wave V (Starr et al., 1994).

These peaks may fuse together into a IV-V complex on the ipsilateral recording channel. This complex can vary between: (a) two peaks which are close but still visibly separate, and (b) a single peak which is completely fused as a tall and wide pyramid. There are also various intermediate stages of trapezoid-shaped figures which represent the partial fusion of the two peaks. On the contralateral recording channel the IV and V peaks tend to be separated more from each other with wave IV being slightly earlier and wave V being slightly later. Comparison of ipsilateral and contralateral peaks can be helpful for distinguishing which peak or shoulder to score as wave V. The wave V is generally followed by a large V trough. Sometimes wave VI appears before the bottom of this trough, and then wave VI can be confused with wave V if the reader is not careful. The fusion of wave VI into

a IV-V-VI complex occurs more often when a 10-30 Hz low filter is used for recording (Nuwer et al., 1994).
The typical IV-V complex has a shape of a somewhat inflated pyramid or trapezoid. The base of this complex should be more than 1.5 msec across. A peak narrower than this is usually a wave IV alone. Wave V is usually most prominent at an intermediate intensity of stimulation. As this stimulus intensity increases further beyond that point, the identification of wave V can actually become more difficult. It is often helpful to have the technician reduce the intensity of stimulation to identify wave V. Wave V is a robust peak that is present despite moderately low intensities of stimulation (and often even despite high frequency hearing impairment, or other types of peripheral auditory changes). Wave V and especially the V trough are often the last deflections to disappear when the stimulus intensity is gradually decreased to threshold (Matsuoka et al., 1994).
Overall there are several ways to help identify wave V when its identity is unclear: the typical contralateral splitting of the IV-V complex; the wide base of a IV-V complex and the preservation of wave V at lower stimulus intensities (Aminoff et al., 1994).

Waves (VI) and (VII)

Are not found in all normal subjects. They are generated in medial geniculate body and auditory radiation from the thalamus to temporal cortex respectively (Row, 1980).
The most constant and most important waves, from the clinical point of view, are waves I, III, V (Rosenhall et al., 1985). Their measurements include absolute latency (stimulus to peak) and interpeak latency (time interval between the peaks). The clinical interpretation is based on the interpeak latencies. Absolute amplitudes are extremely variable in normal subjects (Chiappa, 1983).

3.3 Normal limits and the clinical correlation of changes

There are 5 principle features used to assess routine BAEPs

3.3.1 I-V interpeak interval

This is the primary feature for most BAEP interpretations. It represents conduction from the proximal eighth nerve through pons and into the midbrain. It can be slowed in a variety of disorders, including focal damage (demyelination, ischemia, tumors), or diffuse problems (degenerative disorders, post-hypoxic damage, etc.) (Starr et al., 1994).
A typical upper limit of normal for the I-V interpeak interval is 4.5 msec. That limit is slightly lower for young women and slightly higher for older men. Normal right-left asymmetries for the I-V interpeak interval should be at most 0.5 msec. For full-term infants, the I-V interpeak interval should be less than 5.4 msec (Goodin et al., 1994).

3.3.2 I-III interpeak interval

This interpeak interval represents conduction from the eighth nerve across the subarachnoid space, into the core of the lower pons. The I-III interpeak interval can be increased in any diffuse process that affects the whole I-V interpeak interval. This I-III portion of the pathway is susceptible to a tumor, inflammation or other disorders especially affecting the proximal portion of the eighth nerve, or the ponto-medullary junction where the eighth nerve enters the brain-stem, or impairments in the lower pons around the superior olive or trapezoidal body. Acoustic neuromas or other cerebello-pontine angle tumors can cause a delay at the juncture. Infarction can cause an interruption or a delay here too, although the classical

Wallenberg syndrome is usually too caudal to affect this segment. Inflammation in the subarachnoid space can also increase this I-III interpeak interval (subarachnoid hemorrhage, meningitis and Guillain-Barre syndrome) (Aminoff et al., 1994).
The upper limit of normal for the I-III interpeak interval is about 2.5 msec. The acceptable right-left asymmetry of this interval is less than 0.5msec. An excessively long interpeak interval I-III cannot be considered unless there is an accompanying prolongation of the I-V interpeak interval (Matsuoka et al., 1994).

3.3.3 III-V interval

This interval reflects conduction from the lower to the upper pons and possibly into the midbrain. There is not yet complete agreement about whether this III-V interpeak interval represents conduction along the ipsilateral or contralateral brain-stem, compared to which ear is stimulated. The preponderance of evidence favors a contralateral brain-stem site (Nuwer et al., 1994).
The typical upper limit of normal for a III-V interpeak interval is about 2.4 msec. A right-left asymmetry for these intervals should be less than 0.5 msec. An excessively long III-V interpeak interval is not considered abnormal unless either the I-V interval or the V/I amplitude ratio is also abnormal (Goodin et al., 1994).

3.3.4 V/I amplitude ratio

Absolute amplitudes of BAEP peaks vary widely among normal subjects. In addition, several technical factors influence the absolute amplitudes of BAEP peaks. To reduce this normal intersubject variability, a ratio of amplitudes is usually calculated. For this ratio, the amplitude of IV-V complex is divided by the amplitude of the wave I. The IV-V complex is measured from the highest point of the complex to the trough of the V peak. When V is completely separated from IV, the V amplitude is used In place of the IV-V amplitude. When wave VI is found lying part way down the descending slope of wave V, then the amplitude is measured to the trough following wave VI. The wave I amplitude is measured from the top of the highest part of wave I to the bottom of the trough of I. If wave II is riding on the descending slope of I, then wave I amplitude is measured to the succeeding trough of the wave II (Starr et al., 1994).
The amplitude ratio should be between 50% and 300%. These numbers vary between laboratories and they are especially affected by filter setting changes. When the V/I amplitude ratio is less than 50%, then the IV-V peaks are too small. In that case, suspicion is raised of some central impairment which has diminished the amplitude of the IV-V even if it may have not increased I-V interpeak interval. This is useful criterion for abnormality, especially when the IV-V peaks are so low that they are difficult to distinguish from background noise. Then the record may be interpreted as abnormal because of such low amplitude central peaks, even if the latencies cannot be precisely defined. For full-term infants, the lower limit for V/I is 30% (Goodin et al., 1994).
When the V/I amplitude ratio is greater than 300%, wave I is usually considered to be too small. This raises the suspicion of some peripheral hearing impairment, especially of a high frequency or a sensorineural hearing loss (Aminoff et al., 1994).

3.3.5 Presence of wave I-V

The wave I-V all are seen in most normal individuals. Occasional normal subjects have a wave IV that is so merged into a IV-V complex that it cannot be distinguished as a separate peak, unless extra traces are run at different stimulus rates and intensities. Such a merging of wave IV into a IV-V complex is considered to be a normal variant. Wave II can also be difficult to distinguish when testing some normal subjects. Upon changing stimulus intensities, rates and phase, wave II can be distinguished in essentially all normal subjects. However wave II can appear to be missing at the specific rates and intensities used for simple clinical BAEPs, and this would be considered a normal variant (Matsuoka et al., 1994).

When all waves I-V are absent the BAEP is abnormal, although the cause is usually peripheral (Technical problems must also be considered). It is also abnormal to record a wave I, but not succeeding waves. Finally, it is abnormal if wave I and III are present but IV-V is absent. These roles for the absence of peaks are predicted upon the assumption that technically good quality records have been obtained. The record should be considered technically unsatisfactory if moderate or large amount of background noise are present in the tracing, rather than being interpreted as showing an absence of important peaks (Nuwer et al., 1994).

Waves VI, VII, VIII can normally be present or absent or asymmetrical in latency or amplitude, without any apparent clinical correlation. The main reason for knowing their existence is to prevent confusion with the earlier important waves (Starr et al., 1994).

3.3.6 Absolute latency measurements

The absolute latency measurements of wave I, III and V can be occasionally of clinical value. This is particularly so when some peaks are absent. For example, the absolute latency of wave V can be compared against normal limits when there is no waves I-IV. The absolute latency of wave V is normally less than 6.4 msec. The right-left asymmetry of the wave V absolute latency is normally 0.5 msec or less. Absence of waves I-IV with delayed wave V may be due to a hearing loss. When waves I, III and V are all present, the standard means of interpretation is by the interpeak intervals (Goodin et al., 1994).

The absolute latency of wave I can be used as part of the assessment of hearing. The wave I is often seen around 1.75 msec, but may be seen up to 2.2 msec in some normal subjects. The right-left asymmetry of the wave I absolute latencies is normally 0.4 msec or less. Wave I latency delays or asymmetry suggest a hearing impairment, rather than brain-stem dysfunction (Aminoff et al., 1994).

3.3.7 Reference Values of BAEP (Tandon and Krishna, 1990)

Wave	Mean	Range
Wave I	1.62	1.26-1.98
Wavc II	2.80	2.23-3.37
Wave III	3.75	3.24-4.26
Wave IV	4.84	4.15-5.53
Wave IV/V	5.27	4.61-5.93
Wave V	5.62	4.93-6.31
I-III	2.63	
III-V	2.31	
I-IV/V	4.32	

3.4 Principles of recording of BAEPs

3.4.1 Technical details

The test can be performed under sedation or under general anesthesia; Filter band pass 100-3000 Hz; Standard broadband click stimulation is used on the ear tested; Monoaural stimulation is used; The click intensity should be 60-70 dB above click perception threshold;
The contralateral ear receives masking noise of 30- to 40-dB lesser intensity; The first 10 ms are averaged, and 2-4000 responses may be averaged; At least 2 separate trials should be performed (Leslie et al., 2002).

3.4.2 Stimulation procedures

In neurological practice a sound (Click) generated by pulses through headphones is used as an auditory stimulus. The hearing threshold is determined and the click is applied at an intensity 30,40,50 or 60 decibel (dB) above that hearing threshold. The stimulated ear (in monoaural stimulation) is called ipsilateral ear, the other is the contralateral one (Starr et al., 1976).
To avoid stimulation of the contralateral ear by bone and air conduction on applying the click to the ipsilateral ear, the former should be masked by noise at an intensity of 30 to 40 dB less than of the click stimulus (Leslie et al., 2002).

3.4.3 Electrode montage

The recording montage is at least, and usually, a 2-channel montage channel 1 is ipsilateral ear to vertex and channel 2 is contralateral ear to vertex. The recording electrodes are located, one for each ear lobule and a third electrode is located on the scalp at the vertex at Cz position of 10-20 international system (Stockard et al., 1979a and Leslie et al., 2002).

3.4.4 Interpretation (Poon's, 2003b)

3.4.4.1 Abnormal I-III interpeak latency (IPL): This abnormality suggests the presence of a conduction defect in the brain-stem auditory system between the eighth nerve close to the cochlea and the lower pons.

3.4.4.2 Abnormal III-V IPL: This abnormality suggests the presence of a conduction defect in the brain-stem auditory system between the lower pons and the midbrain.

3.4.4.3 I absent & III-V is normal: Wave I (the eighth nerve activation potential) could not be recorded. This is usually due to a peripheral hearing disorder. Because of this, the state of conduction in the brain-stem auditory pathway between peripheral eighth nerve and lower pons could not be determined. Lower pons to midbrain conduction was normal.

3.4.4.4 IV or V absent or of abnormally low amplitude: This abnormality suggests the presence of a conduction defect in the brain-stem auditory system rostral to the lower pons.

3.4.4.5 Absent II, III, IV and V with normal I: This abnormality indicates a significant lack of function in brain-stem auditory tracts.

3.5 Factors affecting BAEPs

Factors which affect BAEPs are either technical and / or subject related factors

3.5.1 Technical factors

3.5.1.1 Intensity of the stimulus (click)

The intensity of the click stimulus affects the amplitude and absolute latencies of BAEPs peaks. Stockard et al., 1979 reported that absolute latencies increase and amplitudes diminish with decreasing intensity by about 0.03 msec/dB.
Chiappa, (1983) found that waves II, IV and VI diminish more quickly than waves I, III,V with decreasing intensity and also reported that the constancy of the interpeak latency is more reliable in neurologic applications than the use of absolute latency.

3.5.1.2 Rate of the stimulus

Increasing click rate results in increased absolute latency of all BAEPs waves and decrease in the amplitude of most of them. Interpeak latencies increase slightly at higher rates (Stockard et al., 1978 & 1979). Stockard et al., 1980b added that, using rates higher than 30 per second will often worsen pre-existing abnormalities in the BAEP. Some studies used higher rates to reveal the abnormalities. However, Chiappa et al., 1979 mentioned that increasing click rate from 10/second to only 30/second has no value.

3.5.1.3 Stimulus mode

Binaural stimulation produces higher amplitude waves III, IV, V at all stimulus intensities than monoaural stimulation and, because of the monoaural contribution to wave I but binaural contribution to wave IV and V, binaural stimulation logically produces a higher V/I amplitude ratio than monoaural stimulation at a given stimulus intensity. Binaural stimulation should be avoided in routine clinical applications because monoaural abnormalities are common in neurologic disease and may otherwise be masked by the response from the normal ear (Stockard et al.,1978). Separate monoaural stimulation of each ear also allows for comparison of interaural asymmetries in interpeak latency (IPL) and thus may indicate abnormality even when BAEPs from each ear are within normal limits when considered separately (Berlin and Hood, 1984).

3.5.1.4 Filter setting

Filter settings affect relative amplitudes more than interpeak latencies and, in diagnostic applications, should remain fixed at the values used when collecting each laboratory's normative data. The ideal bandpass for clinical purposes is probably 100 to 3,000 Hz or higher. A low frequency filter of much less than 100 Hz allows EMG, EEG and other signals into the average, and a cutoff much higher than 100 Hz distorts the low-frequency BAEP components. A high frequency cutoff of at least 3,000 Hz is necessary to resolve the highest-frequency components of BAEP; settings of less than 1,000 Hz increase the apparent latencies of the BAEPs and decrease their resolution. Increases in high-pass filter above 100 Hz markedly reduce V/I amplitude ratio because of the longer duration of wave V than I. High pass-filtering at 30 Hz or lower is needed in audiologic BAEP applications (Stockard et al., 1978).

3.5.1.5 Site of reference

Using the electrode applied to the contralateral ear as a reference produces a decrease in the II-III interpeak latency and increase the IV-V interpeak latency. Peak latencies of waves II and V are increased when the electrode applied to the contralateral ear is used as a reference in comparison to the use of electrode applied to the ipsilateral ear (Stokard et al., 1978).

De Montes et al., 2002 concluded that BAEP obtained with reference to Cz and Fz are ideal for interpretation, since there is greater constancy, global amplitude and morphological clarity of the first five deflections and less morphological complexity of the other waves.

3.5.2 Subject factors

3.5.2.1 Age

Below the age of 2 years, interpeak latencies are prolonged relative to adult values (Starr et al.,1976). By the age of 2 years, the ranges for adults are reached, the absolute latencies of wave I, III, V increase by 0.1-0.2 msec with age. However, the I-V interpeak latency remains the same (Rosenhall et al., 1985). One obvious explanation for the age-related latency shift is progressive myelination of the auditory tract in infants (Tarantino et al., 1988).
The effects of age on the brain-stem auditory evoked potentials were studied on 156 healthy subjects with ages ranging from 18 to 76 years. There was a small progressive prolongation in the peak latency with increasing age, particularly peak V. Although a correlation between the age and the I-III interval was not observed, there was also a small increase with age in the interpeak latencies of III-V and I-V (Chu, 1985).
Since age effects on central conduction time in the acoustic pathway are still debated, brainstem auditory evoked potentials were recorded in normoacoustic subjects, with no history of neurologic or otologic pathology. Linear regression has been used for statistical analysis. Data obtained show an age-related prolongation of latency values which is particularly marked for wave I, while other waves (particularly wave III) do not show a significant change. Thus, IPL values do not increase with increasing age: in particular IPLs I-II and I-III decrease, showing a negative "r" value, and IPLs I-V and II-V (which is to be considered the true "central conduction time" through the acoustic pathway) do not show a significant change. These data seem to demonstrate that the aging process is essentially a peripheral phenomenon which does not involve the central part of the acoustic pathway (Costa et al., 1990).
Brainstem auditory evoked response (BAER) was recorded in children from birth to 6 years and adults to study the development of wave amplitude. The amplitudes of all BAER waves increased with age, the greatest changes occurring during early infancy. Adult values were reached at 6 months of age for wave I and 2 years for wave V. The two waves continued to increase above the adult values until the highest amplitude value was reached at 3 years for wave I and 5 years for wave V. Subsequently, the amplitudes decreased towards the values in adults. The V/I amplitude ratio, which was slightly lower than the adult value shortly after birth, decreased during the first year of life and reached the minimum value between 1 and 4 years. Thereafter, it increased towards the adult value. Throughout the maturational stages the ratio was smaller than in adults. The amplitude of wave V was relatively stable and its variation was much smaller than those of wave I and V/I amplitude ratio (Jiang et al., 1993).

3.5.2.2 Sex

Females have shorter interpeak latencies than males. This may be explained by shorter corresponding segments of the auditory pathway due to smaller brain size. However, no difference could be detected before the age of 8 years (Stochard et al., 1979).
Sex differences in the amplitudes and latencies of the auditory brain stem potential (BAEP) were investigated using 3 levels of intensity and 3 stimulus presentation rates. The females displayed consistently larger BAEPs for waves IV, V, VI and VII than the males. The only latency differences which reached significance over all the intensities and rates occurred for

wave V. The females showed significantly shorter wave V latencies than the males. Since hearing losses and individually determined click thresholds were comparable between the two groups tested, the exact sources of the uneven distribution of amplitude and latency effects are in question. Differences in the relative distances of the anatomical generators are considered in accounting for the sex differences. Because the precise origin of the sex differences cannot be stated with certainty, attempts to develop normative data for the BAEP should consider the possible influences of sex differences (Michalewski et al., 1980).

3.5.2.3 Hearing disorders

Peripheral hearing disorders give a similar effect on BAEP as decreasing stimulus intensity i.e. the absolute latencies of all waves are increased but no change of the interpeak latencies (Chiappa, 1983).
In patients with sensorineural hearing loss, Coats and Martin, 1977 found an abrupt increase in the latency of wave I at 50 to 60 dB, 4 to 8 kHz hearing loss; this abrupt increase in wave I peak latency was not paralleled by a similar increase in wave V latency, thus the I-V interpeak latencies in these subjects were shorter than in those with normal audiograms.

3.5.2.4 Body temperature

A decrease in body temperature leads to increase in both the absolute and interpeak latencies (Picton et al.,1982).

3.5.2.5 Hypoglycemia

Kern et al., 1994 studied the effects of insulin-induced hypoglycemia on the auditory brainstem response (ABR) in humans. ABRs were examined in healthy men during euglycemia and after 20 minutes and 50 minutes of steady-state hypoglycemia of 2.6 mM induced with insulin. Hypoglycemia increased interpeak latencies III-V and I-V, whereas changes in the latency of wave I were not significant.

3.5.2.6 Medications

3.5.2.6.1 Barbiturate

BAEPs are not affected significantly by barbiturate doses sufficient to render the EEG "flat" (i.e. isoelectric) or by general anesthesia (although it was reported that BAEP has been lost with combined lidocaine and thiopental infusion) (Garcia-Larrea et al., 1988).

3.5.2.6.2 Nicotine (smoking)

Reports of tobacco-induced electrocortical activation have frequently indicated that this effect is mediated via nicotine's action on sub-cortical structures. Twelve regular smokers were tested on two separate sessions involving sham or real smoking. On each session, BAEPs were recorded during a baseline period and immediately after smoking. BAEPs, recorded from Cz, were elicited by presentation of 1,000 monaural, rare fraction click stimuli. Latency and amplitudes of peak components I, III and V were assessed and analyzed. No significant effects were observed for latency measures or for amplitudes of peaks I and III. A significant effect was observed for peak V with tobacco resulting in larger amplitudes relative to sham smoking. Peak V reflects activity from upper pontine-lower midbrain sites (Knott, 1987).

3.5.2.6.3 Aminophylline

To determine the neurophysiological effects of aminophylline on apnea of prematurity, the BAEPs of 30 apnoeic infants and 34 age matched controls were evaluated and compared. After six days of treatment with aminophylline, the brain stem conduction time (interpeak latency of I-V) in apnoeic infants decreased compared with controls of a similar postconceptional age. The mean latencies of the peaks and interpeaks of all waves except wave I were significantly lower in the apnoeic infants after than before receiving aminophylline. No significant differences were found in the latencies of BAEPs between the apnoeic infants who responded and those who did not respond to aminophylline treatment. These results suggest that aminophylline may enhance conduction along central auditory pathways and stimulate the regulatory effect on the respiratory centre of the brain stem (Chen et al.,1994).

3.6 Clinical applications of BAEPs

BAEPs are very resistant to alteration by anything other than structural pathology in the brainstem auditory tracts. Disorders of the peripheral vestibular system do not affect BAEP. Thus, patients who had labyrinthine diseases (i.e. Ménière's disease, labyrinthitis, vestibular neuronitis) had no BAEP interwave latency abnormalities using the limits employed for clinical neurological purposes (Garcia-Larrea et al., 1988).

Brainstem auditory evoked potentials have obtained widespread clinical application in assessing neurologic and audiologic problems. These have maximal clinical utility in evaluating comatose patients, in patients with suspected demyelinating disorders, posterior fossa tumors, or in audiologic evaluation, especially in infants. They are also used for intraoperative monitoring of eighth-nerve and brainstem function during different types of posterior fossa surgery (Markand, 1994).

ABR audiometry is considered an effective screening tool in the evaluation of suspected retrocochlear pathology. However, an abnormal ABR suggestive of retrocochlear pathology indicates the need for MRI or CT scanning. In general, ABR exhibits a sensitivity of over 90% and a specificity of approximately 70-90% (Schmidt et al., 2001).

3.6.1 BAEPs in multiple sclerosis (MS)

An abnormal response may be seen with higher frequency in symptomatic patients; however, a positive test may be recorded in the absence of clinical brainstem symptomatology. BAEPs should be considered if the clinical symptom implicates a lesion outside the brain stem. In this case an abnormal BAEPs would further support the diagnosis of MS. If, however, the clinical sign (e.g., diplopia) points to the brain stem, BAEPs abnormality is merely confirmatory. In various studies about 20% of the population tested for a second lesion have an abnormal BAEPs and about half of these go on to develop MS in the next 1-3 years (Kjaer, 1987).

Purves et al., 1981 reported pattern-shift VEPs to be abnormal in 45%, SSEP abnormal in 35%, and BAEP in 14% of patients without brainstem signs. Combining all 3 modalities, 97% of patients with definite MS, 86% of patients with probable MS, and 63% of patients with possible MS had abnormal findings on at least one of these tests. Similar findings were reported by Ferrer et al., 1993. Kjaer, 1987 reported 38% abnormal BAEPs in patients with silent lesions, while 50% of these patients had an abnormal VEPs and only 13% an abnormal SEP.

Brain-stem auditory evoked responses (BAERs) were examined in 178 patients with multiple sclerosis (MS) and compared to the frequency of abnormalities in visually evoked responses (VERs) and in CSF electrophoresis. In clinically definite MS, BAERs were abnormal in 61% and a significant relationship was noted between disability due to MS and the frequency and severity of BAER abnormalities. In suspected MS, BAERs showed evidence of a second lesion in 14% whereas VERs indicated a second lesion in 24%.

Abnormal BAERs in patients with suspected MS with brain-stem signs were significantly associated with the presence of ataxia. In progressive possible MS, abnormal BAERs were found in 49% but indicated a second lesion in 35% of patients and were significantly related to the duration of illness. In progressive possible MS, abnormal VERs but not abnormal BAERs, were significantly associated with the presence of cerebrospinal fluid (CSF) oligoclonal IgG banding. Normal BAERs in association with clinical brain-stem abnormalities were found in 24% of patients with clinically definite MS, 50% with suspected MS and 33% with progressive possible MS (Hutchinson et al., 1984).

Furthermore, Lehmann and Soukos, 1982 examined patients with certain, probable and possible MS using checkerboard VEP and click-BAEP and concluded that VEPs were clearly more useful than BAEPs in the early diagnostics of MS, however in occasional cases, BAEPs might contribute to the early diagnosis.

Chiappa, 1990 found that the BAEP is positive in 21% of clinically unsuspected cases. Most authors have concluded that BAEP yields the smallest percentage of patients, but it still adds to the detection rate because it is abnormal in a different subset of patients.

3.6.2 CNS tumors

3.6.2.1 Cerebellopontine angle lesions

BAEP may be abnormal when audiometry fails to disclose a lesion. The characteristic findings are increased I-V and increased I-III interpeak latencies ipsilateral to the lesion. Bilateral prolongation of latencies and interpeak latencies may be seen. Gordon and Cohen, 1995 evaluated the efficacy of auditory brainstem response (ABR) as a screening test for small acoustic neuromas by performing a prospective trial to determine the diagnostic sensitivity of brainstem auditory evoked response (BAER) in these tumors. Randomly selected patients with surgically proven acoustic neuromas underwent preoperative BAER tests within 2 months of surgery. A test result was considered abnormal when the interaural I-V interpeak latency difference was greater than 0.2 ms, the absolute wave V latency was abnormally prolonged, or waveform morphology was abnormal or absent. 87.6% Of the tested patients, had an abnormal BAER and 12.4% had completely normal waveforms and wave latencies. Patients with tumors greater than 2 cm in total diameter had abnormal BAER results. Patients with tumors 1.6-2 cm / 1-1.5 cm / 9 mm or smaller, 86% / 85% / 69% had abnormal BAERs respectively. These data show that BAER sensitivity decreases with decreasing tumor size. Therefore, MRI scanning is the preferred study because the accuracy for detection of tumor smaller than 1 cm through BAER is 70%. Nevertheless, BAER is useful in patients who have implanted medical devices (e.g., pacemakers) that prevent MRI scanning.

3.6.2.2 Meningomyelocele

The brainstem auditory evoked potentials (BAEPs) of twenty-seven meningomyelocele (MMC) patients were analyzed and compared with the results of a normal population. The longest wave V or I-V interpeak latencies were seen in patients with shunted hydrocephalus and cranial nerve defects. The shortest wave V and I-V interpeak latencies were found in patients without hydrocephalus. However, these latencies of MMC patients were significantly longer than the latencies of a normal population. It is assumed that I-V interpeak latency prolongation in MMC patients, which is related to the severity of the clinical signs of the Arnold Chiari malformation, is mostly due to an elongation of the brainstem (Lutschg et al., 1985).

It is difficult to estimate the accurate onset of symptoms clinically resulting from Chiari II malformation. Brainstem auditory evoked potentials (BAEPs) may be a useful method in the selection of potential candidates for surgery. BAEPs were studied in asymptomatic infants under 6 months of age with meningomyelocele (MMC). Both the wave latencies and interpeak latencies (IPLs) gradually became shorter during the first 6 months of life in asymptomatic infants with MMC. In particular, shortening of the III-V IPLs and the I-V IPLs was observed from 1 to 4-6 months of age in these infants. These may be characteristic parameters of central auditory function (III-V IPLs) and global auditory function (I-V IPLs). Maturation of brainstem function as viewed by BAEPs in asymptomatic infants with MMC was delayed when compared to data in normal neonates and infants. These data on asymptomatic infants with MMC could potentially be a good reference for selecting the modalities of treatment in infants with symptomatic Chiari II malformation (Fujii et al., 1996).

Taylor et al., 1996 studied BAER in infants with meningomyelocele to determine whether EPs reflect early neurological status and whether BAER have prognostic value in neurological outcome. The infants, aged 1 day to 3 months, were tested while still in hospital after the meningomyelocele repair. Normal BAEPs were found in 41% of patients while abnormal BAEPs were found in all infants studied who had symptomatic Arnold-Chiari malformation. So, BAEPs showed a positive predictive value of 88% and accuracy of 84% in predicting central neurological sequelae.

3.6.3 Brainstem stroke

Brainstem stroke syndromes are primarily determined by clinical criteria. There are few diagnostic procedures which are of benefit for the evaluation of brainstem ischemic events. Brainstem auditory evoked responses are important electrophysiologic technique for assessing brainstem function. The response is variable; some lesions cause abnormal latencies while some do not (Tsuda et al., 1995).

To evaluate the use of BAERs in patients with brainstem ischemic events, 35 individuals with recent brainstem strokes, selected by strict clinical criteria, were evaluated with BAERs. The initial BAER was abnormal in 22 of 35 patients (63%). When the clinical course and site of the lesion are correlated with the BAER results. An unstable course, characterized by progression or remission and relapse, was present in 19/35 (54%) of patients, and 15/19 (79%) of these individuals had an initially abnormal BAER. The other 16 brainstem stroke patients with a stable clinical course had an initially abnormal BAER in 7 instances (44%). This difference is statistically significant at the $P = 0.04$ level. The principal sites of ischemia were mesencephalic in 11/35, pontine in 13/35 and medullary in 11/35. The association of an abnormal BAER with an unstable clinical course seemed independent of the site of the lesion, However, of the 9 deaths that occurred, all were in patients with mesencephalic or pontine lesions, and 8 of these individuals had an initially abnormal BAER. Abnormal BAERs in patients with brainstem ischemic lesions correlate with an unstable clinical course. Furthermore, individuals with ponto-mesencephalic infarction and abnormal BAERs have an especially poor prognosis. The BAER may be of prognostic value in the early evaluation of patients with brainstem ischemic strokes (Stern et al., 1982).

Brain stem auditory evoked potentials were studied in patients with the lateral medullary (Wallenberg's) syndrome. The observed changes included: prolongation of the interpeak latencies from wave I-V and III-V; prolongation of the interaural latency difference for wave V; splitting or absence of wave III and the presence of a broad partly fused wave III-V complex. This study showed that BAEP can be used to confirm the diagnosis of this syndrome and ascertain the site of the lesion (Elwany,1985).

A study of brainstem auditory evoked potentials was carried out in subjects suffering from vertebrobasilar TIA in order to obtain a comparative evaluation of cortical-subcortical functions. The obtained data demonstrate a delay of peak III of the BAEPs in patients with previous vertebrobasilar TIA. These data show that the study of the BAEPs is useful in evaluating the damage produced by anoxia (Benna et al., 1985).

3.6.4 Respiratory insufficiency following encephalitis

Schwarz et al., 1996 showed prolonged interpeak latencies (I-III, I-V, III-V, IV-V) and delayed absolute latencies of waves II, III, V, and I, at least on one side, in the BAEP. The auditory pathways are near the respiratory control centers in the brain stem; therefore, the electrophysiologic abnormalities of wave III and the IV-V complex may be a reflection of the disturbed central control of ventilation.

3.6.5 Prediction of posttraumatic coma in children

BAEP studies were performed within 72 hours of admission in children with severe head injury in order to predict the outcome of posttraumatic coma. Outcomes were categorized as brain death or survival. On first assessment, 40% of comatose children had normal BAEP. About 78% survived and 22% deteriorated and died. 32% 0f children had abnormal findings; 69% of them improved and survived, whilst 31% deteriorated and died. All children who did not have recordable BAEP died. These data suggest that BAER is a useful test in predicting neurological outcome in this setting (Butinar and Gostisa, 1996).

3.6.6 Comatose patient

BAEP can be done while the patient is sedated. It can be used as a prognostic indicator. Survival is unlikely in the absence of BAEP. The brain-dead patient has invariably abnormal BAEPs either the absence of all waveforms or the presence of wave I and the absence of all subsequent waveforms (Goldie et al., 1981).

3.6.7 Intraoperative monitoring

ABR, often used intraoperatively with electrocochleography, provides early identification of changes in the neurophysiologic status of the peripheral and central nervous system. This information is useful in the prevention of neurotologic dysfunction and the preservation of postoperative hearing loss. For many patients with tumors of cranial nerve (CN) VIII or the cerebellopontine angle, hearing may be diminished or completely lost postoperatively, even when the auditory nerve has been preserved anatomically.

Typical uses of intraoperative auditory brainstem response

- **Monitoring cochlear function directed at hearing preservation**

Cerebellopontine angle tumor resection (acoustic neuroma surgery); Vascular decompression of trigeminal neuralgia; Vestibular nerve section for the relief of vertigo; Exploration of the facial nerve for facial nerve decompression; Endolymphatic sac decompression for Ménière's disease.

- **Monitoring brainstem integrity**

Brainstem tumor resection; Brainstem aneurysm clipping or arteriovenous malformation resection (Kileny et al., 1988).

3.6.8 Screening of hearing in newborns

Several clinical trials have shown automated auditory brainstem response (AABR) testing as an effective screening tool in the evaluation of hearing in newborns, with a sensitivity of 100% and specificity of 96-98%. When used as a threshold measure to screen for normal hearing, each ear may be evaluated independently, with a stimulus presented at an intensity level between 35-40 dB. Click-evoked ABR is highly correlated with hearing sensitivity in the frequency range from 1000-4000 Hz. AABRs test for the presence or absence of wave V. No operator interpretation is required (Oudesluys-Murphy et al., 1996).

4. Conclusion

The VEP is preferable in optic nerve and anterior chiasmatic lesions, while MRI is clearly superior in retrochiasmatic disease. Note that the VEP is nonspecific as to the underlying etiology and pathology (Andrew et al., 2002).

The most common uses of BAEP are in MS and in acoustic neuroma. It is a useful screening test, with limitations; MRI scanning may be preferable when a small lesion is under consideration. Increased I-III interpeak latency indicates a lesion from CN VIII to the superior olivary nucleus, while increased III-V interpeak latency suggests a lesion from the superior olivary nucleus to the inferior colliculus ipsilateral to the ear stimulated. Intraoperative monitoring during cerebellopontine angle tumor surgery may be helpful in aiding the surgeon to preserve as much function as possible (Gordon and Cohen, 1995).

Involvement of CNS sensory pathways in hereditary motor and sensory neuropathies has been reported by Carroll et al and Jones et al. However, at that time molecular genetic diagnosis was not yet available and their finding could not be linked to a particular gene defect. Jones et al speculated that the abnormalities might be due to a dying back phenomenon of the affected peripheral nerves. On the other hand, Scaioli et al failed to show central nervous system involvement in patients with Charcot-Marie-Tooth (CMT). Recently, evidence for involvement of the central acoustic pathway was obtained by measuring BAEPs in patients with CMT1X with Cx32 mutations. However, no other CNS pathways were examined in this study (for example, VEPs or transcortical magnetic stimulation measurements) and it remained unclear whether the disorder would also affect structures other than the acoustic pathway.

Bähr et al and Tony et al found that, not only acoustic but also visual and central motor pathways are affected, suggesting a much larger central nervous system involvement than has been presumed from clinical examinations, in which such widespread central nervous system abnormalities have not been reported to date. These findings underscore the necessity of a careful analysis of CNS pathways in patients with CMT and Cx32 mutations. Thus, screening for Cx32 mutations seems to be important in patients with a peripheral neuropathy and abnormalities in motor and sensory central nervous system pathways.

5. References

Aminoff M, Nuwer MR, Goodin D, Matsuoka S and Starr A (1994): IFCN recommended standards for brain-stem auditory evoked potentials. Report of an IFCN committee. Electroencephalography and clinical neurophysiology, February, 91:12-17.

Andrew SB, Leslie H and Francisco T (2002): Clinical Utility of Evoked Potentials. e Medicine, Neurology, Electroencephalography and evoked potentials, May, 30:1-8.

Arden GB, Efaulkner DJ and mair C (1977b): The visual evoked potential in healthy subjects. In: evoked potential in clinical testing edited by A.M. Hallday. Churchill Livingstone New York (first edition), Pp. 72-100.

Asselman P, Chadwick DW and Marsden CD (1975): Visual evoked responses in the diagnosis and management of patients suspected of multiple sclerosis. Exp. Brain Res., Vol. 98: Pp. 261.

Bähr M, Andres F, Timmerman V, Nelis M E, Van Broeckhoven C, Dichgans J (1999): Central visual, acoustic, and motor pathway involvement in a Charcot-Marie-Tooth family with an Asn205Ser mutation in the connexin 32 gene. J Neurol Neurosurg Psychiatry;66:202–206.

Baumgartner J and Epstein CM (1982): Voluntary alteration of visual evoked potential. Ann. Neurol., 12:476.

Benna P, Bianco C, Costa P, Piazza D and Bergamasco B (1985): Visual evoked potentials and brainstem auditory evoked potentials in migraine and transient ischemic attacks. Cephalgia. May;5 Suppl., 2:53-58.

Berlin C and Hood L (1984): Asymmetries in evoked potentials. Hearing Science. San Diego, CA: College-Hill Press. Pp. 73-85.

Berson EL (1994): Visual function testing: Clinical correlations. J. Clin. Neurophysiol., 11:472-481.

Blumhardt LD and Halliday AM (1979): Hemisphere contributions to the composition of the pattern evoked potential waveform. Exp. Brain Res. Vol. 36:53-69.

Bodis-Wollner I, Atkin A, Raab E and Wolkstein M (1977): Visual association cortex and vision in man: Pattern-evoked occipital potentials in a blind boy. Science Nov 11; 198(4317): 629-631.

Brigell M, Kaufman DI and Bobak P (1994): The pattern visual evoked potential. A multicenter study using standardized techniques. Doc. Ophthalmol., 86(1):65-79.

Butinar D and Gostisa A (1996): Brainstem auditory evoked potentials and somatosensory evoked potentials in prediction of post-traumatic coma in children . Pflugers Arch; 431(6 Suppl 2): Pp. 289-290.

Carroll WM, Jones SJ, Halliday AM. Visual evoked potential abnormalities in linked Charcot-Marie-Tooth disease and comparison with Friedreich's ataxia. J Neurol Sci 1983;61:123–33.

Celesia GG (1988): anatomy and physiology of visual evoked potential and electroretinograms. Neurol.Clin., 6:657-665.

Celesia GG and Daly RE (1977): Visual electroencephalographic computer analysis (VECA). Neurology, 27:637-641.

Celesia GG and Kaufman D (1985): Pattern ERGs and visual evoked potentials in maculopathies and optic nerve diseases. Invest. Ophthalmol. Vis. Sci., 26:726.

Celesia GG and Tobimatsu S (1990): Electroretinograms to flash and to patterned visual stimuli in retinal and optic nerve disorders. In Desmedt JE (ed): visual evoked potentials. Elsevier, Amsterdam. Pp.45.

Chen YJ, Liou CS, Tsai CH and Yeh TF (1994): Effect of aminophylline on brainstem auditory evoked potentials in preterm infants. Arch. Dis. Child Fetal Neonatal Ed. Jul., 71(1):Pp. 20-23.

Chiappa KH (1982): Evoked potential in clinical medicine. In clinical neurology edited by AB Baker and LH Baker, JB Lippincott, Philadelphia.

Chiappa KH (1983): Evoked potential in clinical medicine. Edited by KH Chiappa and Con Yiannikas Raven press. New York (1st. ed.).

Chiappa KH (1988): The use of evoked potential in clinical practice with special reference to the diagnosis of multiple sclerosis. In: Evoked Potentials in Clinical Medicine. Chiappa KH, Ravin Press New York Second edition. 1-92.

Chiappa KH (1990): Evoked Potentials in Clinical Medicine. 2nd ed. New York: Raven Press; 37-171, 196-197.

Chiappa KH, Choi S and Young RR (1978): The results of new method for the registration of human short latency somatosensory evoked responses. Neurology, 28:385.

Chiappa KH, Gladston KJ and Young RR (1979): Brainstem auditory evoked responses: Studies of waveform. Arch. Neurol., 36:81-87.

Chiappa KH, Martin JB and Young RR (1987): Diagnostic Methods In Neurology: Disorders of the central nervous system. In Harrison's principles of internal medicine edited by JB Martin Mc Graw-Hill, Inc. Hamburg, Pp. 1913-1921.

Chu NS (1985): Age-related latency changes in the brainstem auditory evoked potentials. Electroencephalogr. Clin. Neurophysiol. Nov., 62(6): 431-436.

Coats AC and Martin JL (1977): Human auditory nerve action potentials and brainstem evoked responses: Effects of audiogram shape and lesion location. Arch. Otolaryngol., 103:105.

Costa P, Benna P, Bianco C, Ferrero P and Bergamasco B (1990): Aging effects on brainstem auditory evoked potentials. Electromyogr. Clin. Neurophysiol. Dec., 30(8):495-500.

Cutler JR, Aminoff MJ and Zawadzki M (1985): Evaluation of patients with multiple sclerosis by evoked potentials and magnetic resonance imaging. Ann. Neurol., 20:645-648.

De Montes C, Manjn M and Viuales M (2002): Morphological study of brainstem auditory evoked potentials. the effect of the position of the reference electrode. Rev. Neurol. Jan 1;34(1):84-88.

Elvin A, Andersson T and Soderstrom M (1998): Optic neuritis. Doppler ultrasonography compared with MR and correlated with visual evoked potential assessments . Acta Radiol. May, 39(3):243-248.

Elwany S (1985): Brainstem auditory evoked potentials in patients with the lateral medullary (Wallenberg's) syndrome. ORL J Otorhinolaryngol Relat. Spec., 47(2):90-94.

Erwin CW (1980): Pattern reversal evoked potentials. Am. J. EEG technol., 20:161-184.

Fenwick PB and Robertson R (1983): Changes in the visual evoked potential to pattern reversal with lithium medication. Electroencephalogr. Clin. Neurophysiol. May., 55(5):538-545.

Ferrer S, Jimenez P, Mellado L and Thieck E (1993): Clinical correlations and evoked potentials in 29 cases of definitive multiple sclerosis. Rev Med Chil Oct; 121(10): 1154-1160.

Fitzgerald PF, Picton TW, Maru J and Wolfe RG (1980): Pattern reversal visual responses. Proceedings from 1st. international workshop and symposium on evoked potentials, Milan.

Fujii M, Tomita T, McLone DG, Grant JA and Mori K (1996): Natural course of brainstem auditory evoked potentials in infants less than 6 months old with asymptomatic meningomyelocele. Pediatr. Neurosurg. Nov., 25(5):227-232.

Garcia-Larrea L, Artru F and Bertrand O (1988): Transient drug-induced abolition of BAEPs in coma. Neurology Sep., 38(9):1487-1489.

Glaser JS (1990): Topical diagnosis: prechiasmal visual pathways. Ophthalmology. 91:255-262.

Goldie WD, Chiappa KH and Young RR (1981): Brainstem auditory and short-latency somatosensory evoked responses in brain death. Neurology Mar., 31(3):248-256.

Goodin D, Nuwer MR, Aminoff M, Matsuoka S and Starr A (1994): IFCN recommended standards for brainstem auditory evoked potentials. Report of an IFCN committee. Electroencephalography and clinical neurophysiology, February; 91:12-17.

Gordon ML and Cohen NL (1995): Efficacy of auditory brainstem response as a screening test for small acoustic neuromas. Am. J. Otol. Mar., 16(2):136-139.

Gottlob I, Weghaupt H, Vass C and Auff E (1989): Effect of levodopa on the human pattern electroretinogram and pattern visual evoked potentials. Graefes. Arch. Clin. Exp. Ophthalmol., 227(5):421-427.

Halliday AM (1982): The Visual EP in clinical testing. Halliday AMI (ed.), Churchill Livingstone, London, (first edition), Pp. 71-120.

Halliday AM, Butler SR and Paul R (Eds) (1987): Visual potential. A textbook of Clinical Neurology. A. Wiley Medical Publication Pp. 348-367.

Halliday AM, Halliday E and Kriss A (1976): The pattern-evoked potential in compression of the anterior visual pathways. Prog. Brain Res. 99:357-374.

Halliday AM, Mc Donald WI and Mushin J (1977): Visual evoked potentials in patients with demyelinating disease . In Desmedt JE (ed): Visual evoked potentials in man: New Developments. Clarendon Press, Oxford. Pp. 438.

Halliday AM, Mconald WI and Mushin J (1973): Delayed pattern responses in optic neuritis in relation to visual acuity. Trans. Ophthalmo. Soc. UK vol. 93:315-324.

Harter MR and White CT (1968): Effects of contour sharpness and check size on visually evoked cortical potentials. Vision Res., 8:Pp. 701-711.

Hutchinson M, Blandford S, Glynn D and Martin EA (1984): Clinical correlates of abnormal brain-stem auditory evoked responses in multiple sclerosis. Acta Neurol. Scand. Aug., 70(2):90-95.

Ikeda H, Nishijo H and Miyamoto K (1998): Generators of visual evoked potentials investigated by dipole tracing in the human occipital cortex. Neuroscience Jun., 84(3):723-739.

Ipata A, Girelli M and Miniussi C (1997): Interhemispheric transfer of visual information in humans: The role of different callosal channels. Arch. Ital. Biol. Mar., 135(2):169-182.

Jiang ZD, Zhang L, Wu YY and Liu XY (1993): Brainstem auditory evoked responses from birth to adulthood: development of wave amplitude. Hear. Res. Jun., 68(1):35-41.

Jones SJ, Carroll WM, Halliday AM. Peripheral and central sensory conduction in Charcot-Marie-Tooth disease and comparison with Friedreich's ataxia J Neurol Sci 1983;61:135–48.

Kaplan PW, Tusa RJ and Shankroff J (1993): Visual evoked potentials in adrenoleukodystrophy: a trial with glycerol trifoliate and Lorenzo oil. Ann. Neurol. Aug., 34(2):169-174.

Kern W, Kerner W and Pietrowsky R (1994): Effects of insulin and hypoglycemia on the auditory brainstem response in humans. J. Neurophysiol. Aug., 72(2):678-683.

Kileny PR, Niparko JK and Shepard NT (1988): Neurophysiologic intraoperative monitoring: I. Auditory function. Am. J. Otol. Dec., 9 Suppl: 17-24.
Kimura J (1985): Abuse and misuse of evoked potentials. Arch. Neuro. 48:78-80.
Kjaer M (1987): Brainstem auditory and visual evoked potentials in multiple sclerosis. Acta Neurol. Scand. Jul., 62(1):14-19.
Knott VJ (1987): Acute effects of tobacco on human brain stem evoked potentials. Addict. Behav., 12(4):375-379.
Kojima S, Hirayama K, Kakisu Y and Adachi E (1990): Magnetic resonance imaging in optic nerve lesions with multiple sclerosis. No To Shinkei, 42:1191.
Kriss A (1980): Setting up an evoked potential laboratory. In evoked potentials in clinical testing edited by AN Halliday (First edition), Churchill Livingstone, New York. Pp. 10-45.
Lehmann D and Soukos I (1982): Visual evoked potentials and click-evoked brainstem potentials in early diagnosis of multiple sclerosis: statistics. Nervenarzt.. Jun., 53(6):327-332.
Lennerstrand G (1982): Delayed visual evoked cortical potentials in retinal disease. Acta Ophthalmol., 60:497.
Leserve N and Romand A (1972): Effects of the diminution of the pattern and density of contrast on evoked potentials. Electroenceph. Clin. Neurophysiol., 35:239-247.
Leslie H, Andrew SB and Francisco T (2002): Clinical Utility of Evoked Potentials. e Medicine, Neurology, Electroencephalography and evoked potentials, May, 30:1-8.
Lutschg J, Meyer E, Jeanneret-Iseli C and Kaiser G (1985): Brainstem auditory evoked potentials in meningomyelocele. Neuropediatrics, Nov., 16(4):202-204.
Mackay DM and Jeffreys DA (1973): Visual evoked potentials and visual perception in man. In: Handbook of sensory physiology. Vol. VII/3 part B. Edited by R Jung Springer, New York, Berlin, Heidelberg. Pp. 647-678.
Markand ON (1994): Brainstem auditory evoked potentials. J. Clin. Neurophysiol. May., 11(3):319-342.
Matsuoka S, Nuwer MR, Aminoff M, Goodin D and Starr A (1994): IFCN recommended standards for brain-stem auditory evoked potentials. Report of an IFCN committee. Electroencephalography and clinical neurophysiology, February; 91:12-17.
Matthews WB, Read DJ and Pountney E (1979): Effects of raising body temperature on visual and somatosensory evoked potentials in patients with multiple sclerosis. J. Neurol. Neurosurg. Psychiatry., 42:250-255.
McDonald WI and Brans D (1992): The ocular manifestations of multiple sclerosis. Abnormalities of the visual system. J. Neurol. Neurosurg. Psychiatry, 55:747-752.
Michalewski HJ, Thompson LW, Patterson JV, Bowman TE and Litzelman D (1980): Sex differences in the amplitudes and latencies of the human auditory brainstem potential. Electroencephalogr. Clin. Neurophysiol. Mar., 48(3):351-356.
Nicholson G, Corbett A. Slowing of central conduction in X-linked Charcot-Marie-Tooth neuropathy shown by brain stem auditory evoked responses. J Neurol Neurosurg Psychiatry 1996;61:43–6.
Nuwer MR, Aminoff M, Goodin D, Matsuoka S and Starr A (1994): IFCN recommended standards for brainstem auditory evoked potentials. Report of an IFCN committee. Electroencephalography and clinical neurophysiology, February., 91:12-17.

Oudesluys-Murphy AM, Van Straaten HL and Bholasingh R (1996): Neonatal hearing screening. Eur. J. Pediatr. Jun., 155(6):429-435.

Phelps ME, Mazziotta JC, Kuhl DE, Nuwer M, Packwood J and Engel J (1981): Tomographic mapping of human cerebral metabolism. Visual stimulation and deprivation. Neurol., 31:517-529.

Picton TW, Hillyard SA, Krauzs HI and Galambos R (1974): Human auditory evoked potentials: I. Evaluation of components. Electroencephalogr. Clin. Neurophysiol. 36:179-190.

Picton TW, Stapells DR and Combell KB (1982): Auditory evoked potentials from the human choclea and brainstem. J. Otolaryngol. Supp 9:1-14.

Poon's M (2003a): Visual Evoked Potentials. Michael Poon's Shrine of Neurology, 12 March, Pp. 1-5.

Poon's M (2003b): Brainstem Auditory Evoked Potentials. Michael Poon's Shrine of Neurology, 14 May., Pp.1- 3.

Purves SJ, Low MD and Galloway J (1981): A comparison of visual, brainstem auditory, and somatosensory evoked potentials in multiple sclerosis. Can. J. Neurol. Sci. Feb., 8(1):15-19.

Richard-Caton (1875): The electric currents of the brain. Br. Med. J.,2: 278.

Rosenhall ULF, Bjorkman G, Pederson K and Kall A (1985): Brainstem auditory evoked potentials in different age groups. Electroenceph. Clin. Neurophysiol. Vol 62:426-430.

Row MJ (1980): The brainstem auditory evoked response (BAER) in patients with vertigo. Electroencephalogr. Clin. Neurophysiol., 49:45.

Row MJ III (1978): Normal variability of the brainstem auditory evoked responses in young and old adult subjects. Electroenceph. Clin. Neurophysiol. 44:428-459.

Russel MH, Murray IJ, Metcalfe RA and Kulikowski L (1991): The visual defect in multiple sclerosis and optic neuritis. Prog. Brain Res., 144, 2419-2435.

Sannita WG, Fatone M and Garbarino S (1995): Effects of physiological changes of serum glucose on the pattern-VEP of healthy volunteers. Physiol. Behav. Nov., 58(5):1021-1026.

Scaioli V, Pareyson D, Avanzini G, et al. F response and somatosensory and brainstem auditory evoked potential studies in HMSN type I and II. J Neurol Neurosurg Psychiatry 1992;55:1027–31.

Schmidt RJ, Sataloff RT and Newman J (2001): The sensitivity of auditory brainstem response testing for the diagnosis of acoustic neuromas. Arch. Otolaryngol. Head & Neck Surg., 127(1):19-22.

Schwarz G, Litscher G and Rumpl E (1996): Brainstem auditory evoked potentials in respiratory insufficiency following encephalitis. Int. J. Neurosci. Feb., 84(1-4):35-44.

Shagass C (1976): Evoked brain potential in man. In: Generally RG and Gabay S (eds). Biological foundations of psychiatry. New York: Raven Press. Pp. 199- 253.

Shearer DE and Dustman RE (1980): The pattern reversal evoked potential, The need for laboratory norms. Am. J. EEG Technol., 20:185-200.

Shibata K, Osawa M and Iwata M (1997): Pattern reversal visual evoked potentials in classic and common migraine. J. Neurol. Sci. Feb., 12; 145(2):177-181.

Sokol S (1980): Visual evoked potential. In electrodiagnosis in clinical neurology edited by M. Aminoff. Churchill Livingstone, New York, Pp. 348-378.

Sokol S, Moskowitz A and Towle LE (1981): Age related changes in the latency of the visual evoked potential. Influence of check size. Electroenceph. Clin. Neurophysiol., 51:559-562.

Starr A, Allen A and Don M (1976): Effect of click rate on the latency of auditory brainstem response in man. Ann. Otol., 86:186-195.

Starr A, Nuwer MR, Aminoff M, Goodin D and Matsuoka S (1994): IFCN recommended standards for brainstem auditory evoked potentials. Report of an IFCN committee. Electroencephalography and clinical neurophysiology, February., 91:12-17.

Stephen W (1983): Brainstem auditory evoked potentials. American Academy of Neurology, Annual course 209:35-52.

Stern BJ, Krumholz A, Weiss HD, Goldstein P and Harris KC (1982): Evaluation of brainstem stroke using brainstem auditory evoked responses. Stroke. Sep-Oct.,13(5):705-711.

Stockard JJ, Hughes JF and Sharbrough FW (1979): Visually evoked potentials to electronic pattern reversal. Latency variations with gender, age technical factors. Am J EEG 19:171-204.

Stockard JJ, Stockard JE and Sharbrough FW (1978): Non pathological factors influencing brain stem auditory evoked potential. Amer. J. EEG Technol. 18:117-209.

Stockard JJ, Stockard JE and Sharbrough FW (1980b): Brainstem auditory evoked potentials in neurology: Methodology interpretation clinical application. In: Electrodiagnosis in clinical neurology edited by Aminoff. Churchill Livingstone, New York Pp. 370-413.

Tandon OP and Krishna SV (1990): Brainstem auditory evoked potentials in children a normative study. Indian Pediatr. Jul.,27(7):737-740.

Tarantino V, Stura M and Vallarino R (1988): Development of auditory evoked potentials of the brainstem in relation to age. Pediatr. Med. Chir. Jan-Feb.,10(1):73-76.

Taylor MJ, Boor R and Keenan NK (1996): Brainstem auditory and visual evoked potentials in infants with myelomeningocele. Brain Dev. Mar-Apr., 18(2): 99-104.

Tony Wu, Hung-Li Wang1, Chun-Che Chu, Jia-Ming Yu2, Jeng-Yeou Chen3, Chin-Chang Huang (2004): Clinical and Electrophysiological Studies of a Family with Probable X-linked Dominant Charcot-Marie-Tooth Neuropathy and Ptosis. Chang Gung Med J Vol. 27 No. 7

Tsuda H, Katsumi Y and Nakamura M (1995): Cerebral blood flow and metabolism in Lafora disease. Rinsho. Shinkeigaku. Feb., 35(2):175-179.

Yiannikas C and Walsh JC (1983): The variation of the pattern shift visual evoked response with the size of the stimulus field. Clin. Neurophysio., 55:427-436.

Yuksel A, Sarslan O and Devranoglu K (1995): Effect of valproate and carbamazepine on visual evoked potentials in epileptic children. Acta. Paediatr. Jpn. Jun., 37(3):358-361.

16

Extraction and Analysis of the Single Motor Unit F-Wave of the Median Nerve

Masafumi Yamada and Kentaro Nagata
Kanagawa Rehabilitation Institute,
Kanagawa Rehabilitation Center,
Japan

1. Introduction

The matrix type multielectrodes have been proved to be useful for getting the information of motor unit (MU) properties (Monster et al., 1980; Reucher et al., 1987; Yamada et al., 1987; Masuda and Sadoyama, 1988; Kleine et al., 2000; Gazzoni et al., 2004). By this electromyography (EMG) technique, we can obtain many essential properties of MU that could not be obtained by conventional surface EMG and/or needle EMG. One of them is the waveform property of motor unit action potential (MUAP) which is enabled by extracting the single propagating MUAP. Another is the two-dimensional location of motor end-plates. There have been many applications of multichannel surface EMG for measuring voluntary muscle activities, but few for evoked EMG responses. However, recent studies have demonstrated the applications of the multichannel surface EMG for the measurement of muscle fiber conduction velocities (MFCVs) (Metani et al., 2005) , for the estimation of firing thresholds (Yamada, 2004), and for the motor unit number estimate (MUNE) (Blok et al., 2005; van Dijk et al., 2008).

The F-wave represents a long latency response detected from a muscle following stimulation of a peripheral nerve at supramaximal intensity. The F-waves are produced by antidromic activation of motor neurons. The latency and the waveform of the F-wave change with each stimulus. The F-wave studies are widely used in clinical neurophysiology as a quantitative estimation method of the objective pathological changes. The F-waves that consist of a single MUAP occur also with submaximal stimulation. Low intensity stimulation could increase the probability of the single MU F-wave (Komori et al., 1991; Doherty et al., 1994; Stashuk et al., 1994; Yamada, 2004), and reduce the discomfort of the subjects. Therefore, different MUAPs can be readily analyzed by classifying F-waves. Many studies concerned with the single MU F-wave were performed for the estimation of the conduction velocity of nerve fibers (Doherty et al., 1994; Felice, 1998; Wang et al., 1999) and the MUNE (Stashuk et al., 1994; Hara et al., 2000). The conventional surface EMG technique was used in these studies, and there were few applications of multichannel surface EMG for F-wave studies.

In a previous study, we investigated the classification and analysis of multichannel bipolar F-waves (Yamada et al., 2007). It is difficult to detect deep MUs from the bipolar EMG. So, in the present study, the thenar MUs F-waves were investigated by extracting single MU F-waves from monopolar multichannel surface EMG signals. By increasing the number of processing data measured under different stimulus conditions, many single MU F-waves could be extracted, and the properties of F-waves and MUs could be analyzed successfully. Then we could find the single MU F-waves with the same waveform but different latencies.

2. Methods

2.1 Subjects and measurements

The subjects were 6 men, aged 22−60 years (mean±S.D., 30.2±14.9 years). None of them had a history of neurological disorders. All subjects gave informed consent prior to participation in the study. The subject sat comfortably on a chair with his right hand supinated. The right median nerve was stimulated at the wrist and the evoked responses were recorded from the thenar muscles with a matrix-type multielectrode. The multielectrode was composed of 32 silver electrodes (8x4 array), 1 mm in diameter, which were arranged on a silicone rubber board (thickness 2 mm) at 4 mm distance in both directions (Fig. 1). This electrode was fixed by bandages with the eight electrode arrays in parallel with the muscle fibers. A small diameter of electrode and a short distance of electrodes enabled the extraction of single MUAP from surface EMG signals. The use of a semi-solid type electrode paste enabled to measure EMG signals for a long period. A reference electrode and a ground electrode, both conventional Ag/AgCl electrodes, were attached to the bone of the dorsal hand. The block diagram of the multichannel surface EMG system is shown in Fig. 2.

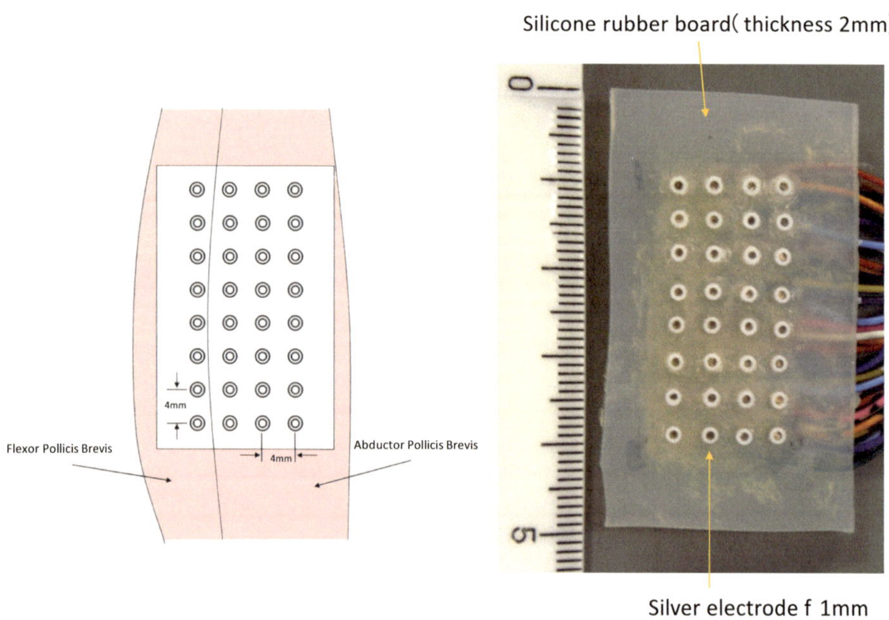

Fig. 1. Thirty-two channel matrix-type multielectrode. Each electrode (1mm in diameter) is arranged on a silicone rubber board at 4 mm distance in both directions.

The 32 channel monopolar evoked potentials (8x4 array) were amplified through a bandwidth of 10-1000 Hz (gain 30dB). The amplified evoked signals were sampled at 10kHz with 16-bit resolution. The stimulation was squarewave pulse of 0.2 ms duration and frequency of 5 Hz or less. The high stimulus rate may cause muscle fatigue, and may change the shape of MUAP. Therefore the low stimulus frequency was selected for recording consecutive evoked responses. The stimulation strength was set to submaximal, approximately 40-80 % of the supramaximal stimulation. Each of the record length was 50ms, and 300 consecutive evoked responses were recorded. Changing the stimulation intensity, several sessions of 300 evoked responses were recorded. The bipolar potentials were obtained by calculating the difference between the monopolar potentials of two adjacent electrodes placed along the muscle fibers.

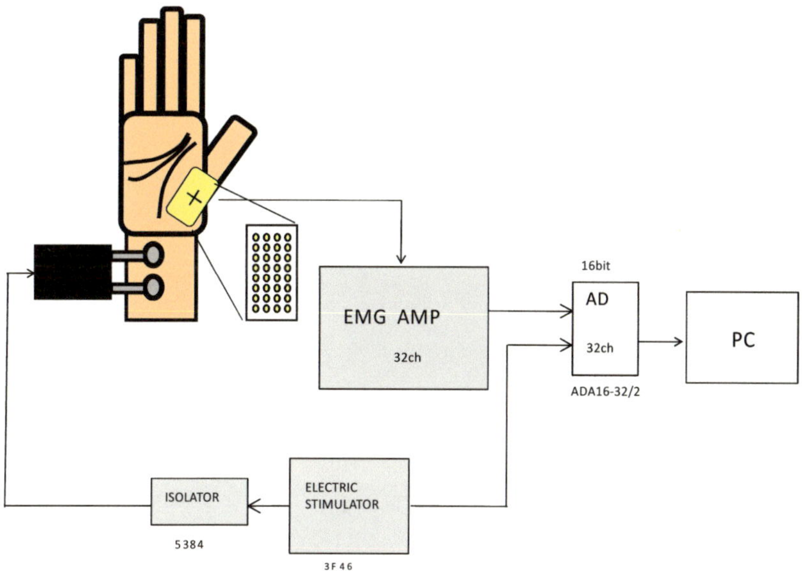

Fig. 2. Block diagram of the multichannel surface EMG system.

As in the case of bipolar signals (Yamada, 2004; Yamada et al., 2007), the origin of the F-wave could be also evaluated by the distribution pattern of monopolar MUAPs. It is presumed that the MUs whose center arrays estimated at array 1 and array 2 are originated from the abductor pollicis brevis (APB), and those estimated at array 3 and array 4 are originated from the flexor pollicis brevis (FPB). In Fig. 3(A), the distribution of 32 channel monopolar evoked potentials recorded in a thenar muscle is shown. This MU is originated from the APB muscle. Fig. 3(B) shows 8 channel records of the center array (array 1).

2.2 Classification of F-waves

The outline of the classification of F-waves is shown in Fig. 4. All channels evoked responses are digitally high-pass filtered in order to remove the late components of the M-waves with a drift filter which barely affects the waveform parameters of the F-waves. The superimposed traces in Fig. 5 show 10 sequentially evoked responses of one electrode array. Although the M-waves are almost uniformed, the F-waves show various patterns. When the evoked response contains the F-wave, the center of the MU in transverse section (center array) is evaluated by the sum of the peak-to-peak amplitude of F-waves in each electrode array. Then we select the records (latency 20-45 ms) in the array for the classification process.

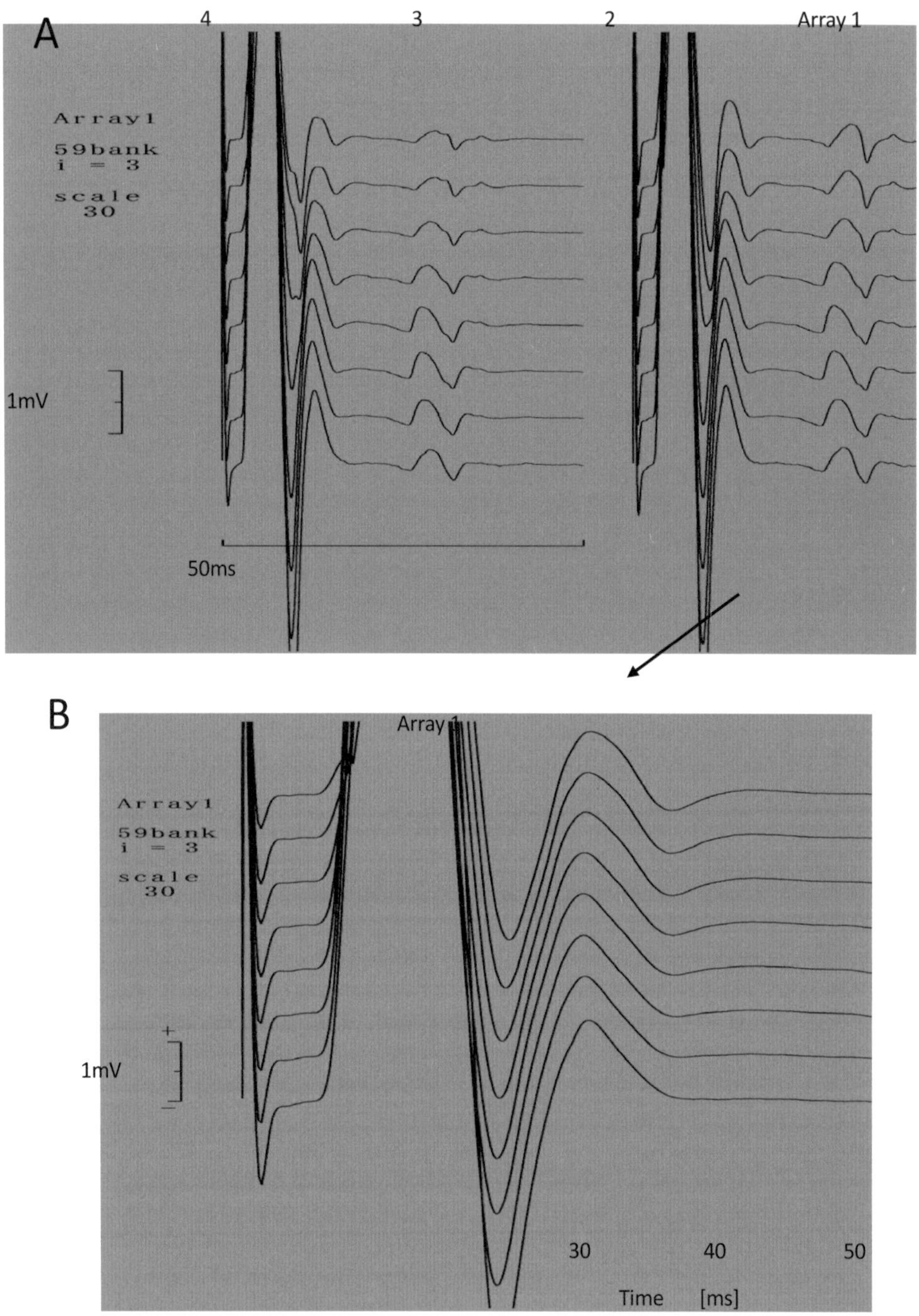

Fig. 3. Distribution of 32 channel monopolar evoked potentials in the thenar muscles at submaximal stimulation (A). Expanded 8 channel monopolar potentials of the center array (B). The signals were digitally high-pass filtered with a drift filter.

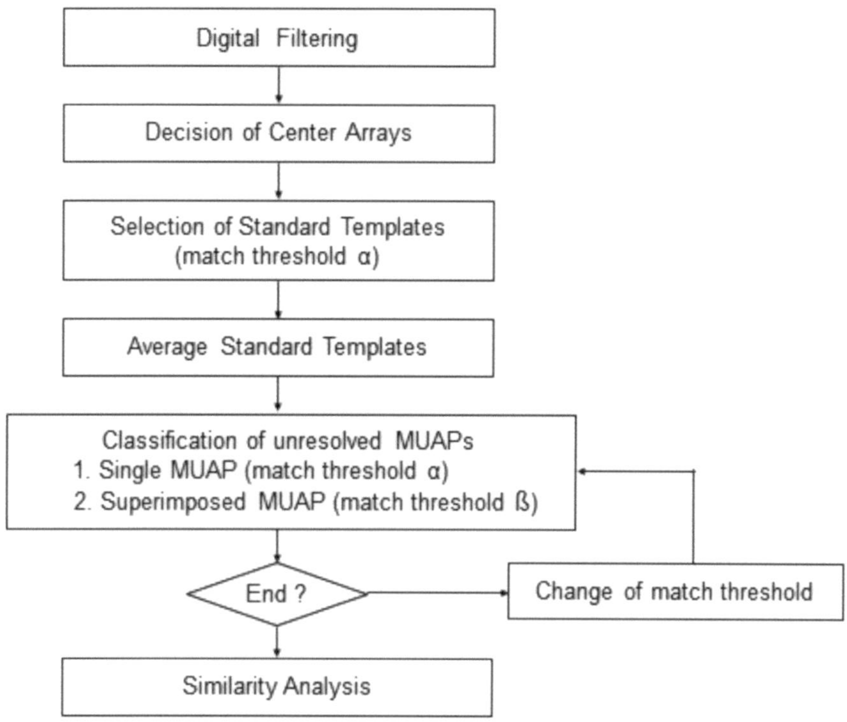

Fig. 4. Flow chart of the classification of F-waves.

Eight channel MUAP waveforms in its center array are classified using a template-matching method based on the least-square error criterion where an initial match threshold α is set to 5% of the objective area value typically. If the F-wave and templates do not match, the waveforms on both sides of the center array are also estimated, because the decision of center arrays is critical and not always proper. After this procedure, the standard templates are selected by the decision rule dependent on the identified number of the corresponding template, and the average waveforms are computed for the next procedure. The group of F-waves, which is not identified as one of the standard templates, is repeatedly classified into an averaged standard template or 2-3 combinations of them by the same method in the selection of standard templates. The match threshold β in case of superposition is initially set to lower than α (typically 4.5% of the objective area value), because high thresholds tend to lead to incorrect combinations of standard templates. After having thresholds α and β gradually increased, the unresolved F-waves are repeatedly processed. By these procedures, the single MU F-waves are classified. Five sessions of recordings measured at different stimulus intensities were processed to extract many single MUs. Fig. 6 shows 38 single MU F-waves extracted and classified from the thenar muscles of a subject.

2.3 Estimation of F-wave parameters

The amplitude of a single MUAP was evaluated from measuring the largest peak-to-peak amplitude in 8 channel MUAP waveforms in its center array, and the latency was obtained

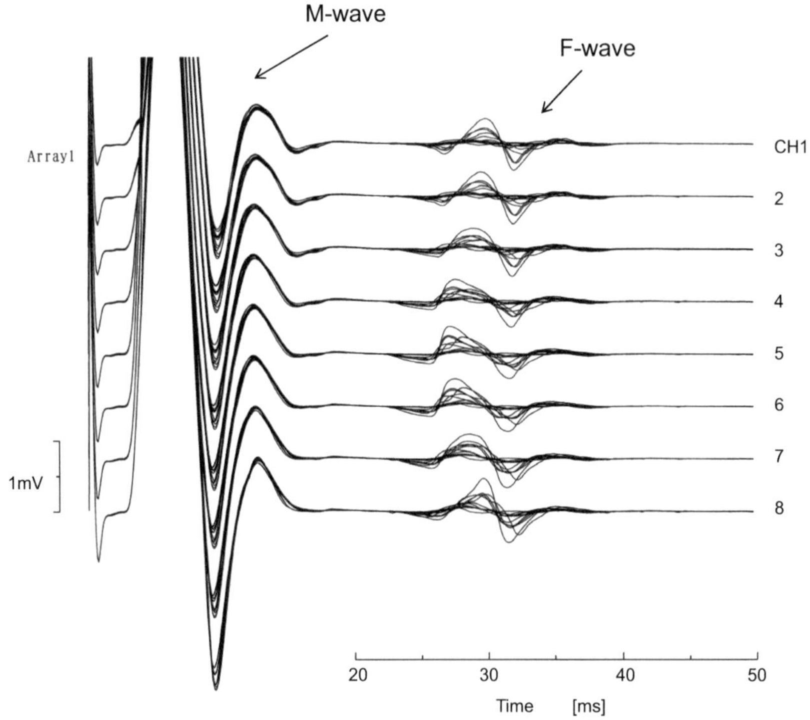

Fig. 5. Superimposed 10 evoked responses of one electrode array.

from measuring the fastest onset of MUAP in the array. In the case of MUAPs showing propagating time delays, the MFCV was calculated from the time delay of a single pair of MUAPs in the array. The MUAPs in the region of the motor end-plates band indicated non-linear propagating time delays, and we estimated the conduction velocity in the area a small distance on either side of the band, where the conduction velocity was uniform along the length of the muscle. The muscle fiber conduction velocities of all classified MUAPs, excepting superimposed ones, were computed according to the above considerations, and other parameters were estimated automatically as well.

Statistical analysis was carried out for F-wave parameters. The correlation coefficients among amplitudes, latencies and MFCVs were calculated in each subject. The level of statistical significance was set at $p<0.05$.

2.4 Detection of single MU F-waves with the same waveform but different latencies

From these classified F-waves, the F-waves with the same waveform but different latencies (latency differences above 0.5 ms) were searched using 8 channel and 32 channel similarity values between the two averaged F-waves.

In the case of similarity values higher than 0.8, the comparison of two F-waves was performed by examining 8 channel propagation patterns of MUAPs in its center array and 32 channel distribution patterns of MUAPs in a superimposed form and in an averaged form. In addition, bipolar waveforms were also compared for reference. The F-wave analysis is planned to execute interactively, or automatically. At present, the operator is required in some processes to obtain reliable and accurate results.

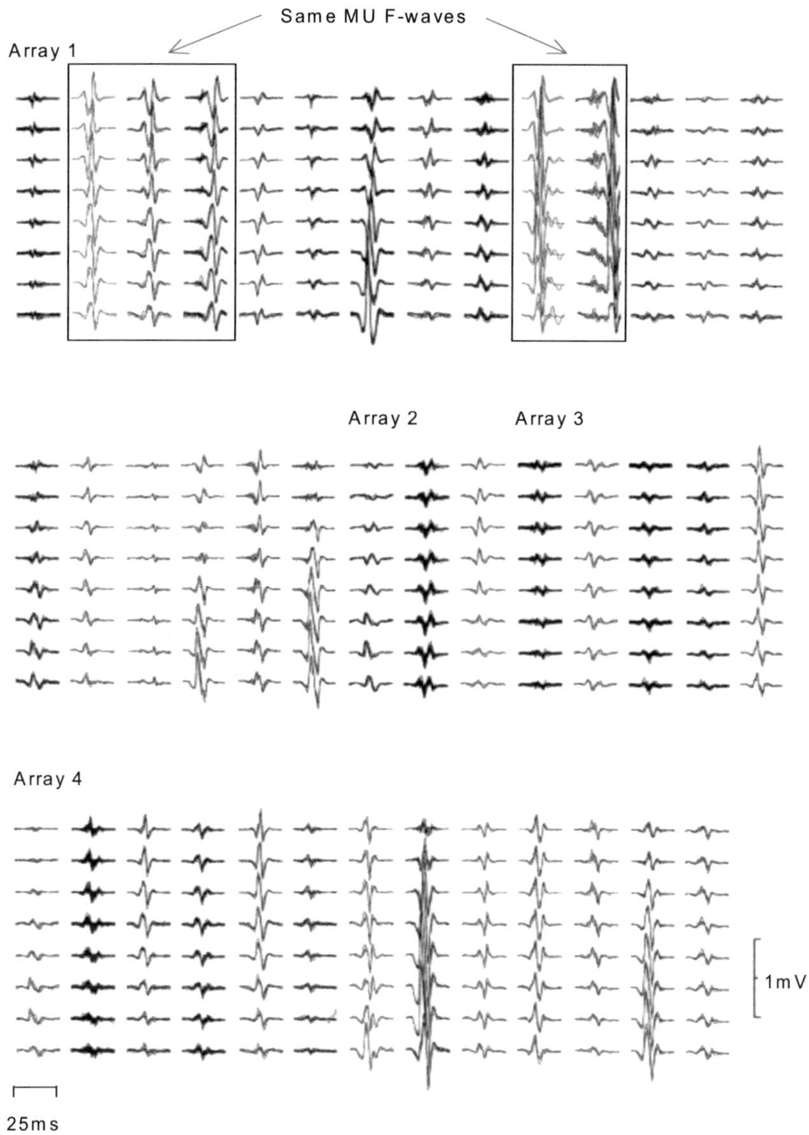

Fig. 6. Thirty-eight single MU F-waves extracted and classified in the thenar muscles of one subject. Two APB MUs with the same waveform but different latencies are shown in the top traces.

3. Results

Single MU F-waves were classified by using the template-matching method. The classification results and estimated F-wave parameters of thenar MUs in 6 normal subjects are shown in Table 1 and Fig. 7. The mean F-wave persistence (occurrence rate) was high (88.8%), and a total of 7724 F-waves were detected in the evoked responses. The numbers of MUs extracted from 5 sessions of data (1500 responses) were increased by 75-116%

Subjects	F-wave (n=1500)	MU				
		n(APB+FPB) (FPB)	Amplitude Mean ± SD. (mV)	Latency Mean ± SD. (ms)	MFCV Mean ± SD. (m/s)
1	1376(91.7%)	38(18)	0.367±0.304	28.07±2.08	5.369±1.065(11)
2	1279(85.3%)	41(22)	0.179±0.130	27.20±1.63	5.425±1.096(2)
3	1413(94.2%)	35(10)	0.317±0.222	25.99±2.95	6.200±0.000(3)
4	1080(90.0%)*	30(6)	0.142±0.107	25.30±0.97	3.832±1.331(5)
5	1236(82.4%)	31(15)	0.250±0.188	26.20±2.25	4.112±1.020(10)
6	1340(89.3%)	26(3)	0.183±0.186	27.90±1.23	4.753±1.56(3)
Total	7724(88.8%)	201(74)	0.251±0.222	26.74±2.25	4.800±1.237(35)

*n=1200

Table 1. Classification results for the F-waves in 6 normal subjects: the numbers of F-waves, the numbers of MUs and the estimated MU parameters.

(mean±S.D., 92±15%) compared with those from the maximum sessions (300 responses). The numbers of MU in 6 subjects were 38, 41, 35, 30, 31 and 26, respectively. The total of 201 thenar MUs were extracted from the F-wave data.

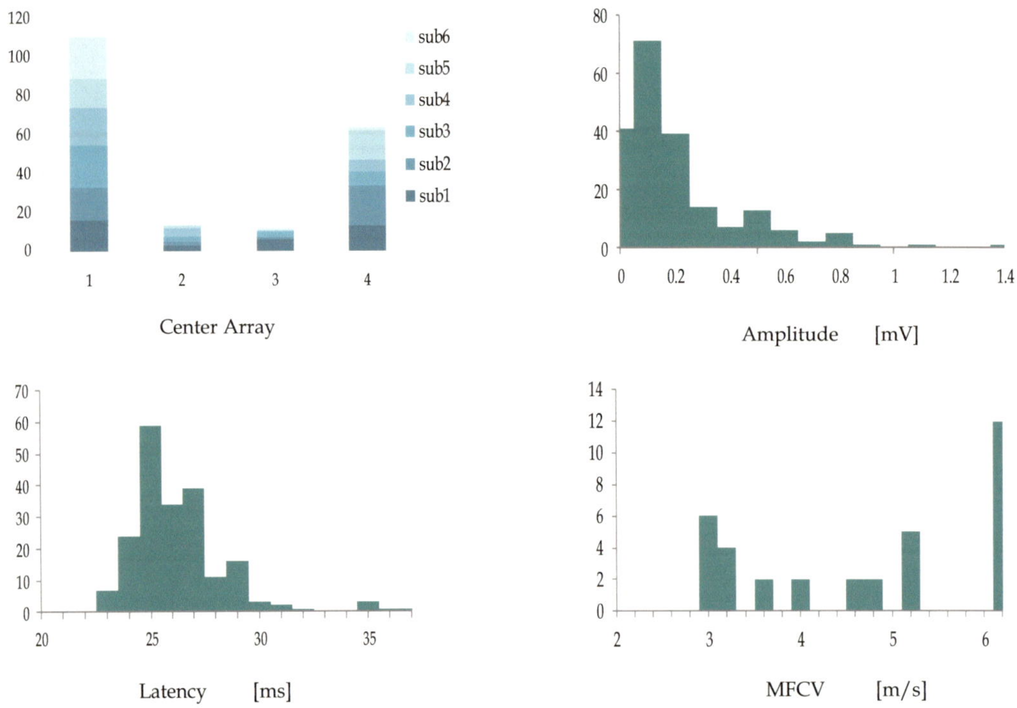

Fig. 7. Estimated parameters of single MU F-waves: Center array, Amplitude, Latency and MFCV.

The numbers of MUs originated from the APB and FPB were 127 (63.2%) and 74 (36.8%). In 5 out of 6 subjects, the numbers of APB MUs were larger than those of FPB MUs. Fig. 6(a) shows the histogram of the center arrays of 201 MUs. Thirty-eight single MU F-waves classified in a subject are shown in Fig. 7. This example shows 20 APB MUs and 18 FPB MUs. The mean peak-to-peak amplitudes, latencies, and MFCVs were 0.251±0.222 mV, 26.74±2.25 ms and 4.80±1.24 m/s. The long latencies greater than 30 ms were detected in 11 MUs (5 subjects). The numbers of MUs in which MFCVs could be evaluated in 6 subjects were 11, 2, 4, 5, 10 and 3, respectively. The total was 35 MUs (17.4%). The significant correlations were not found between amplitudes, latencies and MFCVs in all subjects.

An example of single MU responses (FPB MU) with the same waveform but different latencies is shown in Fig. 8. The latencies of the two responses were (a) 25.7 ms and (b) 36.1 ms, and the latency difference was 10.4 ms. The similarity values for 8 channel and 32 channel signals were high, namely 0.91 and 0.90 respectively.

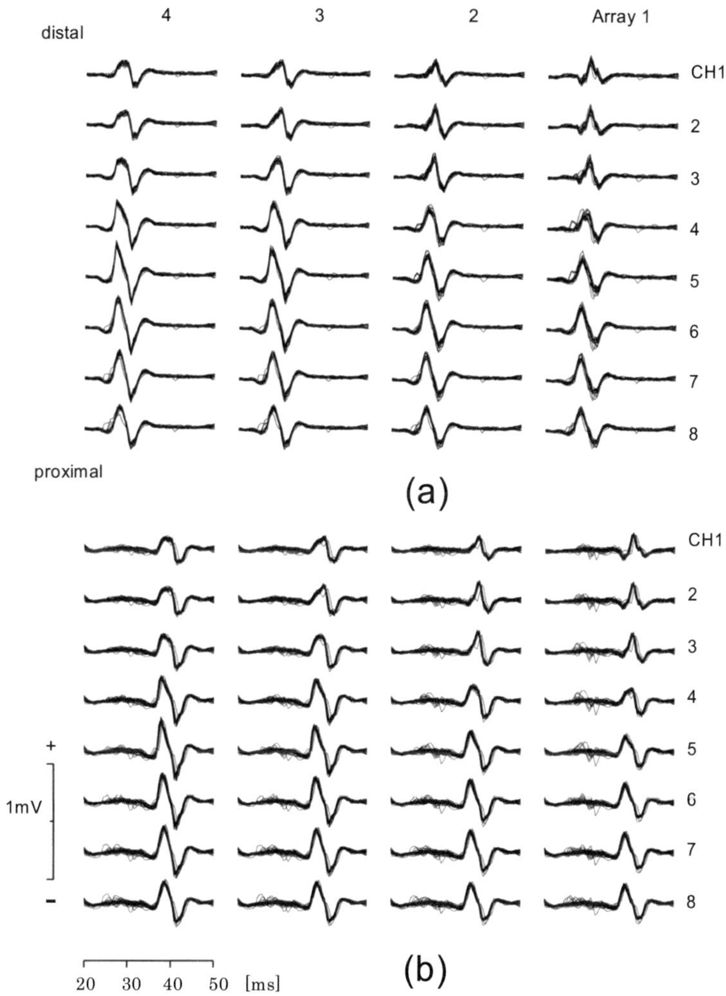

Fig. 8. Distributions of 32 channel MUAPs with the same waveform but different latencies. The latencies were (a) 25.7 ms and (b) 36.1 ms, and the latency difference was 10.4 ms.

The single MU F-waves with the same waveform but different latencies were detected in 5 out of 6 subjects, the total number was 12 MUs (8 APB MUs and 4 FPB MUs, 6%). The estimated F-wave parameters of these MUs are summarized in Table 2.
The latency differences of the two responses ranged 0.9 to 10.4 ms (mean 2.82±3.22 ms), and half of them were around 1 ms. There was no significant relationship between the stimulus intensities and the latencies in these MUs. Figs. 9(a) and 9(b) show the examples of the single MU F-waves (a: FPB MU, b: APB MU) with 0.9 ms and 1.2 ms latency differences. One of the MUs with 3 different latencies (APB MU, 26.3, 29.4 and 32.2 ms) is shown in Fig. 10(a)-(c). The waveforms in Fig. 10(b) differ slightly from those in Figs. 10(a) and 10(c), because the F-waves in Fig. 10(b) are overlapped by the FPB MU with small amplitude MUAPs. These results were confirmed by the distribution and propagation patterns of the MUAPs.

Subject	Array	Amplitude (mV)	Latency 1 (ms)	Latency 2 (ms)	Latency 3 (ms)	Similarity (8CH)	Similarity (32CH)
1	1	1.08	24.0	33.5(9.5)		0.96	0.95
	1	0.57	26.3	29.4(3.1)	32.2(5.9)	0.94	0.91
2	4	0.18	23.9	26.0(2.1)		0.92	0.83
	1	0.68	24.4	25.3(0.9)		0.86	0.89
	4	0.53	24.8	26.0(1.2)		0.90	0.87
	4	0.56	25.7	36.1(10.4)		0.91	0.90
3	1	0.12	25.3	26.3(1.0)		0.87	0.89
	2	0.21	25.7	27.0(1.3)		0.81	0.79
	1	0.26	25.7	27.0(1.7)		0.82	0.72
4	4	0.41	24.8	26.0(1.2)		0.94	0.94
	1	0.19	24.8	26.6(1.8)		0.85	0.83
5	1	0.12	27.1	28.0(0.9)		0.88	0.93
Mean		0.41±0.29	25.2±0.95	28.0±3.23 (2.82±3.22)		0.89±0.05	0.87±0.07

Table 2. Estimated parameters of single MU F-waves with the same waveform but different latencies.

4. Discussion

The F-wave persistence in monopolar recordings was high compared with that in bipolar signals, because it is thought that the deep MUs, which could not be detected from bipolar waveforms, might be detectable from monopolar waveforms. Accordingly, the numbers of MUs that were extracted and classified from evoked responses were increased than those in the previous study (Yamada et al., 2007). In the case of bipolar signals, the noise and interference are lower than those in the monopolar signals. Then, the MUAPs can be classified precisely, and the superimposed MUAPs can be decomposed into its constituent MUAPs. On the other hand, in the case of monopolar signals, the decomposition processing of superimposed MUAPs had a little problem with the classification accuracy.
By using the distribution and propagation patterns of the MUAPs measured by the multichannel surface EMG technique, the single MU F-waves could be extracted and

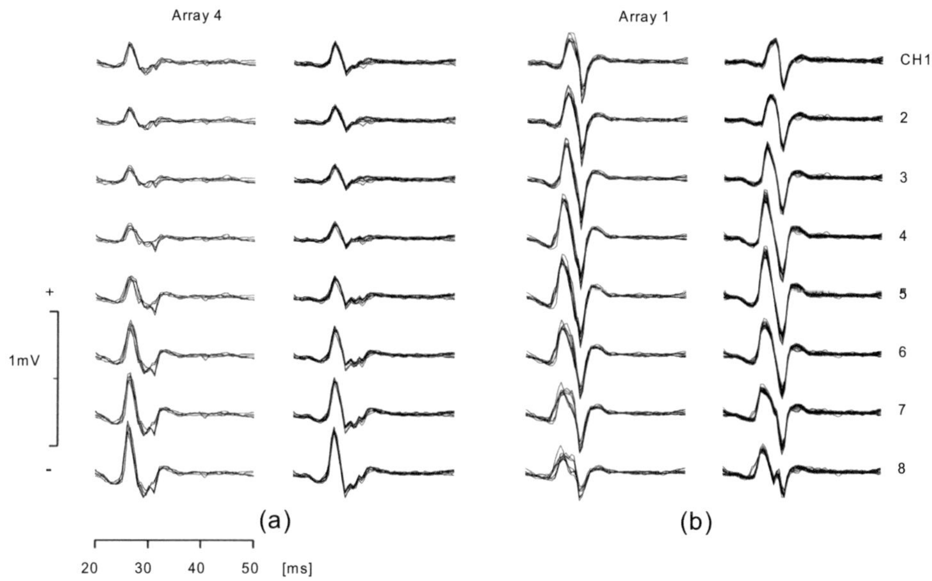

Fig. 9. Single MU F-waves (a: FPB MU, b: APB MU) with 0.9 ms and 1.2 ms latency differences.

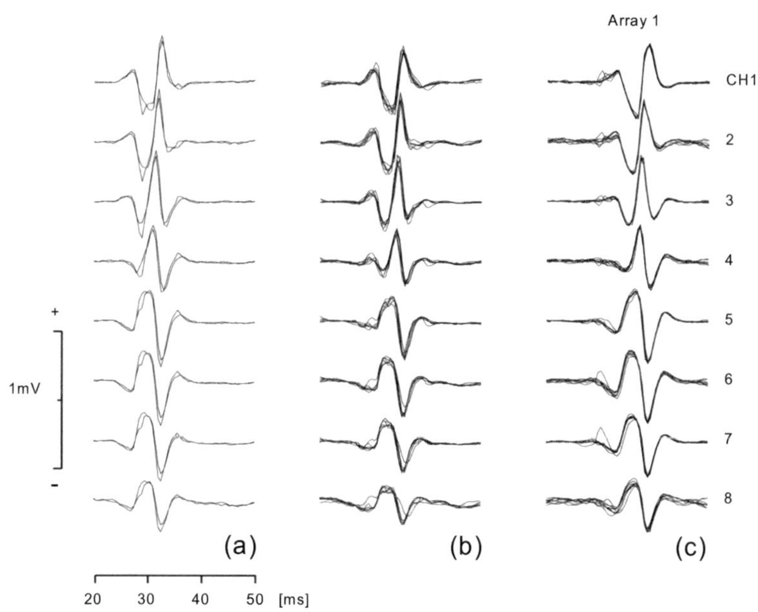

Fig. 10. Single MU F-waves with 3 different latencies ((a) 26.3 ms, (b) 29.4 ms and (c) 32.2 ms). The latency differences were (b)-(a) 3.1 ms and (c)-(a) 5.9 ms.

classified precisely, and the origin of the F-wave is evaluated easily. In the case of bipolar signals, the extracted numbers of APB MUs were larger than those of FPB for all the subjects, and most of the MUs (84.5%) were originated from the APB muscle (Yamada et al., 2007). In this study, 127 APB MUs (63.2%) were extracted from monopolar signals. These results suggest that the number of APB MU is greater than that of FPB MU.

The F-wave amplitude and persistence were increased with increasing the stimulus intensity (Yamada et al., 2007; Fisher et al., 2008). On the other hand, low intensity stimulation increased the probability of single MU F-wave (Komori et al., 1991; Doherty et al., 1994; Shefner, 2001; Yamada et al., 2007). By investigating in detail the relationship between stimulus intensity and the properties of the extracted MUs, it seems that the experimental conditions of stimulus intensity and the combination of intensities, from which more MUs can be extracted, may be determined.

The latency of F-wave is useful to detect alterations in peripheral nerves (Fisher, 1992; Panayiotopoulos and Chroni, 1996; Toyokura and Murakami, 1997; Nobrega et al., 2001). Moreover the latency varies in each MU, so this parameter is useful for classifying individual F-waves. By using the multichannel surface EMG technique, the latency may be measured precisely than other methods, because the locations of motor end-plates, where the MUAPs begin to propagate along muscle fibers in both directions, are readily identified in the two-dimensional plane (Yamada et al., 1991; Yamada, 2004).

The single MU responses with the same waveform but different latencies were detected in 12 MUs out of 201 extracted MUs (6%). Though the latency differences of the two single MUAPs ranged 0.9 to 10.4 ms (Table 2), many of the differences were around 1 ms (50%). In these examples, it suggests that the prolonged latencies occurred due to synaptic delays in the spinal interneuronal network. The synaptic delay is usually of about 0.5 ms (Guyton and Hall, 1996). Therefore, in the case of one interneuron in the pathway, the time delay will be about 1 ms. The long-latency reflexes (LLRs) can be elicited by electric stimulation of the median nerve at the wrist during voluntary contraction of the thenar muscles (Upton et al., 1971; Conrad et al., 1977; Deuschl et al., 1989; Burke et al., 1999). As shown in Figs. 8 and 10 (10.4 ms, 3.1, 5.9 ms), it was confirmed that single MUAP LLRs with prolonged latencies were included in F-wave data. In the present study, the record length was set to 50 ms. By using a longer record length, single MUAP LLRs with longer latencies may be detected further.

In the MUNE by the F-wave method, the same MUs with prolonged latencies should be excluded from the calculation of the mean MUAP. In particular, the MUs with long latencies, which were due to supraspinal or transcortical pathways, should not be included in the MUNE process, because they will affect the MUNE values more sensibly than in the case of small latency differences.

5. Conclusions

The extracted number of single MU F-waves could be increased by increasing the number of processing data measured under different stimulus conditions, then the properties of many MUs could be analyzed easily, and we could find the single MU responses with the same waveform but different latencies. The similarity analysis was useful to search the same waveform pair from many pairs of single MU responses. It is suggested that the prolonged latencies occurred due to spinal interneuronal pathways, in the case of large differences in latencies, supraspinal pathways, or transcortical pathways.

6. References

Blok, JH.; van Dijk, JP.; Zwarts, MJ. & Stegeman, DF. (2005). Motor unit action potential topography and its use in motor unit number estimation, *Muscle Nerve,* Vol.32, pp. 280-291

Burke, D.; Hallet, M.; Fuhr, P. & Pierrot-Deseilligny, E. (1999). H reflexes from the tibial and median nerves. In Recommendations for the Practice of Clinical Neurophysiology: guidelines of the International Federation of Clinical Neurophysiology. *Electroenceph. Clin. Neurophysiol.* (Suppl. 52), pp. 259-262

Conrad, B.; & Aschoff, JC. (1977). Effects of voluntary isometric and isotonic activity on late transcortical reflex components in normal subjects and hemiparetic patients. *Electroencephalogr. Clin. Neurophysiol.*, Vol.42(1), pp. 107-116

Deuschl, G.; Ludolph, A.; Schenck, E. & Lücking, CH. (1989). The relations between long-latency reflexes in hand muscles, somatosensory evoked potentials and transcranial stimulation of motor tracts, *Electroencephalogr. Clin. Neurophysiol.*, Vol.74, pp. 425-430

Doherty, TJ.; Komori, T.; Stashuk, DW.; Kassam, A. & Brown, WF. (1994). Physiological properties of single thenar motor units in the F-response of younger and older adults, *Muscle Nerve,* Vol.17, pp. 860-872

Felice, KJ. (1998). Nerve conduction velocities of single thenar motor axons based on the automated analysis of F waves in amyotrophic lateral sclerosis. *Muscle Nerve,* Vol.21, pp. 756-761

Fisher, MA. (1992). AAEM Minimonograph #13: H reflexes and F waves: physiology and clinical indications, *Muscle Nerve*, Vol.15, pp. 1223-1233

Fisher, MA.; Zhu, JQ.; Uddin, MK. & Grindstaff, P. (2008). Submaximal stimulation and f-wave parameters, *J. Clin. Neurophysiol.* , Vol.25, No.5, pp. 299-303

Gazzoni, M.; Farina, D. & Merletti, R. (2004). A new method for the extraction and classification of single motor unit action potentials from surface EMG signals, *J Neuroscience Methods*, Vol.136, pp. 165-177

Guyton, AC. & Hall, JE. (1996). *Human Physiology and Mechanisms of disease*, 6th ed., Saunders, Philadelphia , USA

Hara, Y.; Akaboshi, K.; Masakado, Y. & Chino, N. (2000). Physiologic decrease of single thenar motor units in the F-response in stroke patients, *Arch. Phys. Med. Rehab.*, Vol.81, pp. 418-423

Kleine, BU.; Schumann, NP. Stegeman, DF. & Scholle, HC. (2000). Surface EMG mapping of the human trapezius muscle: the topography of monopolar and bipolar surface EMG amplitude and spectrum parameters at varied forces and in fatigue, *Clin. Neurophysiol.*, Vol.111, pp. 686-693

Komori, T.; Watson, BV. & Brown, WF. (1991). Characteristics of single 'F' motor units at different stimulus intensities, *Muscle Nerve, Vol.*14 pp. 875

Masuda, T. & Sadoyama, T. (1988). Topographical map of innervation zones within single motor units measured with a grid surface electrode, *IEEE Trans. biomed. Engng.*, Vol.BME-35, pp. 623-628

Metani, H.; Tsubahara, A. Hiraoka, T.; Aoyagi, Y. & Tanaka, Y. (2005). A new method using F-waves to measure muscle fiber conduction velocity (MFCV), *Electromyogr. Clin. Neurophysiol.*, Vol.45, pp. 245-253

Monster, AW.; Pittore, J. & Barrie, W. (1980). A system for the rapid acquisition of surface potential maps of human skeletal muscle motor units, *IEEE Trans. biomed. Engng.* Vol.BME-27, pp. 110-112

Nobrega, JAM.; Manzano, GM. & Monteagudo, PT. (2001). A comparison between different parameters in F-wave studies, *Clin. Neurophysiol.*, Vol.112, pp. 866-868

Panayiotopoulos, CP. & Chroni, E. (1996). F-waves in clinical neurophysiology: a review, methodological issues and overall value in peripheral neuropathies, *Electroencephalogr. Clin. Neurophysiol.*, Vol.101, pp. 365-374

Reucher, H.; Rau, G. & Silny, J. (1987). Spatial filtering of noninvasive multielectrode EMG: Part I- Introduction to measuring technique and applications, *IEEE Trans. biomed. Engng.* Vol.BME-34, pp. 98-105

Shefner, JM. (2001). Motor unit number estimation in human neurological diseases and animal models, *Clin. Neurophysiol.*, Vol.112, pp. 955-964

Stashuk, DW.; Doherty, TJ.; Kassam, A. & Brown, WF. (1994). Motor unit number estimates based on the automated analysis of F-responses. *Muscle Nerve* Vol.17, pp881-890

Toyokura, M. & Murakami, K. (1997). F-wave study in patients with lumbosacral radiculopathies, *Electromyogr. Clin. Neurophysiol.*, Vol.37, pp. 19-26

Upton, ARM.; McComas, AJ. & Sica, REP. (1971). Potentiation of «late» responses evoked in muscles during effort, *J Neurol. Neurosurg. Psychiatry.*, Vol.34, pp. 699-711

van Dijk, JP.; Blok, JH.; Lapatki, BG.; van Schaik, IN.; Zwarts, MJ. & Stegeman, DF. (2008). Motor unit number estimation using high-density surface electromyography, *Clin. Neurophysiol.*, Vol.119, pp. 33-42

Wang, FC.; de Pasqua, V. & Delwaide, PJ. (1999). Age-related changes in fastest and slowest conducting axons of thenar motor units. *Muscle Nerve,* Vol.22, pp.1022-1029

Yamada, M.; Kumagai, K. & Uchiyama, A. (1987). The distribution and propagation pattern of motor unit action potentials studied by multi-channel surface EMG, *Electroencephalogr. clin. Neurophysiol.* Vol.67, pp. 395-401

Yamada, M.; Kumagai, K. & Uchiyama, A. (1991). Muscle fiber conduction velocity studied by the multi-channel surface EMG. *Electromyogr. Clin. Neurophysiol.*, Vol.31, pp. 251-256

Yamada, M. (2004). Comparison of F-waves and motor unit action potentials activated during voluntary contraction. *Electromyogr Clin Neurophysiol,* Vol.44, pp. 29-34

Yamada, M.; Nakazawa, T.; Kyoso, M. & Ishijima, M. (2007). Single motor unit F-waves in the thenar muscles studied by the multichannel surface EMG, *Electromyogr. Clin. Neurophysiol.*, Vol.47, pp. 43-48

17

EMG and Evoked Potentials in the Operating Room During Spinal Surgery

Induk Chung and Arthur A. Grigorian
Georgia Neurosurgical Institute and Mercer University School of Medicine, Macon, GA, USA

1. Introduction

EMG is an important clinical electrodiagnostic tool to assess function of neuromuscular tissue. It assesses spinal motor nerve roots and determines correct placement of hardware in surgical procedures, including cervical, thoracic, and lumbosacral spinal decompression, instrumentation, and fixation of spinal deformity. Evoked potentials provide information on vascular compromise of the spinal cord and nerves. Hence, concurrent recordings of EMG and evoked potentials can assess function integrity of the spinal cord and nerve more accurately. In this chapter, we will discuss application of EMG and evoked potentials in spinal surgery.

2. EMG recording techniques in the operating room (OR)

2.1 Recording electrodes

Surface, intramuscular, and subdermal needle electrodes are used to record EMG activity in the OR. Surface electrodes may not be used because of their inability to detect neurotonic discharges in spine surgery (Skinner et al., 2008). In addition, sweat causes electrodes to detach from the skin, preventing stable recording during lengthy surgery (Chung, unpublished data). Both intramuscular and subdermal needle electrodes are sufficient to detect neurotonic discharges (Skinner et al., 2008). Intramuscular needle electrodes may have an advantage to record EMG activity when the subcutaneous tissue is thick. Subdermal needle electrodes (13 mm length and 0.4 mm diameter) are generally used to record EMG in the OR, and we also routinely use subdermal needle electrodes in our practice.

2.2 Recording parameters

EMG is a simple and reliable technique which does not interfere with the surgical procedure. It is important to use proper recording parameters to achieve EMG recordings to obtain high signal-to-noise ratio. Recommended parameters of routine free-run EMG are low-frequency filter (LFF) of 20-30 Hz, high frequency filter (HFF) of 1-3 KHz, a gain of 500-5,000, a sensitivity of 50-500 μV, and a sweep speed of 10-200 msec per division (Toleikis et al., 2000; Bose et al., 2002; Chung et al., 2009). LFF of greater than 50 Hz and HFF of less than 3 KHz should be avoided. Impedance of subdermal needle electrodes is recommended to be less than 5 KΩ, for impedance greater than 5 KΩ may mask real EMG activity. If impedance of all electrodes is too high, ground electrode should be replaced. If a particular electrode gives high impedance, the electrode should be replaced.

2.3 Muscle group selections and electrode placement

EMG in spinal surgery should cover all nerve roots at risk innervated by surgical levels. In routine EMG, depending on the surgical levels and number of channels available, bipolar electrodes (an active and a reference) are placed subdermally over the belly of each muscle group of interest. Electrodes should be placed ~1 cm apart with care and secured with tape to prevent dislodgement. EMG should be recorded from the bilateral muscle groups to increase specificity of nerve root activation. If fewer channels are available in the monitoring equipment, an active electrode is placed in one muscle and a reference electrode is placed in other muscle. Multiple nerve roots can be monitored with this montage, but it may be difficult to identify specific nerve root at risk. Table 1 indicates representative muscle groups to be recorded during spinal surgery (Leppanen, 2008).

Cervical	Muscle
C2, C3, C4	Trapezius, Sternomastoid (spinal portion of the spinal accessory nerve)
C5, C6	Deltoid, Biceps
C6	Triceps, Extensor Carpi Radialis
C7	Flexor Carpi Radialis
C8, T1	Abductor Pollicis Brevis, Abductor Digiti Minimi
Thoracic	
T5, T6	Upper Rectus Abdominis
T7, T8	Middle Rectus Abdominis
T9, T10, T11	Lower Rectus Abdominis
T12	Inferior Rectus Abdominis
Lumbar	
L2, L3, L4	Vastus Medialis, Adductor Magnus
L4. L5, S1	Vastus Lateralis, Tibialis Anterior
L5, S1	Proneous Longus, Gastrocnemius
Sacral	
S1, S2	Gastrocnemius
S2, S3, S4	External anal sphincter

Table 1. Representative muscle groups innervated by the cervical, thoracic, lumbar, and sacral nerve roots.

3. EMG recording

3.1 Neuromuscular junction (NMJ) recording

Blockade of NMJ significantly attenuates motor activity. Short acting muscle relaxants may be used to facilitate intubation, but long acting muscle relaxants should be avoided. If pre-existing nerve root injury should be identified, succinylcholine, an NMJ blocking agent, is recommended to use. However, succinylcholine should not be used for patients with malignant hyperthermia (Minahan et al., 2000).

There are electrical stimulation techniques to monitor status of NMJ, and these are single twitch, train-of-four (TOF) twitch ratio, tetanus, post-tetanic stimulation, and pulse or double burst technique (Leppanen, 2008). TOF twitch ratio is routinely used during surgery. Electrical stimulation (stimulation frequency of 1 Hz, duration of 300~500 msec, and intensity of 10~40 mA) is delivered to a peripheral nerve 4 times, and 4 resulting compound muscle action potentials (CMAPs) are recorded. TOF is monitored from the thenar eminence following stimulation of the median nerve, the abductor pollicis brevis following stimulation of the ulnar nerve at the wrist, the tibialis anterior following stimulation of the peroneal nerve at the knee, or the abductor hallucis following stimulation of the posterior tibial nerve. It is recommended that TOF should be monitored in a muscle of the extremity where EMG activity is being monitored (Minahan et al., 2000; Leppanen, 2008). Four of four twitch ratio is obtained if less than 75% of NMJ is blocked. Three of four twitch ratio is obtained with 75% blockade, 2 of 4 with 80% blockade, and 1 of 4 with 90% blockade. No twitch is obtained if 100% of NMJ is blocked (Leppanen, 2008). It is not desirable to use muscle relaxants during surgical procedures where direct stimulation of pedicle screws and nerve roots are required (Minahan et al., 2000).

3.2 Free-run EMG

The dorsal and ventral roots spit into rootlets and minirootlets. The nerve root is susceptible to mechanical injury at the area that the split is present. The axons at this point are enclosed by a thin root sheath and cerebrospinal fluid meninges, but lack epineurim and perineurim. Hypovascularity at the junction of the proximal and middle 1/3 of the dorsal and ventral roots place nerve roots more susceptible to injury (Berthold et al., 1984). Intraoperative free-run EMG is utilized to detect motor nerve root compromise during decompression for spinal stenosis and spondylosis, correction of spinal deformity, radiculopathy secondary to disc herniation, and removal of tumor involving neural tissue in anterior and posterior surgical approaches (Holmes et al., 1993; Beatty et al., 1995; Maguire et al., 1995; Welch et al., 1997; Balzer et al., 1998; Toleikis et al., 2000; Bose et al., 2002; Chung et al., 2011).

To determine any pre-existing nerve root injury, baseline EMG recording is made before surgery starts. EMG recording is then made continuously throughout the surgical procedure. Pre-existing nerve root injury will be shown as spontaneous activity with low amplitude and periodic activity, whereas a normal free-run EMG response is absence of activity. If small amplitude, low frequency, or isolated discharge occurs at times which do not correlate with surgical manipulation of nerve roots, the EMG may not be pathologic. Mechanically elicited activity is characterized as polyphasic or a burst pattern consisting of single or nonrepetitive asynchronous potentials (Fig. 1A). Tonic or train activity consisting of multiple or repetitive synchronous discharges may last for several minutes (Fig. 1B). Burst potentials are associated with direct nerve trauma such as tugging, displacement, free irrigation, electrocautery, and application of soaked pledgets, but may not be associated with neural insult. Train activity is related to sustained traction and compression of nerve roots, and it is more associated with neural injury. When these patterns occur, the surgeon should be notified and corrective maneuver should occur. Audio and visual signal recognitions are available in most monitoring equipment. For communication with the operating surgeon, it is recommended to use audio signal through loud speakers for immediate feedback.

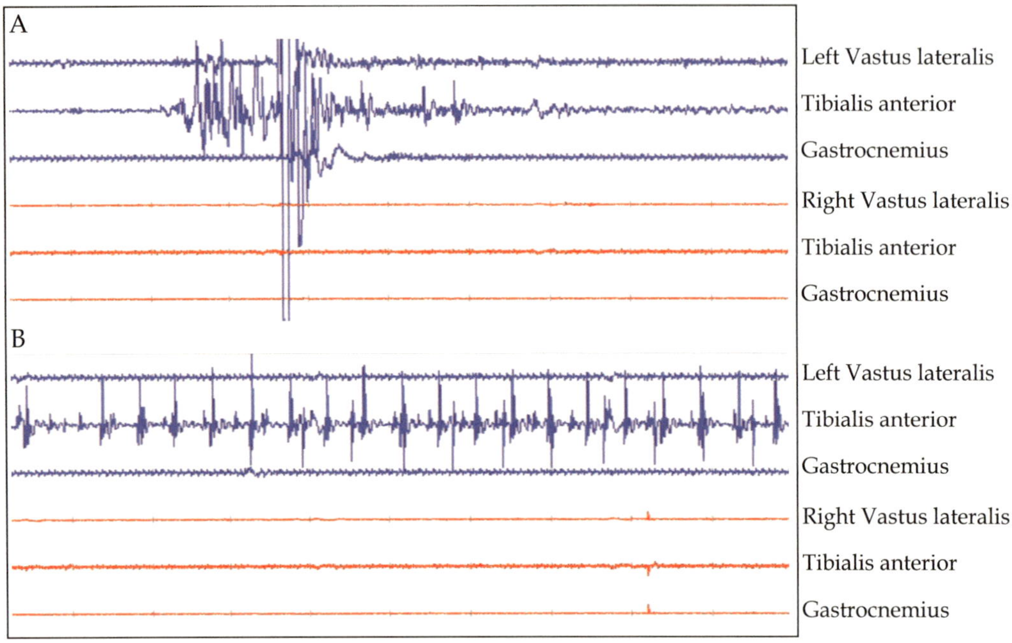

Fig. 1. Free-run EMG. EMG activity was recorded from the vastus lateralis, tibialis anterior, and gastrocnemius muscles during posterior spinal decompression. Bursts (A) and prolonged trains (B) of EMG activity are present in the left tibialis anterior muscle during decompression of nerve roots. Sensitivity 100 μV, time base 2 sec.

3.3 Stimulated EMG

3.3.1 Monitoring segmental motor nerve root function

Segmental nerve root monitoring involves monitoring of function of the motor unit axon. This is achieved by recording free-run and electrically stimulated EMG activity from the muscle fibers of the motor units. When EMG activity is recorded with needle electrodes, the activity recorded may be the result of activation of only a few motor units innervating that muscle. Other motor units may be activated, but this activation will go undetected because of the location of the recording electrodes. A monopolar EMG needle records the summated activity of 9 to 17 muscle fibers (Leppanen, 2008).

Motor nerve root stimulation technique is applied when motor axons and non-neural tissue (tumor, scar) should be identified and differentiated between motor and sensory roots. When scar tissue is present from previous surgical procedures, electrical stimulation can identify where the motor axons lie within the scar tissue. The direct nerve root stimulation technique is also used to determine a degree of decompression of compressed nerve roots. A nerve root is stimulated using an insulated ball-tip probe, and a reference needle electrode placed around the site of incision. The current (duration of 0.1 msec, frequency of 1-3 Hz) is gradually increased until stimulus evoked EMG responses or CMAPs are recorded from the muscle innervated by the nerve root. Stimulation threshold should not be greater than several milliamperes for uninjured motor nerve roots when neural tissue is directly stimulated. If tumor or scar is stimulated and threshold is greater than this value, viable neural tissue lies within the tumor or scar or no neural tissue is involved (Holland et al., 1998; Leppanen, 2008).

3.3.2 Evaluation of pedicle screws

3.3.2.1 Pedicle screw stimulation technique

Electrophysiological pedicle screw stimulation technique has been developed to assess whether the screws have been placed within the pedicle bone. The principle of the pedicle screw stimulation technique is that the electrical resistance of bone is higher than that of surrounding fluid and soft tissue. If an implanted pedicle screw is completely surrounded by bone, the screw is electrically shielded and electrical stimulation of the screw will fail to activate the nerve (Fig. 2A). However, if there is a breach in the medical wall of the pedicle, a low resistance pathway is formed between the screw and the adjacent tissue (Fig. 2B and C). Application of electrical current to the screw will result in stimulation of the nerve root and a subsequent muscle contraction, which is recorded as a CMAP. Constant current or constant voltage stimulations can be used, and constant current stimulation appears less variable than constant voltage stimulation. For direct screw stimulation, monopolar, cathodal, constant current stimulation (duration of 0.2 msec, frequency of 1~3 Hz) is delivered using an insulated ball-tip probe, and the anodal reference needle electrode is placed in or around the site of incision. The current is gradually increased until CMAPs are elicited (Leppanen, 2008).

3.3.2.2 Evaluation of lumbosacral pedicel screws

Spinal instrumentation technique with pedicle screws and rods has long been used correct spinal instability and deformity, for it provides rigidity for the vertebral motion segment. However, incorrect placement of screws results in considerable radicular pain or postoperative neurological deficits (Matsuzaki et al., 1990; West et al., 1991). Although intraoperative fluoroscopy or postoperative radiography guide screw placement, these image studies may not detect functional integrity of pedicle screws. For instance, pedicle screw stimulation technique was 93% sensitive, whereas radiography was 63% sensitive to detect drill bits and screws that had breached the cortex (Maguire et al., 1995). Pedicle screw stimulation could detect incorrect screw placement in 8 out of 90 patients that was not identified on radiograph (Glassman et al., 1995). With 102 pedicle screws placed in 18 patients, 7 mA was delivered to test correct placement of screws. Electrophysiological evidence of a perforation was seen in 13% of the patients, but palpation or visualization could not detect this perforation (Calancie et al., 1994).

It appears that there is close correlation between the intensity of screw stimulation to elicit CMAPs and the risk for neurological injury associated with the screw placement. A stimulation threshold of 10~15 mA was associated with adequate screw position in 512 pedicle screws implanted to 90 patients, but exploration of the pedicle was recommended. A stimulation threshold of greater than 15 mA indicated adequate screw position. A threshold of 5~10 mA was used as an indicator of abnormal thresholds (Glassman et al., 1995). With 3,409 pedicle screws placed in 662 patients, a threshold of 7~10 mA was associated with pedicle breach or a slight medial exposure of the screw. With threshold of 5~7 mA, there was a 58% likelihood that the screw should be removed and redirected. A stimulation threshold of less than 5 mA was associated with a significant cortical perforation and direct contact with a nerve root (Toleikis et al., 2000). A stimulus threshold of less than 6 mA correlated with misplaced drill bits and screws that breached the cortex in 144 screws and 95 drill bits tested in 29 patients (Maguire et al., 1995).

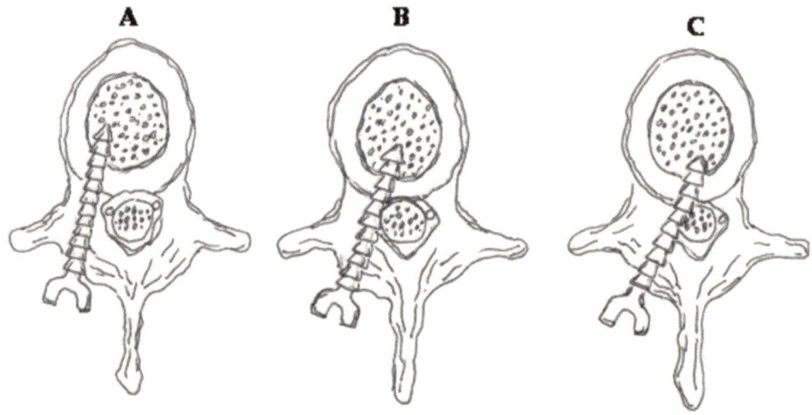

Fig. 2. Placement of pedicle screws. Screws are placed within the pedicle (A), close to the medical wall of the pedicle (B), or breach the cortex to make a direct contact with a nerve root (C).

Fig. 3 is a representative trace of CMAPs following stimulation of a pedicle screw. CMAPs were recorded mostly from the right vastus lateralis and tibialis anterior muscles with a stimulation threshold of 17 mA, indicating that the pedicle screw was placed securely within the pedicle bone.

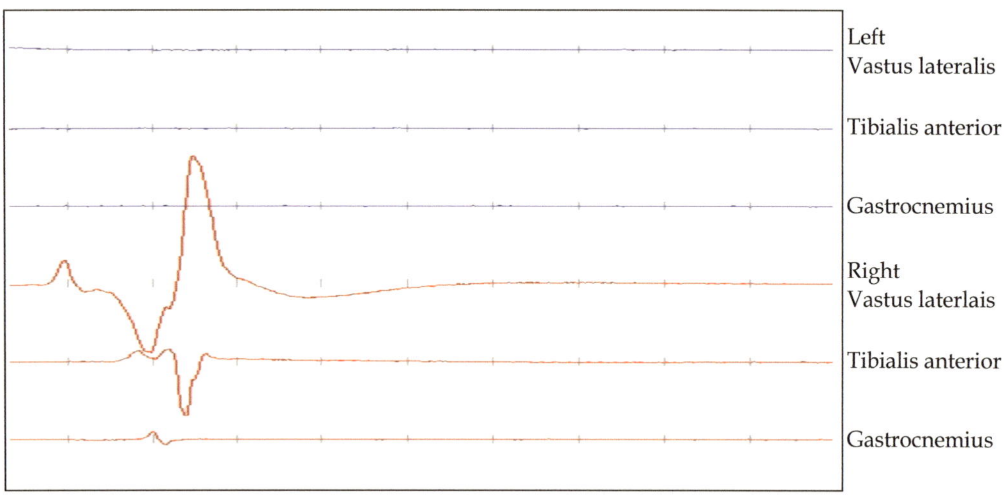

Fig. 3. CMAPs were elicited following electrical stimulation of the pedicle screw. EMG was recorded from the bilateral vastus lateralis, tibialis anterior, and gastrocnemius muscles. Current (duration of 0.2 msec, frequency of 1 Hz) was slowly increased to right L4 pedicle screw head via monopolar ball-tip probe. CMAPs were recorded mostly from the right vastus lateralis and tibialis anterior muscles at the current threshold of 17 mA. Sensitivity 200 μV, timebase 0.1 sec.

3.3.2.3 Evaluation of cervical pedicle screws

C5 nerve root palsy is most commonly attributed to direct nerve root injury secondary to manipulation or traction of the nerve root and a segmental spinal cord injury secondary to ischemia. Free-run EMG monitoring could detect potential injury to single nerve root (Fan et al., 2002; Bose et al., 2004; Hillbrand et al., 2004; Khan et al., 2006). Simulated EMG technique for posterior cervical screws is also a useful tool to guide screw placement. Djurasovic and colleagues (2005) tested the lateral mass and pedicle screws (122 lateral mass screws and 25 C7 pedicle screws) implanted in 26 patients. A stimulation threshold of 15 mA provided a 99% positive predictive value (89% sensitivity and 87% specificity) that the screw was within the lateral mass or pedicle. A stimulation threshold of 10~15 mA provided a 13% predictive value (66% sensitivity and 90% specificity) that the screw was within the lateral mass or pedicle. A stimulation threshold of less than 10 mA provided a 100% predictive value that the screw was malpositioned (70% sensitivity and 100% specificity).

3.3.2.4 Evaluation of thoracic pedicle screws

Placement of thoracic pedicle screws is a considerable technical challenge because of the smaller pedicle size (Cinotti et al., 1999). The risk of misplacement of screws in the thoracic spine ranged between 16% and 41% even with careful probing of the pedicle wall (Vaccaro et al., 1995; Xu et al., 1999). Simulation threshold values did not seem to reflect whether the screws were correctly positioned nor predict postoperative outcomes associated with the screw placement (Danesh-Clough et al., 2001). With 87 thoracic pedicle screws placed in 22 patients, 81 screws had a stimulus threshold >11 mA and 6 screws had thresholds ≤11 mA, of which 3 showed cortical breakthrough. However, new postoperative neurologic complications did not result in any of the 22 patients (Shi et al., 2003). Two hundred and nine thoracic pedicle screws were placed in 29 patients. Five of 6 screws penetrated cortical bone in one patient, but no new postoperative neurologic deficit, visceral injuries, or pedicle screw instrumentation failure was developed in this patient (Kuntz et al., 2004). Six hundred and seventy-seven thoracic pedicle screws were placed in 92 patients, and 27 screws had a stimulation threshold of <6.0 mA and 6 of 27 screws had medial wall perforations. There were no new postoperative neurologic deficits or radicular chest wall complaints (Raynor et al., 2002). One hundred and sixteen thoracic pedicle screws were placed in 7 patients. There were medical wall defects in 19 screws, and average stimulus thresholds of these pedicle screws were 19.8±5.3 mA. Eight of these 19 screws had thresholds 25~30 mA (Donohue et al., 2008).

4. Evoked potentials

Free-run and stimulated EMG can detect injury to neural tissue during surgical manipulations. However, the same technique fails to detect malpositioned thoracic pedicle screws and predict postoperative outcomes. Literature indicates that evoked potential monitoring assesses integrity of the spinal cord and nerve roots and improve clinical efficacy of EMG monitoring.

4.1 Somatosensory evoked potential (SSEPs) and recording technique

SSEP is an evoked response generated from nerve tracts and nuclei in the brain after peripheral nerve stimulation. Typically, the median or ulnar nerves at the wrist is stimulated to acquire SSEPs from the upper extremities and the posterior tibial nerve at the ankle or the peroneal nerve at the fibular head to acquire SSEPs from the lower extremities. The ascending sensory volley enters the spinal cord through dorsal nerve roots at several segmental levels and ascends to the sensory cortex. SSEPs are mediated by primarily through the dorsal column (Nuwer, 1999) or dorsal spinocerebellar tracts (York,

1985). SSEPs are used to assess the functional status of somatosensory pathways during surgical procedures which affect peripheral nerve or plexus (Prielipp et al., 1999; Chung et al., 2009), spinal cord (deformity correction, traumatic spinal fracture, tumor removal, Duffau, 2008), and brain (carotid endarterectomy, aneurysm repair, Friedman et al., 1991; Lam et al., 1991).

For upper extremity SSEP recordings, cortical (C3, C4 of the international 10-20 system, reference to Fz) and subcortical SSEPs (cervical spinous process, reference to Fz) are monitored upon alternate stimulation of the median or ulnar nerve at the wrist (stimulation intensity of ~20 mA, stimulation frequency of 3.1 Hz, stimulation duration of 0.5 msec) through surface electrodes (Fig. 4, left panel). For lower extremity SSEP recordings, cortical (Cz, reference to Fz) and subcortical SSEP (cervical spinous process, reference to Fz) are monitored upon alternate stimulation of the posterior tibial nerve at the ankle or peroneal nerve at the popliteal fossa (stimulation intensity of ~30 mA, stimulation frequency of

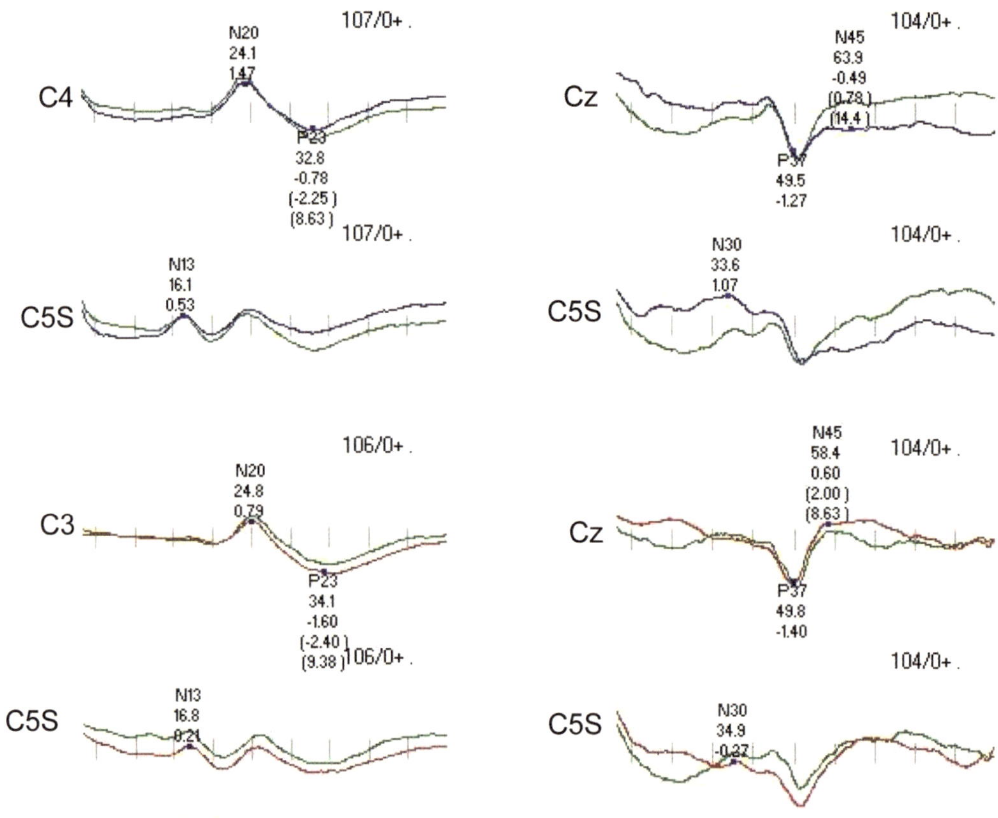

Fig. 4. Representative traces of SSEPs. Traces on the left column are upper-extremity SSEPs recorded from C3, C4 for cortical response and C5 spinous process for subcortical response following alternate stimulation of the ulnar nerve at the wrist (Timebase 50 msec). Lower-extremity SSEPs are shown in the right column. SSEPs were recorded from Cz and C5 spinous process following alternate stimulation of the posterior tibial nerve at the ankle (Timebase 100msec). The number of averaged samples, latency (msec), and amplitude (μV) are indicated in the trace. Parentheses indicate interpeak latency and interpeak amplitude.

3.1 Hz, a stimulation duration of 0.5 msec) through surface electrodes (Fig. 4, right panel). A few hundreds of samples (sampling rate of 8 kHz) are required to average to increase a signal-to-noise ratio. Signals were amplified (gain of 5,000~20,000) and filtered (LFF of 30 Hz, HFF of 300 Hz,). Impedance of electrodes should be ~5 KΩ. All of these electrical connections are grounded at patient's shoulder (Balzer et al., 1998; Chung et al., 2009).

4.2 Motor evoked potentials (MEPs) and recording technique

MEPs assess functional integrity of the anterolateral column of the spinal cord. MEPs provide information about long tract function, segmental interneurons, and anterior gray matter function. Epidural stimulation of the spinal cord and transcranial electrical (TES) or magnetic stimulation (TMS) of the motor cortex of the brain are the techniques used to obtain MEPs. TES is the most favorite technique utilized in the OR (McDonald, 2002, 2006). TES technique involves eliciting CMAPs after transcranial electrical stimulation of motor area at 1~2cm anterior to C3 and C4, referenced to C4 and C3 (Calalncie et al., 1998; Chung et al., 2011) or C1 and C2, reference to C2 and C1 (Bose et al., 2004; Drake et al., 2010). For electrical stimulation, an internal or external stimulator can be used. Some monitoring equipment has its own internal stimulator. An external cortical stimulator is also used for this purpose. Digitimer™ D185 Multipulse stimulator (Digitimer Ltd., Welwyn Garden City, UK) is the only FDA approved stimulator for this clinical use. It has capabilities to control inter-stimulation interval (ISI) and stimulation intensity up to 1,000 volts. Multipulse stimulation technique (4~6 repetitive stimulations and ISI of 1~2 msec) is usually applied (Calalncie et al., 1998; Bose et al., 2004; Drake et al., 2010; Chung et al., 2011). Stimulation thresholds range between a few hundreds and several hundreds of volts to elicit CMAPs depending on pathophysiological status of the spinal cord, depth of anesthesia, and bone thickness. Evoked CMAPs are recorded from the muscles of upper and lower extremities as indicated in Table 1.

Representative traces of MEPs are shown in Fig. 5. After TES, evoked CMAPs were recorded from the muscles of upper and lower extremities during placement of thoracic pedicle screws. Stable CMAPs were present in all the muscles during pedicle screw placement, and the patient did not develop new postoperative complication. We have been routinely testing MEPs during all cervical and thoracic spine surgery for the past over ten years, and the presence of stable MEPs is the most reliable indicator to assess cervical and thoracic spinal cord and nerve root function, instead of stimulation of mass and pedicle screws (Chung, unpublished data).

There are safety concerns to test MEPs for patients. High voltage transcranial electrical stimulation causes jaw movement, resulting in tong laceration and mandibular fracture in 0.2% of the patients undergoing TES. Bite blocks should be placed to prevent these complications. MEPs should not be tested for patients with pre-existing history of seizure, intracranial injury, or presence of intracranial metal implants (McDonald, 2002, 2006).

4.3 Dermatomal somatosensory evoked potentials (DSSEPs) and recording technique

Researchers have demonstrated that SSEPs increase specificity of EMG during lumbosacral (Holmes et al., 1993; Balzer et al., 1998; Chung, unpublished data) and anterior spine surgery (Chung et al., 2011). However, one can argue that SSEPs can not detect injury in a single nerve root because multiple nerve roots contribute to generate SSEPs. Dermatomal somatosensory evoked potentials (DSSEPs) are suggested to use when assessing function of individual nerve roots. Stimulation is achieved with paired patch paste skin electrode placed 3-4 cm apart at dermatomal sites such as L3 at anterior mid-thigh, L4 at medial

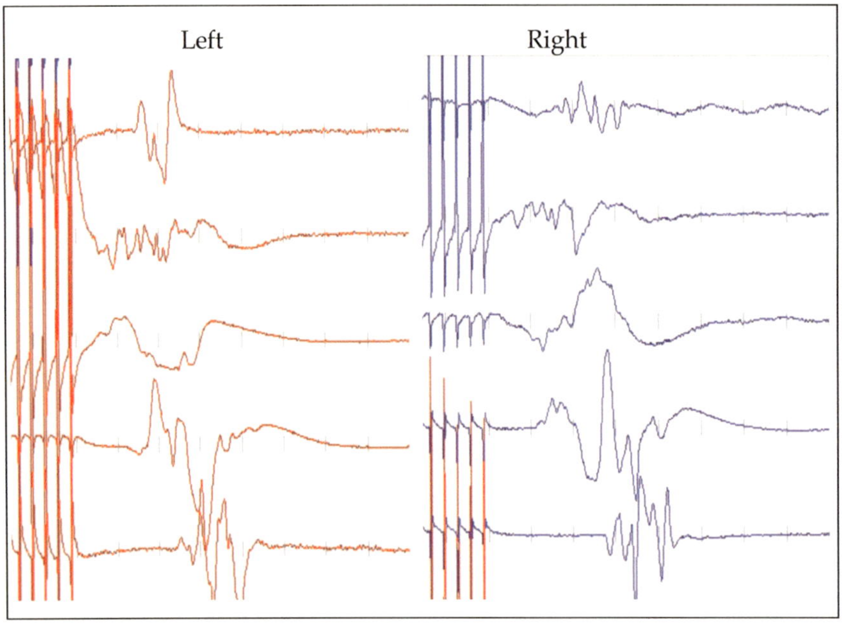

Fig. 5. MEPs were obtained after transcranial electrical stimulation (325V, ISI of 2 msec, 5 repetitive pulse trains). CMAPs were recorded from the abductor pollicis brevis/abductor digiti minimi, external anal sphincter, vastus laterlais, tibialis anterior/gastrocnemius, and abductor hallucis muscles bilaterally. Timebase 100 msec, 100msec, vertical scales 50-200 μV.

midcalf, L5 at the dorsum of the foot, and S1 at the lateral aspect of the foot. Responses are recorded from cervical spinous process. Recording parameters are stimulation intensity of ~40 mA, duration of 0.3 msec, frequency of 5.1 Hz, LFF of 30 Hz, and HFF of 1 KHz. Each trial usually consists of 500 samples (Tsai et al., 1997). Clinical efficacy of intraoperative DSSEPs appears controversial. DSSEPs are sensitive to detect nerve root compression and mechanical manipulation, but insensitive to nerve root decompression. DSSEPs can detect a misplaced pedicle screw only when the screw directly contacts and mechanically injures a nerve root (Toleikis, 1993). DSSEPs are difficult to record and often require averaging ~500 samples to increase a signal-to-noise ratio, indicating that DSSEPs can not detect mechanical insult immediately. Even with averaging more samples, Tsai and colleagues (1997) could obtain baseline in only 57.6% of the patients. Hence, it is suggested that DSSEPs may be an adjunct to improve the sensitivity and specificity for detecting individual nerve injury when free-run and/or stimulated EMG is concurrently recorded.

4.4 Clinical efficacy of SSEPs and MEPs

Research for over the past three decades supports that SSEPs can detect and prevent spinal cord injury in cervical and thoracic, lumbosacral spinal surgeries. No quadriplegia resulted in a group of 100 patients with SSEP monitoring, compared with 8 quadriplegic patients from a group of unmonitored 218 patients (Epstein et al., 1993). Five patients with persistent SSEP changes were associated with postoperative motor deficit among 20 patients undergoing cervical and thoracic intramedullary cervical cord tumor removal (Kearse et al., 1993). SSEPs could detect ischemia in 44 out of 210 patients undergoing anterior cervical surgery. With simultaneous monitoring of SSEPs and EMG during posterior lumbar spinal fusion, bursts and trains of EMG activity were associated with a concurrent decrease in amplitudes of SSEPs (Chung, unpublished data).

However, SSEPs may not be sensitive to predict postoperative clinical status in anterior cervical spine surgery. Significant SSEP amplitude changes were observed in 33 out of 191 patients, and 50% of the patients developed postoperative neurological deterioration in anterior and/or posterior cervical spinal surgery (May et al., 1996). In a study with 871 patients undergoing anterior cervical deformity surgery, 26 patients had significant SSEP changes, and only 5 patients had postoperative neurological deficit (Leung et al., 2005). In 508 patients undergoing anterior cervical discectomy and fusion (ACDF) with corpectomy, 8 patients had postoperative deficits with preserved SSEPs (Khan et al., 2006). Seven patients developed new postoperative neurological deficit with preserved SSEPs in 758 patients undergoing ACDF. SSEPs showed 35% sensitivity and 100% specificity to predict postoperative neurological functions (Chung et al., 2011). A retrospective study with 1,055 patients demonstrated that SSEPs had a sensitivity of 52% and a specificity of 100% to predict postoperative neurological status in cervical spine and spinal cord surgery (Kelleher et al., 2008). Quadriparesis and paraplegia still resulted in patients with preserved SSEPs in anterior cervical fusion (Ben-David et al., 1987; Bose et al., 2004; Smith et al., 2007; Taunt et al., 2005).

Simultaneous monitoring of SSEPs and MEPs has proven that MEP monitoring is more reliable than SSEP monitoring to predict postoperative motor deficits. Hillbrand and colleagues (2004) reported that 12 out of 427 patients undergoing cervical surgery had substantial or complete MEP loss. Ten patients restored MEPs with surgical intervention, and did not develop new postoperative deficit. Two patients with persistent MEP loss developed new postoperative motor weakness. This study claimed that MEP monitoring showed 100% sensitivity and 100% specificity to predict postoperative neurological status, whereas SSEP monitoring had 25% sensitivity and 100% specificity (Hillbrand et al, 2004). Six patients with persistent MEP loss had new postoperative deficits, whereas significant SSEP loss without MEP changes observed in 2 patients did not have postoperative deficit in 69 intracranial and spinal surgeries (Weinzierl et al., 2007). MEPs were also more sensitive than SSEPs for detection of ischemia. MEPs were lost due to fluctuating blood pressure, and an increase in the mean arterial pressure above 90 mmHg restored them in 1 patient, but SSEPs were preserved during the entire surgical course in this patient (Wee et al., 1989). MEPs were superior to SSEPs for detection and prediction of postoperative neurological status. Whereas MEPs showed 100% sensitivity and 77% specificity, SSEPs had 35% sensitivity and 100% specificity to predict postoperative neurological outcomes in 758 patients receiving ACDF (Chung et al., 2011).

5. Anesthesia

Although EMG is minimally sensitive to anesthesia, muscle relaxants should not be used during EMG recordings (Minahan et al., 2000). Evoked potentials, especially MEPs are highly sensitive to anesthesia, but monitoring was still feasible with propofol/fentanyl/nitrous oxide and partial neuromuscular blocking agents. In animal studies, inhalant anesthetics significantly increased onset latency and amplitudes of MEPs (Haghighi et al., 19990a, 1990b, 1996). Under general anesthesia with fentanyl/propofol/ nitrous oxide, 20% and 40~60% nitrous oxide attenuated MEPs by 40~60% and 50~70%, respectively (vanDongen et al., 1999), and 66% of nitrous oxide completely abolished MEPs

(Zentner & Ebner, 1989). Narcotics were also shown to depress MEPs. Following administration of equipotent intravenous bolus of fentanyl, alfentanil, or sufentanil, amplitudes of MEPs were decreased to 34%, 43%, and 53% of baseline values, respectively (Thees et al., 1999). Total intravenous anesthetic or TIVA technique comprising remifentanil with minimally depressive agents such as ketamine and etomidate improved MEP recordings (Ghaly et al., 1999, 2001). Compared with sufentanil or fentanyl, remifentanil infusion could always produce stable MEPs with faster emergence (Chung, unpublished data).

6. Conclusion

Free-run and stimulated EMG assesses spinal motor nerve roots and determines correct placement of hardware in cervical, thoracic, and lumbosacral spinal surgeries. Because SSEPs and MEPs provide additional information on functional integrity of the spinal cord and nerves, SSEPs and MEPs together with free-run and stimulated EMG should provide more accurate assessment of spinal cord and nerve function during spinal surgery.

7. References

Balzer, JR.; Rose, RD.; Welch, WC.; Sclabassi, RJ. (1998) Simultaneous somatosensory evoked potential and electromyographic recordings during lumbosacral decompression and instrumentation. *Neurosurgery* 42:1318-1324

Beatty, RM.; McGuire, P.; Moroney, JM.; Holladay, FP. (1995) Continuous intraoperative electromyographic recording during spinal surgery. *J Neurosurg* 82:401-405

Ben-David, B.; Haller, G.; Taylor, P. (1987) Anterior spinal fusion complicated by paraplegia. A case report of a false-negative somatosensory evoked potential. *Spine* 12:536-539

Berthold, CH.; Carlstedt, T.; Coeneliuson, O. 1984. Anatomy of the root at the central-peripheral transitional region, In: *Peripheral neuropathy,* Dyck PJ, Thomas PK, Lambert EH, Bunge R (Eds.), pp 156-170, W. B. Saunders, Philadelphia.

Bose, B.; Sestokas, AK.; Schwartz, DM. (2004) Neurophysiological monitoring of spinal cord function during instrumented anterior cervical fusion. *Spine J* 4:202-207

Bose, B.; Wierzbowski, LR.; Sestokas, AK. (2002) Neurophysiologic monitoring of spinal nerve root function during instrumented posterior lumbar spine surgery. *Spine* 27:1444-1450

Calancie, B.; Harris, W.; Broton, JG.; Alexeeva, N.; Green, BA. (1998) "Threshold-level" multipulse transcranial electrical stimulation of motor cortex for intraoperative monitoring of spinal motor tracts: description of method and comparison to somatosensory evoked potential monitoring. *J Neurosurg* 88:457-470

Calancie, B.; Madsen, P.; Lebwohl, N. Stimulus-evoked EMG (1994) monitoring during transpedicular lumbosacral spine instrumentation: Initial clinical results. *Spine (Phila Pa 1976)* 19:2780-2786

Chung, I.; Glow, JA.; Dimopoulos, V.; Walid, S.; Smisson, HF.; Johnston, KW., et al (2009) Upper-limb somatosensory evoked potential monitoring in lumbosacral spine surgery: a prognostic marker for position- ulnar nerve injury. *Spine J* 9:287-295

Chung, I.; Glow, JA.; Grigorian, AA.; Smisson, HF.; Johnston, KW.; Robinson, JS. (2011) Clinical efficacy of intraoperative somatosensory and motor evoked potential monitoring during anterior cervical discectomy and fusion (ACDF): A review of 758 cases. Submitted to *Global Spine J*

Cinotti, G.; Gumina, S.; Ripani, M.; Postacchini ,F. (1999) Pedicle instrumentation in the thoracic spine. A morphometric and cadaveric study for placement of screws. *Spine (Phila Pa 1976)* 15; 24:114-119

Danesh-Clough, T.; Taylor, P.; Hodgson, B.; Walton, M. (2001) The use of evoked EMG in detecting misplaced thoracolumbar pedicle screws. *Spine (Phila Pa 1976)* 26:1313-1316

Djurasovic, M.; Dimar, JR.; Glassman, SD.; Edmonds, HL.; Carreon, LY. (2005) A prospective analysis of Intraoperative electromyographic monitoring of posterior cervical screw fixation. *J Spinal Disord Tech* 18:515-518

Donohue, M.; Murtagh-Schaffer, C.; Basta, J.; Moquin, RR.; Bashir, A.; Calancie, B. (2008) Pulse-train stimulation for detecting medical malpositioning of thoracic pedicle screws. Spine 33:E378-385

Drake, J.; Zeller, R.; Kulkarni, AV.; Strantzas, S.; Holmes, L. (2010) Intraoperative neurophysiological monitoring during complex spinal deformity cases in pediatric patients: methodology, utility, prognostication, and outcome. *Childs Nerv Syst* 26:523-544

Duffau, H. (2008) Intraoperative neurophysiology during surgery for cerebral tumors, In: *Intraoperative monitoring of neural function,* Nuwer, MR. (Ed.), pp 491-507, Elsevier, ISBN 978-0-444-51824-8, ISBN 1567-4231, Amsterdam, The Netherlands

Epstein, NE.; Danto, J.; Nardi, D. (1993) Evaluation of intraoperative somatosensory-evoked potential monitoring during 100 cervical operations. *Spine* 18:737-747

Fan, D. & Schwartz, DM.(2002) Intraoperative neurophysiologic detection of iatrogenic C5 nerve root injury during laminectomy for cervical compression myelopathy. *Spine* 22:2499-2502

Friedman, WA.; Chadwick, GM.; Verhoeven, FJ.; Mahla, M.; Day, AL. (1991)Monitoring of somatosensory evoked potentials during surgery for middle cerebral artery aneurysms. *Neurosurgery* 29:83-88

Ghaly, RF.; Lee, JJ.; Ham, JH.; Stone, JL.; George, S.; Raccforte, P. (1999) Etomidate dose-response on somatosensory and transcranial magnetic induced spinal motor evoked potentials in primates. *Neurol Res* 21:714-720

Ghaly, RF.; Ham, JH.; Lee, JJ. (2001) High-dose ketamine hydrochloride maintains somatosensory and magnetic motor evoked potentials in primates. *Neurol Res* 23:881-886

Glassman, DS.; Dimar, JR.; Puno, RM.; Johnson, JR.; Shields, CB.; Linden, RD. (1995) A prospective analysis of Intraoperative electromyographic monitoring of pedicle screw placement with computed tomographic scan configuration. *Spine* 20:1375-1379

Haghighi, SS.; Green, KD.; Oro, JJ.; Drake, RK.; Kracke, GR. (1990) Depressive effect of isoflurane anesthesia on motor evoked potentials. *Neurosurgery* 26:993-997

Haghighi, SS.; Madsen, R.; Green, KD.; Oro JJ.; Kracke GR. (1990) Suppression of motor evoked potentials by inhalation anesthetics. *J Neurosurg Anesthesiol* 2:73-78

Haghighi, SS.; Sirintrapun, SJ.; Keller, BP.; Oro, JJ.; Madsen, R. (1996) Effect of desflurane anesthesia on transcortical motor evoked potentials. *J Neurosurg Anesthesiol* 8:47-51

Hillbrand, AS.; Schwartz DM.; Sethurman, V.; Vaccaro, AR.; Albert, TJ. (2004) Comparison of transcranial electric motor and somatosensory evoked potential monitoring during cervical spine surgery. *J Bone Joint Surg* 86:1248-1253

Holland, NR.; Lukaczyk, TA.; Kostuik, JP. (1998) A comparison of the stimulus thresholds required to evoke myogenic response from normal and chronically compressed nerve roots: implications for intraoperative testing during transpedicular instrumentation. *Spine* 23:224-227

Holmes, JT. & Chappuis, JL. (1993) Monitoring of lumbosacral nerve roots during spinal instrumentation. *Spine* 18:2059-2062

Kearse, LA, Jr.; Lopez-Bresnahan, M.; McPeck, K.; Tambe, V. (1993) Loss of somatosensory evoked potentials during intramedullary spinal cord surgery predicts postoperative neurologic deficits in motor function. *J Clin Anesth* 5:392-398

Kelleher, MO.; Tan, G.; Sarjeant, R.; Fehlings, MG. (2008) Predictive value of intraoperative neurophysiological monitoring during cervical spine surgery: a prospective analysis of 1055 consecutive patients. *J Neurosurg Spine* 8:215-221

Khan, MH.; Smith, PN.; Balzer, JR.; Crammond, D.; Welch, WC.; Gerszten, P. et al. (2006) Intraoperative somatosensory evoked potential monitoring during cervical spine corpectomy surgery: experience with 508 cases. *Spine* 15:E105-113

Kuntz, C,; Maher, C.; Levine, N.; Kurokawa, R. (2004) Prospective evaluation of thoracic pedicle screw placement using fluoroscopic imaging. *J Spinal Disord Tech* 17:206-214

Lam, AM.; Lam, AM.; Manninen, PH.; Ferguson, GG.; Nantau, W. (1991) Monitoring electrophysiologic function during carotid endarterectomy: a comparison of somatosensory evoked potentials and conventional electroencephalogram. *Anesthesiology* 75:15-21

Leppanen, RE. (2008) Intraoperative monitoring of segmental nerve root function with free-run and electrically triggered electromyography and spinal cord function with reflexes and F-responses. In: *Position Statement by American Society of Neurophysiological Monitoring*, pp 1-46

Leung, YL.; Grevitt, M.; Henderson, L.; Smith, J. (2005) Cord monitoring changes and segmental vessel ligation in the "at risk" cord during anterior spinal deformity surgery. *Spine* 30:1870-1874

Maguire, J.; Wallace, S.; Madiga, R.; Leppanen, R.; Draper, V. (1995) Evaluation of intrapedicular screw position using intraoperative evoked electromyography. *Spine* 20:1068-1074

May, DM.; Jones, SJ.; Crockard, A. (1996) Somatosensory evoked potential in cervical surgery: identification of pre- and intraoperative risk factors associated with neurological deterioration. *J Neurosurg* 85:566-573

Matsuzaki, H.; Toiyama, Y.; Matsumoto, F.; Hoshino, M.; Kiuchi, T.; Toriyama, S. (1990) Problems and solutions of pedicle screw plate fixation of lumbar spine. *Spine* 15:1159-1165

McDonald, DB. (2002) Safety of intraoperative transcranial electrical stimulation motor evoked potential monitoring. *J Clin Neurophysiol* 19:416-429

McDonald, DB. (2006) Intraoperative motor evoked potential monitoring: overview and update. *J Clin Neurophysiol* 20:347-377

Minahan, RE.; Riley, III LH.; Lukacyk, T.; Cohen, DB.; Kostuik, JP. (2000) The effect of neuromuscular blockade on pedicle screw stimulation thresholds. *Spine* 25:2526-2530

Naito, M.; Owen, JH.; Bridwell, KH.; Sugioka, Y. (1992) Effects of distraction on physiologic integrity of the spinal cord, spinal cord blood flow, and clinical status. *Spine* 17:1154-1158

Nuwer, MR. (1999) Spinal cord monitoring. *Muscle Nerve* 2:620-1630

Prielipp, RC.; Morell, RC.; Walker, FO.; Santos, CC.; Bennett, J.; Butterworth, J. (1999) Ulnar nerve pressure: influence of arm position and relationship to somatosensory evoked potentials. *Anesthesiology* 91:345-354

Raynor, BL.; Lenke, LG.; Kim, Y.; Hanson, DS.; Wilson-Holden, TJ.; Bridwell, KH., et al. (2002) Can triggered electromyograph thresholds predict safe thoracic pedicle screw placement? *Spine (Phila Pa 1976)* 27:2030-2035

Sebastián, C.; Raya, JP.; Ortega, M.; Olalla, E.; Lemos, V.; Romero, R. (1997) Intraoperative control by somatosensory evoked potentials in the treatment of cervical myeloradiculopathy. *Eur Spine J* 6:316-323

Shi, YB.; Binette, M.; Martin, WH.; Pearson, JM.; Hart, RA. (2003) Electrical stimulation of intraoperative evaluation of thoracic pedicle screw placement. *Spine* 28:595-601

Skinner, SA.; Transfeldt, EE.; Savik, K. (2008) Surface electrodes are not sufficient to detect neurotonic discharges: observations in a porcine model and clinical review of deltoid electromyographic monitoring using multiple electrodes. *J Clin Monit Comput* 22:131-139

Smith, PN.; Balzer, JR.; Khan, MH.; Davis, RA.; Crammond, D.; Welch, WC., et al. (2007) Intraoperative somatosensory evoked potential monitoring during anterior cervical discectomy and fusion in nonmyelopathic patients - a review of 1,039 cases. *Spine J* 7:83-87

Taunt, CJ.; Sidhu, KS.; Andrew, SA. (2005) Somatosensory evoked potential monitoring during anterior cervical discectomy and fusion. *Spine* 30:1970-1972

Tew, JM Jr. & Mayfield, FH. (1976) Complications of surgery of the anterior cervical spine. *Clin Neurosurg* 23:424-434

Thees, C.; Scheufler, KM.; Nadstawek, J.; Pechstein, U.; Hanisch, M.; Juntke, R., et al. (1999) Influence of fentanyl, alfentanil, and sufentanil on motor evoked potentials. *J Neurosurg Anesthesiol* 11:112-118

Thompson, JP. & Rowbotham, DJ. (1996) Remifentanil-an opioid for the 21st century. *Br J Anaesth* 76:341-343

Toleikis, JR.; Carlvin, AO.; Shapiro, DE.; Schafer, MF. (1993) The use of dermatomal evoked responses during surgical procedures that use intrapedicular fixation of the lumbosacral spine. *Spine* 18:2401-2407

Toleikis, JR.; Skelly, JP.; Carlvin, AO.; Toleikis, AC.; Bernard, TN.; Burkus, KJ., et al. (2000) The usefulness of electrical stimulation for assessing pedicle screw placements. *J Spinal Disorders* 13:283-289

Tsai, RYC.; Yang, R.; Nuwer MR.; Kanim, LEA.; Delamarter, RB.; Dawson EG. (1997) Intraoperative dermatomal evoked potential monitoring fails to predict outcome from lumbar decompression surgery. *Spine* 17:1970-1975

Ueta, T.; Owen, JH.; Sugioka, Y. (1992) Effects of compression on physiologic integrity of the spinal cord on circulation, and clinical status in four different directions of compression: posterior, anterior, circumferential, and lateral. *Spine* 17:S217-S226

Vaccaro, AR.; Rizzolo, SJ.; Balderston, RA.; Allardyce, TJ.; Garfin, SR.; Dolinskas, C., et al. (1995) Placement of pedicle screws in the thoracic spine. Part II: An anatomical and radiographic assessment. *J Bone Joint Surg Am* 77:1200-1206

van Dongen, EP.; ter Beek, HT.; Schepens, MA.; Morshuis, WJ.; de Boer, A.; Aarts, LP., et al. (1999) Effect of nitrous oxide on myogenic motor potentials evoked by a six pulse train of transcranial electrical stimuli: a possible monitor for aortic surgery. *Br J Anesth* 82:323-328

Wee, AS. & Ashley, RA. (1989) Cortical somatosensory evoked potentials during acute hemorrhagic hypotension. *Eur Neurol* 29:284-286

Weinzierl, MR.; Reinacher, P.; Gilsbach, JM.; Rohde, V. (2007) Combined motor and somatosensory evoked potentials for intraoperative monitoring: intra- and postoperative data in a series of 69 operations. *Neurosurg Rev* 30:109-116

Welch, WC.; Rose, RD.; Balzer, JR.; Jacobs, GB. (1997) Evaluation with evoked and spontaneous electromyography during lumbar instrumentation: a prospective study. *J Neurosurg* 87:397-402

West, JL III.; Ogilvie, JW.; Bradford, DS. (1991) Complications of the variable screw plate pedicle screw fixation. *Spine* 16:576-579

Xu, R.; Ebraheim, NA.; Shepherd, ME.; Yeasting, RA. (1999) Thoracic pedicle screw placement guided by computed tomographic measurements. *J Spinal Disord* 12:222-226

York, DH. (1985) Somatosensory evoked potentials in man: differentiation of spinal pathways responsible for conduction from forelimbs vs. hindlimb. *Prog Neurbiol* 25:1-25

Zentner, J. & Ebner, A. (1989) Nitrous oxide suppresses the electromyographic response evoked by electrical stimulation of the motor cortex. *Neurosurgery* 24:60-62

18

Combination of Transcranial Magnetic Stimulation with Electromyography and Electroencephalography: Application in Diagnosis of Neuropsychiatric Disorders

Faranak Farzan[1], Mera S. Barr[1],
Paul B. Fitzgerald[2] and Zafiris J. Daskalakis[1]
[1]*Centre for Addiction and Mental Health,*
University of Toronto, Toronto
[2]*Monash Alfred Psychiatry Research Centre,*
The Alfred and Monash University School of Psychology and Psychiatry, Melbourne
[1]*Canada*
[2]*Australia*

1. Introduction

Transcranial magnetic stimulation (TMS) is a non-invasive brain stimulation technique that allows for in vivo examination of cortical processes. In 1985, Barker et al. introduced TMS as a tool for investigating the functional state of the motor pathways in patients with neurological disorders as well as in healthy human subjects (Barker et al., 1985). It was shown that a single TMS pulse applied to the motor cortex could activate cortical tissues associated with the hand or leg muscles and this activation could elicit a motor evoked potential (MEP) at the periphery captured through electromyography (EMG) recordings. The amplitude, area, latency and duration of this TMS induced MEP could then be used to investigate the integrity of the corticospinal pathways and the activation threshold of human motor cortex. Since this discovery, the combination of single and multi-pulse TMS with peripheral EMG recordings has allowed for examining various other processes in the human motor cortex such as excitability, plasticity, cortico-cortical connectivity, as well as the interaction between excitatory and inhibitory cortical processes. The integration of EMG with TMS has, therefore, offered a valuable tool for assessment of pathological processes that underlie neurological and psychiatric disorders such as Parkinson's disease, dystonia, stroke, Alzheimer's disease, schizophrenia, and depression.

The combination of paired pulse TMS with EMG recordings, for example, permits altering the excitability of the motor cortex and observing the effect of this alteration on subsequent stimulation. In paired pulse TMS, the first TMS pulse (conditioning stimulus) inhibits or facilitates the MEP response to the second TMS pulse (test stimulus). The nature and the strength of this modulatory effect depend on the intensity of the conditioning stimulus and the latency (i.e. interstimulus interval (ISI)) at which it is delivered with respect to the test stimulus. It has been demonstrated that the TMS induced modulation of MEPs are selectivity impaired in several neurological conditions (e.g. schizophrenia, Alzheimer's disease) when compared to the measures obtained in the age- and sex-matched healthy subjects. In this regard, the TMS induced MEP modulation has been associated with the activation and interaction between specific inhibitory and excitatory mechanisms at the cortical level, which provides insight on the specific cortical processes that may underlie the neuropsychopathology of such disorders. However, evidence for the cortical origin of MEP modulation is relatively scarce and has often been collected from rather invasive procedures such as epidural recordings in patients with implanted electrodes and by demonstrating that MEP modulation is not due to the refractoriness of the corticospinal tract.

In recent years, it has become possible to combine TMS-EMG with simultaneous electroencephalography (EEG) recordings. The combination of TMS with EEG, however, has not been easy. Simultaneous EEG recording during TMS stimulation was previously unattainable because of the technological shortcomings of EEG amplifiers that would saturate for a long duration due to the large artifact produced by the magnetic stimulation. For example, application of a single TMS pulse would result in artifact lasting for several seconds after the pulse. Such long lasting artifact blocked the window of time during which neurophysiological processes such as cortical inhibition occur. Through advances in EEG amplifier technology, researchers have conducted series of studies to examine TMS paradigms in the motor cortex through simultaneous EEG and EMG recordings and in non-motor regions of the cortex through EEG recordings.

The integration of EEG recordings with TMS-EMG will generate important neurophysiological leads in both the healthy and diseased states. First, it allows for non-invasive examination of the origin and the mechanisms through which MEPs are modulated. For example, using the TMS-EEG technology we have recently examined the EEG substrate of the MEP modulation induced by the paired pulse paradigm long interval cortical inhibition (LICI). In LICI, a conditioning stimulus precedes the test stimulus by 100 ms and suppresses the amplitude of the MEP response to the test stimulus by about 50% (Daskalakis et al., 2002a; Valls-Sole et al., 1992), a processes which is thought to be mediated by the activity of cortical GABAergic inhibitory interneurons and more specifically the activation of $GABA_B$ receptors (McDonnell et al., 2006; Sanger et al., 2001). Through concurrently recording MEP and EEG responses, we were able to show that the LICI induced suppression of MEPs at the periphery is positively correlated with the suppression of cortical evoked potentials at the site of TMS stimulation, therefore, providing further evidence for the cortical origin of the MEP modulation in the LICI paradigm (Daskalakis et al., 2008).

A second advantage of online EEG recording is the possibility to evaluate the effects of electromagnetic induction on cortical oscillatory activity in order to identify the cortical oscillations that more closely underlie the TMS induced MEP generation and modulation. Indeed, we have recently demonstrated that following LICI application to the motor cortex, cortical oscillations in the frequency range of 1 Hz to 30 Hz are significantly suppressed, while higher frequencies (e.g. gamma oscillations (30-50 Hz)) are not affected (Farzan et al., 2009). Identifying the cortical oscillatory activities that underlie TMS induced MEP modulation may provide further insight into the neurophysiology of the human motor cortex and would be valuable in improving the diagnostic and therapeutic strategies in several neuropsychiatric disorders.

Furthermore, a major advantage of combined TMS-EMG and EEG is the possibility to evaluate the cortico-cortical connectivity between motor cortices. Functional connectivity between cortical regions (e.g. left and right motor cortices) can be more easily probed through measuring the propagation of TMS induced cortical responses across cortical mantles, as opposed to evaluating the modulation of the peripheral activity. In this regard, we have recently demonstrated that by monitoring the propagation of TMS induced cortical evoked potentials from the site of stimulation to the contralateral motor area, it may be possible to evaluate the extent of cross talk between the left and right motor areas in healthy subjects at rest (Voineskos et al., 2010). The propagation of TMS induced cortical activity can be also investigated during various motor tasks. Such cortical indices would be of great value in several clinical populations, first for understanding the underlying pathology, for example by comparing the topographical map of signal propagation in stroke patients compared to healthy subjects, and second for optimizing more individually tailored treatment approaches.

One of the most important features of the TMS-EEG combination, however, is the ability to study the neurophysiology of non-motor regions of the cortex where a peripheral response may not be available. For example, examining the modulatory effect of LICI in the prefrontal cortex would enhance our understanding of the inhibitory mechanisms in a cortical area that is more closely associated with the pathophysiology of psychiatric disorders such as schizophrenia and depression. Indeed, using TMS-EEG technology, we have been able to demonstrate selective differences between the modulations of gamma oscillations in the dorsolateral prefrontal (DLPFC) of patients with schizophrenia in comparison to both healthy subjects and patients with bipolar disorder (Farzan et al., 2010a). This is while no deficits were observed in the MEP modulation or modulation of the cortical oscillations in the motor cortex. Therefore, TMS-EEG-EMG combination offers the possibility to monitor subtle changes in the non-motor regions of the cortex which previously were not available through examinations of the peripheral responses.

In this chapter, we provide a brief overview of the past, present and the future status of the TMS-EMG-EEG research. First, we provide a description of the working principle of TMS. We proceed by introducing commonly used TMS-EMG paradigms while providing evidence for the cortical mechanisms that are thought to be involved in the generation and modulation of the TMS evoked MEPs in each TMS paradigm. Then, the way in which TMS-EMG and EEG can be integrated are described along with examples of recent findings which illustrate the validity, reliability and thus the power of combined measurements. Finally, we highlight the application of these techniques in healthy and diseased states, and conclude by briefly discussing the future directions for the TMS-EMG-EEG research.

2. Examining motor pathways through cortical stimulation

2.1 In vitro and animal studies

In vivo examination of the mammalian motor pathways can be traced back to electrical stimulation of the motor cortex of cats under anesthesia (Adrian & Moruzzi, 1939). In these studies, electric shocks were delivered to an exposed area of the cat motor cortex and the potential changes in the pyramidal tracts were recorded through thin wire electrodes inserted into the dorsal surface of the medulla (Adrian & Moruzzi, 1939). Such direct recordings from the pyramidal tracts demonstrated that the stimulation of the motor area results in an excitatory response followed by a period of complete inactivity of the pyramidal tract (Adrian & Moruzzi, 1939). In subsequent experiments, it was further shown that the excitatory response lasted up to 20 ms which was succeeded by a silent period that would last about 200 ms (Krnjevic et al., 1964). It was also shown that the repetitive application of electrical stimulation with a frequency of 5 to 10 pulses per second (i.e. 5-10 Hz) would prolong the duration of the inhibitory period (Adrian & Moruzzi, 1939), while at higher stimulation frequencies (e.g. 20-50 Hz) convulsive firing would be generated followed by even a longer period of inhibition. This long lasting inhibitory phase, which was unlikely to be a result of the refractory period that lasts only about 4 ms, was associated with activation of cortical GABAergic inhibitory interneurons (Krnjevic et al., 1964). Similarly, later in vitro stimulation of human neocortical slices demonstrated similar findings (McCormick, 1989). In this regard, the intracellular recordings from the human temporal lobe slices showed three distinct response phases: an initial fast excitatory post synaptic potential (EPSP) followed by a fast inhibitory post synaptic potential (IPSP) and finally a slow IPSP (McCormick, 1989). It has been suggested that glutamate may underlie the initial EPSP and pharmacological assessments have associated the fast inhibitory response with activation of $GABA_A$ receptors and the second slow acting response with activation of $GABA_B$ receptors (McCormick, 1989).

2.2 Cortical stimulation in humans

Transcranial electrical stimulation (TES) can be regarded as the first technique that permitted the focal stimulation of the human motor cortex by the placement of external electrodes on the scalp (Merton & Morton, 1980). In TES, the electrical stimulation is delivered through a set of two electrodes, one positioned over the motor cortex, and the other 4 cm anterior to the first electrode. Merton and Morton demonstrated that TES applied to the motor cortex through these electrodes could generate a MEP at the periphery that could be captured through EMG recordings. It has been suggested that the activation of cortex through TES is similar to the direct electrical stimulation of the exposed motor cortex of non-human primates (for a review see (Day et al., 1989)). However, TES is a painful procedure, owing to the dissipation of a significant amount of current over the skin before it reaches the brain tissue. For example, to evoke a peripheral response a capacitor that is charged up to 2000 V has to be discharged within a very short time of about 10 μs. As such, TES is mostly used to examine motor pathways in patients with spinal cord injuries and it is often administered during anesthesia. Since the introduction of TMS in 1985, it has now become possible to non-invasively examine the excitability of the motor pathways in awake healthy humans.

2.2.1 Working principles of TMS

Activation of neurons through TMS technique is based on the Faraday's law of induction of electric current via a time-varying magnetic field (Hallett, 2000). In TMS, a magnetic coil is placed tangential to the subject's scalp over the motor area, and intense time-varying current pulses of about 8 kA run though the coil. The time-varying current in the coil induces a time-varying magnetic field perpendicular to the plane of the coil, and hence the surface of brain tissue, which in turn induces an electric field parallel to the plane of the coil in the brain tissue. The duration of a single pulse TMS is typically within a range of 200 to 600 μs. Unlike TES, the induced magnetic field passes through skin, scalp and skull unimpeded, and as such, TMS is less painful than TES. The maximum magnetic field induced by a magnetic stimulator is about 2.5 Tesla which can induce electric field and tissue current of magnitude 500 volt/m and 15 mA/cm^2, respectively. Furthermore, the strength of the induced magnetic field falls exponentially with increasing distance from the surface. Thus, TMS activates the brain tissue in the outer most 2-2.5 cm.

Due to the horizontal orientation of TMS induced current in the cortex, TMS activates horizontally-oriented interneurons with a higher probability compared to the vertically-oriented pyramidal neurons. Therefore, focal TMS activates pyramidal neurons transynaptically, rather than at the axon of pyramidal tract neurons (Rothwell, 1997). For example, when the handle of the magnetic coil is pointed backward, approximately 45° to the mid-sagittal line, the induced current in the brain is perpendicular to the presumed direction of the central sulcus (Day et al., 1989). The indirect activation of pyramidal neurons by TMS is supported by epidural recordings of descending volleys following application of TMS and TES in patients who have spinal stimulators implanted in the epidural space. The results of epidural recordings have demonstrated that TES produces an early descending volley (referred to as direct wave or D-wave) which at a high intensity of stimulation is followed by indirect multiple waves (I-waves) that peak with a delay period of 1.5 ms from one another. By contrast, focal monophasic TMS results primarily in I-waves, and the number of these I-waves and their amplitude increase with the intensity of stimulation. It is reported that TMS may also generate a D-wave at very high intensities (Di Lazzaro et al., 1999b). D-wave and I-waves were originally observed following electrical stimulation of pyramidal tracts of cats. I-waves have been associated with the synaptic activation of pyramidal neurons through excitatory interneurons while D-waves are associated with a direct activation at the axon of pyramidal neurons (reviewed in (Ziemann & Rothwell, 2000)).

2.2.2 Factors affecting the TMS induced current

Several factors affect the depth and pattern of tissue activation and shape of the TMS induced MEP at the periphery. The geometry of the coil (e.g. circular, figure-8, double-cone, H-coil), the shape of the magnetic pulse generated by the coil (e.g. monophasic or biphasic pulse), and the type of material used to construct the core (e.g. solid-core or air-core) affect the characteristics of the induced current. In regards to the coil geometry, a figure-of-8 coil has a greater focality than a circular coil while the newer generations of deep coils, such as H-coil, have the greatest depth of stimulation. The shape of the induced current also varies between each coil type. For example, the induced electrical field is maximal under the rim of the circular coil, and the strength reduces in the centre, while in the figure-eight coil, the maximum field is in the centre of the coil at the junction of the two circular wings. In addition, biphasic TMS pulses are suggested to be more powerful than monophasic pulses and they generate a more complex pattern of neural activation (Di Lazzaro et al., 2001). Finally, solid-core coil are more efficient than air-core coils in transferring the electrical energy to magnetic field and as a result dissipate less heat. In addition to these parameters, the intensity of the pulse and the positioning of the coil affect the induced current and consequently the activation pattern. Consequently, by changing the intensity and the orientation of the coil different populations of neurons can be activated.

3. TMS combined with electromyography

TMS has been used for both therapeutic and diagnostic purposes (Rossini & Rossi, 2007). In relation to its diagnostic application, TMS-EMG provides a tool to assess the timing of cortical processes, cortico-cortical connectivity, cortical inhibition and facilitation, and the interaction between cortical processes (Anand & Hotson, 2002; Chen, 2004; Daskalakis et al., 2004; Di Lazzaro et al., 2004; Pascual-Leone et al., 2000; Sanger et al., 2001). In this section, several of these TMS paradigms will be discussed in more details, and wherever applicable, evidence supporting their neurophysiological mechanisms will be provided.

3.1 Motor threshold

Motor threshold is often determined by applying single pulse TMS to the motor cortex while the coil is placed at the optimal position for eliciting MEPs from a target muscle. The two muscles which are more easily accessible by TMS stimulation are the abductor pollicis brevis (APB) and the first dorsal interosseous (FDI) muscles. Resting motor threshold (RMT) for a target muscle can be determined through applying single pulse TMS to an area of the motor cortex that generates the largest MEP amplitude for the target muscle, and it is defined as the minimum stimulus intensity that can elicit an MEP of more than 50 μV in at least five out of ten trials in the target muscle (Rossini et al., 1994). It has been demonstrated that NMDA antagonists such as ketamine reduce motor threshold, the block of voltage-gated sodium channels increases motor threshold, and GABA has no influence on motor threshold (for a review refer to (Ziemann, 2004)).

3.2 Short interval cortical inhibition

In short interval cortical inhibition (SICI), a subthreshold conditioning stimulus delivered 1 to 5 ms prior to a suprathreshold test stimulus suppresses the MEP response to the test stimulus compared to the MEP response to a test stimulus delivered alone (Kujirai et al., 1993). It has been suggested that suppression of MEP occurs at the cortical level and is not due to the refractoriness of corticospinal tract (Di Lazzaro et al., 1998; Kujirai et al., 1993). For example, epidural recordings have shown that a preceding subthreshold stimulus that does not produce an I-wave by itself, suppresses the late I-waves of a suprathreshold stimulus that is delivered after 1 to 5 ms (Di Lazzaro et al., 1998). In addition, it was shown that magnetic conditioning stimulus did not suppress the response to an electrical test stimulus which activates the axon of the corticospinal tract (Kujirai et al., 1993). Finally, an electrical conditioning stimulus was less effective in suppressing the response to a magnetic test stimulus suggesting that the inhibition observed in SICI is not due to the refractoriness of corticospinal tract (Kujirai et al., 1993). SICI has been associated with the activity of $GABA_A$ receptor mediated inhibitory neurotransmission, as $GABA_A$ agonists such as lorazepam have been shown to enhance SICI as well as the suppression of the late I-waves (Di Lazzaro et al., 2000).

3.3 Intracortical facilitation

In this paradigm, a subthreshold conditioning stimulus delivered 7 to 20 ms prior to a test stimulus, facilitates the MEP response to the test stimulus (Kujirai et al., 1993). It has been suggested that intracortical facilitation (ICF) is an index of the excitability of the excitatory circuits in motor cortex (Ziemann et al., 1996). Pharmacological studies by Ziemann et al. demonstrated that some NMDA antagonists (such as dextrometorphan) and $GABA_A$ agonists (such as lorazepam) reduce ICF, while $GABA_B$ agonists (such as baclofen) increase ICF (Ziemann, 2004). The reduction of ICF by NMDA antagonist suggests that glutamate may play a role in mediating the cortical response observed in ICF.

3.4 Long interval cortical inhibition

In long interval cortical inhibition (LICI), a suprathreshold conditioning stimulus, delivered within 50 to 200 ms prior to a suprathreshold test stimulus, suppresses the response to the test stimulus compared to the response to the test stimulus delivered alone (Valls-Sole et al., 1992). Epidural recordings suggest that this suppression has a cortical origin at ISI of 100 to 200 ms (Chen et al., 1999; Di Lazzaro et al., 2002a; Nakamura et al., 1997). For example, it was shown that LICI at ISI of 100, 150 and 200 ms resulted in suppression of descending volleys, in particular the late I-waves (Chen et al., 1999; Di Lazzaro et al., 2002a; Nakamura et al., 1997). Several lines of evidence suggest that the LICI induced suppression of MEP responses is related to the activity of $GABA_B$ receptor mediated inhibitory neurotransmission ((McDonnell et al., 2006; Sanger et al., 2001); also reviewed in (Kapogiannis & Wassermann, 2008)). It has been suggested that in LICI, activation of the $GABA_B$ receptors by the conditioning stimulus, inhibits excitation of the motor cortex to the test stimulus that would have otherwise excited the cortex if delivered alone. The $GABA_B$ receptor activation is suggested to peak around 150 to 200 ms post stimulus (McCormick, 1989), and interestingly LICI is optimal when conditioning stimulus precedes the test stimulus by 100 to 150 ms (Sanger et al., 2001).

3.5 Cortical silent period

Cortical silent period (CSP) involves a transient suppression of EMG activity following delivery of a single suprathreshold TMS pulse to the motor cortex during voluntary contraction of the target muscle. Previous studies suggest that early part (i.e. first 50 ms) of CSP is due to spinal mechanism, while the later part is mediated by cortical inhibition (Chen et al., 1999; Inghilleri et al., 1993). Similar to LICI, CSP is also associated with $GABA_B$ receptor mediated inhibitory neurotransmission (Chen et al., 1999; Nakamura et al., 1997; Siebner et al., 1998; Werhahn et al., 1999). For example, Siebner et al. reported a significant prolongation of the CSP duration following a continuous intrathecal administration of baclofen in a patient with generalized dystonia (Siebner et al., 1998). Also, tiagabine, a GABA uptake inhibitor, was shown to enhance LICI and prolong CSP duration (Werhahn et al., 1999). Furthermore, administration of vigabatrin, a selective GABAergic drug that increases the availability of GABA in the brain, has also been shown to enhance LICI and CSP (Pierantozzi et al., 2004). In addition, we have recently shown a significant positive relationship between the suppression of MEP amplitudes in LICI (with an ISI of 100 ms), and the duration of the silent period in the CSP paradigm in healthy subjects (Farzan et al., 2010b).

3.6 Interhemispheric inhibition

Interhemispheric inhibition (IHI), also known as transcallosal inhibition, refers to a phenomenon in which a suprathreshold TMS pulse delivered to one hemisphere can inhibit the MEP response to a suprathreshold TMS pulse that is delivered within 6 to 50 ms to the opposite hemisphere (Ferbert et al., 1992; Gerloff et al., 1998). IHI is conventionally measured at an ISI of 6 to 12 ms, however MEP modulation at an ISI of 40 ms has also been demonstrated but suggested to be mediated by different mechanisms (Chen et al., 2003; Ni et al., 2009). By demonstrating the suppression of the late I-waves, epidural recordings have confirmed that IHI is mediated cortically and most likely through transcallosal pathways (Di Lazzaro et al., 1999a). Furthermore, it was shown that the magnetic conditioning stimulation of contralateral hemisphere did not significantly inhibit the response to an electrical test stimulus (Ferbert et al., 1992). Moreover, triple pulse TMS studies have demonstrated that IHI modulates the MEP response to SICI and LICI which, as previously described, are cortically mediated phenomenon, providing further evidence that IHI itself has a cortical origin (Daskalakis et al., 2002b). Moreover, recently a positive association was found between IHI and the integrity of callosal motor fibers (Wahl et al., 2007). The integrity of callosal motor fiber was examined through diffusion tensor imaging and by measuring the fractional anisotropy, a measure of white matter tract integrity. The results of this study suggest that TMS-EMG combination may also provide useful information about the integrity of the callosal motor fibers.

3.7 Sensory afferent inhibition

Sensory afferent inhibition (SAI) involves the modulation of motor cortex excitability by means of an afferent input produced by the electrical stimulation of digital or medial nerve at the wrist (Tokimura et al., 2000). In SAI, a preceding electrical stimulation of the peripheral nerve suppresses the MEP amplitude elicited by the application of a single pulse TMS to the contralateral motor cortex. There are two forms of SAIs that are suggested to be mediated by slightly different mechanisms: short latency SAI, and long latency SAI. Short SAI, which is investigated more thoroughly, occurs when the peripheral stimulation is delivered about 25 ms prior to the TMS pulse, while long SAI is observed when the sensory input is delivered about 200 ms prior to the TMS pulse. Comparison of TMS and TES and recordings of descending volleys suggest that SAI occurs at the cortical level (Tokimura et al., 2000). The molecular underpinnings of SAI are complex and SAI likely relates to an interaction between several neurotransmitter systems with the possible involvement of the cholinergic neurotransmission (Di Lazzaro et al., 2005; Di Lazzaro et al., 2007; Di Lazzaro et al., 1999c).

3.8 Repetitive TMS

It has been demonstrated that repetitive delivery of TMS pulses (rTMS) as well as repetitive application of TMS pulses paired with electrical peripheral nerve stimulation results in an MEP modulation which would outlast the duration of TMS delivery. Conventionally, rTMS is administered through application of TMS pulses at a frequency of 0.5 Hz (ISI of 2 s) to 50 Hz (ISI of 20 ms). It is thought that the repetitive administration of TMS pulses results in summation of TMS induced alteration of cortical activity, thereby causing an effect which may outlast the stimulation period (Chen et al., 1997; Pascual-Leone et al., 1994). The alteration of cortical activity by rTMS has been typically indexed as a suppression or potentiation of MEP responses to the standard single pulse TMS paradigm before and after an active rTMS session or sometimes by comparing the after effects of active versus sham rTMS. A few studies have also evaluated the effect of rTMS on intracortical inhibition by measuring the changes in CSP and MEP modulation by paired pulse TMS before and after rTMS administration (Daskalakis et al., 2006; Fitzgerald et al., 2004). The results of these studies have demonstrated that on average low frequency rTMS (< 5 Hz) applied to the motor cortex suppresses the MEP amplitudes for about 30 min following the end of the rTMS administration ((Chen et al., 1997); reviewed in (Fitzgerald et al., 2006)). The effect of fast frequency rTMS (> 5 Hz) has been shown to be the facilitation of the MEP amplitudes, however results have been somewhat inconsistent across laboratories (Daskalakis et al.,

2006; Fitzgerald et al., 2006; Maeda et al., 2000), perhaps suggestive of a biphasic effect of fast rTMS with a short period of increased excitability followed by a phase of increased inhibition.

It has been suggested that rTMS combined with EMG may be an effective tool for probing and modifying cortical plasticity. Neural plasticity, a mechanism thought to be critical for learning and memory, represents synaptic strength and the degree of signal transmission between coactive cells which can be weakened (long term depression, LTD) or strengthened (long term potentiation, LTP) in response to the presentation of a strong or weak synchronous synaptic stimulation. The lasting effect of rTMS, reflected through suppression and facilitation of TMS induced MEPs, has been suggestive of the potential value of TMS in probing and inducing LTP and LTD like plasticity in the cortex (reviewed in (Pell et al., 2010)). Owing to this lasting effect, application of rTMS to different brain regions may cause behavioural changes that would outlast the duration of rTMS stimulation (For a review refer to (Ridding & Rothwell, 2007)). This aspect of rTMS has been used to improve and restore functional impairments in several disorders such as stroke, movement disorders, addiction, cognitive as well as psychiatric disorders, with the most promising outcomes observed in the treatment of depression (for a review see (Slotema et al., 2010; Wassermann & Lisanby, 2001)).

Plasticity may also be induced through repeated presentation of a pair of somatosensory afferent stimulation and cortical simulation. This can be achieved through the TMS paradigm paired associative stimulation (PAS) which involves pairing of the peripheral electrical nerve stimulation and single pulse TMS of the contralateral motor cortex repeated at a frequency of 0.1 Hz (Classen et al., 2004; Stefan et al., 2002; Stefan et al., 2000). Choosing an appropriate ISI between peripheral and cortical stimulation (e.g. 25 ms), PAS has been shown to induce a potentiation of MEPs in the target muscle which would last about 40 min following the end of the stimulation (Tsuji & Rothwell, 2002). Moreover, pharmacological studies showed that NMDA antagonists suppressed the PAS induced MEP facilitation, while $GABA_A$ receptor antagonist had no effect (Stefan et al., 2002). Some experimental findings suggest that PAS induced effects have a cortical origin. First, following the PAS intervention and in the presence of facilitated MEPs, the F waves recorded from the median nerve stimulation reflected no change in the excitability of α- motor neurons of the median nerve (Stefan et al., 2002). Second, the MEPs evoked by the electrical stimulation of the brainstem remained unchanged following PAS intervention, while the MEP responses to single pulse TMS were increased compared to the baseline MEP responses (Stefan et al., 2000). These findings along with the transynaptic activation of pyramidal neurons by TMS suggest that PAS-induced MEP potentiation is likely mediated through transynaptic mechanisms in the motor cortex (Stefan et al., 2000), seemingly related to the associative (i.e. Hebbian) LTP of synaptic efficacy (Stefan et al., 2002). According to animal studies and in vitro recordings from neocortical slices, associative LTP occurs at an input to a postsynaptic cell which is conditioned by a synchronous activation of another input to that same cell (Buonomano & Merzenich, 1998). Given that PAS induced MEP potentiation is ISI-dependant, it is inferred that the PAS induced plasticity is likely due to the synchronous arrival of the somatosensory afferent input and the TMS induced activation of horizontally oriented interneurons in the sensorimotor cortex (Classen et al., 2004; Stefan et al., 2002; Stefan et al., 2000).

Recently, it was shown that the delivery of repetitive TMS through a protocol named theta burst stimulation (TBS) may be a more efficient way of altering cortical excitability and probing LTP and LTD like cortical responses (Huang et al., 2005). Theta burst stimulation involves application of 3 bursts of 50 Hz rTMS repeated every 200 ms either continuously for a total of 40 s, or intermittently (every 8 s) for a total of 3 min. The continuous (cTBS) and intermittent delivery of TBS (iTBS) have been shown to result in suppression and facilitation of cortical excitability, respectively, as indexed through suppression and facilitation of MEPs at the periphery (Huang et al., 2005). More importantly, it has been shown that despite the relatively short duration of TBS administration (40 s in cTBS and ~ 3 min in iTBS) compared to the conventional rTMS (~ 25 min), the alteration of cortical excitability by TBS can last for about 70 min which is more than twice as long as the duration of the after effects reported in the conventional rTMS approaches (Di Lazzaro et al., 2011; Thut & Pascual-Leone, 2010).

While the combination of TMS with EMG has been instrumental in assessment of several cortical processes, measuring the effect of cortical stimulation at the periphery has several limitations. First, and foremost and as the motor cortex is concerned, the exact mechanism underlying the generation and modulation of the TMS evoked MEPs remains unclear. While TMS-EMG studies in combination with epidural recordings and electrical stimulation can to some extent confirm the cortical origin of MEP responses, such recordings are invasive and only possible in specific subgroups of patients suffering from neurological disorders. To examine the cortical mechanisms involved in the generation of MEPs in healthy human subjects, therefore, a reliable non-invasive recording from the intact brain is desirable. In the next two sections, we will address how a direct but non-invasive recording of cortical activity would complement the conventional TMS-EMG measures.

4. Recording cortical activity in humans through electroencephalography

Recording electrical activity from the intact surface of mammalian cortex dates back to recordings from the dog's skull in 1870s and to the works of Richard Caton and Vladimir Pravdich-Neminski. Later in 1920s, Hans Berger recorded brain waves from the surface of human scalp and named the technique electroencephalography (EEG) (Buzsáki, 2006; Swartz & Goldensohn, 1998). To date, EEG is still the cheapest and the most widely used neurophysiological technique for measuring cortical local field potentials (Buzsáki, 2006). In EEG, electrical activity of the cerebral cortex is monitored by placing multiple electrodes on the scalp. While TMS induced MEPs, for example, are an outcome of an action potential generated by the activation of pyramidal neurons, cortical potentials recorded from the scalp are not a measure of action potential but they represent the activity of slow and fact acting EPSPs and IPSPs mostly originating from the surface of the cortex (Buzsáki, 2006). Cortical potentials recorded through EEG, therefore, represent the oscillatory activity of the underlying brain tissue. Comparison between monozygotic and dizygotic twins has revealed a high heritability for the temporal structure of amplitude fluctuations in EEG oscillations, implying that EEG may be a reliable neurophysiological technique (Linkenkaer-Hansen et al., 2007).

4.1 Generation and function role of cortical oscillations

While the typical firing rate of a motor unit does not exceed the frequency range of 6-35 Hz, neuronal tissues are capable of oscillating within a wide frequency band ranging from less than 1 Hz to as high as 600 Hz. The results of in vivo and in vitro recordings suggest that the brain generates finite number of discrete frequency bands which are conventionally categorized as delta (1-4 Hz), theta (4-7 Hz), alpha (8-12 Hz), beta (12-28 Hz) and gamma (30-50 Hz) oscillations (Buzsáki, 2006), with some recent experimental findings suggestive of the presence of slower (0.02 Hz to 1 Hz) and faster oscillations (up to 600 Hz) (Buzsáki, 2006). Several factors can affect the frequency of cortical oscillations in humans. In particular, the amplitude and frequency of cortical oscillations have been shown to vary between the mental states of sleep, resting, wakefulness, movement or engagement in complex cognitive functioning. Furthermore, it has been shown that each cortical region may have a specific frequency, with slower alpha oscillations observed more prominently over the posterior and parietal lobes and higher gamma frequencies predominant in the anterior region of the brain (i.e. prefrontal cortex)(Rosanova et al., 2009).

The exact mechanisms underlying the generation of cortical oscillations are not yet fully understood. It is suggested that the presence of various channels in the cell membrane provides neurons with intrinsic properties that allow them to oscillate at various frequencies (Buzsáki, 2006). There are several channels in the cell membrane of neurons through which ions move in and out of the cell. The state of these channels (i.e. open versus close state) is regulated by several mechanisms which are collectively referred to as gating. Four gating mechanisms have been identified: voltage gating, ligand gating, ion-dependent gating, and second-messenger gating. It is suggested that a change in the membrane voltage, release of neurotransmitters, or a change in the concentration of ions can change the state of membrane channels and give rise to an oscillatory activity (Buzsáki, 2006). It is further demonstrated that different population of neurons may selectively respond to inputs of different frequencies (Hutcheon & Yarom, 2000; Pike et al., 2000). For example, in hippocampus of rats, fast spiking GABAergic interneurons respond with highest temporal precision to frequencies in the gamma band, whereas pyramidal cells respond to lower frequency rhythmic inputs (Pike et al., 2000). Furthermore, it has been demonstrated that there may be an inverse relation between the size of the neuronal pool and the frequency of oscillations. That is, low frequency oscillations are generated by a larger population of neurons while higher frequency oscillations may be generated by a smaller number of neurons (Buzsáki, 2006).

The functional role of various cortical oscillations is currently under investigation. The functional role of slow frequency delta oscillations, which in healthy subjects are typically observed during deep sleep, is associated with learning and motivational processes (Knyazev, 2007). The cortical activity within the theta-band has been linked to memory functions, and emotional regulations (Knyazev, 2007). Alpha-band oscillations which are predominant during wakeful resting state are suggested to arise from cortical operations in the absence of sensory inputs, and also may reflect the disengagement of task-irrelevant brain areas (Palva & Palva, 2007). Cortical oscillations within the beta range are shown to be more dominant in the central region of the human cortex, suggestive of their functional role in movement execution and control. It has recently been hypothesized that the functional role of beta oscillations may be related to the maintenance of sensorimotor and cognitive state. That is, oscillations within beta band may be a signal for maintenance of status quo (Engel & Fries, 2010). Consistent with this view, it has been suggested that prolongation of beta oscillations may result in deterioration of flexible behaviour (Engel & Fries, 2010). Finally, the functional role of gamma oscillations has been more closely associated with cognitive control. In this regard, results of several EEG studies have found an association between the oscillataory acitivity in the gamma range and perceptual binding such as the construction of object representations, basic information processing such as sensory processing, and complex cognitive processes such as working memory (Buzsáki, 2006; Engel & Singer, 2001; Fries et al., 2007; Howard et al., 2003; Tallon-Baudry & Bertrand, 1999; Tallon-Baudry et al., 1996; Tallon-Baudry et al., 1998).

Recordings of brain activity through EEG suggest that cortical potentials are a result of summation of different oscillatory activities. Several theories and experimental findings exist to explain why different oscillations may be active at the same time. It has been hypothesized that presence of various oscillations may provide the brain with the ability to function through multiple time scales (Buzsáki, 2006). For example, it has been proposed that different frequencies (e.g. slow versus fast oscillations) may favor different types of computation or different level of connectivity. Based on experimental findings, it was hypothesized that middle-frequency oscillations, such as theta and alpha, may represent top-down processes, while high frequency oscillations, such as gamma, may be related to bottom-up processes (von Stein et al., 2000). Furthermore, the interaction between frequency bands has been proposed to be an essential mechanism for optimal information processing (Roopun et al., 2008). One form of frequency-band interaction is frequency concatenation (Roopun et al., 2008). In this regard, two local networks that are co-activated and oscillate at two different frequency bands may interact and generate a third frequency of oscillations. The period of the new oscillation is the concatenation sum of the original two (Roopun et al., 2008). Another form of frequency-band interaction is nesting. In nesting, phase of a lower frequency band (e.g. theta) may modulate the amplitude of a higher frequency band (e.g. gamma). The theta modulation of gamma oscillations has been observed in the hippocampus ((Bragin et al., 1995); reviewed in (Roopun et al., 2008)). The oscillatory modulation of neuronal responses is suggested to play a key role in information processing perhaps by providing a temporal frame with respect to which neurons may communicate with each other (Fries et al., 2007).

4.2 Cortical oscillations in the motor cortex

The presence of beta oscillations over the precentral region was first reported by Jasper and Andrews EEG recordings from healthy human subjects in 1938 (Jasper and Andrews 1938). It is believed that beta frequency can be further subdivided into narrower frequency bands of low- (12-15 Hz), mid- (15-18 Hz) and high-range (18-30 Hz) beta oscillations, each subserving a distinct functional mechanism. A number of previous studies have attempted to explore the cortical correlate of the EMG signals in order to examine the connectivity between the peripheral muscle and the homologous motor area. This has been typically achieved through computing the coherence between the cortical oscillations measured from the motor cortex through EEG or magnetoencephalography and the EMG recordings from the corresponding peripheral muscle often obtained during voluntary isometric hand contraction (for a review see (Mima & Hallett, 1999)). The findings of these cortico-peripheral coherence studies suggest that beta oscillatory activity in the contralateral motor cortex may underlie the generation of EMG signals in the corresponding body part (Brown et al., 1998). For example, tonic hand muscle contraction has been shown to induce beta oscillations (~15-30 Hz) in the contralateral hemisphere which are coherent with the EMG recordings at the periphery (Brown et al., 1998; Salenius et al., 1997).

The modulation of cortical oscillatory activity before, during and after motor task execution, imagination and observation has been well documented. Several studies have reported on desynchronization of alpha and beta oscillations prior to self-paced hand or finger movement often measured through C3 EEG electrode in the left hemisphere and C4 in the right hemisphere (Pfurtscheller et al., 2000). Following self-paced hand movement, desynchronization of alpha oscillations are observed over the contralateral motor cortex (Pineda, 2005) while beta oscillations (~14-32 Hz) are induced shortly (within one second) after the movement termination (Pfurtscheller et al., 2000). Observation and imagination of motor movement also result in suppression of alpha oscillations in motor areas corresponding to that body part (Pfurtscheller et al., 2000). Furthermore, the peak frequency of the induced beta oscillations may differ between motor areas associated with different body parts. For example, hand movement was shown to induce an oscillatory activity within a frequency range of 16-22 Hz over the hand area, while slightly higher frequency oscillatory activity (19-26 Hz) were recorded in the foot area following foot movement (Neuper & Pfurtscheller, 2001).

The combination of TMS with EMG has offered the possibility to trigger and quantify the magnitude of an involuntary movement, and evoke or slow down activation of a target muscle. As previously described, this is achieved through transynaptic manipulation of corticospinal pathway through application of TMS to the motor area that optimally represents the target muscle on the periphery. However, the specific cortical oscillations that underlie these TMS induced motor responses cannot be clearly identified through only EMG recordings. In the following section, it will be demonstrated that combination of online EEG recording with TMS-EMG would permit examining the functional role of cortical oscillations in each TMS paradigm. The advancement in the EEG amplifier technology that has led to the combination of these modalities will be first briefly described.

5. Combining TMS-EMG with concurrent EEG recording

Simultaneous EEG recording during TMS stimulation was previously unattainable because of the technological shortcomings of EEG amplifiers that would saturate for a long duration due to the large artifact produced by the magnetic stimulation. For example, application of a single monophasic TMS pulse would result in artifact lasting for several seconds after the pulse. Such long lasting artifact blocked the window of time during which neurophysiological processes such as cortical inhibition occur (the first 250 ms following TMS). The newer generation of EEG systems, however, can recover from the TMS artifact within a time window of 10 to 70 ms.

The newer generations of EEG systems offer several strategies to minimize the saturation of amplifiers following TMS. In a majority of TMS-EEG systems, the saturation of EEG amplifiers is avoided by virtue of a sample and hold circuit that pins the amplifier output to a constant level starting from a few milliseconds prior to the TMS application to a few milliseconds after the pulse (Nexstim Ltd., Helsinki, Finland). Some systems are equipped with a magnetic shielding technology in which the EEG electrodes and the amplifiers are shielded from the magnetic artifact (Advanced Neuro Technology, Enschede, Netherland). It is also possible to minimize amplifier saturation and the TMS related artifact through a combination of a wide dynamic range (e.g. recording potentials ranging from -200 to 200 mV in amplitude and with a resolution much lower than 1 μV), high frequency sampling rate (e.g. 20 KHz) and DC filtering (NeuroScan, Compumedics, USA). By employing any of the above strategies, EEG recording can become TMS compatible. Therefore, it is possible to continuously record EEG during TMS stimulation (for a review refer to (Ilmoniemi & Kicic, 2009)).

5.1 Single pulse TMS

Ilmoniemi and colleagues were one of the first research groups that used the interleaved TMS-EEG technique to investigate the effect of TMS on cortical excitability (Ilmoniemi et al., 1997). It was demonstrated that TMS applied to the hand representation area of the human motor cortex elicited a cortical response that spread to the adjacent ipsilateral area as well as to the homologous regions in the opposite hemisphere. It was further shown that the application of TMS to the visual cortex resulted in similar pattern of signal propagation to the contralateral areas, therefore providing evidence that the cortical potentials following motor cortex stimulation were less likely to be a result of peripheral sensory activation. This original experiment resulted in a series of studies that further characterized the EEG substrate of cortical excitability, plasticity and connectivity in healthy subjects (Esser et al., 2006; Kahkonen et al., 2001; Kahkonen et al., 2003; Komssi et al., 2002; Komssi & Kahkonen, 2006; Nikulin et al., 2003; Paus et al., 2001; Thut et al., 2003).

In a number of previous studies it was demonstrated that single pulse TMS applied to the motor cortex generated several EEG peaks within the first 300 ms of TMS stimulation. The EEG components that are commonly replicated across TMS-EEG studies are a negativity at 15 ms (N15), a positivity at 30 ms (P30) followed by N45, P55, N100, P180, and N280 (Komssi & Kahkonen, 2006). Comparing these EEG peaks with the size of MEP responses may permit examining the cortical origin of the TMS induced MEPs. In this regard, it has been shown that TMS induced MEP amplitudes positively correlate with the amplitude of the TMS induced early evoked potential, measured as the peak-to-peak amplitude of the N15-P30 component (Maki & Ilmoniemi, 2010b). In a study by the same group, the relationship between the TMS induced MEPs and the cortical oscillatory activity was explored. It was shown that in the motor cortex, the power of mid-range beta oscillatory activity (12-18 Hz) was weaker before large MEPs as compared to smaller MEPs. Furthermore, the phase of the mid-range beta oscillations recorded over the occipital cortex correlated with the MEP amplitudes (Maki & Ilmoniemi, 2010a). Similarly, Schutter and Hortensius examined the association between cortical oscillatory activity and MEP amplitudes during isometric hand contraction. It was reported that MEP amplitudes could be modeled by the activity of theta (4-7 Hz) and beta (13-30 Hz) cortical oscillations in the right and left primary motor cortex (Schutter & Hortensius, 2011). These authors went a step further and applied this finding to selectively control the therapeutic outcome of transcranial alternative current stimulation (tACS) (for detailed description of tACS readers may refer to (Kanai et al., 2008)). In this experiment, they applied the tACS with two different frequency settings of theta-beta and alpha-alpha configuration which were administered on two separate days. It was shown that the theta-beta tACS significantly increased cortical excitability compared to the alpha-alpha stimulation (Schutter & Hortensius, 2011).

A few studies have also examined the inhibitory components of TMS induced cortical potential. For example, Nikulin et al. demonstrated that following visually triggered hand movement, the N100 component of EEG response was suppressed while the MEP amplitudes were increased (Nikulin et al., 2003). This inverse relationship between the amplitudes of N100 and MEP is thought to reflect the inhibitory nature of N100. Consistent with this finding, the duration of silent period in the CSP paradigm was shown to be positively correlated with the amplitude of the N100 component (Kimiskidis et al., 2008). Interestingly, in a TMS study that investigated the effect of alcohol on TMS evoked cortical potentials, it was shown that following alcohol intake, which is thought to affect the activity of GABAergic neurotransmission, the amplitude of N100 response to single pulse TMS was significantly decreased (Kahkonen & Wilenius, 2007). Finally, the effect of age, TMS intensity, sensory attention and response preparation on TMS induced N100 response was investigated in a TMS study conducted in motor cortex of healthy children within an age range of 6-10 years. It was shown that N100 response was attenuated following a task that required a fast response, providing further evidence that N100 was likely related to an inhibitory process (Bender et al., 2005). In addition, N100 response was reported to be larger in children compared to N100 responses of adults in previous studies and a negative correlation was found between N100 response and age in children, suggesting that N100 response may undergo maturation (Bender et al., 2005). Collectively, these findings suggest that GABAergic inhibitory mechanism may underlie the N100 generation. If proved a reliable measure, N100 may be used as a marker for investigating the integrity of the inhibitory responses in healthy and pathological conditions.

5.2 Paired Pulse TMS

5.2.1 Short interval cortical inhibition and intracortical facilitation

One of the first studies evaluating the modulatory effect of paired pulse TMS on cortical evoked potentials is the experiments conducted by Paus et al. (Paus et al., 2001). In this study, SICI and ICF paired pulse paradigms were applied to the left motor cortex of healthy subjects and the amplitude and frequency of EEG responses were compared between single and paired pulse conditions. In this study, three prominent EEG peaks were observed following the singe pulse TMS: N45, P55 and N100. Furthermore, it was shown that single pulse TMS resulted in synchronization of beta oscillations which lasted for several hundred milliseconds after the TMS delivery. Following the ICF paired pulse paradigm, which as discussed before is designed to examine intracortical facilitation, the presence of a subthreshold conditioning stimulus (at an ISI of 12 ms) significantly reduced the amplitude of the EEG N45 component. In addition, the beta oscillatory activity that was recorded following ICF was reported to be smaller as compared to the oscillatory activity following the single pulse condition. By contrast, a conditioning stimulus delivered at an ISI of 3 ms (SICI paradigm) had no effect on either the N45 or beta oscillatory activity.

In a recent study, similar paired pulse experiments were conducted to further confirm and expand the above mentioned findings (Ferreri et al., 2010). In this study, SICI (ISI of 3 ms) and ICF (ISI of 11 ms) paradigms were applied to the left motor cortex of healthy subjects. Several EEG components were observed following single pulse TMS including: N7, P13, N18, P30, N44, P60, N100, P190 and N280. These EEG components were further identified for each stimulation condition and each EEG electrode (19 electrodes). The authors then examined the correlation between the MEP amplitudes and the amplitude of each EEG components in each electrode, after the three TMS conditions of suprathreshold single pulse and the paired pulse conditions of SICI and ICF. It was observed that depending on the stimulation condition (single pulse, SICI or ICF), MEP amplitudes correlated with different EEG components and at a different cortical region. For example, a positive correlation was observed between the MEP amplitude and the P30 component over the non-stimulated motor cortex following the single pulse condition and in the F4 (contralateral prefrontal cortex) following the paired pulse condition. Moreover, N44 peak was attenuated in the contralateral cortex more prominently in the ICF condition, a finding consistent with the earlier report of attenuation of N45 flowing ICF (ISI of 12 ms) as described above (Paus et al., 2001). Furthermore, it was noted that the N100 component was strongest over the stimulation area (C3 electrode) and its amplitude was larger following the paired pulse conditions as compared to the single pulse condition. Collectively these findings suggest that TMS-EEG offers the possibility to examine not only the MEP-EEG relationship but also the connectivity between cortical regions as it may be evident by comparing the TMS induced EEG activity at the stimulation site with the EEG components recorded in the remaining electrodes.

5.2.2 Long interval cortical inhibition

As briefly described in the introduction, the cortical correlate of LICI has been recently investigated through the combination of TMS-EMG with simultaneous EEG recording. That is, we demonstrated that EMG measures of LICI, measured as the suppression of MEPs in the paired pulse condition compared to the single pulse conditions, were positively correlated with the suppression of the cortical evoked potentials at the site of stimulation (C3 electrode) in the paired pulse condition compared to the single pulse conditions (Daskalakis et al., 2008). In this study, however, instead of examining the peak-to-peak amplitude of EEG components separately, the TMS induced cortical response was identified as the area under the rectified EEG response following the single and paired pulse conditions within the time window of 50 ms (the earliest reliable recording without TMS artifact) to 150 ms (the maximum peak of $GABA_B$ receptor activation). Similarly, the potentiation of MEP response was also examined by comparing the area under the rectified MEP response between the single and paired pulse condition.

Furthermore, in a separate study we found a positive correlation between the duration of the silent period indexed through the CSP paradigm and the extent of EEG and EMG suppression following LICI in a subset of subjects who received both LICI and CSP in their left motor cortex (Farzan et al., 2010b). A key observation was that the silent period seemed to be more strongly correlated with the EEG measures of LICI as compared to the EMG measures of LICI (Farzan et al., 2010b). This observation suggests that EEG measures of LICI maybe a more precise technique for evaluating and comparing the cortical mechanisms that may be common across TMS-EMG paradigms. For instance, it has been suggested that the early (< 50 ms) part of the silent period in the CSP paradigm may originate from spinal mechanism (Chen et al., 1999; Inghilleri et al., 1993). Therefore, by comparing CSP with both EEG and EMG measures of LICI (and other paired pulse paradigms), it may be possible to approximate to what degree each of these paradigms originate from the cortical rather than spinal mechanisms and also to what extent they are mediated by similar processes.

Furthermore, using the above methods, for the first time we examined the modulatory effect of LICI in the DLPFC, a non-motor region of the cortex which is implicated in a number of neurological and psychiatric illnesses (Daskalakis et al., 2008). We were able to show that similar to the motor cortex, LICI applied over the left DLPFC resulted in significant suppression of cortical evoked potentials (30% suppression) in the vicinity of TMS application (i.e. AF3 electrode). However, it was also shown that the extent of EEG suppression following LICI in the DLPFC was not correlated with the EEG or EMG suppression following the application of LICI to the motor cortex (Farzan et al., 2010b), a finding which may further reflect the valuable integration of EEG and paired pulse TMS which allow us to both measure and compare the neurophysiology of motor and non-motor regions of the cortex.

In line with this view, we also examined the effect of LICI on cortical oscillatory activity at the site of TMS stimulation following the LICI application in both the motor cortex and the

DLPFC (Farzan et al., 2009). Interestingly, it was observed that LICI applied over the motor cortex had a different modulatory effect on the cortical oscillations as compared to the LICI applied to the DLPFC (Farzan et al., 2009). In the motor cortex, delta, theta and alpha oscillations were suppressed without any suppression of beta and gamma oscillations. By contrast, all cortical oscillations were significantly suppressed following the application of LICI to the left DLPFC. The differential effect of LICI on fast cortical oscillations (e.g. gamma oscillations) in the prefrontal and motor cortices provides more insight about the functional roles of these cortical oscillations in each cortical mantel.

5.2.3 Interhemispheric inhibition

Through TMS-EEG it is possible to examine the correlation between functional and structural interhemispheric connectivity in both motor and non-motor regions of the cortex. This is possible through application of suprathreshold single pulse TMS to one hemisphere and examining the propagation of TMS induced cortical evoked activity to the contralateral hemisphere, a cortical process which we suggest may be mediated by similar mechanisms that underlie MEP suppression observed in the conventional IHI paradigm (Voineskos et al., 2010). Using TMS-EEG and diffusion tensor imagining, we investigated the extent of interhemispheric signal propagation from the stimulated site to the contralateral hemisphere as a function of integrity of callosal fibers (Voineskos et al., 2010). We showed that following suprathreshold TMS applied to the left motor cortex, the amount of cortical evoked activity that reached the contralateral hemisphere was inversely correlated with the integrity of callosal motor fibers but not with the integrity of anterior callosal fibers, suggesting an anatomically specific structural-functional relationship. Similarly, we found an anatomically-specific relationship between the extent of interhemispheric propagation of TMS-induced cortical activity from the left DLPFC to the right DLPFC and the fractional anisotropy of anterior callosal fibers (genu) connecting left and right DLPFC, and not with the integrity of callosal motor fibers. That is, in subjects that fractional anisotropy of callosal motor fibers was larger, the propagation of suprathreshold TMS induced activity to the contralateral motor cortex was of smaller magnitude, and in subjects that fractional anisotropy of genu fibers was larger, the extent of propagation of suprathreshold TMS induced activity to the contralateral DLPFC was of a smaller value. These results collectively suggest that in the presence of suprathreshold stimulus, callosal fibers may regulate the cross talk between hemispheres perhaps through similar mechanism that underlie the inhibition of MEPs in the contralateral hand muscle in the conventional IHI paradigm.

5.2.4 Sensory afferent inhibition

The interleaved TMS-EEG was also used to examine the correlation between the cortical and peripheral effects of SAI. In a study conducted by Bikmullina et al., it was demonstrated that the suppression of MEPs following SAI was positively correlated with the attenuation of the amplitude of the EEG N100 component (Bikmullina et al., 2009). This finding supports the findings of earlier studies that suggested a cortical origin for the suppression of MEPs in SAI paradigm. Furthermore, the attenuation of N100 is an interesting observation by itself as it may be a further support for a link between N100 and activity of $GABA_B$ receptor mediated inhibitory mechanism. In this regard, in a triple pulse study, it was demonstrated that SAI had an inhibitory effect on LICI (Udupa et al., 2009). As previously mentioned, suppression of MEPs in LICI has been associated with the activity of slow acting $GABA_B$ receptors.

Therefore, the attenuation of N100 component following SAI is a further support for the inhibitory effect of SAI on GABAergic mechanism and the plausible involvement of $GABA_B$ receptors in generation of N100 component.
Moreover, spectral analysis of EEG response following SAI in rat somatosensory cortex has demonstrated that the extent of SAI varies with the cortical state and the frequency of the underlying cortical oscillations. In particular SAI was enhanced following increases in delta oscillations (Funke & Benali, 2009). The findings of this animal experiment provides further support to reiterate the importance of online EEG recording during TMS-EMG, as some of the inter-subject and inter-laboratory variance that are observed across studies may be explained by the dependence of TMS-EMG measures on cortical states and cortical oscillatory activity immediately before or at the time of TMS stimulation.

5.3 Repetitive TMS

A key advantage of concurrent EEG recording is the ability to directly evaluate the effect of rTMS on cortical excitability. As previously mentioned, slow and fast frequency rTMS applied to the motor cortex may have a differential effect on the cortical excitability. As described earlier, the alteration of cortical excitability by rTMS is conventionally probed through evaluating the changes in MEP responses to single pulse of TMS applied to the motor cortex before and after rTMS session. However, brain is a network of interconnected cortical regions and it is unlikely that rTMS effect would remain solely within the stimulated region. In fact, as described above, the TMS induced cortical evoked activity propagates across cortical mantels and may differentially affect the interconnected local and distant brain regions (Ferreri et al., 2010; Voineskos et al., 2010). Furthermore, evaluation of MEP modulations is limited to investigating the cortical activity of the motor cortex while rTMS treatment is often administered in non-motor regions of the cortex such as the DLPFC in the treatment of depression. Finally, the origin of rTMS mediated modulation of MEP remains a matter of debate. Therefore, recording both cortical and peripheral response before, during and after rTMS would enhance our understanding of the effect of rTMS on both motor and non-motor regions of the cortex and would be critical in examining the exact mechanisms through which rTMS exerts its therapeutic effect. In this vein, research examining the cortico-peripheral effect of rTMS is expanding, some of which will be discussed here.
In one of the earlier studies examining the cortical signature of rTMS induced MEP potentiation, the cortical and peripheral response to single pulse TMS were evaluated before and after 5 Hz rTMS of motor cortex in healthy human subjects (Esser et al., 2006). It was reported that following rTMS, the TMS induced EEG components in response to subthreshold single pulse TMS were selectively potentiated within a time window of 15 to 55 ms. In a similar study, the effect of slow frequency rTMS (0.6 Hz) was assessed by examining the amplitude of EEG N45 response to subthreshold single pulse TMS before and after 15 minutes of rTMS administration (Van Der Werf & Paus, 2006). In this study, it was reported that despite the lack of any rTMS induced MEP modulation, the amplitude of N45 response was reduced. This finding may suggest that EEG response is a more sensitive indicator of rTMS effect as compared to MEP. In another study, the effect of 1 Hz rTMS on cortical oscillations was examined and compared with the suppression of MEPs at the periphery (Brignani et al., 2008). In this study, three 10-min blocks of 1 Hz rTMS was applied to the left primary motor cortex of healthy subjects. Spectral analysis was performed and the power of alpha and beta band oscillations was obtained during each three rTMS blocks. It was shown that the power of cortical oscillations, more prominently alpha oscillations, increased with increase in TMS

duration. The increase in power of cortical oscillations was inversely correlated with the suppression of MEP amplitudes at the periphery. It was suggested that the increase of oscillatory activity may be a representation of altered cortical excitability, possibly related to an increase in the activity of inhibitory mechanism (Brignani et al., 2008). Interestingly, the increase in alpha and beta band cortical oscillations was also documented in a recent study that examined cortical response to 20 Hz rTMS applied to the left primary motor cortex (Veniero et al., 2011). It was demonstrated that synchronization of alpha and beta band cortical oscillations recorded from the C3 electrode was also positively related to the number of delivered stimuli. Furthermore, there was an inverse correlation between the MEP amplitude and synchronization of beta band oscillations, showing that smaller MEP amplitudes were related to higher power of beta oscillations (Veniero et al., 2011).

Theta burst stimulation is a relatively new rTMS approach that has attracted a lot of interest due to its long lasting effect relative to the short administration period. While 25 minutes of 1 Hz rTMS may induce changes lasting for about 30 minutes, only 40 seconds of TBS may result in MEP modulation lasting for more than 60 minutes (Huang et al., 2005). Previous TMS-EMG studies had shown that application of cTBS over the motor cortex results in suppression of MEPs at the periphery. Through combination of TMS-EMG with concurrent EEG recording, it has been demonstrated that the cortico-peripheral effect of cTBS involves a reduction in the cortico-muscular coherence within the cortical beta band oscillations measured thorough EEG C3 electrode in the primary motor cortex (Saglam et al., 2008).

The effect of PAS on cortical evoked potentials has recently been investigated to also examine the cortical origin and EEG substrate of PAS induced LTP in the motor cortex of healthy subjects. In an interesting study by Hubert et al it was shown that the EEG changes following PAS, as opposed to MEP changes, could predict the modification of slow wave (0.5-4.7 Hz) activity during sleep (Huber et al., 2008). In this study, PAS was administered to healthy subjects at two ISIs of 10 ms and 25 ms. Authors then evaluated the cortical evoked potentials in response to single pulse of TMS applied to the motor cortex before and after PAS intervention. Subjects were then allowed to sleep shortly after PAS and their sleep EEG was recorded and analyzed. It was reported that on average PAS at 25 ms resulted in potentiation of TMS-evoked MEPs and PAS at 10 ms resulted in suppression of MEP responses, although the reverse was also observed in a few subjects. The study yielded three interesting findings. First, it was shown that there was a weak but significant correlation between the MEP amplitudes measured through EMG and the cortical evoked potentials measured through EEG. Second, interestingly, the location of maximum cortical activation was over the sensorimotor cortex near the site of stimulation where the effect of afferent and cortical stimulation would most likely overlap, thus further supporting the LTP like mechanisms that underlie PAS-induced MEP potentiation. Finally, in subjects that showed a potentiation of cortical evoked potentials in response to PAS intervention (regardless of the ISI or MEP modulation) the power of slow wave activity was increased during sleep that followed the PAS intervention. By contrast, in subjects that cortical evoked potentials were suppressed following PAS intervention (again, regardless of the ISI or MEP modulation), a relative reduction of slow wave activity was observed. The finding that the modulation of cortical evoked potentials was a better predictor of subsequent changes during sleep is a further support for the significance of probing plasticity and modulation of cortical excitability directly from the cortex.

Furthermore, utilizing the cortical evoked potentials to index PAS induced LTP and LTD like plasticity, a recent study has attempted to examine the PAS induced plasticity in both the motor cortex and DLPFC of healthy subjects. Application of PAS in the DLPFC was achieved by pairing the afferent peripheral stimulation with single pulse TMS applied to the contralateral DLPFC. The preliminary results of this study, currently presented in an abstract form (Rajji TK et al., 2011), shows that in line with findings of Hubert et al. following PAS intervention in the motor cortex, there was a significant correlation between the cortical evoked potentials recorded at the stimulation site and the MEP response at the periphery. It was noted that while all subjects demonstrated potentiation of cortical evoked potentials, MEPs were not potentiated in a subset of subjects. Finally, it was shown that PAS applied to the DLPFC results in significant potentiation of cortical evoked potentials recorded from the DLPFC which is perhaps, if not the first, one of the first studies directly probing LTP like plasticity in the DLPFC of healthy subjects, a cortical region more closely associated with learning and memory.

Similarly, the effect of rTMS on non-motor regions of the cortex can also be evaluated through TMS-EEG. The observation that LICI modulated cortical oscillations differently in the motor compared to the prefrontal cortex (Farzan et al., 2009) suggests that fast versus slow rTMS and cTBS versus iTBS may have differential modulatory effect on cortical oscillations of motor compared to non-motor regions of the cortex such as DLPFC. In fact, in a recent study published by our group it was demonstrated that one session of 20 Hz rTMS applied bilaterally to the left and right DLPFC results in increased power of gamma cortical oscillations during cognitive performance in healthy subjects (Barr et al., 2009) and reduced gamma oscillations in patients with schizophrenia (Barr et al. 2011). Future studies should more systematically investigate the effect of rTMS with different stimulation parameters (e.g. frequency) on motor and non-motor regions of the cortex. Such studies would enhance the efficacy of rTMS therapy.

6. Reproducibility and reliability of TMS-EEG-EMG measures

Research experiments systematically examining the test-retest reliability of TMS induced MEPs are relatively scarce. In this regard, one study has examined the reliability of TMS in identifying the APB muscle motor map between two separate sessions (Corneal et al., 2005). It was also shown that increasing the number of delivered stimuli in TMS paradigms would reduce the intersession variability (Boroojerdi et al., 2000). There are also a few studies that have demonstrated the reliability of TMS induced MEP modulation in the paired pulse paradigms of SICI and ICF (Boroojerdi et al., 2000; Maeda et al., 2002). For example, Maeda et al. reported that SICI was reproducible and correlated between two sessions separated by two weeks (Maeda et al., 2002).

Given the increasing popularity of TMS-EEG-EMG approach as both a therapeutic and diagnostic tool, the number of research experiments examining the reliability and validity of cortical and peripheral indices of TMS is on the rise. The reproducibility of TMS induced cortical responses to single pulse TMS were recently demonstrated in the motor cortex and DLPFC of healthy subjects (Lioumis et al., 2009). Lioumis et al. reported generation of six EEG peaks in the ipsilateral (at latencies 13, 32, 54, 66, 111, 172 ms post TMS) and contralateral (12, 31, 50, 73, 111, 176 ms post TMS) motor cortex following the application of suprathreshold single pulse to the left motor cortex, and six peaks were defined in the ipsilateral DLPFC (first one contaminated by noise, 25, 49, 64, 113, 170 ms post TMS) and contralateral DLPFC (21, 32, 48, 63, 113, and 174 ms post TMS) following suprathreshold TMS to the left DLPFC. It was reported that the amplitudes of TMS evoked cortical potentials at various stimulation intensities were highly reliable in both the ipsilateral DLPFC and motor cortex between sessions separated by a one-week interval (test-retest correlation >0.83), while considering the contralateral response, contralateral DLPFC response was more reliable than motor cortex perhaps reflecting the stronger interhemispheric connectivity of the prefrontal cortices (Lioumis et al., 2009).

In a study conducted by our group, we extended the results of previous reports by demonstrating the reliability of cortical and peripheral indices of LICI, as well as the reliability of LICI mediated modulation of each cortical oscillation in both the left motor cortex and left DLPFC (Farzan et al., 2010b). In the motor cortex, we showed that all EEG and EMG measures of LICI were highly reliable, and in the DLPFC all EEG indices of LICI were highly reliable between sessions separated by one-week (Cronbach's alpha ranging from 0.7 to 0.9). Furthermore, we replicated the correlation between EEG measures of LICI and EMG measures of LICI in an extended sample size of 36 subjects. Finally, for the first time we demonstrated a positive correlation between the EEG measures of LICI and the duration of cortical silent period, as indexed through the CSP paradigm. Previous pharmacological studies had linked the cortical silent period and MEP suppression by LICI to the activity of $GABA_B$ receptor mediated inhibitory neurotransmission. Collectively, these findings further confirm the validity and reliability of EEG measures of LICI as indices of GABAergic inhibitory mechanism, and also provide evidence for the cortical origin of MEP modulation and the silent period in the LICI and CSP paradigms, respectively. In the next section, we will discuss how some of these measures can be used to enhance the diagnostic and therapeutic efficacy of TMS.

7. TMS-EEG-EMG in diagnosis and treatment of neuropsychiatric disorders

Since the introduction of TMS in 1985, deficits of TMS induced MEPs have been reported in a number of neurological and psychiatric conditions. Among movement disorders, reduction of SICI (Hanajima et al., 1996; Pierantozzi et al., 2001; Ridding et al., 1995; Strafella et al., 2000), prolongation of silent period, and increases in LICI has been reported in the motor cortex of patients with Parkinson's disease (Berardelli et al., 2008; Berardelli et al., 1996). In another study, impairment of both SICI and ICF was observed in early Parkinson's disease patients not treated with dopamine agonists (Bares et al., 2003). Among neuropsychiatric disorders, reduction of CSP, IHI and SICI was reported in unmedicated patients with schizophrenia, while these measures of cortical inhibition were not significantly impaired in medicated patients with schizophrenia (Daskalakis et al., 2002a). Similarly, the reduction of SICI, IHI and CSP was also demonstrated in the motor cortex of patients with bipolar disorder (Levinson et al., 2007). Application of TMS-EMG in cognitive disorders has shown that patients with Alzheimer's disease have reduced SAI measures (Di Lazzaro et al., 2002b), and it was reported that an oral dose of rivastigmine enhanced SAI in a subgroup of patients (Di Lazzaro et al., 2002b). Reduction of SAI has also been reported in early Alzheimer's disease (Nardone et al., 2008). While these TMS-EMG indices have moved us a step closer to the underlying source of some of these disorders, the exact mechanisms underlying the generation of MEPs and thus the sources of such impairments have remained a matter of debate. Furthermore, the pathophysiology of neuropsychiatric illnesses such as schizophrenia, bipolar disorder and Alzheimer's disease is more closely associated with impairment of non-motor regions of the cortex which are not easily accessible through the conventional TMS-EMG indices of cortical processes.

The combination of TMS-EMG with concurrent EEG recordings permits the assessment of cortical origin of MEP impairments. For example, the cortico-muscular coherence and EEG spectral analysis, discussed in previous sections, can be used to understand the origin of MEP impairments in movement disorders and neurological diseases that have abnormalities of the corticospinal pathway and the cortical oscillatory activity of the motor cortex such as in Parkinson's disease and dystonia (Di Lazzaro et al., 2009; Levy et al.). Furthermore, the combination of TMS with EEG allows for examining cortical processes in neuropsychiatric disorders which are closely associated with impairments of cortical oscillatory activity in the non-motor regions of the cortex. For example, impairments in gamma oscillations have been reported during cognitive performance in the prefrontal cortex in patients with schizophrenia (Basar-Eroglu et al., 2007; Cho et al., 2006). In this regard, we have recently replicated previous studies, such as those by Basar-Eroglu et al. by demonstrating that patients with schizophrenia exhibit excessive power of gamma oscillations during working memory performance (Barr et al., 2010). Given these frontal gamma deficits, we conducted a TMS-EEG-EMG experiment to examine the integrity of LICI induced modulation of gamma oscillations in the DLPFC of patients with schizophrenia compared to healthy subject in whom, as described previously, LICI resulted in a significant inhibition of gamma oscillations following paired pulse stimulation of DLPFC(Farzan et al., 2009). Utilizing these EEG measures of LICI, which were shown to have high test-retest reliability (Farzan et al., 2010b), we have in fact demonstrated that inhibition of gamma oscillations was selectively impaired in the DLPFC of patients with schizophrenia compared to both healthy subjects and patients with bipolar disorder (Farzan et al., 2010a). Interestingly, we observed no deficits in the EEG or EMG measures of LICI in the motor cortex or in modulation of any other frequency bands in the DLPFC. Patients with bipolar disorder were similar to patients with schizophrenia in relation to severity of symptoms, illness duration, and history of psychosis, and about half of them were on antipsychotic medications. In addition, the extent of gamma inhibition did not correlate with the medication dosage, suggesting that the specificity of gamma inhibition deficits to schizophrenia and the DLPFC is less likely to be part of a generalized deficit that is simply related to psychotropic medications and it may represent a candidate endophenotype for schizophrenia. Combining these finding with evidence of impaired gamma modulation during cognitive performance in patients with schizophrenia, it may be hypothesized that the impairments of LICI induced modulation of gamma oscillations in the DLPFC may, at least partly, underlie the excessive power of gamma oscillations that has been reported during working memory performance and perhaps the frontal cognitive deficits in this illness.

In line with these findings, cognitive impairments and the deficits in learning and memory, a process thought to be related to cortical plasticity, constitute one of the core deficits of schizophrenia (Gold & Harvey, 1993). Indeed, in a previous TMS-EMG study, TMS paradigm PAS was used to investigate the integrity of LTP-like plasticity in the motor cortex of patients with schizophrenia (Frantseva et al., 2008). In this study, the effect of PAS in patients with schizophrenia and healthy subjects was evaluated through evaluating the TMS induced MEP response to single pulse of TMS after PAS, and also through examining the effect of PAS on learning a subsequent motor task (rotary pursuit motor task). It was demonstrated that not only patients with schizophrenia had significantly less MEP facilitation in response to PAS, but there was also a correlation between the PAS induced potentiation of MEPs and performance on the motor learning task (Frantseva et al., 2008). That is, patients with schizophrenia who had less MEP potentiation following PAS compared to healthy subjects, also performed poorly on the subsequent motor task compared to healthy subjects. Consistent with these finding, both medicated and unmedicated patients with schizophrenia demonstrated a reduced plastic response to 15 min of 1 Hz rTMS applied to the motor cortex compared to healthy subjects (Fitzgerald et al., 2004). It was also shown that the duration of CSP at baseline correlated positively with the rTMS response. That is, patients who had less plastic response to rTMS also had a shorter CSP duration at baseline. The results of these studies would be significantly complemented by examining LTP like plasticity in the DLPFC of patients with schizophrenia through PAS or rTMS combined with EEG. In fact, such experiments are currently underway. Preliminary results of a recent experiment has so far shown that following application of PAS in the DLPFC, patients with schizophrenia demonstrate a deficit in potentiation of cortical evoked potentials recorded from the DLPFC compared to the healthy subjects (Rajji TK et al., 2011).

Furthermore, similar to PAS and LICI, EEG measures of SAI can be used to assess the cortical origin and the cortical oscillatory activity underlying the SAI deficits in Alzheimer's disease. The combination of TMS-EMG with EEG would further permit assessing the effect of afferent sensory stimuli on the prefrontal cortex, which is perhaps more closely associated with the impairment of cognitive disorders. Similar to PAS, this can be conducted through combination of peripheral nerve and single pulse TMS applied to the DLPFC, as opposed to the motor cortex, and examining the amplitude and frequency components of the cortical evoked activity in the DLPFC as well as the spread of the signal to the interconnected cortical regions.

Finally, the neurophysiological measures obtained through TMS-EEG-EMG studies would significantly enhance our understanding of the mechanism through which repetitive TMS exerts its effect, and would further enable us to optimally select stimulation parameters that would benefit individual patients based on their underlying impairment. To this day, the outcomes of repetitive TMS therapy have been inconsistent across studies. There are several reasons for this variability. First, certain stimulation patterns such as intensity, frequency, and number of stimuli delivered can significantly influence the outcome measures. Second, emerging lines of evidence suggest that rTMS effects are highly state dependent (Silvanto et al., 2008a; Silvanto et al., 2008b). That is the level of underlying cortical activity prior to rTMS treatment may influence the rTMS effect and could even be used to predict whether rTMS would suppress or facilitate cortical excitability. However, the classical rTMS treatments, not equipped with any concurrent EEG recordings, have not evaluated or controlled such baseline activities, which explains some of the variability observed in the rTMS studies.

Therefore, online EEG recording during rTMS therapy can improve the efficacy of TMS therapy in several ways. First, proof of concept studies similar to some of the rTMS-EEG experiments described before (Barr et al., 2010; Esser et al., 2006; Saglam et al., 2008; Van Der Werf et al., 2006) should be expanded to more systematically examine the effect of various stimulation parameters (e.g. intensity and frequency) on the cortical evoked potentials that seem to be a better predictor of subtle changes that take place in the cortex, as compared to the conventional MEP responses (Farzan et al., 2010b; Ferreri et al., 2010; Huber et al., 2008; Van Der Werf & Paus, 2006). Second, the results of these studies can then be utilized to custom design rTMS treatment sessions though carefully selecting parameters that would induce a specific response in the cortex (e.g. increased or reduced cortical excitability) similar to the tACS frequency adjustments in a recent study by Schutter and Hortensius (Schutter & Hortensius, 2011). Finally, a major advancement in EEG and TMS technology would hopefully give rise to the design of reliable EEG triggered TMS machines in which continuous online monitoring of underlying cortical potential would trigger the rTMS stimulation whenever the cortical activity reaches a state which would be more prone to be affected by the therapeutic efficacy of a specific rTMS therapy (e.g. low vs. fast frequency) (Rotenberg, 2009). Finally, in an even more advanced design, an EEG-triggered TMS system would be capable of updating the rTMS parameters (e.g. changing the rTMS frequency) during the treatment and based on the online analysis of changes in the cortical activity. Such advances in cortical stimulation technology could revolutionize the TMS field and would be a major step toward making the cortical stimulation a standard treatment approach for several neuropsychiatric disorders.

8. Conclusion

Advances in cortical stimulation and cortical recording techniques over the past few decades have allowed researchers to more systematically and non-invasively investigate the neurophysiological processes from the intact cortex of awake humans. Among such advancements, the concurrent TMS and EMG recordings has been instrumental in identifying and probing cortical processes that underlie generation and modulation of motor evoked potentials. The ability to evaluate cortical processes such as inhibition, excitation and plasticity in healthy subjects has further led to the discovery of pathophysiological processes in various neuropsychiatric disorders. In recent years, the introduction of TMS compatible EEG systems has brought about a significant advancement to the TMS field, enhancing both the diagnostic and therapeutic aspects of TMS. This is achieved through the superior temporal, spatial and spectral precision of TMS-EEG combination in identifying subtle changes of cortical activity before, during and post TMS delivery in both motor and non-motor regions of the cortex. In addition, the integration of EEG data with EMG recordings has provided further confirmation for the cortical origin of the classical TMS-EMG paradigms and has provided new information about the cortical oscillatory activity that underlies the generation and modulation of the peripheral effects. Although today there are only a few number of studies that have systematically investigated the reliability of EEG measures of TMS, the results are promising and suggest that TMS does have a potential for reliably identifying biological markers for several neuropsychiatric disorders. In regards to the future prospect of TMS-EEG-EMG research, it is expected that the integration of online EEG recording during rTMS therapy and advancements of EEG triggered cortical stimulation technology would significantly enhance the therapeutic outcomes of TMS and increase the certainty with which its therapeutic efficacy is predicated for each clinical condition. Such advancement would ultimately assist physicians in selecting patients who would benefit from rTMS therapy.

9. References

Adrian ED, Moruzzi G. (1939). Impulses in the pyramidal tract. *J Physiol,* 97, pp 153-199

Anand S, Hotson J. (2002). Transcranial magnetic stimulation: neurophysiological applications and safety. *Brain Cogn,* 50, pp 366-386

Bares M, Kanovsky P, Klajblova H, Rektor I. (2003). Intracortical inhibition and facilitation are impaired in patients with early Parkinson's disease: a paired TMS study. *Eur J Neurol,* 10, pp 385-389

Barker AT, Jalinous R, Freeston IL. (1985). Non-invasive magnetic stimulation of human motor cortex. *Lancet,* 1, pp 1106-1107

Barr MS, Farzan F, Arenovich T, Chen R, Fitzgerald PB, Daskalakis ZJ. (2011). The effect of repetitive transcranial magnetic stimulation on gamma oscillatory activity in schizophrenia. *PLoS One*, 6, p e22627

Barr MS, Farzan F, Rusjan PM, Chen R, Fitzgerald PB, Daskalakis ZJ. (2009). Potentiation of gamma oscillatory activity through repetitive transcranial magnetic stimulation of the dorsolateral prefrontal cortex. *Neuropsychopharmacology*, 34, pp 2359-2367

Barr MS, Farzan F, Tran LC, Chen R, Fitzgerald PB, Daskalakis ZJ. (2010). Evidence for excessive frontal evoked gamma oscillatory activity in schizophrenia during working memory. *Schizophr Res*, 121, pp 146-152

Basar-Eroglu C, Brand A, Hildebrandt H, Karolina Kedzior K, Mathes B, Schmiedt C. (2007). Working memory related gamma oscillations in schizophrenia patients. *Int J Psychophysiol*, 64, pp 39-45

Bender S, Basseler K, Sebastian I, Resch F, Kammer T, Oelkers-Ax R, et al. (2005). Electroencephalographic response to transcranial magnetic stimulation in children: Evidence for giant inhibitory potentials. *Ann Neurol*, 58, pp 58-67

Berardelli A, Abbruzzese G, Chen R, Orth M, Ridding MC, Stinear C, et al. (2008). Consensus paper on short-interval intracortical inhibition and other transcranial magnetic stimulation intracortical paradigms in movement disorders. *Brain Stimul*, 1, pp 183-191

Berardelli A, Rona S, Inghilleri M, Manfredi M. (1996). Cortical inhibition in Parkinson's disease. A study with paired magnetic stimulation. *Brain*, 119 (Pt 1), pp 71-77

Bikmullina R, Kicic D, Carlson S, Nikulin VV. (2009). Electrophysiological correlates of short-latency afferent inhibition: a combined EEG and TMS study. *Exp Brain Res*, 194, pp 517-526

Boroojerdi B, Kopylev L, Battaglia F, Facchini S, Ziemann U, Muellbacher W, et al. (2000). Reproducibility of intracortical inhibition and facilitation using the paired-pulse paradigm. *Muscle Nerve*, 23, pp 1594-1597

Bragin A, Jando G, Nadasdy Z, Hetke J, Wise K, Buzsaki G. (1995). Gamma (40-100 Hz) oscillation in the hippocampus of the behaving rat. *J Neurosci*, 15, pp 47-60

Brignani D, Manganotti P, Rossini PM, Miniussi C. (2008). Modulation of cortical oscillatory activity during transcranial magnetic stimulation. *Hum Brain Mapp*, 29, pp 603-612

Brown P, Salenius S, Rothwell JC, Hari R. (1998). Cortical correlate of the Piper rhythm in humans. *J Neurophysiol*, 80, pp 2911-2917

Buonomano DV, Merzenich MM. (1998). Cortical plasticity: from synapses to maps. *Annu Rev Neurosci*, 21, pp 149-186

Buzsáki G (2006). *Rhythms of the Brain*, Oxford University Press, 13 978-0-19-530106-9, New York

Chen R. (2004). Interactions between inhibitory and excitatory circuits in the human motor cortex. *Exp Brain Res*, 154, pp 1-10

Chen R, Classen J, Gerloff C, Celnik P, Wassermann EM, Hallett M, et al. (1997). Depression of motor cortex excitability by low-frequency transcranial magnetic stimulation. *Neurology*, 48, pp 1398-1403

Chen R, Lozano AM, Ashby P. (1999). Mechanism of the silent period following transcranial magnetic stimulation. Evidence from epidural recordings. *Exp Brain Res*, 128, pp 539-542

Chen R, Yung D, Li JY. (2003). Organization of ipsilateral excitatory and inhibitory pathways in the human motor cortex. *J Neurophysiol*, 89, pp 1256-1264

Cho RY, Konecky RO, Carter CS. (2006). Impairments in frontal cortical gamma synchrony and cognitive control in schizophrenia. *Proc Natl Acad Sci U S A*, 103, pp 19878-19883

Classen J, Wolters A, Stefan K, Wycislo M, Sandbrink F, Schmidt A, et al. (2004). Paired associative stimulation. *Suppl Clin Neurophysiol,* 57, pp 563-569

Corneal SF, Butler AJ, Wolf SL. (2005). Intra- and intersubject reliability of abductor pollicis brevis muscle motor map characteristics with transcranial magnetic stimulation. *Arch Phys Med Rehabil,* 86, pp 1670-1675

Daskalakis ZJ, Christensen BK, Chen R, Fitzgerald PB, Zipursky RB, Kapur S. (2002a). Evidence for impaired cortical inhibition in schizophrenia using transcranial magnetic stimulation. *Arch Gen Psychiatry,* 59, pp 347-354

Daskalakis ZJ, Christensen BK, Fitzgerald PB, Roshan L, Chen R. (2002b). The mechanisms of interhemispheric inhibition in the human motor cortex. *J Physiol,* 543, pp 317-326

Daskalakis ZJ, Farzan F, Barr MS, Maller JJ, Chen R, Fitzgerald PB. (2008). Long-interval cortical inhibition from the dorsolateral prefrontal cortex: a TMS-EEG study. *Neuropsychopharmacology,* 33, pp 2860-2869

Daskalakis ZJ, Moller B, Christensen BK, Fitzgerald PB, Gunraj C, Chen R. (2006). The effects of repetitive transcranial magnetic stimulation on cortical inhibition in healthy human subjects. *Exp Brain Res,* 174, pp 403-412

Daskalakis ZJ, Paradiso GO, Christensen BK, Fitzgerald PB, Gunraj C, Chen R. (2004). Exploring the connectivity between the cerebellum and motor cortex in humans. *J Physiol,* 557, pp 689-700

Day BL, Dressler D, Maertens de Noordhout A, Marsden CD, Nakashima K, Rothwell JC, et al. (1989). Electric and magnetic stimulation of human motor cortex: surface EMG and single motor unit responses. *J Physiol,* 412, pp 449-473

Di Lazzaro V, Dileone M, Pilato F, Capone F, Musumeci G, Ranieri F, et al. (2011). Modulation of motor cortex neuronal networks by rTMS: comparison of local and remote effects of six different protocols of stimulation. *J Neurophysiol,* 105, pp 2150-2156

Di Lazzaro V, Oliviero A, Mazzone P, Insola A, Pilato F, Saturno E, et al. (2001). Comparison of descending volleys evoked by monophasic and biphasic magnetic stimulation of the motor cortex in conscious humans. *Exp Brain Res,* 141, pp 121-127

Di Lazzaro V, Oliviero A, Mazzone P, Pilato F, Saturno E, Insola A, et al. (2002a). Direct demonstration of long latency cortico-cortical inhibition in normal subjects and in a patient with vascular parkinsonism. *Clin Neurophysiol,* 113, pp 1673-1679

Di Lazzaro V, Oliviero A, Meglio M, Cioni B, Tamburrini G, Tonali P, et al. (2000). Direct demonstration of the effect of lorazepam on the excitability of the human motor cortex. *Clin Neurophysiol,* 111, pp 794-799

Di Lazzaro V, Oliviero A, Pilato F, Saturno E, Dileone M, Mazzone P, et al. (2004). The physiological basis of transcranial motor cortex stimulation in conscious humans. *Clin Neurophysiol,* 115, pp 255-266

Di Lazzaro V, Oliviero A, Profice P, Dileone M, Pilato F, Insola A, et al. (2009). Reduced cerebral cortex inhibition in dystonia: direct evidence in humans. *Clin Neurophysiol,* 120, pp 834-839

Di Lazzaro V, Oliviero A, Profice P, Insola A, Mazzone P, Tonali P, et al. (1999a). Direct demonstration of interhemispheric inhibition of the human motor cortex produced by transcranial magnetic stimulation. *Exp Brain Res,* 124, pp 520-524

Di Lazzaro V, Oliviero A, Profice P, Insola A, Mazzone P, Tonali P, et al. (1999b). Direct recordings of descending volleys after transcranial magnetic and electric motor cortex stimulation in conscious humans. *Electroencephalogr Clin Neurophysiol Suppl,* 51, pp 120-126

Di Lazzaro V, Oliviero A, Saturno E, Dileone M, Pilato F, Nardone R, et al. (2005). Effects of lorazepam on short latency afferent inhibition and short latency intracortical inhibition in humans. *J Physiol,* 564, pp 661-668

Di Lazzaro V, Oliviero A, Tonali PA, Marra C, Daniele A, Profice P, et al. (2002b). Noninvasive in vivo assessment of cholinergic cortical circuits in AD using transcranial magnetic stimulation. *Neurology,* 59, pp 392-397

Di Lazzaro V, Pilato F, Dileone M, Profice P, Ranieri F, Ricci V, et al. (2007). Segregating two inhibitory circuits in human motor cortex at the level of GABAA receptor subtypes: a TMS study. *Clin Neurophysiol,* 118, pp 2207-2214

Di Lazzaro V, Restuccia D, Oliviero A, Profice P, Ferrara L, Insola A, et al. (1998). Magnetic transcranial stimulation at intensities below active motor threshold activates intracortical inhibitory circuits. *Exp Brain Res,* 119, pp 265-268

Di Lazzaro V, Rothwell JC, Oliviero A, Profice P, Insola A, Mazzone P, et al. (1999c). Intracortical origin of the short latency facilitation produced by pairs of threshold magnetic stimuli applied to human motor cortex. *Exp Brain Res,* 129, pp 494-499

Engel AK, Fries P. (2010). Beta-band oscillations--signalling the status quo? *Curr Opin Neurobiol,* 20, pp 156-165

Engel AK, Singer W. (2001). Temporal binding and the neural correlates of sensory awareness. *Trends Cogn Sci,* 5, pp 16-25

Esser SK, Huber R, Massimini M, Peterson MJ, Ferrarelli F, Tononi G. (2006). A direct demonstration of cortical LTP in humans: A combined TMS/EEG study. *Brain Res Bull,* 69, pp 86-94

Farzan F, Barr MS, Levinson AJ, Chen R, Wong W, Fitzgerald PB, et al. (2010a). Evidence for gamma inhibition deficits in the dorsolateral prefrontal cortex of patients with schizophrenia. *Brain,* 133, pp 1505-1514

Farzan F, Barr MS, Levinson AJ, Chen R, Wong W, Fitzgerald PB, et al. (2010b). Reliability of Long Interval Cortical Inhibition in Healthy Human Subjects: A TMS-EEG Study. *J Neurophysiol,*

Farzan F, Barr MS, Wong W, Chen R, Fitzgerald PB, Daskalakis ZJ. (2009). Suppression of gamma-oscillations in the dorsolateral prefrontal cortex following long interval cortical inhibition: a TMS-EEG study. *Neuropsychopharmacology,* 34, pp 1543-1551

Ferbert A, Priori A, Rothwell JC, Day BL, Colebatch JG, Marsden CD. (1992). Interhemispheric inhibition of the human motor cortex. *J Physiol,* 453, pp 525-546

Ferreri F, Pasqualetti P, Maatta S, Ponzo D, Ferrarelli F, Tononi G, et al. (2010). Human brain connectivity during single and paired pulse transcranial magnetic stimulation. *Neuroimage,* 54, pp 90-102

Fitzgerald PB, Brown TL, Marston NA, Oxley T, De Castella A, Daskalakis ZJ, et al. (2004). Reduced plastic brain responses in schizophrenia: a transcranial magnetic stimulation study. *Schizophr Res,* 71, pp 17-26

Fitzgerald PB, Fountain S, Daskalakis ZJ. (2006). A comprehensive review of the effects of rTMS on motor cortical excitability and inhibition. *Clin Neurophysiol,* 117, pp 2584-2596

Frantseva MV, Fitzgerald PB, Chen R, Moller B, Daigle M, Daskalakis ZJ. (2008). Evidence for impaired long-term potentiation in schizophrenia and its relationship to motor skill learning. *Cereb Cortex,* 18, pp 990-996

Fries P, Nikolic D, Singer W. (2007). The gamma cycle. *Trends Neurosci,* 30, pp 309-316

Funke K, Benali A. (2009). Short-latency afferent inhibition varies with cortical state in rat somatosensory cortex. *Neuroreport,* 20, pp 1313-1318

Gerloff C, Cohen LG, Floeter MK, Chen R, Corwell B, Hallett M. (1998). Inhibitory influence of the ipsilateral motor cortex on responses to stimulation of the human cortex and pyramidal tract. *J Physiol,* 510 (Pt 1), pp 249-259

Gold JM, Harvey PD. (1993). Cognitive deficits in schizophrenia. *Psychiatr Clin North Am,* 16, pp 295-312

Hallett M. (2000). Transcranial magnetic stimulation and the human brain. *Nature,* 406, pp 147-150

Hanajima R, Ugawa Y, Terao Y, Ogata K, Kanazawa I. (1996). Ipsilateral cortico-cortical inhibition of the motor cortex in various neurological disorders. *J Neurol Sci,* 140, pp 109-116

Howard MW, Rizzuto DS, Caplan JB, Madsen JR, Lisman J, Aschenbrenner-Scheibe R, et al. (2003). Gamma oscillations correlate with working memory load in humans. *Cereb Cortex,* 13, pp 1369-1374

Huang YZ, Edwards MJ, Rounis E, Bhatia KP, Rothwell JC. (2005). Theta burst stimulation of the human motor cortex. *Neuron,* 45, pp 201-206

Huber R, Maatta S, Esser SK, Sarasso S, Ferrarelli F, Watson A, et al. (2008). Measures of cortical plasticity after transcranial paired associative stimulation predict changes in electroencephalogram slow-wave activity during subsequent sleep. *J Neurosci,* 28, pp 7911-7918

Hutcheon B, Yarom Y. (2000). Resonance, oscillation and the intrinsic frequency preferences of neurons. *Trends Neurosci,* 23, pp 216-222

Ilmoniemi RJ, Kicic D. (2009). Methodology for combined TMS and EEG. *Brain Topogr,* 22, pp 233-248

Ilmoniemi RJ, Virtanen J, Ruohonen J, Karhu J, Aronen HJ, Naatanen R, et al. (1997). Neuronal responses to magnetic stimulation reveal cortical reactivity and connectivity. *Neuroreport,* 8, pp 3537-3540

Inghilleri M, Berardelli A, Cruccu G, Manfredi M. (1993). Silent period evoked by transcranial stimulation of the human cortex and cervicomedullary junction. *J Physiol,* 466, pp 521-534.

Kahkonen S, Kesaniemi M, Nikouline VV, Karhu J, Ollikainen M, Holi M, et al. (2001). Ethanol modulates cortical activity: direct evidence with combined TMS and EEG. *Neuroimage,* 14, pp 322-328

Kahkonen S, Wilenius J. (2007). Effects of alcohol on TMS-evoked N100 responses. *J Neurosci Methods,* 166, pp 104-108

Kahkonen S, Wilenius J, Nikulin VV, Ollikainen M, Ilmoniemi RJ. (2003). Alcohol reduces prefrontal cortical excitability in humans: a combined TMS and EEG study. *Neuropsychopharmacology,* 28, pp 747-754

Kanai R, Chaieb L, Antal A, Walsh V, Paulus W. (2008). Frequency-dependent electrical stimulation of the visual cortex. *Curr Biol,* 18, pp 1839-1843

Kapogiannis D, Wassermann EM. (2008). Transcranial magnetic stimulation in Clinical Pharmacology. *Cent Nerv Syst Agents Med Chem,* 8, pp 234-240

Kimiskidis VK, Papagiannopoulos S, Kazis DA, Vasiliadis G, Oikonomidi A, Sotirakoglou K, et al. (2008). Silent period (SP) to transcranial magnetic stimulation: the EEG substrate. Brain Stimulation 1. Abstracts from the 3rd international conference on transcranial magnetic simulation and direct current stimulation, pp 315–316

Knyazev GG. (2007). Motivation, emotion, and their inhibitory control mirrored in brain oscillations. *Neurosci Biobehav Rev,* 31, pp 377-395

Komssi S, Aronen HJ, Huttunen J, Kesaniemi M, Soinne L, Nikouline VV, et al. (2002). Ipsi- and contralateral EEG reactions to transcranial magnetic stimulation. *Clin Neurophysiol,* 113, pp 175-184

Komssi S, Kahkonen S. (2006). The novelty value of the combined use of electroencephalography and transcranial magnetic stimulation for neuroscience research. *Brain Res Brain Res Rev,* 52, pp 183-192

Krnjevic K, Randic M, Straughan DW. (1964). CORTICAL INHIBITION. *Nature,* 201, pp 1294-1296

Kujirai T, Caramia MD, Rothwell JC, Day BL, Thompson PD, Ferbert A, et al. (1993). Corticocortical inhibition in human motor cortex. *J Physiol,* 471, pp 501-519

Levinson AJ, Young LT, Fitzgerald PB, Daskalakis ZJ. (2007). Cortical inhibitory dysfunction in bipolar disorder: a study using transcranial magnetic stimulation. *J Clin Psychopharmacol,* 27, pp 493-497

Levy R, Lozano AM, Lang AE, Dostrovsky JO. (2010). Event-related desynchronization of motor cortical oscillations in patients with multiple system atrophy. *Exp Brain Res,* 206, pp 1-13

Linkenkaer-Hansen K, Smit DJ, Barkil A, van Beijsterveldt TE, Brussaard AB, Boomsma DI, et al. (2007). Genetic contributions to long-range temporal correlations in ongoing oscillations. *J Neurosci,* 27, pp 13882-13889

Lioumis P, Kicic D, Savolainen P, Makela JP, Kahkonen S. (2009). Reproducibility of TMS-Evoked EEG responses. *Hum Brain Mapp,* 30, pp 1387-1396

Maeda F, Gangitano M, Thall M, Pascual-Leone A. (2002). Inter- and intra-individual variability of paired-pulse curves with transcranial magnetic stimulation (TMS). *Clin Neurophysiol,* 113, pp 376-382

Maeda F, Keenan JP, Tormos JM, Topka H, Pascual-Leone A. (2000). Interindividual variability of the modulatory effects of repetitive transcranial magnetic stimulation on cortical excitability. *Exp Brain Res,* 133, pp 425-430

Maki H, Ilmoniemi RJ. (2010a). EEG oscillations and magnetically evoked motor potentials reflect motor system excitability in overlapping neuronal populations. *Clin Neurophysiol,* 121, pp 492-501

Maki H, Ilmoniemi RJ. (2010b). The relationship between peripheral and early cortical activation induced by transcranial magnetic stimulation. *Neurosci Lett,*

McCormick DA. (1989). GABA as an inhibitory neurotransmitter in human cerebral cortex. *J Neurophysiol,* 62, pp 1018-1027

McDonnell MN, Orekhov Y, Ziemann U. (2006). The role of GABA(B) receptors in intracortical inhibition in the human motor cortex. *Exp Brain Res,* 173, pp 86-93

Merton PA, Morton HB. (1980). Stimulation of the cerebral cortex in the intact human subject. *Nature,* 285, p 227

Mima T, Hallett M. (1999). Electroencephalographic analysis of cortico-muscular coherence: reference effect, volume conduction and generator mechanism. *Clin Neurophysiol,* 110, pp 1892-1899

Nakamura H, Kitagawa H, Kawaguchi Y, Tsuji H. (1997). Intracortical facilitation and inhibition after transcranial magnetic stimulation in conscious humans. *J Physiol,* 498 (Pt 3), pp 817-823

Nardone R, Bergmann J, Kronbichler M, Kunz A, Klein S, Caleri F, et al. (2008). Abnormal short latency afferent inhibition in early Alzheimer's disease: a transcranial magnetic demonstration. *J Neural Transm,* 115, pp 1557-1562

Neuper C, Pfurtscheller G. (2001). Evidence for distinct beta resonance frequencies in human EEG related to specific sensorimotor cortical areas. *Clin Neurophysiol,* 112, pp 2084-2097

Ni Z, Gunraj C, Nelson AJ, Yeh IJ, Castillo G, Hoque T, et al. (2009). Two phases of interhemispheric inhibition between motor related cortical areas and the primary motor cortex in human. *Cereb Cortex,* 19, pp 1654-1665

Nikulin VV, Kicic D, Kahkonen S, Ilmoniemi RJ. (2003). Modulation of electroencephalographic responses to transcranial magnetic stimulation: evidence for changes in cortical excitability related to movement. *Eur J Neurosci,* 18, pp 1206-1212

Palva S, Palva JM. (2007). New vistas for alpha-frequency band oscillations. *Trends Neurosci,* 30, pp 150-158

Pascual-Leone A, Valls-Sole J, Wassermann EM, Hallett M. (1994). Responses to rapid-rate transcranial magnetic stimulation of the human motor cortex. *Brain,* 117 (Pt 4), pp 847-858

Pascual-Leone A, Walsh V, Rothwell J. (2000). Transcranial magnetic stimulation in cognitive neuroscience--virtual lesion, chronometry, and functional connectivity. *Curr Opin Neurobiol,* 10, pp 232-237

Paus T, Sipila PK, Strafella AP. (2001). Synchronization of neuronal activity in the human primary motor cortex by transcranial magnetic stimulation: an EEG study. *J Neurophysiol,* 86, pp 1983-1990

Pell GS, Roth Y, Zangen A. (2010). Modulation of cortical excitability induced by repetitive transcranial magnetic stimulation: influence of timing and geometrical parameters and underlying mechanisms. *Prog Neurobiol,* 93, pp 59-98

Pfurtscheller G, Neuper C, Pichler-Zalaudek K, Edlinger G, Lopes da Silva FH. (2000). Do brain oscillations of different frequencies indicate interaction between cortical areas in humans? *Neurosci Lett,* 286, pp 66-68

Pierantozzi M, Marciani MG, Palmieri MG, Brusa L, Galati S, Caramia MD, et al. (2004). Effect of Vigabatrin on motor responses to transcranial magnetic stimulation: an effective tool to investigate in vivo GABAergic cortical inhibition in humans. *Brain Res,* 1028, pp 1-8

Pierantozzi M, Palmieri MG, Marciani MG, Bernardi G, Giacomini P, Stanzione P. (2001). Effect of apomorphine on cortical inhibition in Parkinson's disease patients: a transcranial magnetic stimulation study. *Exp Brain Res,* 141, pp 52-62

Pike FG, Goddard RS, Suckling JM, Ganter P, Kasthuri N, Paulsen O. (2000). Distinct frequency preferences of different types of rat hippocampal neurones in response to oscillatory input currents. *J Physiol,* 529 Pt 1, pp 205-213

Pineda JA. (2005). The functional significance of mu rhythms: translating "seeing" and "hearing" into "doing". *Brain Res Brain Res Rev,* 50, pp 57-68

Rajji TK, Sun Y, Farzan F, D'Souza R, Wass C, Mulsant BH, et al. (2011). Assessing plasticity in the dorsolateral prefrontal cortex in patients with schizophrenia. Conference Abstract. The International Congress on Schizophrenia Research, April 2011.

Ridding MC, Rothwell JC. (2007). Is there a future for therapeutic use of transcranial magnetic stimulation? *Nat Rev Neurosci,* 8, pp 559-567

Ridding MC, Sheean G, Rothwell JC, Inzelberg R, Kujirai T. (1995). Changes in the balance between motor cortical excitation and inhibition in focal, task specific dystonia. *J Neurol Neurosurg Psychiatry,* 59, pp 493-498

Roopun AK, Kramer MA, Carracedo LM, Kaiser M, Davies CH, Traub RD, et al. (2008). Temporal Interactions between Cortical Rhythms. *Front Neurosci,* 2, pp 145-154

Rosanova M, Casali A, Bellina V, Resta F, Mariotti M, Massimini M. (2009). Natural frequencies of human corticothalamic circuits. *J Neurosci,* 29, pp 7679-7685

Rossini PM, Barker AT, Berardelli A, Caramia MD, Caruso G, Cracco RQ, et al. (1994). Non-invasive electrical and magnetic stimulation of the brain, spinal cord and roots: basic principles and procedures for routine clinical application. Report of an IFCN committee. *Electroencephalogr Clin Neurophysiol,* 91, pp 79-92

Rossini PM, Rossi S. (2007). Transcranial magnetic stimulation: diagnostic, therapeutic, and research potential. *Neurology,* 68, pp 484-488

Rotenberg A. (2009). Prospects for clinical applications of transcranial magnetic stimulation and real-time EEG in epilepsy. *Brain Topogr,* 22, pp 257-266

Rothwell JC. (1997). Techniques and mechanisms of action of transcranial stimulation of the human motor cortex. *J Neurosci Methods,* 74, pp 113-122

Saglam M, Matsunaga K, Murayama N, Hayashida Y, Huang YZ, Nakanishi R. (2008). Parallel inhibition of cortico-muscular synchronization and cortico-spinal excitability by theta burst TMS in humans. *Clin Neurophysiol,* 119, pp 2829-2838

Salenius S, Portin K, Kajola M, Salmelin R, Hari R. (1997). Cortical control of human motoneuron firing during isometric contraction. *J Neurophysiol,* 77, pp 3401-3405

Sanger TD, Garg RR, Chen R. (2001). Interactions between two different inhibitory systems in the human motor cortex. *J Physiol,* 530, pp 307-317

Schutter DJ, Hortensius R. (2011). Brain oscillations and frequency-dependent modulation of cortical excitability. *Brain Stimul,* 4, pp 97-103

Siebner HR, Dressnandt J, Auer C, Conrad B. (1998). Continuous intrathecal baclofen infusions induced a marked increase of the transcranially evoked silent period in a patient with generalized dystonia. *Muscle Nerve,* 21, pp 1209-1212

Silvanto J, Cattaneo Z, Battelli L, Pascual-Leone A. (2008a). Baseline cortical excitability determines whether TMS disrupts or facilitates behavior. *J Neurophysiol,* 99, pp 2725-2730

Silvanto J, Muggleton N, Walsh V. (2008b). State-dependency in brain stimulation studies of perception and cognition. *Trends Cogn Sci,* 12, pp 447-454

Slotema CW, Blom JD, Hoek HW, Sommer IE. (2010). Should we expand the toolbox of psychiatric treatment methods to include Repetitive Transcranial Magnetic Stimulation (rTMS)? A meta-analysis of the efficacy of rTMS in psychiatric disorders. *J Clin Psychiatry,* 71, pp 873-884

Stefan K, Kunesch E, Benecke R, Cohen LG, Classen J. (2002). Mechanisms of enhancement of human motor cortex excitability induced by interventional paired associative stimulation. *J Physiol,* 543, pp 699-708

Stefan K, Kunesch E, Cohen LG, Benecke R, Classen J. (2000). Induction of plasticity in the human motor cortex by paired associative stimulation. *Brain,* 123 Pt 3, pp 572-584

Strafella AP, Valzania F, Nassetti SA, Tropeani A, Bisulli A, Santangelo M, et al. (2000). Effects of chronic levodopa and pergolide treatment on cortical excitability in patients with Parkinson's disease: a transcranial magnetic stimulation study. *Clin Neurophysiol,* 111, pp 1198-1202

Swartz BE, Goldensohn ES. (1998). Timeline of the history of EEG and associated fields. *Electroencephalogr Clin Neurophysiol,* 106, pp 173-176

Tallon-Baudry C, Bertrand O. (1999). Oscillatory gamma activity in humans and its role in object representation. *Trends Cogn Sci,* 3, pp 151-162

Tallon-Baudry C, Bertrand O, Delpuech C, Pernier J. (1996). Stimulus specificity of phase-locked and non-phase-locked 40 Hz visual responses in human. *J Neurosci,* 16, pp 4240-4249

Tallon-Baudry C, Bertrand O, Peronnet F, Pernier J. (1998). Induced gamma-band activity during the delay of a visual short-term memory task in humans. *J Neurosci,* 18, pp 4244-4254

Thut G, Northoff G, Ives JR, Kamitani Y, Pfennig A, Kampmann F, et al. (2003). Effects of single-pulse transcranial magnetic stimulation (TMS) on functional brain activity: a combined event-related TMS and evoked potential study. *Clin Neurophysiol,* 114, pp 2071-2080

Thut G, Pascual-Leone A. (2010). A review of combined TMS-EEG studies to characterize lasting effects of repetitive TMS and assess their usefulness in cognitive and clinical neuroscience. *Brain Topogr,* 22, pp 219-232

Tokimura H, Di Lazzaro V, Tokimura Y, Oliviero A, Profice P, Insola A, et al. (2000). Short latency inhibition of human hand motor cortex by somatosensory input from the hand. *J Physiol,* 523 Pt 2, pp 503-513

Tsuji T, Rothwell JC. (2002). Long lasting effects of rTMS and associated peripheral sensory input on MEPs, SEPs and transcortical reflex excitability in humans. *J Physiol,* 540, pp 367-376

Udupa K, Ni Z, Gunraj C, Chen R. (2009). Interactions between short latency afferent inhibition and long interval intracortical inhibition. *Exp Brain Res,* 199, pp 177-183

Valls-Sole J, Pascual-Leone A, Wassermann EM, Hallett M. (1992). Human motor evoked responses to paired transcranial magnetic stimuli. *Electroencephalogr Clin Neurophysiol,* 85, pp 355-364

Van Der Werf YD, Paus T. (2006). The neural response to transcranial magnetic stimulation of the human motor cortex. I. Intracortical and cortico-cortical contributions. *Exp Brain Res,* 175, pp 231-245

Van Der Werf YD, Sadikot AF, Strafella AP, Paus T. (2006). The neural response to transcranial magnetic stimulation of the human motor cortex. II. Thalamocortical contributions. *Exp Brain Res,* 175, pp 246-255

Veniero D, Brignani D, Thut G, Miniussi C. (2011). Alpha-generation as basic response-signature to transcranial magnetic stimulation (TMS) targeting the human resting motor cortex: A TMS/EEG co-registration study. *Psychophysiology,*

Voineskos AN, Farzan F, Barr MS, Lobaugh NJ, Mulsant BH, Chen R, et al. (2010). The role of the corpus callosum in transcranial magnetic stimulation induced interhemispheric signal propagation. *Biol Psychiatry,* 68, pp 825-831

von Stein A, Chiang C, Konig P. (2000). Top-down processing mediated by interareal synchronization. *Proc Natl Acad Sci U S A,* 97, pp 14748-14753

Wahl M, Lauterbach-Soon B, Hattingen E, Jung P, Singer O, Volz S, et al. (2007). Human motor corpus callosum: topography, somatotopy, and link between microstructure and function. *J Neurosci,* 27, pp 12132-12138

Wassermann EM, Lisanby SH. (2001). Therapeutic application of repetitive transcranial magnetic stimulation: a review. *Clin Neurophysiol,* 112, pp 1367-1377

Werhahn KJ, Kunesch E, Noachtar S, Benecke R, Classen J. (1999). Differential effects on motorcortical inhibition induced by blockade of GABA uptake in humans. *J Physiol,* 517 (Pt 2), pp 591-597

Ziemann U. (2004). TMS and drugs. *Clin Neurophysiol,* 115, pp 1717-1729

Ziemann U, Rothwell JC. (2000). I-waves in motor cortex. *J Clin Neurophysiol,* 17, pp 397-405

Ziemann U, Rothwell JC, Ridding MC. (1996). Interaction between intracortical inhibition and facilitation in human motor cortex. *J Physiol,* 496 (Pt 3), pp 873-881

Part 5

EMG in Combination with Other Technologies

19

Muscle Force Analysis of Human Foot Based on Wearable Sensors and EMG Method

Enguo Cao, Yoshio Inoue, Tao Liu and Kyoko Shibata
Kochi University of Technology,
Japan

1. Introduction

Sports injuries, traffic accident, childhood diseases and life-style related diseases may cause movement disorder, and especially in aged persons, physical deterioration may leads to high risk of degeneration of motor function and falling in movement problems. Nowadays, in the trend of population aging of many countries, a large proportion of movement disorder patients are difficult to recover completely in the recent medical condition. Therefore, muscle strength and motor function recovery have aroused general concern from the society, musculoskeletal analysis and rehabilitation activities have been greatly progressed in many countries (Yoon et al., 2010), (Vallery et al., 2007), (Peshkin et al., 2005). Furthermore, modern robots are on high speed developing, but multiple-units foot has seldom caught scientists' attention, robot feet are generally treated as a single rigid part which makes gait seems clumsiness (Park et al., 2009), (Ishida et al., 2003). The human walking style is adequate for various situations compared with wheeled mobile robot, and understanding the muscle works of human limb is implemental for medical diagnosis. It is valuable to develop a multiple-units foot for flexible walking robots and rehabilitation training robots. With economical considerations, developing an easy-operating muscle diagnostic system of multiple-units foot is practical for clinical applications.

Muscle force estimation is not easy because some muscles are locating at inner part of limbs and human foot is a complex musculoskeletal system. For direct measurement of muscle forces, electromyography (EMG) method has been frequently applied as a standard clinical tool in identifying activation level of muscles, but in the EMG method the muscle activity result is relative large or small with the unit of % rather than quantitative values with the unit of Newton (Lee et al., 2008), (Merlo et al., 2003). Moreover through surface EMG method only activities of surface muscles could be estimated, but through needle EMG method the invasiveness of needles may cause reluctance of patients (Kizuka et al., 2009). For indirect estimation method, the quantitative muscle forces of human foot could be calculated, but acquirements of motions of limbs, forces applied on limbs, and the construction of musculoskeletal model are essential (Hou et al., 2007).

Up to the present there are various methods to measure human motion and ground reaction force (GRF) for limb dynamics analysis. But many of them are restricted to laboratory environment and sick to adapt to different situations. The commercial motion camera system, which is regarded as the most popular instrument and a standard tool in measuring movement of human limb, could be performed only in laboratory environment and expensive for implements (Ferreira et al., 2009). The force plate, which is the widely used in measuring GRF with high accuracy in various fields, is limited in single stride measurement (Moustakidis et al., 2008). In this situation, wearable sensor systems based on miniature type force sensors, acceleration sensitive units and gyroscopes play more important role in the applicability for continuously walking and climbing stairs or slopes (Liu et al., 2009), (Boonstra et al., 2006). For construction of musculoskeletal dynamic model, the AnyBody Modeling System, which works in a minimum fatigue criterion way, could be introduced in various applications of variable situation. The geometric data of the model could be decided based on measurements of human anatomy model, and through inverse dynamics method quantitative results of muscle forces of human foot could be calculated. Furthermore, the EMG system could be introduced to validate the calculated muscle force results.

In this chapter, muscle forces of human foot were estimated through inverse dynamics method in AnyBody Modeling System based on wearable sensors and EMG method. A wearable sensor system was developed to measure rotational angles, GRF and centres of pressure (COP) of human limbs. Moreover one group of measured GRF and COP data are transferred into two group of GRF on two loading points in the musculoskeletal model. In AnyBody Modeling System a model of multiple-units foot was established to calculate quantitative muscle forces by inverse dynamics analysis. The shank was also built in the model for attaching muscles between foot and shank, and for the angular acceleration of the shank has influence on these muscles in inverse dynamics method. To make the model suit to different individuals, the size factor was indicated based on the length of human foot. To validate our estimation results of muscle forces, a personal surface EMG system was adopted in the experiment and the muscle activation level of Anterior Tibialis (ANT TIB), Peroneus Longus (PL), Gastrocnemius (GAST) and Soleus (SOL) were directly measured. The raw EMG result measured by hard type sensor system was filtered and rectified into integral EMG results, and the integral EMG results were introduced in the validation with the muscle force results of AnyBody Modeling System.

2. Methods

2.1 Wearable sensor system for measuring angular motion, GRF and COP

Angular motions of shank and thigh were measured by two wearable sensors with acceleration sensitive units and gyroscopes. And angular motions, GRF and COP of multiple-units foot were measured by a pair of developed instrument shoes with both force sensors and motion sensors. The measured data were expressed in a general coordinate system which was aligned with the orientation of the shoe, and located on the contacting plane between the shoe and the floor. As shown in Fig. 1, the *Z*-axis was made vertical, and the *Y*-axis was chosen to represent the anterior-posterior direction of the shoe on the interface plane contacting with the ground, while the X-axis was chosen such that the global coordinate system would be right-handed (Liu et al., 2008). Accurate location of the sensors is not necessary because the limb segments are regarded as rigid bodies in the study.

In this way the dispersion force on the bottom of shoe was expressed by concentrated GRF and COP, and the measured electrical data of angular motion, GRF and COP of multiple-units foot were transmit into a signal process box, which took the responsibility for wave filtering, data consolidation and transmission, as shown in Fig. 2. The signal process box also played a role of signal synchronization by sending a start pulse to the wearable sensor system combined on the leg, as all the sensors have the same sampling frequency. The

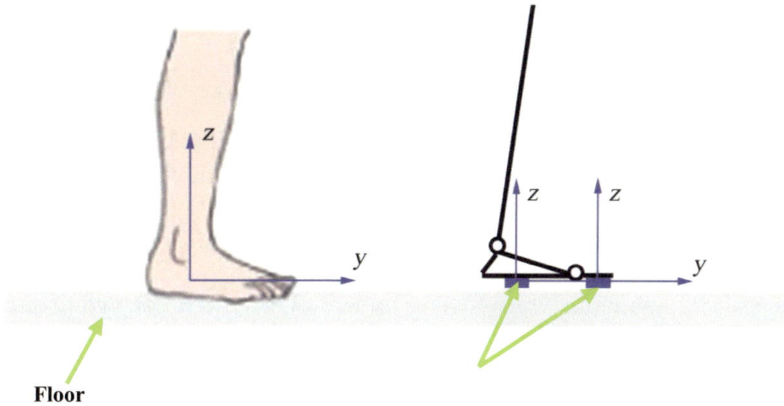

Fig. 1. Ordinate system of an instrument shoe with multiple sensors to obtain GRF, COP and angular motion of multiple-units foot.

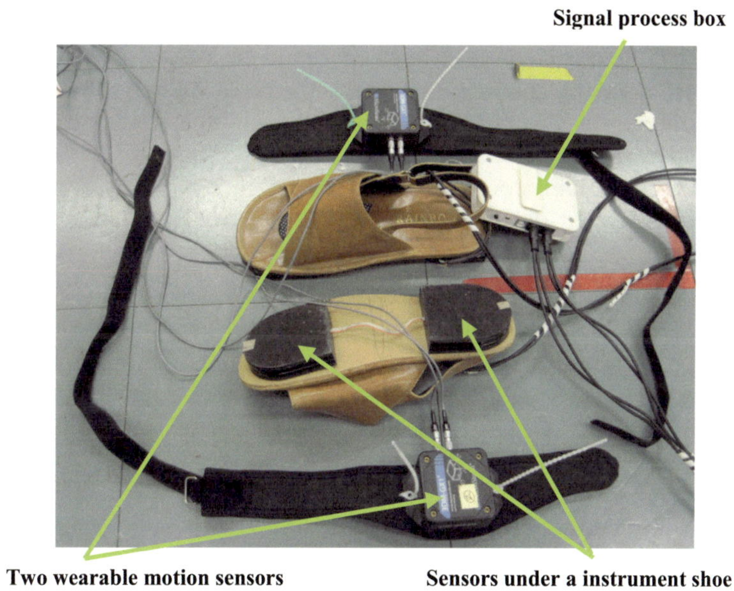

Fig. 2. The instrument shoes and two wearable sensors designed to obtain GRF, COP and angular motions of lower limbs during successive walking trial.

motion of shank was measured because muscles joint points in shank have non-separable relationship with the muscles driving the foot, and the process of gait is relied on the co-operation of these muscles. The angular motion of thigh was not involved in the calculation of muscle forces of the foot because there are no muscles connect from thigh to the foot directly, although the motion of thigh was measured in this experiment for the future research. In the wearable motion and GRF sensor system, all the sensors had the sampling frequency of 100 Hz, and the GRF, COP, multiple-units foot and shank rotations had the units of Newton (N), millimeter (mm) and degree (°) respectively. Totally four groups of

GRF, two group of COP and four groups of angular of multiple-units foot were measured by the instrument shoes, moreover one groups of angular of shank and one groups of angular of thigh were measured by the wearable sensors.

2.2 AnyBody modeling system for establishing multiple-units foot model

In human body muscles are activated by the central nervous system (CNS) base on a complicated electro-chemical process. Determining the activation that realizes a desired movement requires an extremely intricate control algorithm. The AnyBody Modeling System is not only a professional musculoskeletal modeling system, but also a kinematics and kinetics analysis system, in which inverse dynamics method is adapted to quantitatively estimate muscle forces. AnyBody imitates the workings of the CNS by computing backwards from the movement and load specified by the user to the necessary muscle forces in a process known as inverse dynamics. Maximum synergism would be the case where all muscles capable of a positive contribution to balancing the external load work together, in such a way that the maximum relative load of any muscle in the system is as small as possible. It means that the body would maximize its endurance and precisely, this criterion might decide survival of the fittest in an environment where organisms are competing with each other for limited resources. So in AnyBody a minimum fatigue criterion way is employed because fatigue is likely to happen first in the muscle working on the maximum relative load, and it makes physiological sense that the body might work that way.

To implement dynamic analysis of human foot, a multiple-units foot and shank model was created in AnyBody Modeling System. As shown in Fig. 3, the coordinates of knee, ankle, and toe joints and muscle joint points were determined by measuring datum of the human lower limb (McMinn et al., 1982). The shank was also built in the model for attaching

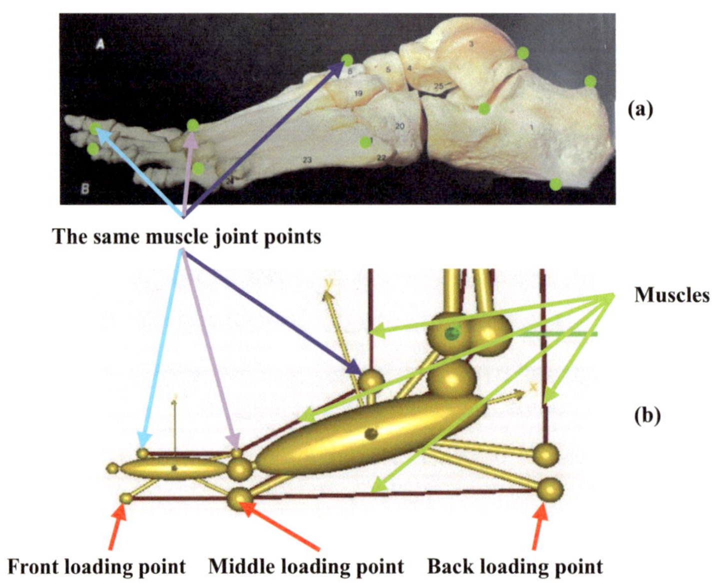

Fig. 3. Method for obtaining coordinates of multiple-units foot model in AnyBody System.
(a) Human anatomy sscannogram for obtaining geometric data of human foot.
(b) Musculoskeletal multiple-units foot model in AnyBody Modeling System.

muscles between foot and shank; furthermore the angular acceleration of the shank has influences on these muscles in the inverse dynamics method. To simulate the true situation of human walking, the GRF were implemented on three loading points locating on the bottom of foot model, and the loads applied on loading points contain both pressure and tangential forces as shown in Fig. 3 (b). The main working muscles involved in the model were ANT TIB, GAST, SOL, PL, Peroneus Brevis (PB), Posterior Tibialis (POST TIB), Extensor Digitorum Longus (EDL) and Flexor Digitorum Longus (FDL), that were built with the maximum strength of 5000 N. Totally seventeen muscle points were created to join muscles, four joints of hip, knee, ankle and toe were created to restrict the activity freedom degree, and three loading points were created to load the GRF and COP. The model worked as an integrated kinetics system after all the units were combined by joints and muscles. The foot model was established based on a rigid barefoot as the instrument shoes nearly have no elasticity, and to make the model suit for different individuals, the model size factor was indicated based on the length of human foot.

2.3 Inverse dynamics method for calculating muscle forces

The GRF, COP and angular motion data measured by the wearable sensor system were imported into the developed multiple-units foot and shank model in AnyBody Modeling System to calculate muscle forces of human foot through an inverse dynamic method. To simulate the true situation of human walking, one group of GRF and COP was transferred into two forces on different locations based on Eq. (1) and Eq. (2), in this way the measured two groups of GRF and COP data were transferred into three groups of force data applied on three loading points on the bottom plane of foot model. In single gait cycle, loads were transferred from posterior foot to the anterior foot continuously and the whole force process was simulated. This transformation can perfectly imitate the GRF variation and COP shifting because the multiple-units foot is regarded as a rigid body system, furthermore real human foot receives GRF mainly on similar three points too. The loads applied on loading points contain both pressure and tangential forces. The pressure force of GRF was expressed on the Z-direction, and the COP_z (x_0, y_0, z_0) on this dirction is defined by Eq. (1), and the tangential force of GRF was expressed on the Y-direction, and the COP_y (x_0, y_0, z_0) on this direction is defined by Eq. (2).

$$x_0 = 0, \quad y_0 = \frac{\sum F_z \bullet y}{\sum F_z}, \quad z_0 = 0 \tag{1}$$

$$x_0 = 0, \quad y_0 = \frac{\sum F_y \bullet y}{\sum F_y}, \quad z_0 = 0 \tag{2}$$

F_z — A force on Z-direction.
F_y — A force on Z-direction.
x — X-axis coordinate values of the force.
y — Y-axis coordinate values of the force.

As shown in Fig. 4, the angular motion data of shank, the posterior foot and the anterior foot were measured in general coordinate system as ϕ_{shank}, ϕ_{heel}, ϕ_{toe}. Because all the parts in the model were regarded as rigid bodies, the relative angular motion ($\Delta\phi_{\text{shank}}$, $\Delta\phi_{heel}$, $\Delta\phi_{\text{toe}}$)

could be calculated by quantitative subtraction. Furthermore in AnyBody Modeling System, the shank, the posterior foot and the anterior foot were driven by $\Delta\phi_{\text{shank}}$, $\Delta\phi_{heel}$, $\Delta\phi_{\text{toe}}$ respectively as shown in Eq. (3), (4), (5). After all the model units were combined by joints and driven by imported motion data, the AnyBody musculoskeletal model worked as an integrated kinetics system and quantitative muscle forces were calculated out through inverse dynamic process.

$$\Delta\phi_{\text{shank}} = \phi_{\text{shank}} \tag{3}$$

$$\Delta\phi_{\text{heel}} = \phi_{\text{heel}} - \phi_{\text{shank}} \tag{4}$$

$$\Delta\phi_{\text{toe}} = \phi_{\text{toe}} - \phi_{\text{heel}} \tag{5}$$

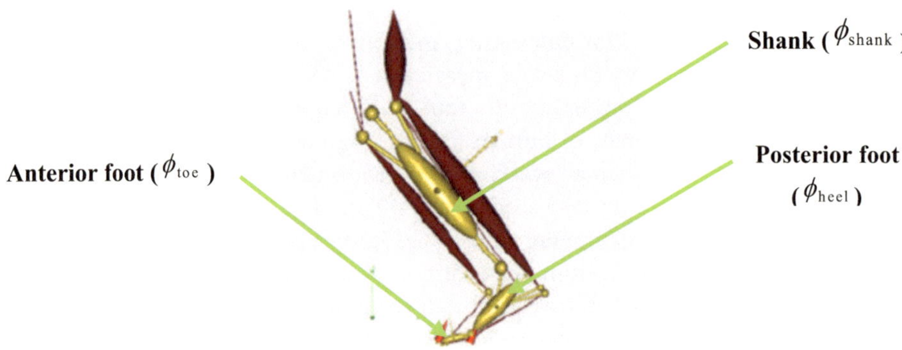

Fig. 4. Angular motion data of shank, the posterior foot and the anterior foot were measured in general coordinate system as ϕ_{shank}, ϕ_{heel}, ϕ_{toe}.

2.4 EMG method for validating muscle force results

The main muscles of human shank and foot were illustrated in Fig. 5, the motions of human limb are motivated by complex teamwork of these muscles, but only several of these muscles were involved in the EMG experiment, that because only the muscles visible in skin surface and offering primary motive power in walking process are possible and worthy for directly analysing. As shown in Fig. 6, the personal-EMG system (P-EMG-0403A01) includes hard type sensor system, filter box and data process system, and based on this system the EMG method was adopted to directly measure muscle activation level of ANT TIB, PL, GAST and SOL. The raw EMG results were filtered and rectified by the filter box and the data process system into integral EMG results that could represent the muscle activation levels. Both the raw EMG and the integral EMG were real time recorded and displayed by the data process system, furthermore the integral EMG results were introduced in the validation with muscle force results calculated by AnyBody Modeling System. Furthermore, one hundred percent standard voluntary contractions (100%SVC) were defined as standard isolation of muscle activity in the respective muscle tests for the normalization of EMG signal (Perry et al., 1986).

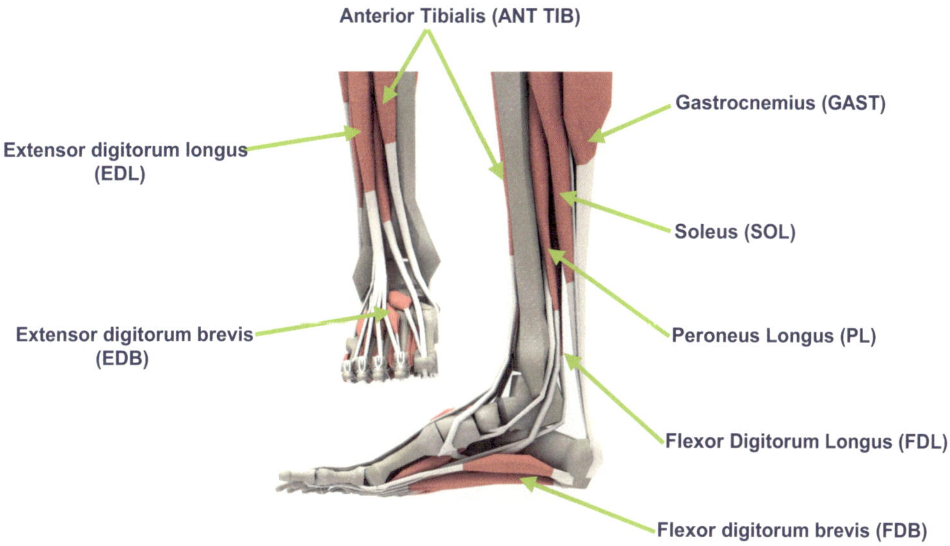

Fig. 5. Illustration of main muscles of human shank and foot.

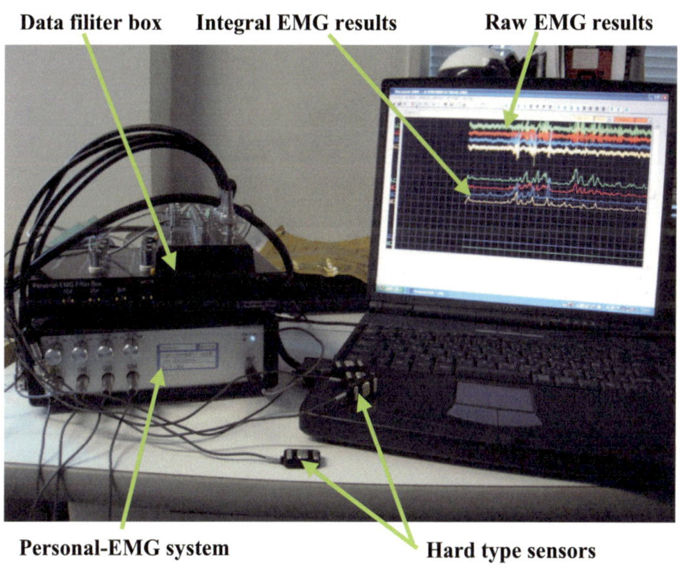

Fig. 6. Personal-EMG system adopted to directly measure muscle activation levels in human lower limb.

3. Experimental study

3.1 Experiment method

The first experiment step is acquisition motion and GRF information of human lower limbs in gait cycle, five adult volunteers (age: 28.5±5 years, weight: 75±6.5 kg.) who had no musculoskeletal disease history were requireed to performed their normal gait in the experiment. The distance of the performance was four meters, duration time was ten seconds. As shown in Fig. 7, three-dimensional angular motion of thigh, shank, posterior part and anterior part of the multiple-units foot were measured with the unit of degree (°), and three-dimensional GRF and two-dimensional COP were measured by the instrument shoes with the unit of Newton (N) and millimeter (mm) respectively. Because all the limb parts were regarded as rigid segments, precise location of wearable sensors which attached on human limbs was unnecessary, so was the size adjustable of the instrumented shoes for the same reason. The sampling frequency of all sensors were regulated as 100 Hz, signal synchronization was realized by the signal process box which would send a pulse to wearable sensors attached on shank and thigh. To remove noise, low-pass filtering was performed on obtained signals with the cut-off frequency of 10 Hz.

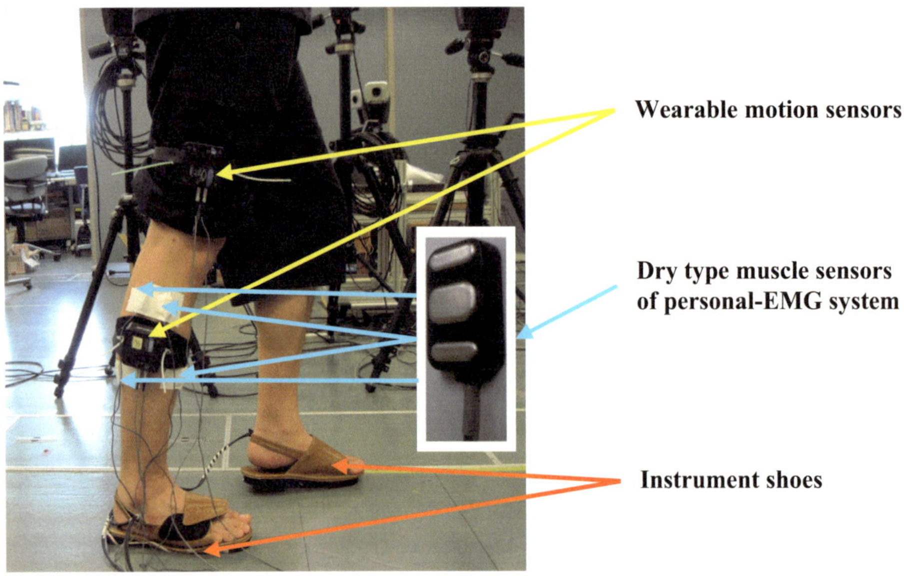

Fig. 7. Prototype of a volunteer wearing instrument shoes, wearable motion sensors and muscle sensors of personal-EMG in the experiment.

To directly measure muscle activation levels of ANT TIB, PL, GAST and SOL, the personal-EMG system and dry type muscle sensors were adopted in the experiment. The dry type muscle senors, which works on a myoelectricity difference principle, could sensing the muscle activation level while being pasted on the eneurosis zone of muscle surface. Furthermore the measured raw EMG results were real time filtered and rectified into integral EMG results by the personal-EMG application system, and both raw EMG results and integral EMG results were real time displayed for easy checking and adjusting. As shown in Fig. 8, we divided one gait cycle into four steps: contacting step, supporting step, leaving step and swing step. The contacting step starts from the heel contacting the ground and ends in the whole foot bottom plane stamping on the ground, the supporting step represents the process of gravity movement from posterior to anterior while one foot supporting the whole weight, the leaving step stands for the action from the heel leaving the ground to the whole foot leaving the ground, and the swing step means the foot swing forward process without contacting the floor.

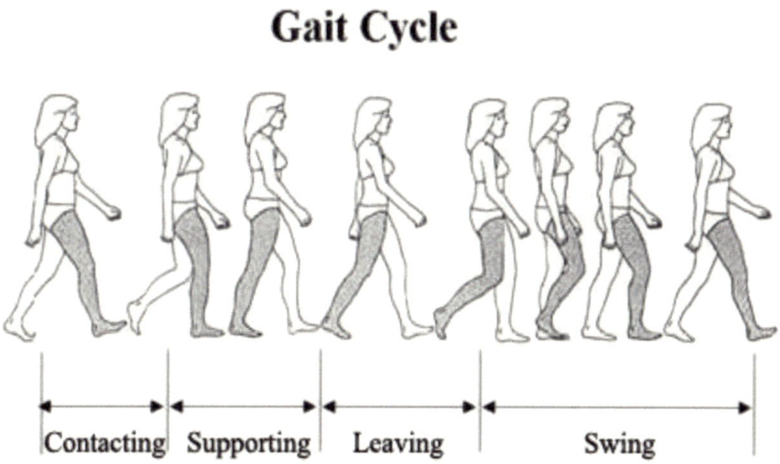

Fig. 8. One gait cycle was divided into contacting step, supporting step, leaving step and swing step.

The second experiment step was calculating the muscle forces in AnyBody Modeling System. For preparation, the measured motion and GRF data of lower limb were transferred into the form that is adequate to the AnyBody system. As a rigid body system, the relative angular motion data ($\Delta\phi_{\text{shank}}$, $\Delta\phi_{heel}$, $\Delta\phi_{\text{toe}}$) were imported into the model to drive the movement of the shank and the multiple-units foot. The measured GRF data were transformed into three forces on three loading points to imitate GRF variation and COP shifting. As shown in Fig. 9, in Z-axis the entire pressure GRF data measured by sensors was drawn as F_z, and GRF

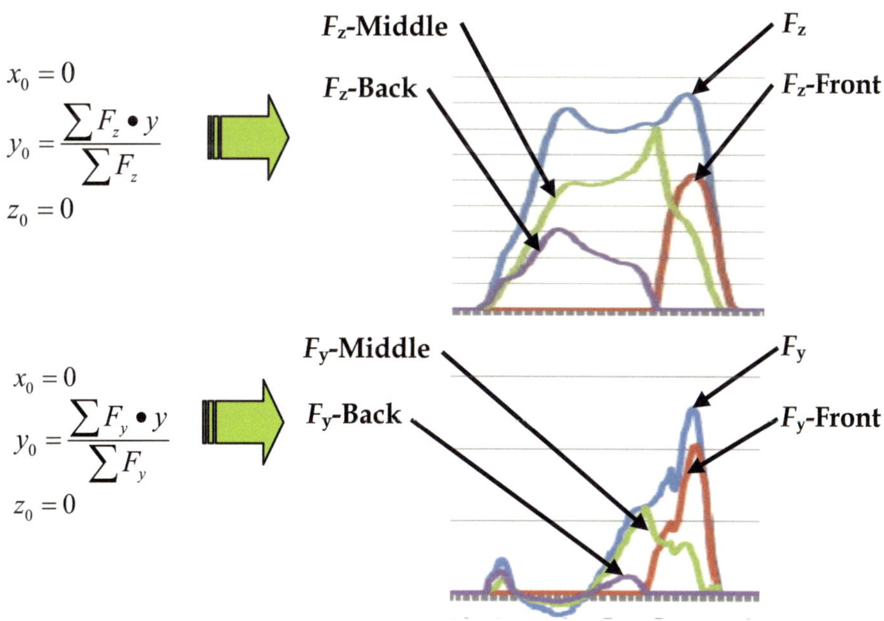

Fig. 9. The GRF were transferred into three forces on three loading points to imitate GRF variation and COP shifting in gait cycle.

transformation data applied on three loading points were drawn as F_z-Front, F_z-Middle and F_z-Back. Futhermore in *Y*-axis, the entire tangential GRF data were transformed into F_y-Front, F_y-Middle and F_y-Back with the same algorithm. In order to make the foot model suitable for diferent individual, the size factors of foot length were dopted. As shown in Table 1, the size fators of five volunteers were summarized. Finally, the muscle forces and joint moment, while ankle joint muscles collaborating with each other in normal walking, were calculated through the inverse dynamics method in AnyBody Modeling System. This experiment has been approved by the ethics committee of the Department of Intelligent Mechanical System Engineering, Kochi University of Technology.

Subject	Size factor of AnyBody foot model (mm)
1	245
2	240
3	265
4	260
5	235

Table 1. List of size factors of the five subjects in the experiment.

3.2 Experimental results

The muscle force results through indirect AnyBody method and direct EMG method were summarized in this section. In AnyBody Modeling System the complex walking kinematic system requires high collaborations of all units, so the muscle forces of human foot were calculated based on a minimum fatigue criterion way. As shown in Fig. 10, the established AnyBody model, which can demonstrate the walking process and the muscle activation video, made the whole process easier to understand in a visualized way. The muscle activity level could be identified by the muscle bulge level, the value and direction of GRF could be discerned by the length and direction of the arrow in the AnyBody gait process video. The quantitative results of ANT TIB, POST TIB, GAST, SOL, EDL and FDL of five subjects in their normal gait were shown in Fig. 11, in Y-axis the quantitative muscle forces were expressed while in *X*-axis the time was represented. The muscles connecting shank and foot were classified in foot muscle analysis because these muscles would offer foot driven power, whereas the muscle from thigh to shank were excluded because those muscles could only drive the movement of shank in the gait dynamitic system.

To validate the muscle forces calculated by the musculoskeletal multiple-units foot model, contradistinctive analysis was implemented between AnyBody results and EMG results. Only ANTTIB, PL, SOL and GAST were involved in the analysis becasue these four muscles are powerful muscles for driving the movements of human limbs in normal gait, futhermore these muscles are easy to find in skin surface for surface EMG measurement. As shown in Fig. 12, the AnyBody results were drawn in blue while the EMG results were expressed in shadow, in comparison diagrams the *X*-axis represented percentage of gait cycle (%GC) while the left Y-axis indicated the muscle force with the unit of Newton, and the right *Y*-axis indicated the percentage of standard voluntary contraction (%SVC) of muscles. Futhermore for making the discussion clearly, the step division figure of gait cycle was expressed on the top of each diagram.

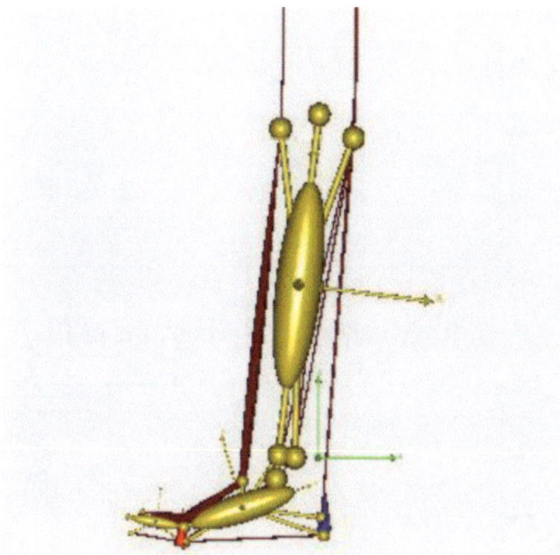

(a) Screenshot in contacting step

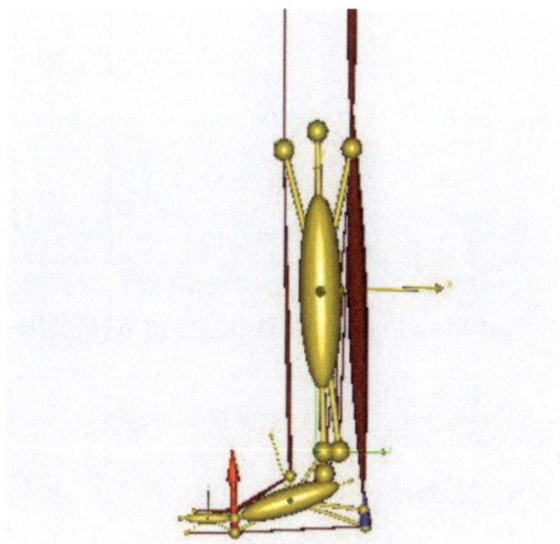

(b) Screenshot in supporting step

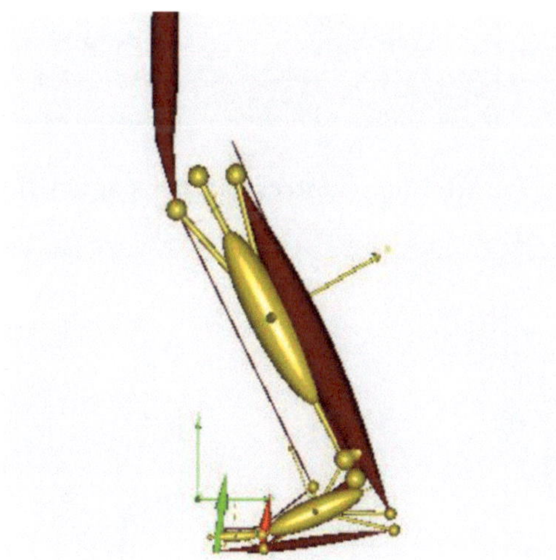

(c) Screenshot in leaving step

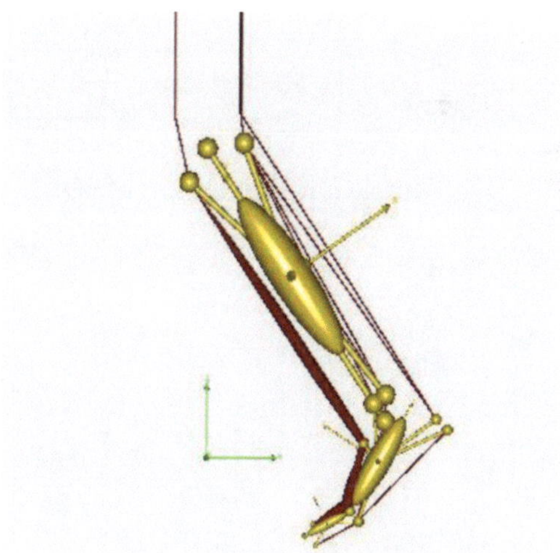

(d) Screenhots in swing step

Fig. 10. Screenshots of gait video in AnyBody Modeling System, four postures in one gait cycle were shown.

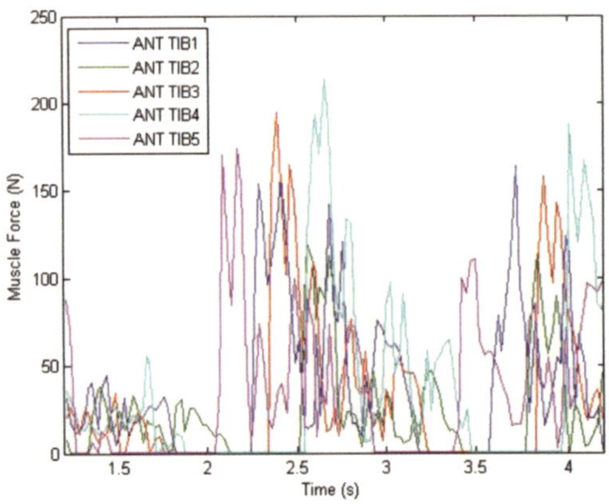

(a) Muscle forces diagrams of ANT TIB

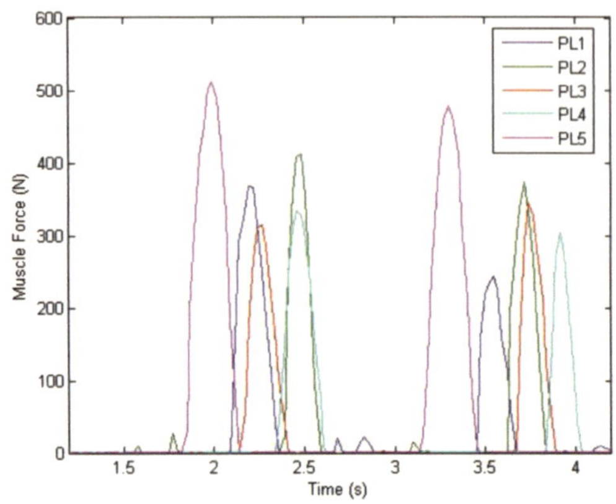

(b) Muscle forces diagrams of PL

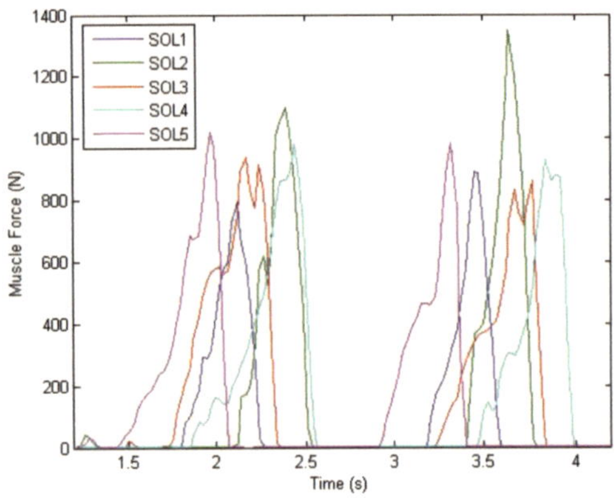

(c) Muscle forces diagrams of SOL

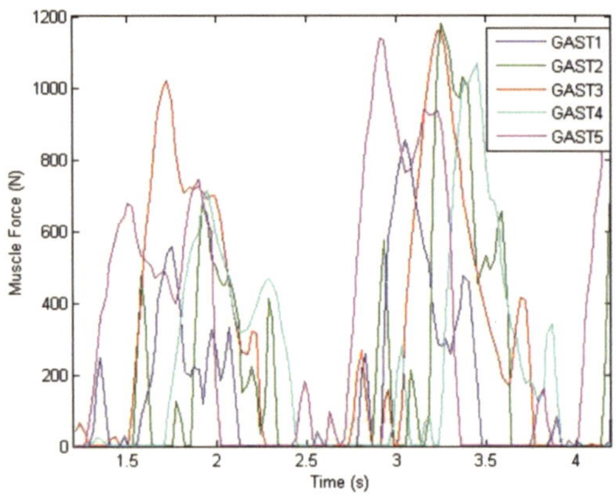

(d) Muscle forces diagrams of GAST

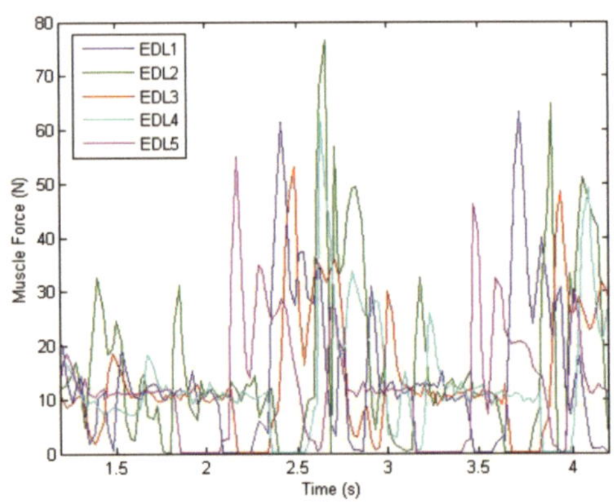

(e) Muscle forces diagrams of EDL

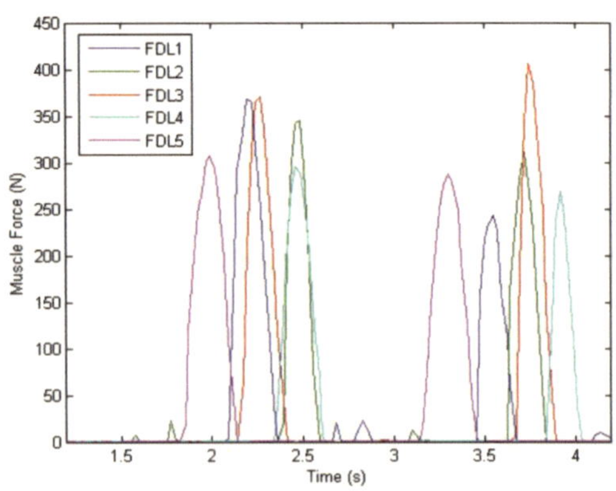

(f) Muscle forces diagrams of FDL

Fig. 11. Muscle forces diagrams of ANT TIB, PL, SOL, GAST, FDL and EDL of five subjects obtained in AnyBody Modeling System.

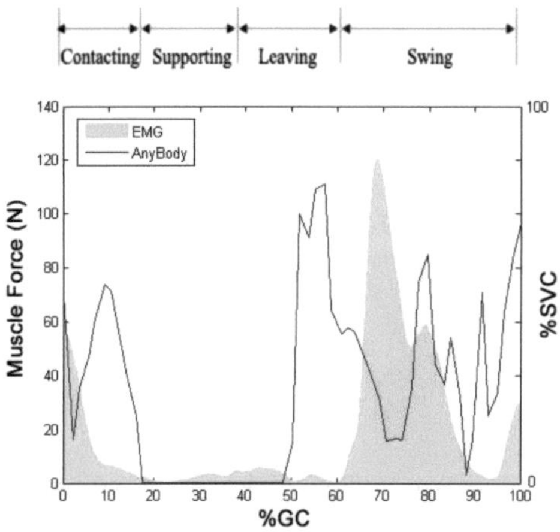

(a) ANT TIB 1

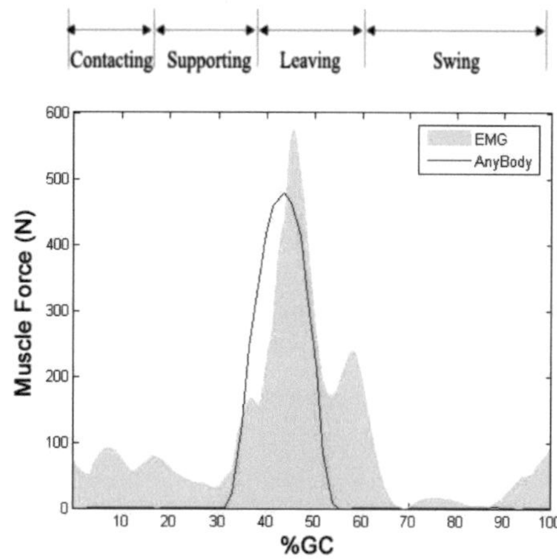

(b) PL 1

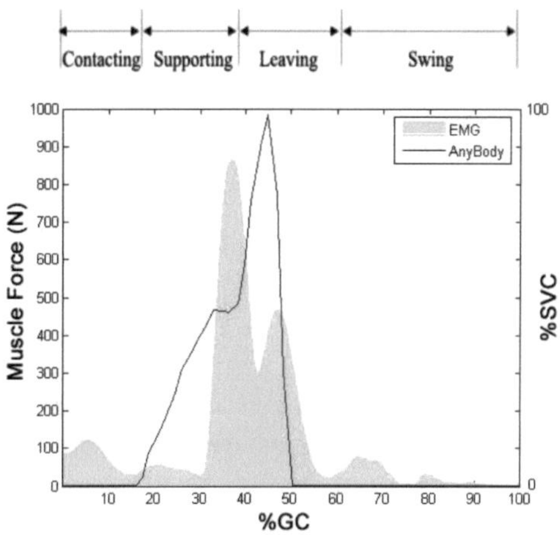

(c) SOL 1

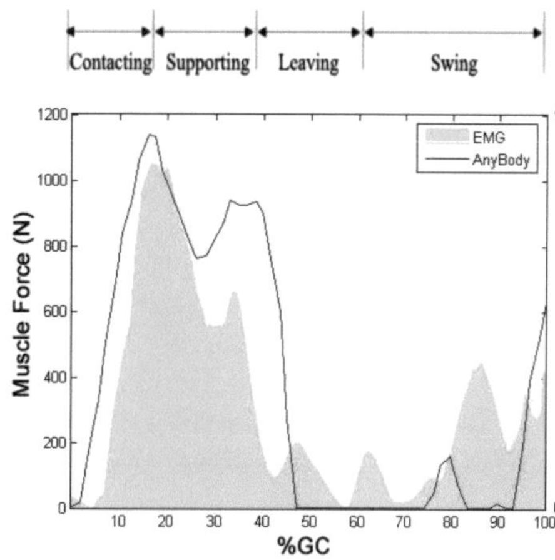

(d) GAST 1

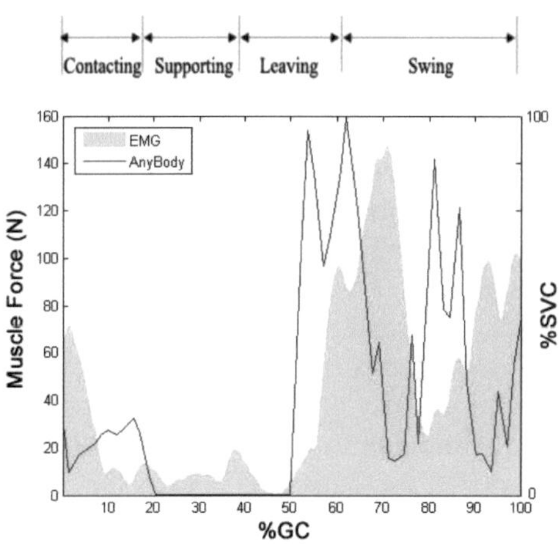

(e) ANT TIB 2

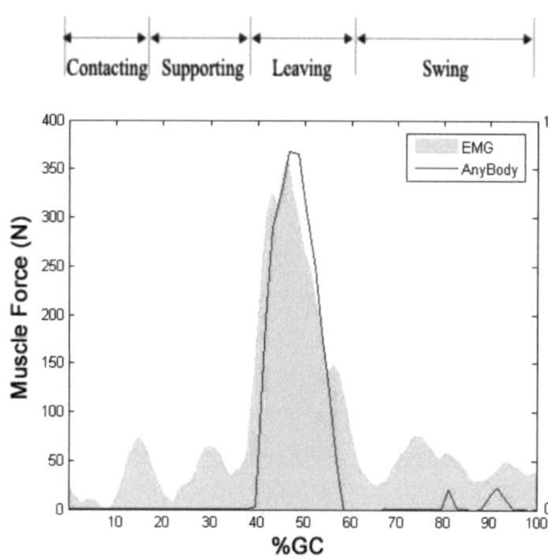

(f) PL 2

Fig. 12. (Continued)

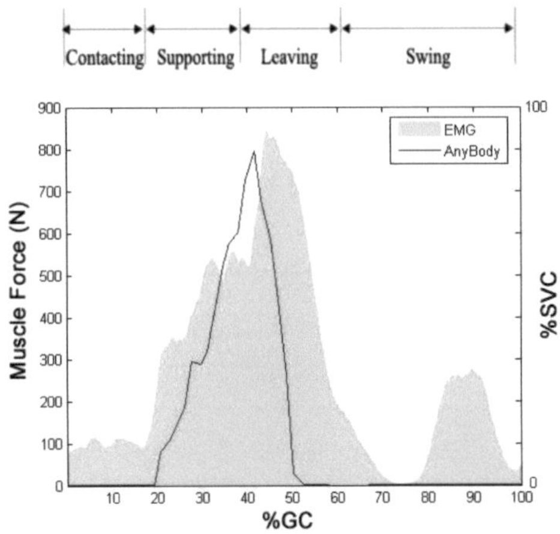

(g) SOL 2

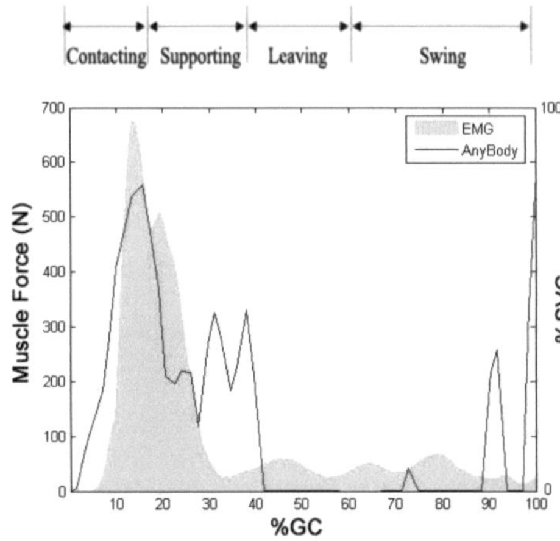

(h) GAST 2

Fig. 12. Comparison diagrams of muscle activation of ANT TIB, PL, SOL and GAST in one gait cycle. The results of AnyBody Modeling System were drawn in blue while the results of EMG method were expressed in shadow.

4. Discussions

As muscle force results were estimated base on wearable sensor system and AnyBody Modeling system, EMG results had been used to do the comparison as in EMG method the muscle activity result is relatively large or small. As shown in Fig. 11, AnyBody results of five volunteers was exhibited, futhermore reality sense for walking process and similarty could be found among different indivaduals. And in Fig. 12, contradistinctive analysis was implemented between calculated results of AnyBody method and measured results of EMG method, obviously similar comparability could be found although the two results had many differences.

As shown in Fig. 11 (a), (e), the muscle force of ANT TIB and EDL were relatively larger in the first contacting step because the muscles in fronter of shank need to grow up to balance the moment of ankle joint while the heel contacting the floor. And in the last swing step ANT TIB and EDL were larger because they offered forces to drive the limb swing till next gait cycle started. Whereas the values of ANT TIB and EDL were keeping nearly zero in the other steps of gait cycle. As shown in Fig. 12 (a), (e), the value of ANT TIB was relatively high in both AnyBody results and EMG results in the beginning and ending period of one gait cycle, but in the middle steps the AnyBody results were keeping nearly zero while the EMG results were only keeping relatively smaller values.

As shown in Fig. 11 (c), (d), the tensile forces of SOL and GAST increased obviously in the supporting step when the GRF were transfered from posterior foot to anterior foot, moreover the peak value of GAST occurred in this step too. And in the leaving ground step, the SOL continued to increase for pushing human body moving forward and upward till the whole foot separated from the ground and start to swing, moreover the peak value of SOL occurred in this step. The peak Achilles tendon forces occured in the leaving step of our results that ranging from 1.07 kN to 1.66 kN, which were in good agreement with the reported peak Achilles tendon forces of 1430±500 N (Finni et al., 1998). The SOL and GAST were keeping small vaules in the contacting step because the center of gravity were behind the ankle joint. As shown in Fig. 12 (c), (d), (g), (h), the AnyBody results and EMG results were not in high agreement but the variation tendencies were similar.

As shown in Fig. 11 (b), (f), FDL and PL had similar rising period and descending period, and peak values of PL and FDL both occurred in the leaving step, that because the two muscles are both located in the posterior of shank and play a similar role of pushing human body moving forward and upward in the normal human gait. As shown in Fig. 12 (b), (f), in contacting, supporting and swing steps the EMG results of PL showed relatively higher values while the AnyBody results were keeping nearly zero, but in the whole gait cycle obvious comparability could be found between the two results.

5. Conclusions

Muscle forces of human foot were estimated through the inverse dynamics method in AnyBody Modeling System based on wearable sensors and EMG method. The angular motions, GRF and COP of human limb segments could be measured by the developed wearable motion and force sensors with acceleration sensitive units and gyroscopes in various situations. AnyBody Modeling System that professional concerns on musculoskeletal kinematics and kinetics analysis could imported the sensor measured data into a bionic dynamic model. And through invise dynamic method the quantitative muscle forces of human foot could be estimated in AnyBody system. The EMG method was adopted to directly measure muscle activition levels for validation, and the muscle activation results of EMG method have certain comparability with the muscle force results of AnyBody model, futhermore the tendency curves of these muscle forces have reality sense for walking process analysis. This reserch method for human foot appears to be a practical means to determine muscle forces in musculoskeletal analysis and in on-the-spot medical applications. In the future, the muscle force can be made into vector quantity instead of scalar quantity by 3D technology in AnyBody Modeling System as the angular motion and GRF sensors own the capability of 3D measurement.

6. Acknowledgement

The authors wish to acknowledge the support of the volunteer subjects of Robotics and Dynamics Research Lab in Kochi University of Technology.

7. References

Yoon, J.; Novandy, B.; Yoon, C. H. & Park, K. J. (2010). A 6-DOF Gait Rehabilitation Robot With Upper and Lower Limb Connections That Allows Walking Velocity Updates on Various Terrains, *IEEE/ASME Trans. on Mechatronics*, Vol. 15, No. 2, pp. 201–215, ISSN 1083-4435

Vallery, H.; Ekkelenkamp, R.; Buss, M. & Kooij, H. (2007). Complementary Limb Motion Estimation based on Interjoint Coordination: Experimental Evaluation, *Proc. of IEEE 10th Intl. Conf. on Rehabilitation Robotics*, pp. 798–803, ISBN 978-1-4244-1320-1, Noordwijk. Netherlands

Peshkin, M.; Brown, D. A.; Santos-Munné, J. J.; Makhlin, A.; Lewis, E.; Colgate, J. E.; Patton, J. & Schwandt, D. (2005). KineAssist: A Robotic Overground Gait and Balance

Training Device, *Proc. of IEEE 9th Intl. Conf. on Rehabilitation Robotics,* pp. 241–246, ISBN 0-7803-9003-2, Chicago, USA

Park, J.H. & Kim, E.S. (2009). Foot and Body Control of Biped Robots to Walk on Irregularly Protruded Uneven Surfaces, *IEEE Transactions on Systems, Man, and Cybernetics, Part B: Cybernetics,* Vol. 39, No. 1, pp. 289-297, ISSN 1083-4419

Ishida, T.; Kuroki, Y. & Yamaguchi, J. (2003). Mechanical System of a Small Biped Entertainment Robot, *Proceedings of IEEE/RSJ International Conference on Intelligent Robots and Systems,* pp. 1129-1134, ISBN 0-7803-7860-1, Las Vegas, Nevada, USA

Lee, K.S. (2008). EMG-Based Speech Recognition Using Hidden Markov Models With Global Control Variables, *IEEE Transactions on Biomedical Engineering,* Vol. 55, No. 3, pp. 930-940, ISSN 0018-9294

Merlo, A.; Farina, D. & Merletti, R. (2003). A Fast and Reliable Technique for Muscle Activity Detection From Surface EMG Signals, *Transactions On Biomedical Engineering,* Vol. 50, No. 3, pp. 316-323, ISSN 0018-9294

Kizuka T.; Masuda, T.; Kiryu, T. & Sadoyama, T. (2009). *Biomechanism Library Practical Usage of Surface Electromyogram,* Publisher of Tokyo Denki University, ISBN 4-501-32510-0, Tokyo, Japan

Hou, Y.F.; Zurada, J.M.; Karwowski, W.; Marras, W.S. & Davis, K. (2007). Estimation of the Dynamic Spinal Forces Using a Recurrent Fuzzy Neural Network, *IEEE Transactions on Systems, Man, and Cybernetics – Part B: Cybernetics,* Vol. 37, No. 1, pp. 100-109, ISSN 1083-4419

Ferreira, J.P.; Crisostomo, M.M. & Coimbra, A.P. (2009). Human Gait Acquisition and Characterization, *IEEE Transactions on Instrumentation and Measurement,* Vol. 58, No. 9, pp. 2979-2988, ISSN 0018-9456

Moustakidis, S.P.; Theocharis, J.B. & Giakas, G. (2008). Subject Recognition Based on Ground Reaction Force Measurements of Gait Signals, *IEEE Transactions on Systems, Man, and Cybernetics – Part B: Cybernetics,* Vol. 38, No. 6, pp. 1476-1485, ISSN 1083-4419

Liu, K.; Liu, T.; Shibata, K.; Inoue, Y. & Zheng, R.C. (2009). Novel Approach to Ambulatory Assessment of Human Segmental Orientation on A Wearable Sensor System, *Journal of Biomechanics,* Vol. 42, No. 16, pp. 2747-2752, ISSN 0021-9290

Boonstra, M.C.; Slikke, R.M.; Keijsers, N.L.; Lummel, R.C.; Malefijt, M.C. & Verdonschot, N. (2006). The Accuracy of Measuring the Kinematics of Rising from a Chair with Accelerometers and Gyroscopes, *Journal of Biomechanics,* Vol. 39, No. 2, pp. 354-358, ISSN 0021-9290

Liu, T.; Inoue, Y. & Shibata, K. (2008). New Method for Assessment of Gait Variability Based on Wearable Ground Reaction Force Sensor, *30th Annual International IEEE EMBS Conference Vancouv*er, pp. 2341-2344, ISSN 1557-170X

McMinn, R.M.H.; Hutchings, R.T. & Logan, B.M. (1982). *Colour Atlas of Foot and Ankle Anatomy,* Year Book Medical Publishers, ISBN 0-815-15829-7, Chicago, USA

Perry, J.; Ireland, M.; Gronley, J. & Hoffer, M. (1986). Predictive Value of Manual Muscle Testing and Gait Analysis in Normal Ankles by Electromyography, *Foot Ankle,* Vol. 6, No. 5, pp. 254-259, ISSN 1071-1007

Finni, T.; Komi, P.V. & Lukkariniemi, J. (1998). Achilles Tendon Loading During Walking: Application of a Novel Optic Fiber Technique, *Eur J Appl Physiol Occup Physiol,* Vol. 77, No. 3, pp. 289-291, ISSN 0301-5548

20

Affective Processing of Loved Familiar Faces: Contributions from Electromyography

Pedro Guerra, Alicia Sánchez-Adam, Lourdes Anllo-Vento and Jaime Vila
University of Granada, Spain

1. Introduction

Human faces stand among the most unique stimuli in social and emotional communication. By looking at faces we can access a broad range of significant information about the other, such as personal identity, emotional state (facial expression), sex, age, race, attractiveness, attitudes (whether they are friendly or hostile), intentions, and thoughts (Dekowska et al., 2008; Adolphs, 2009). Because of its relevance in everyday interactions, the face has been the target of much study throughout the past decades. Most studies on the psychology of face perception and recognition have focused on emotional facial expressions, following the pioneering work of Tomkins (1962), Izard (1971, 1977, 1994), and Ekman (1984, 1992) (see Russell, 1994; Dimberg, 1997; Whalen et al., 1998; Öhman et al., 2001; Adolphs, 2002; Eimer & Holmes, 2007; Vuilleumier & Pourtois, 2007; Li et al., 2010), based on the evolutionary perspective outlined by Darwin in his book *The expression of emotions in man and animals* (1872). More recently, a large body of research has been devoted to delineate the brain mechanisms involved in face perception and identity recognition (see Adolphs, 2002; Faihall & Isahi, 2006; Dekowska et al., 2008; Li et al., 2010). In this context, studies using central electrophysiological techniques, such as electroencephalography (EEG), event-related potentials (ERPs), or magnetoencephalography (MEG), and metabolic techniques, such as positron emission tomography (PET) or functional magnetic resonance imaging (fMRI), have proven particularly useful in describing the chain of events taking place in the processing of facial information and the neural circuitry responsible for face recognition, respectively. Thus, several event-related components such as P1, N170, N250r, P300, and N400, have been used to determine the temporal sequence that goes from pictorial/structural encoding to retrieval of biographical/emotional information (Bentin et al., 1996; Bruce & Young, 1986; Eimer, 2000a; Herrmann et al., 2005; Schweinberger, 2011). Imaging techniques, on their part, have helped identify the specific brain areas involved in face perception and recognition, including recognition of emotional expression and personal identity (Adolphs, 2002; Gobbini & Haxby, 2007; Zeki, 2007, Haxby & Gobbini, 2011). These brain areas constitute a distributed network with a core system responsible for the analysis of visual appearance (posterior superior temporal sulcus, inferior occipital and fusiform gyri), and an extended system that underlies the retrieval of person knowledge (medial prefrontal cortex, temporo-parietal junction, anterior temporal cortex, precuneus, and posterior cingulate), action understanding (inferior temporal and frontal operculum, and intraparietal sulcus), and emotion (amygdala, insula, and striatum/reward system).

In the context of this broad literature, a subset of studies has looked into the emotional processing associated with recognition of familiar loved faces (i.e., relatives, friends, own children, or romantic partner) by using electrophysiological or fMRI indices of brain activity (Aron et al., 2005; Baçar et al., 2008; Bartels & Zeki, 2000, 2004; Bobes et al., 2007; Fisher et al., 2005; Grasso et al., 2009; Grasso & Simons, 2011; Herzmann et al., 2004; Langeslag et al., 2007; Xu et al., 2011). A major shortcoming in this literature, besides the need to integrate it with research on the neural mechanisms of social and cultural cognition (Tomasello et al., 2005; Amodio & Frith, 2006; Herrmann et al., 2007), is the lack of evidence regarding the elicitation of a genuine positive emotional response to loved familiar faces. This is in part due to the presence of two significant confounding factors in most experimental studies: emotional arousal and familiarity.

Emotional arousal refers to the intensity of an emotion, regardless of its affective valence (positive or negative). Arousal-related ERP modulation is a robust phenomenon that primarily affects long-latency components (Oloffson et al., 2008). Those studies focusing on the modulation of brain responses (ERPs) associated with processing of loved familiar faces have consistently found enhanced P300 and Late Positive Potential (LPP) amplitudes when comparing loved familiar faces to control familiar (newly-learned) and neutral faces. However, similar amplitude increases have been reported in response to highly unpleasant stimuli such as mutilated faces or attacking animals, thus casting doubt on whether the larger late positivity evoked by loved faces reflects activation of positive emotional mechanisms or plain emotional arousal (Palomba et al., 1997; Cuthbert et al., 2000; Schupp et al., 2000, 2004; Sabatinelli et al., 2007; Bradley, 2009).

On its part, familiarity has been defined as a form of explicit or declarative memory (Gobbini & Haxby, 2007; Voss & Paller, 2006, 2007) that is affected by factors such as length of time spent with an individual, number of previous encounters, duration of the relationship, or information accumulated about that individual. Attempts to control for familiarity effects include viewing faces of acquaintances, famous people, or newly learned faces. However, familiarity of loved faces will always exceed that of control faces because of the amount of time spent with them (Grasso et al., 2009). Studies on ERP modulation associated with familiarity have consistently found increases in late positivities at posterior locations (Eimer, 2000a, b; Voss and Paller, 2006; Yovel and Paller, 2004). Interestingly, these same effects have been reported in studies of loved familiar faces (Bobes et al., 2007; Grasso et al., 2009; Herzmann et al., 2004; Langeslag et al., 2007).

Here we propose that studies on the processing of loved familiar faces would benefit from the use of those tools developed in the context of emotional processing research, with special emphasis on the potential contribution of electromyographic recordings.

The picture-viewing paradigm used by Lang and colleagues (Bradley & Lang, 2007; Codispoti, Bradley, & Lang, 2001; Lang, 1995; Lang & Davis, 2006; Lang, Davis, & Öhman, 2000) allows us to disentangle those effects attributable to picture valence (either positive or negative) from those elicited by emotional arousal (intensity of emotion, regardless of its affective valence). In this paradigm, a broad set of central and peripheral measures are simultaneously recorded while participants view pleasant, neutral, and unpleasant pictures taken from the International Affective Picture System (IAPS; Lang, Bradley, & Cuthbert, 2008), an instrument that provides normative ratings of valence, arousal, and dominance for each picture. Research conducted within this framework has consistently shown that highly pleasant pictures are associated with (a) a pattern of accelerative changes in the heart rate, (b) reduced eye-blink startle responses, (c) increases in zygomatic muscle activity, and (d) decreases in corrugator supercilii muscle activity. The inverse pattern is observed with highly arousing unpleasant pictures. Moreover, highly arousing pleasant and unpleasant pictures, when compared to neutral ones, provoke (a) increases in skin conductance, and (b) larger amplitudes for both P3 and LPP components obtained at central-parietal locations (Bradley et al., 2001; Lang & Bradley, 2010). Therefore, two different sets of measures can be identified: one that consistently responds to affective valence, and a second one that is most sensitive to variations in emotional arousal.

Both eye-blink startle and facial EMG have been extensively investigated in the context of emotional processing (see Bradley & Lang, 2007, for a review), and their ability to differentiate affective states has been repeatedly established. The startle reflex consists of a chain of extensor-flexor movements that spread throughout the body (Landis & Hunt, 1939) in response to intense and abrupt stimulation (i.e., an intense white noise). Rapid closing of the eyes constitutes one of the most stable components of this reflex in humans and it can be easily measured by placing electrodes over the orbicularis muscle under the eye. In studies of emotional modulation of the startle reflex using the picture-viewing paradigm, startle eye-blink is consistently potentiated when viewing highly arousing unpleasant pictures, and inhibited when facing highly arousing pleasant pictures, compared to neutral ones (Bradley & Lang, 2007). This valence-mediated effect has been interpreted in terms of the *motivational priming hypothesis* (Lang et al., 1997). According to this model, perceptual stimuli that engage the aversive motivational system potentiate the reflex, whereas those stimuli that engage the appetitive motivational system provoke startle inhibition. The same linear relationship between startle amplitude and affective valence is observed in a large variety of perceptual settings: using pictures (Bradley et al., 2001), films (Jansen & Fridja, 1994), sounds (Bradley & Lang, 2000), and odors (Miltner, 1994).

Facial EMG also provides reliable indices of affective engagement. Special attention has been given to the activation of the corrugator supercilii and zygomatic major muscles in different induction contexts, such as perception, anticipation, and imagery (Bradley & Lang, 2007). The corrugator supercilii muscles are located above and between the eyes and are responsible for drawing down the eyebrows. The zygomatic major muscles originate in the cheeks bones and exert their action by lifting the corner of the mouth obliquely and upwards. Activity in these two sets of muscles is associated with frowning and smiling, respectively.

Since the pioneering work of Schwartz and colleagues (Brown & Schwartz, 1980; Schwartz et al., 1976a, b) and until recently, corrugator supercilii and zygomatic major EMG have been often used to study emotional processing. Processing of unpleasant material elicits larger corrugator activity than neutral or pleasant stimuli (Bradley et al., 2001; Cacioppo et al., 1986; Lang et al., 1993; Larsen et al., 2003). Lang and colleagues (1993) found a linear relationship between activity of the corrugator muscle and the hedonic valence of the pictures, with unpleasant slides eliciting the largest contraction, and pleasant pictures causing inhibition of the corrugator muscles. This same linear gradation was obtained by Larsen, Norris, and Cacioppo (2003) in a study that measured facial EMG in response to three different kinds of stimuli: pictures, sounds, and words. When looking at corrugator activity as a function of emotional picture contents (Bradley et al., 2001), slides depicting mutilations and contamination-related scenes elicit the largest activity in this muscle compared to other unpleasant material.

The relationship between zygomatic activity and affective valence is somewhat more complex. Lang and colleagues (1993) obtained a quadratic relationship between emotional valence and zygomatic activity, with highly pleasant pictures eliciting the largest responses, when compared to either neutral or unpleasant material. However, significant zygomatic activation was also found for unpleasant pictures, compared to neutral stimuli. Larsen and colleagues (2003) confirmed this finding for emotional pictures and sounds, but not for affective words. Because the zygomatic major is involved in smiling and smiling has an unquestionable communicative function in humans, it has been argued that its activity is malleable according to rules of social display. Ekman, Davidson, and Friesen (1990), however, noted that a true smile (the so-called Duchenne smile) is accompanied by simultaneous activation of the zygomatic and orbicularis muscles, while social smiles devoid of positive emotion involve only zygomatic activity.

In this chapter, we summarize the results of three studies aimed at unraveling the mechanisms underlying the processing of loved familiar faces, while distinguishing the relative effects of affective valence, undifferentiated emotional arousal, and familiarity, with special emphasis on zygomatic and orbicularis activity. All three studies combine the following elements: (a) an experimental paradigm that allows differentiation of valence versus arousal effects, (b) simultaneous recording of a broad set of psychophysiological measures, and (c) different sets of stimuli that differ in valence, arousal, and familiarity ratings.

2. Methodology

2.1 Experiment 1

Experiment 1 was aimed at investigating the neurophysiological mechanisms associated with the affective processing of loved familiar faces by combining peripheral and central electrophysiological measures while separating the relative contributions of valence (i.e., positive vs. negative affect), arousal (i.e., more vs. less activation), and familiarity (i.e., known vs. unknown faces). Event-related potentials, skin conductance, heart rate, and electromyography of the *zygomatic major* muscle were obtained along with subjective ratings of valence, arousal, and dominance for each picture. Because of the scope of the present chapter, we will focus on the activity of the zygomatic muscle.

2.1.1 Participants

Thirty female undergraduate students, ranging between 20 and 27 years of age, took part in the study. Subjects were required to have a current romantic relationship (between 6 months and 6 years in duration) and to live in close proximity to five loved ones, including the partner, so as to be able to take their photographs. None of the participants reported current physical or psychological problems and none were under pharmacological treatment. All were right-handed and had normal or corrected to normal vision. All subjects signed informed consent forms and received course credit for their participation.

2.1.2 Materials and design

Participants viewed faces belonging to one of five categories in two separate blocks that differed in picture presentation rate and were administered in counterbalanced order. The slow block, whose results are presented here, consisted of an initial 5-min baseline period, followed by 50 trials with the following structure per trial: 4-sec baseline, 4-sec picture presentation, and 4-sec post-picture period. Inter-trial intervals (ITI) varied randomly between 8 and 12 seconds. The study included 5 photographs of faces in each of 5 categories: loved ones, neutral, unknown, famous, and baby faces. In addition to the partner, faces of loved ones could include parents, siblings, second-degree relatives, and friends. Neutral faces were selected from Ekman and Friesen's (1978) "Facial Action Coding System". Unknown faces were selected among the photographs of loved ones provided by some other participant, after ensuring that those pictures did not depict anyone known to that participant. Famous faces were selected by each participant prior to the experimental session, from a set of 9 photographs portraying people that frequented Spanish media. Participants were asked to identify famous people as such, and were expected not to feel strong attraction or rejection towards them. Finally, faces of babies were selected from the IAPS (Lang et al., 2008) among those with valence scores over 7 (rating scale ranging from 1 to 9) according to Spanish norms (Moltó et al., 1999; Vila et al., 2001). Pictures of loved ones were provided by each participant a few days before the experiment and after they had followed full detailed instructions on how to take the photographs (i.e., loved ones had to look straight at the camera with neutral expression in front of a light background). All pictures were edited using Corel-Draw Photopaint software (version 7). Photographs were matched in size, color, and background. All were cropped down to 650 x 650 pixels, transformed into gray scale (8 bits), and surrounded by a black background.

Each picture was presented twice following a double Latin Square design. The first Latin Square included a 5x5 matrix, where each row and each column contained only one picture belonging to the same category. The second Latin Square was an inverted mirror of the first one. Participants, in groups of 5, were randomly assigned to 5 different sequences (each of those starting with a different picture category) to ensure that all categories were equally distributed within the complete sample. In addition, 15 participants had the slow presentation block followed by the fast presentation block, while the other 15 participants had the inverse order.

Subjects were instructed to simply look at the pictures for the entire time they were on the screen, while trying to withhold from blinking or, if necessary, blinking during the ITI. After the second block, participants evaluated the valence, arousal, and dominance of each single picture according to the Self-Assessment Manikin (Bradley & Lang, 1994).

2.1.3 Apparatus

A Coulbourn polygraph, model V-Link, was used for the recording of zygomatic activity. Stimulus control and peripheral physiological data acquisition were accomplished using an IBM-compatible computer running VPM data acquisition and reduction software (Cook III, 1997). E-Prime software (Psychological Tools, Pittsburgh) controlled the actual presentation of the pictures using a second Pentium 4 computer connected to the master computer through the serial port. Finally, a digital camera, model Kodak Easy Share DX6490, was used to obtain the photographs of loved ones.

2.1.4 Zygomatic EMG recording

Zygomatic EMG activity was recorded using miniature In Vivo Metrics silver/silver chloride electrodes. The raw EMG was amplified by 5000 and band-pass filtered (90-1000 Hz) by means of a Coulbourn V75-04 bioamplifier. The signal was subsequently rectified and integrated using a Coulbourn V75-23A integrator. Time constant for zygomatic activity was 500 ms. The integrated EMG was sampled at 100 Hz and averaged every one half-second for the length of the trial. Each value was expressed in terms of differential scores with respect to the averaged EMG activity during the 4 sec preceding stimulus onset.

2.1.5 Statistical analysis

Zygomatic EMG data were averaged across trials within the same face category and order of block presentation, and analyzed by means of repeated measures ANOVA, using a 5 x 16 design, with the first factor being Face Category (Loved, Neutral, Unknown, Famous, and Babies faces), and the second factor being Time, expressed in 16 one half-second bins following stimulus onset. The Greenhouse-Geisser epsilon correction was applied to correct for sphericity. Analysis of significant interactions was performed identifying the levels of the interacting factors explaining the significant effects, followed by post-hoc pairwise comparisons using Bonferroni test.

2.1.6 Results

Figure 1 shows changes in zygomatic activity during face presentation when the slow block was presented in first and second place, respectively. Regardless of task order, only loved familiar faces evoked a clear response, starting right after stimulus onset and continuing until the end of the 8-sec recording period. Although less pronounced, a response can also be observed for baby faces. The ANOVA revealed significant effects of Face Category ($F(4,116)=9.74$, $p<0.002$, $\eta p^2=0.251$), Time ($F(15, 435)=3.56$, $p<0.04$, $\eta p^2=0.109$), and Face Category x Time ($F(60, 1740)=3.59$, $p<0.007$, $\eta p^2=0.110$).

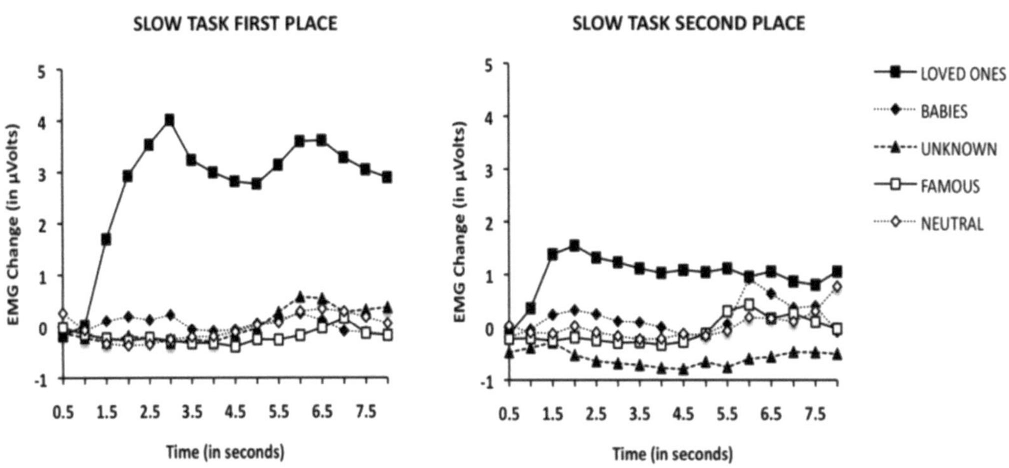

Fig. 1. Zygomatic activity across categories in the slow task as a function of task order.

Analysis of the Face Category x Time interaction yielded significant Face Category effects for all Time points from second 1.5 to second 8 (all p-values < 0.02). Except for seconds 6 and 6.5, loved familiar faces prompted a larger response than all other categories (all p-values < 0.04). Significant differences were also found between babies and neutral faces in seconds 2.5 and 3 (both p-values < 0.05). No differences were found between famous and unknown faces.

Figure 2 displays the average zygomatic response across the four subcategories of loved faces. Separate ANOVAs for each pair of subcategories yielded significant differences between partner and friend ($F(1, 18)=4.015$, $p<0.05$, $\eta p^2=0.157$), though only in the first trial. Differences between partner and parent ($F(1, 21)=3.75$, $p<0.07$, $\eta p^2=0.160$), and partner and sibling (F(1,19)=3.346, $p<0.08$, $\eta p^2=0.165$), also during the first trial, were marginally significant. No other significant differences were found.

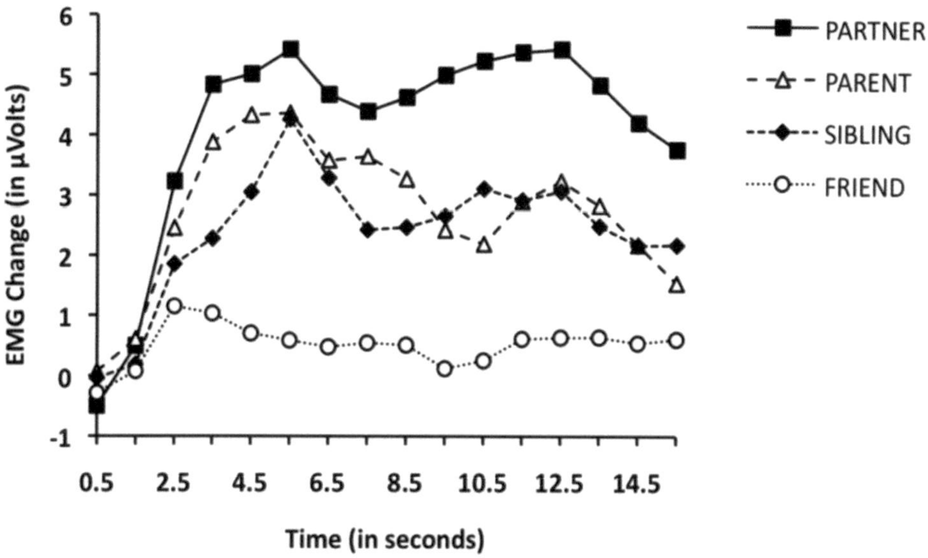

Fig. 2. Zygomatic activity as a function of subcategory of loved familiar faces.

2.2 Experiment 2

In Experiment 1, familiarity of the faces was indirectly controlled by comparing loved faces with famous faces and, additionally, by examining the responses to loved faces differing in their familiarity (partner, parents, friends, and siblings) among themselves. The findings of the experiment above suggest that familiarity is not a major determinant of the substantial zygomatic activity differences obtained in that study. However,, two problems affect the familiarity issue in Experiment 1: on the one hand, the degree of familiarity of loved faces and famous faces is not comparable, since the former will always exceed any other category; on the other hand, the first experiment did not equate subcategories of loved faces in number or order of presentation. In fact, of the 30 participants, 15 included both parents among the 5 loved faces; 6 included only the father, and 8 did not include any parent. Similarly uneven numbers were associated with the rest of loved familiar faces (siblings, second-degree relatives, and friends) freely chosen by participants.

In this second experiment, we examined psychophysiological responses in a design that controlled for familiarity differences among pictures and that included five different face categories: boyfriend, father, control-boyfriend, control-father, and baby faces.

2.2.1 Participants

Thirty-five female undergraduate students, ranging in age between 20-29 years, took part in this study. Inclusion criteria were the same as in Experiment 1. None of the participants reported current physical or psychological problems and none were under pharmacological treatment. All were right-handed and had normal or corrected-to-normal vision. All subjects signed informed consent forms and were given course credit for their participation.

2.2.2 Materials and design

Subjects viewed faces belonging to one of five categories in a passive picture viewing paradigm: boyfriend, father, control-boyfriend, control-father and baby. A few days before the experimental session, participants provided photographs of their boyfriend and their father according to detailed instructions provided by the experimenters (i.e., neutral expression, face looking straight at the camera, and subject standing in front of a light background). Control-boyfriend and control-father pictures were selected among the boyfriend and father photographs provided by other participants, once the experimenter ensured that the pictures did not depict someone known to the participant. The baby picture was selected from the IAPS (Lang et al., 2008) and had a valence score over 7 (rating scale from 1 to 9) according to the Spanish norms (Moltó et al., 1999; Vila et al, 2001). Pictures provided by participants were taken using a Nikon D-60 camera. All pictures were edited using Corel-Draw Photopaint software (version 7). All of them were matched in size, color, and background. All photographs had 650 x 650 pixels, were transformed to a gray scale (8 bits), and inserted into a circle surrounded by a black background. Pictures were presented by using Presentation software (Neurobehavioral Systems, CA) on a 19-in flat monitor located approximately 0.6 m from the participant.

Each picture was presented 20 times following a quadruple Latin Square design. The first Latin Square consisted of a 5x5 matrix that included one picture category in each row and each column. The rest of the Latin Squares were inverted mirrors of the first one. Five different sequences of pictures were created, each one starting with a different category, so as to be equally distributed within the 35 participants. Participants, in groups of five, were randomly assigned to one of the five sequences. After a 5-min baseline period, 100 picture trials were presented with the following structure per trial: 4-sec baseline, 4-sec picture presentation, and 4-sec additional recording period. The inter-trial interval varied randomly from 1 to 3 seconds (with an average of 2 sec). No recording was obtained during that period.

Participants were instructed to simply look at the pictures for the entire time they were projected on the screen.

2.2.3 Physiological measures

Zygomatic major EMG activity was obtained using miniature In Vivo Metrics silver/silver chloride electrodes. EMG activity was sampled at 100 Hz. The raw EMG signals were amplified by 5000 and band-pass filtered (13-1000 Hz) with a Coulbourn V75-04 bioamplifier. They were subsequently rectified and integrated using a Coulbourn V75-23A integrator. Time constant for zygomatic activity was 500 ms. Activity in the orbicularis muscle was recorded by placing two miniature In Vivo Metrics silver/silver chloride electrodes under the left eye. The raw EMG signal was amplified by 5000 and band-pass filtered (28-500 Hz) with a Coulburn V75-04 bioamplifier and a V75-48 High Performance Filter. Orbicularis EMG was subsequently integrated by a V75-23A integrator with a time-constant of 20 ms. Integrated EMG was recorded with a sampling rate of 100 Hz and averaged every one half-second during the period of face presentation. Subsequently, each value was expressed in terms of differential scores with respect to the averaged EMG during the 4 sec preceding stimulus onset.

Stimulus control and peripheral physiological data acquisition were accomplished using an IBM-compatible computer running VPM data acquisition and reduction software (Cook III, 1997).

2.2.4 Data reduction and analysis

Both zygomatic and orbicularis EMG data were averaged across trials within the same face category. Zygomatic activity was analyzed by repeated measures ANOVA using a 5x16 design, with the first factor being Category (boyfriend, father, control-boyfriend, control-father, and baby), and the second factor being Time (the 16 one half-second bins following picture onset). Post-hoc pairwise comparisons were performed using the same procedure than in the previous study. For correlation analysis between zygomatic and orbicularis EMG, the maximum amplitude values during the whole period of picture presentation were obtained across categories and the Pearson bivariate correlation calculated.

2.2.5 Results

Figure 3 shows changes in zygomatic activity for each of the 5 face categories. Only boyfriend and father pictures prompted visible responses starting right after stimulus onset. In addition, the face of the romantic partner elicited a larger response compared to the face of the father.

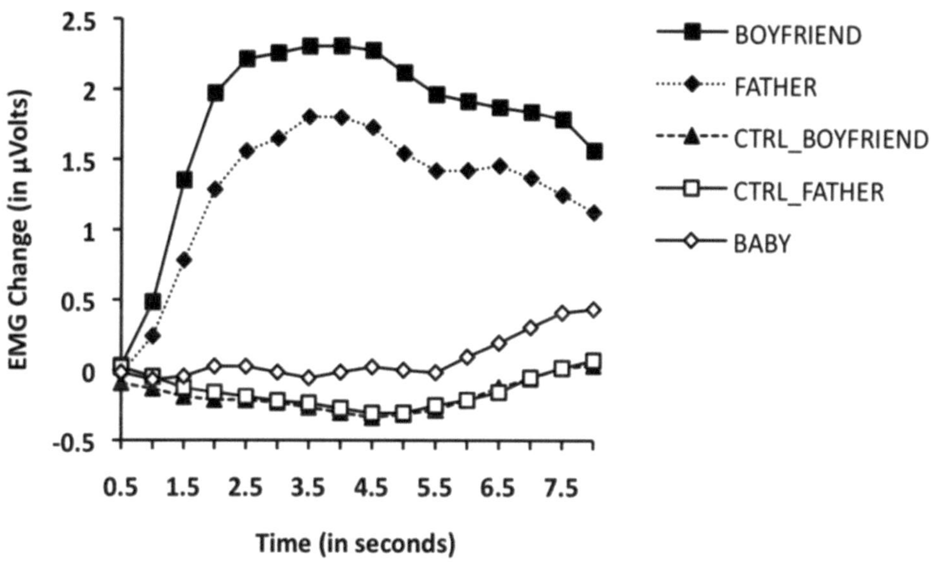

Fig. 3. Zygomatic activity across categories in study 2.

The ANOVA results yielded significant effects for Category ($F(4,136) = 12.825$, $p < 0.0001$, $\eta p^2 = 0.274$), Time ($(15,510) = 4.889$, $p < 0.017$, $\eta p^2 = 0.126$), and Category x Time ($F(60,2040) = 7.307$, $p < 0.001$, $\eta p^2 = 0.177$). Planned comparisons revealed the following results: (a) loved faces produced a significantly larger EMG response than control ($p < 0.001$) and baby ($p < 0.001$) faces, and (b) the face of the boyfriend produced a significantly larger EMG response than the different of the father ($p < 0.02$).

Significant positive correlations were found between the zygomatic and orbicularis muscle activity evoked by loved familiar faces, but not by unknown or baby faces (see Figure 4), thus suggesting that the Duchenne smile effect was present in these data.

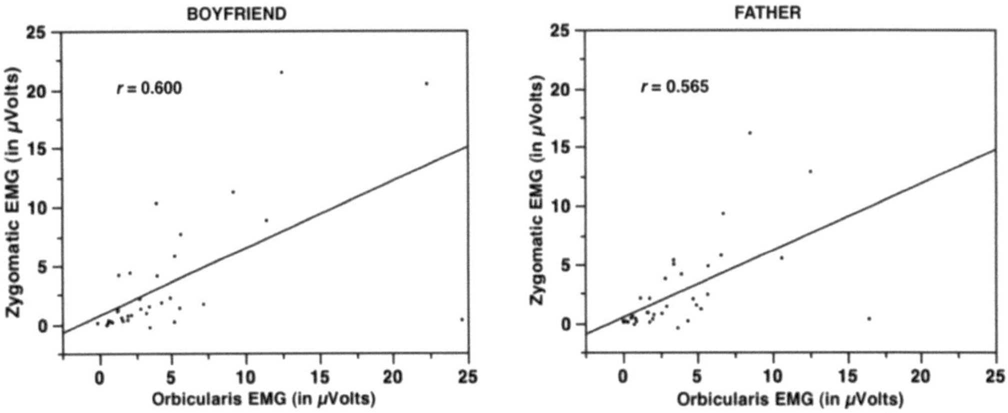

Fig. 4. Correlation between zygomatic major and orbicularis oculii activity for boyfriend and father faces.

2.3 Experiment 3

Experiments 1 and 2 have shown that processing of loved familiar faces elicits a pattern of responses that are indicative of a positive emotional state. Further evidence supporting the view that loved familiar faces engage the appetitive motivational system would be available if the same loved familiar faces proved to be efficient inhibitors of some defensive response (e.g., the startle reflex). Consequently, this third experiment was conducted to explore whether faces perceived as highly positive (i.e., loved familiar faces) were able to inhibit the startle reflex when compared to either neutral (i.e., unknown) or unpleasant (i.e., mutilated) faces. Additionally, Experiment 3 was designed so as to replicate previous findings regarding central and peripheral physiological reactions to loved familiar faces

2.3.1 Participants

Forty-two undergraduate students (12 males) participated in this experiment. Inclusion criteria were the same as in Experiments 1 and 2. None of the participants reported current physical or psychological problems and none were under pharmacological treatment. All were right-handed and had normal or corrected-to-normal vision. All subjects signed informed consent forms and received course credit for their participation

2.3.2 Materials and design

Participants viewed faces in a passive picture viewing paradigm, which belonged to three face categories: loved familiar faces (partner, father, mother, and best-friend), neutral faces (control-boyfriend, control-father, control-mother, and control-best-friend), and unpleasant faces[1]: This latter category included pictures from the IAPS (Lang, Bradley, & Cuthbert, 2008) that were present in the Spanish normative ratings (Moltó et al., 1999; Vila et al., 2001). The participants provided photographs of loved familiar persons a few days before the experiment and according to full detailed instructions on how to take the photographs (i.e.,

[1] International codes for unpleasant pictures were: 3000, 3051, 3060, and 3080)

pictures could not be taken by the participant him/herself, and people in the pictures should look straight at the camera with a neutral expression in front of a light background). Neutral pictures were selected among the loved familiar pictures provided by other participants after ensuring those pictures did not depict anyone known to that participant. Photographs of loved familiar persons were taken using a Nikon D-3000 camera. All pictures were edited using Corel Draw Photopaint (version 7). They were matched in size, color, and background. All photographs were cropped to 650 x 650 pixels, transformed to a gray scale (8 bits), and inserted into a circle surrounded by a black background. Pictures were presented using Presentation Software (Neurobehavioral Systems, CA) on a 19-in flat monitor located at approximately 60 cm from the participant.

Participants were randomly assigned to 6 different picture-presentation sequences that were created following a set of eight 3x3 Latin Squares. In each of those 3x3 matrices, one out of the four pictures included in each category was discarded so that, in total, each picture was presented 6 times during the whole task. To control for order effects, each sequence started with a different category.

The task started with a 5-min baseline period, followed by 72 trials with the following structure per trial: 4-sec baseline, 6-sec picture presentation, and 4-sec post-picture interval. Two-thirds of the pictures (48) were presented together with a startle probe (a burst of white noise at 105dBs, 50-ms duration and nearly instantaneous rise time) at 4, 4.5, 5, or 5.5 sec after picture onset. The same number of startle probes was assigned to each picture (n=4). In addition, 8 startle probes were delivered during the inter-trial interval in order to minimize noise predictability. The inter-trial interval varied randomly between 2 and 4 sec (with an average of 3 sec). Throughout the whole task a fixation point was presented in the centre of the screen to minimize eye movements. Participants were instructed to simply look at the pictures for the entire time they were on the screen.

2.3.2 Physiological measures

Zygomatic and orbicularis EMG activity were both measured using miniature silver chloride electrodes, and acquired using two Coulbourn V75-04 bioamplifiers. Band-pass filter settings for zygomatic and orbicularis raw signals were 13-1000 Hz, and 28-500 Hz, respectively. Both signals were amplified by 5000 and then rectified and integrated using a Coulbourn V76-24 integrator. Time constants for zygomatic and orbicularis muscles were 500 and 20 ms, respectively. Both raw signals were acquired at a sampling rate of 100 Hz during baseline with an increase in sampling rate for orbicularis muscle activity to 1000 Hz from 500 ms before the onset of the startle probe up to 500 ms after probe onset.

2.3.3 Data reduction and analysis

Zygomatic EMG activity was determined by subtracting the activity in the 3 sec before picture onset from that occurring at each half-second after picture presentation. Amplitude of the startle reflex was defined as the difference in microvolts between the peak and the onset of the orbicularis muscle response in a time window between 20 and 120 ms after stimulus onset, computed following the algorithm described by Balaban et al. (1986). To control for between-subject variability, startle magnitudes for each subject were converted to *t* scores.

Zygomatic activity was analyzed by repeated measures ANOVA using a 3x12 design with the first factor being Category (loved familiar faces, unknown faces, and unpleasant faces) and the second factor being Time (the 12 half-second increments following stimulus onset). Startle reflex magnitude was analyzed using repeated measures ANOVA with Face Category as single factor.

Finally, correlational analysis between zygomatic and orbicularis muscle activity was conducted as in the previous study, except that the maximum amplitude values were obtained during the first 4 seconds of picture presentation in order to avoid orbicularis EMG contamination by the startle probe.

2.3.4 Results

As can be observed in Figure 5, loved familiar faces prompted a clear zygomatic response, starting right after picture presentation and continuing until the end of the picture-presentation interval. No activation of the zygomatic muscle was observed for all other picture categories.

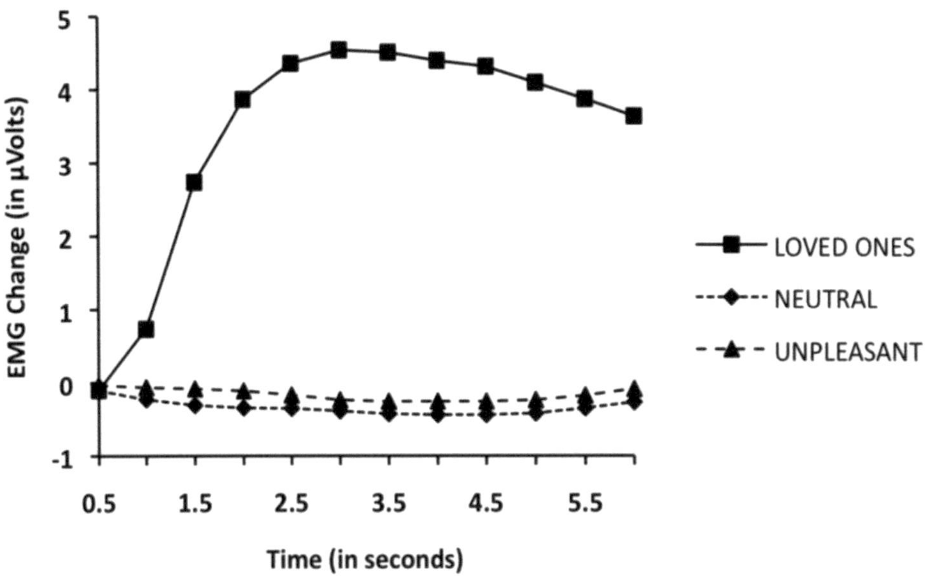

Fig. 5. Zygomatic activity response across face category.

The ANOVA yielded significant effects for Face Category ($F(2,82) = 16.629$, $p < 0.001$, $\eta p^2 = 0.289$), Time ($F(11,451) = 13.065$, $p < 0.001$, $\eta p^2 = 0.242$), and Face Category x Time ($F(22,902) = 15.594$, $p < 0.001$, $\eta p^2 = 0.276$).

Analysis of the Face Category x Time interaction revealed significant Face Category effects for all Time points from the second 1.5 to the end of the picture presentation. At all these Time points, loved familiar faces differed significantly from all others (all p-values < 0.007). No significant effects were found between neutral and unpleasant faces at any Time point.

The correlational analysis revealed a significant positive covariation between zygomatic and orbicularis EMG only for loved familiar faces, as can be seen in Figure 6.

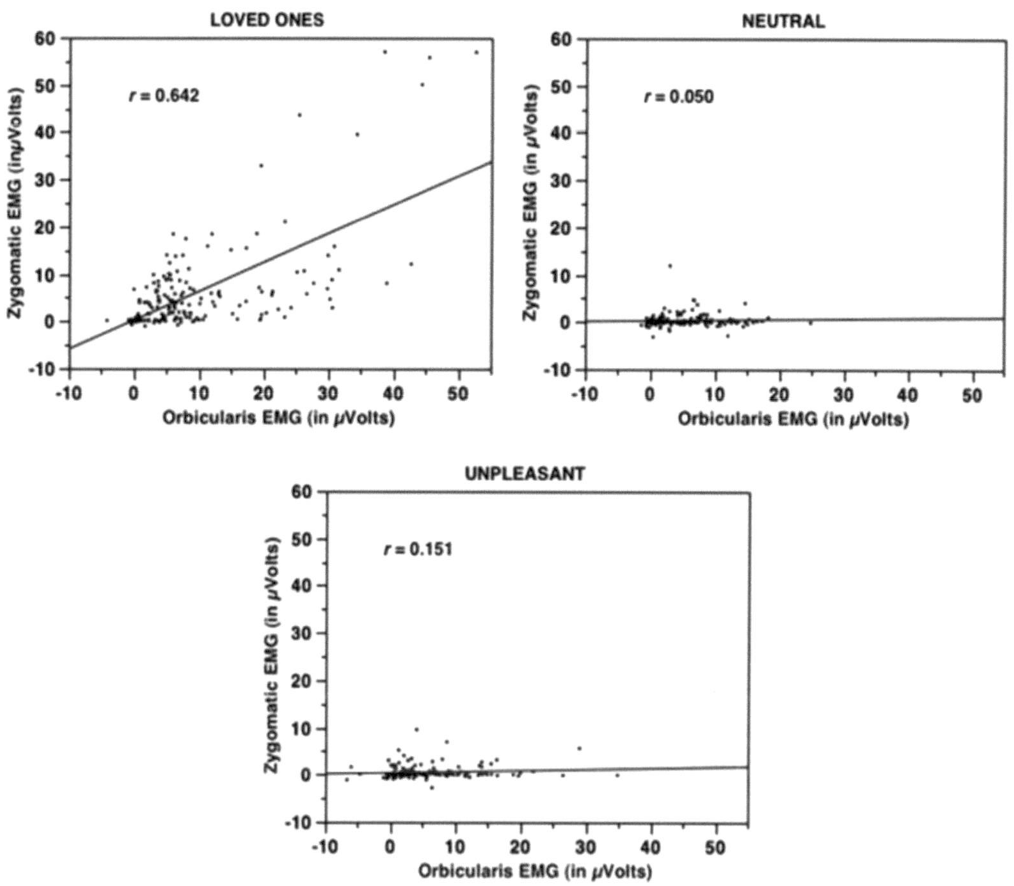

Fig. 6. Correlation between zygomatic major and orbicularis oculii across face category.

Finally, a clear modulation of the startle response was observed: loved familiar faces inhibited the startle response whereas mutilated faces potentiated the startle response, compared to neutral (unknown) faces, as can be seen in Figure 7. The ANOVA results yielded a significant main effect of Face Category ($F(2,82) = 25.135$, $p < 0.0001$, $\eta p^2 = 0.380$). Planned comparisons revealed significant differences (a) between loved familiar and neutral faces (($p<0.01$)), (b) between neutral and unpleasant faces ($p<0.002$), and (c) between loved familiar and unpleasant faces ($p<0.0001$).

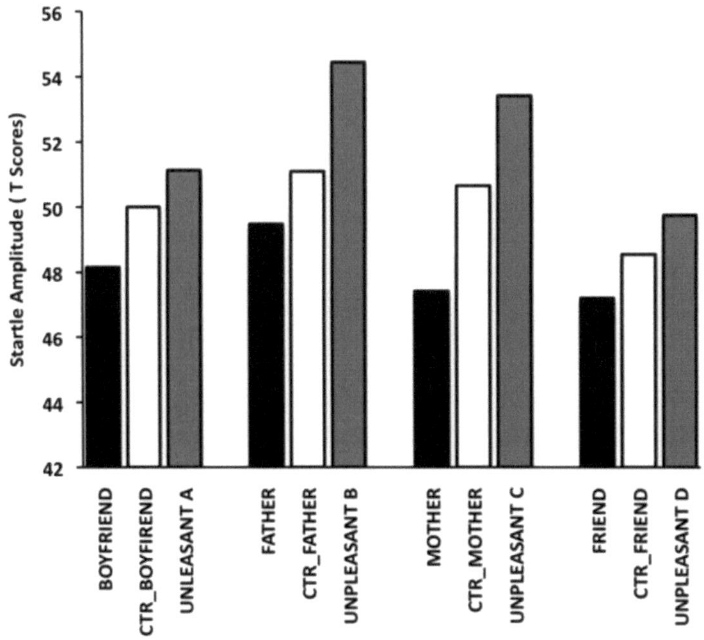

Fig. 7. Startle eyblink modulation for the different subcategories of loved familiar faces.

3. Discussion

The results of the three studies highlight the relevance of including electromyographic measures to advance knowledge on the psychological and physiological mechanisms underlying the affective processing of faces associated with identity recognition. The three studies were highly consistent in showing a large zygomatic major response to faces of loved ones, a response that starts around one second after picture onset and lasts for several seconds after picture offset. This response was totally absent or greatly diminished to all other categories of faces used as control in our three studies: unknown, famous, baby, neutral, and unpleasant faces. In all cases, the faces were photographs in black and white and with no emotional expression. Moreover, in the three studies, loved and unknown faces were physically identical since they were interchangeable across participants, guaranteeing that the observed differences among faces in physiology and subjective ratings were due to identity recognition and not to differences in emotional expression or physical features of the faces.

The sequence of the three studies was also highly consistent in confirming that the processing of loved familiar faces involves activation of an intense positive emotional response that cannot be explained by undifferentiated emotional arousal or familiarity. In the first study, the arousal effect was controlled by simultaneously recording heart rate and skin conductance. In the context of Lang's picture-viewing paradigm (Bradley & Lang, 2007), heart rate is an unambiguous index of emotional valence (positive versus negative emotion), whereas skin conductance is an index of emotional arousal (the intensity of the emotion, regardless of its positive or negative valence). Both indices confirmed that the zygomatic response to the loved faces was reflecting the presence of an intense positive emotional response. In this study, the familiarity effect was indirectly controlled by comparing famous versus unknown faces, as well as loved faces with different levels of familiarity among themselves. No differences were found between famous and unknown faces, and the few differences found among loved faces were contrary to the familiarity explanation: larger responses to the less familiar (partner) than to the more familiar (parent and siblings) faces.

In the second and third study, the confounding arousal and familiarity effects were further controlled by including a second electromyographic measure (the orbicularis muscle activity) and by using an experimental design that better controlled for familiarity. The simultaneous recording of the zygomatic and orbicularis muscles provides two additional specific indices of emotional valence: the Duchenne smile and the eye-blink startle response. As mentioned in the introduction, the Duchenne or true smile is characterized by simultaneous activation of the zygomatic and orbicularis muscles, whereas social smile devoid of positive emotion involves only zygomatic activation (Ekman et al., 1980). The significant correlation found between zygomatic and orbicularis muscle activity only for loved faces in our second and third study is another piece of evidence supporting the conclusion that viewing faces of loved ones induces a feeling of genuine positive affect that cannot be explained in terms of arousal or familiarity.

On the other hand, the eye-blink startle response is perhaps the most robust physiological response showing emotional modulation by affective valence. Numerous studies (see Bradley & Lang, 2007, for a review) have consistently demonstrated that viewing highly pleasant pictures (e.g., erotica or sport images) reduces the magnitude of the eye-blink startle response, whereas viewing highly unpleasant pictures (e.g., mutilation or threatening images) increases its magnitude, compared to neutral pictures (e.g., household objects or non-emotional faces). In these studies, however, the startle magnitude while viewing neutral pictures not always occupies an intermediate position with significant differences with respect to both pleasant and unpleasant images. The results of our third study, showing significant differences between our three categories of faces (loved, neutral, and unpleasant), are not only an independent confirmation of Lang's *motivational priming hypothesis* (startle inhibition during activation of the appetitive motivational system by pleasant pictures and startle potentiation during activation of the aversive motivational system by unpleasant pictures, compared to neutral ones). They are also an unambiguous demonstration that viewing loved familiar faces induces an intense positive emotion capable of inhibiting defensive reflexes.

The electromyographic results of our second and third study also contribute to disentangle the confounding effects of familiarity in the processing of loved familiar faces. The control of familiarity has always been a major methodological problem in this type of studies. Although difficult to separate, emotional valence and familiarity are not inevitably confounded. In studies using the picture-viewing paradigm with pleasant, neutral, and unpleasant pictures from the IAPS, the enhanced zygomatic response while viewing pleasant pictures has been interpreted in terms of positive affect, rather than familiarity, since all pictures are new and there is no explicit memory involvement. But in studies on loved familiar faces, familiarity is necessarily confounded with emotion, since both memory and emotion are involved in their processing. Our second and third study controlled for familiarity by comparing the face of the romantic partner (with less than 6 years relationship) with the face of the parent of same sex (with more than 18 years relationship). Therefore, two categories of loved familiar faces, differing in amount of familiarity, were compared. Both studies (although the details of the third one are not reported here) replicated the results of the first study revealing larger zygomatic responses to the less familiar face (i.e., the romantic partner) than to the more familiar face (i.e., the parent), thus disconfirming the familiarity hypothesis.

It should be noted, however, that the three studies reported here not only recorded EMG responses. A broad set of autonomic (heart rate and skin conductance), electromyographic (zygomatic and orbicularis muscle activity), and brain (N100, P200, P3, and LPP) responses was recorded, in addition to subjective indices of valence, arousal, and dominance, the three general dimensions of emotional reactions (see Osgood, Suci & Tannenbaum, 1957; Mehrabian & Russel, 1974; Bradley & Lang, 2007). The results of the three studies revealed a very consistent pattern of physiological and subjective responses to loved familiar faces: (a) increases in heart rate, skin conductance, zygomatic activity, and the event-related potentials P3, and LPP; (b) decreases in eye-blink startle magnitude and the event-related potential N200; and (c) higher ratings of positive valence and arousal, but lower ratings of dominance. This set of physiological and subjective responses suggests that the processing of loved familiar faces involves a complex pattern of psychophysiological mechanisms that single physiological measures, whether central or peripheral, would fail to capture accurately. The use of both central and peripheral measures to investigate the affective processing of familiar faces contrasts with the dominant trend in current cognitive and affective neuroscience, almost limited to central physiological measures (EEG, ERP, MEG, PET, or fMRI). In the context of studies on emotional processing, the neglect of peripheral physiological measures, such as facial EMG or heart rate, has the shortcoming of not providing unambiguous evidence of the type of response being elicited, confounding emotional valence, undifferentiated emotional arousal, and familiarity.

But the shortcoming of a neuroscience approach that ignores peripheral physiological measures has much wider implications. It assumes a model of brain function apparently unrelated to efferent motor components. As Robert Sperry emphasized in 1952, the human brain primarily evolved not to contemplate and understand the world but to facilitate behavioral adaptation: *The primary function of the brain is essentially the transformation of sensory patterns into patterns of motor coordination* (Sperry, 1952, p. 297)... *Cerebration, essentially, serves to bring into motor behavior additional refinement, increased direction toward distant, future goals, and greater over-all adaptiveness and survival value. The evolutionary increase in man's capacity for perception, feeling, ideation, imagination, and the like, may be regarded, not so much as an end in itself, but as something that has enabled us to behave, to act, more wisely and efficiently* (Sperry, 1952, p. 299). Sperry's neuroscience approach implies that mental and motor processes are intimately associated and that research on brain mechanisms of psychological processes should integrate both central and peripheral physiological measures.

This approach not only has distinguished roots in early behaviorism and motor theory of thought and emotion (Watson, 1913; Washburn, 1928; Jacobson, 1929). It also has relevant defendants among more recent psychophysiologists and cognitive neuroscientists. McGuigan published in 1978 a book entitled *Cognitive Psychophysiology: Principles of covert behavior* gathering together a bulk of experimental studies showing the close covariation between electromyographical measures at different muscle locations and numerous cognitive processes. Based on these data, he suggested that all brain circuits are basically neuromuscular circuits, a proposal not too different from Sperry's ideas on mind-body interactions. More recent developments within cognitive and affective neuroscience are also beginning to suggest the need to integrate brain and bodily responses in order to fully comprehend the brain mechanisms underlying psychological processes. The embodied cognition (Lenggenhager et al., 2006; De Vega, Glenberg & Graesser, 2008; Niedenthal et al., 2009) and social cognition (Tomasello et al., 2005; Amodio & Frith, 2006; Herrmann et al., 2007; Losin et al., 2010) groups are perhaps the most relevant cognitive movements of this new approach within neuroscience research. The basic idea of both movements is that bodily responses and affective social interactions are integral part of our cognitive representations in the brain and that both, central and peripheral responses, play a crucial role in successful behavioral adaptation and survival.

In summary, the present chapter summarizes a set of three studies aimed at investigating the affective processing of loved familiar faces using a set of central and peripheral physiological measures, including electromyographic recordings of the zygomatic major and orbicularis oculii muscle, in the context of Lang's picture-viewing paradigm. The results of the three studies support the conclusion that viewing the faces of familiar loved ones elicits an intense positive emotional reaction that cannot be explained either by familiarity or arousal alone. The three studies highlight the relevance of integrating central and peripheral measures to advance knowledge on the brain mechanisms underlying affective processing.

4. Ackowledgements

This research was supported by a grant from the Junta de Andalucía (Project P07-SEJ-02964).

5. References

Adolphs, R. (2009). The social brain: neural basis of social knowledge. *Annual Review of Psychology*, Vol. 60, (September 2008), pp. 693–716, ISSN: 0066-4308.

Adolphs, R. (2002). Neural systems for recognizing emotion. *Current Opinion in Neurobiology*, Vol. 12, No. 2, (April 2002), pp. 169-177, ISSN: 0959-4388

Amodio, D.M., & Frith, C.D. (2006). Meeting minds: The medial frontal cortex and social cognition. Nature Reviews/Neuroscience, Vol. 7, (April 2006), pp. 268-277, ISSN: 1471-003X.

Aron, A., Fisher, H., Mashek, D.J., Strong, G., Li, H., & Brown, L.L. (2005). Reward, motivation, and emotion systems associated with early-stage intense romantic love. *Journal of Neurophysiology*, Vol. 94, No. 1, (March 2005), pp. 327-337, ISSN: 0022-3077.

Baçar, E., Schmiedt-Fehr, C., Örniz, A., & Baçar-Eroglu, C. (2008). Brain oscillations evoked by face of a loved person. *Brain Research*, Vol. 1214, (June 2008), pp. 105-115, ISSN: 00068993.

Balaban, M.T., Losito, B.D., Simons, R.F., & Graham, F.K. (1986). Off-line latency and amplitude scoring of the human reflex eye blink with Fortran IV. Psychophysiology, 23, 612.

Bartels, A. & Zeki, S. (2000). The neural basis of romantic love. *NeuroReport*, Vol. 11, No. 17, (November 2000), pp. 3829-2834, ISSN: 0959-4965.

Bartels, A. & Zeki, S. (2004). The neural correlates of maternal and romantic love. *NeuroImage*, Vol. 21, No. 3, (March 2004), pp. 1155-1166, ISSN: 10538119.

Bentin, S., Allison, T., Puce, A., Perez, E., McCarthy, G., 1996. Electrophysiological studies of face perception in humans. *Journal of Cognitive Neuroscience*, Vol. 8, No. 6, (November 1996), pp. 551–565, ISSN: 0898-929X.

Bobes, M.A., Quiñonez, I., Perez, J., Leon, I., & Valdés-Sosa, M. (2007). Brain potentials reflect access to visual and emotional memories for faces. *Biological Psychology,* Vol. 75, No. 2, (May 2007), pp. 146-153, ISSN: 0301-0511.

Bradley, M.M., & Lang, P.J. (2007). Emotion and Motivation. In: *Handbook of Psychophysiology, Third Edition,* John T. Cacioppo, Louis G. Tassinary, & Gary Berntson, pp. 581-607.

Bradley, M.M. (2009). Natural selective attention: orienting and emotion. *Psychophysiology,* Vol. 46, No. 1, (January 2009), pp. 1–11, ISSN: 0048-5772.

Bradley, M.M., Codispoti, M., Cuthbert, B.N., Lang, P.J. (2001). Emotion and motivation I: defensive and appetitive reactions in picture processing. *Emotion,* Vol 1, No. 3, (September 2001), pp. 276–298, ISSN: 1528-3542.

Bradley, M.M., Lang, P.J. (2000.) Measuring emotion. behavior, feeling, and physiology. In: Lane, R.D., Nadel, L. (Eds.), *Cognitive Neuroscience of Emotion.* Oxford University Press, New York, pp. 242– 276.

Brown, S. L., & Schwartz, G. E. (1980). Relationships between facial electromyography and subjective experience during affective imagery. *Biological Psychology,* Vol. 11, No. 1, (August 1980), pp. 49–62, ISSN: 0301-0511.

Bruce, V., & Young, A. (1986). Understanding face recognition. *British Journal of Psychology,* Vol. 77, No. 3, (August, 1986), pp. 305-327, ISSN: 2044-8295.

Cacioppo, J. T., Petty, R. E., Losch, M. E., & Kim, H. S. (1986). Electromyographic activity over facial muscle regions can differentiate the valence and intensity of affective reactions. *Journal of Personality and Social Psychology,* Vol. 50, No. 2, (February 1986), pp. 260–268, ISSN: 0022-3514.

Codispoti, M., Bradley, M.M., Lang, P.J., 2001. Affective reactions to briefly presented pictures. *Psychophysiology,* Vol. 38, No. 3, (April 2001), pp. 474–478, ISSN: 0048-5772.

Cook III, E.W. (1997). VPM Reference Manual [Computer Software]. Author, Birmingham, Alabama.

Cuthbert, B. N., Schupp, H. T., Bradley, M. M., Birbaumer, N., & Lang, P. J. (2000). Brain potentials in affective picture processing: Covariation with autonomic arousal and affective report. *Biological Psychology,* Vol. *52,* No. 2, (March 2000),pp. 95-111, ISSN: 0301-0511.

Dekowska, M., Kuniecki, M., & Jaskowski, P. (2008). Facing facts: Neuronal mechanisms of face perception. *Acta Neurobiologiae Experimentalis,* Vol. 68, No. 2, pp. 229-252.

De Vega, M., Glenberg, A.M., & Graesser, A.C. (2008). *Symbols and embodiment: debates on meaning and cognition.* Oxford University Press: New York.

Dimberg, U. (1997). Psychophysiological reactions to facial expressions. In U. Segerstrale and P. Molnar (Eds.), *Nonverbal communication: Where nature meets culture* (pp.27-60). Mahwah, NJ: Erlbaum.

Eimer, H., & Holmes, A. (2007). Event-related potential correlates of emotional face processing. *Neuropsychologia,* Vol. 45, No. 1, pp. 15-31, ISSN: 0028-3932.

Eimer, M. (2000a). Event-related brain potentials distinguish processing stages involved in face perception and recognition. *Clinical Neurophysiology,* Vol. 111, No. 4, (April 2000), pp. 694–705, ISSN: 1388-2457.

Eimer, M. (2000b). Effects of face inversion on the structural encoding and recognition of faces: evidence from event-related brain potentials. *Cognitive Brain Research,* Vol. 10, No. 1-2, (September 2000), pp. 145–158, ISSN: 0926-6410.

Ekman, P. (1980). Face of man: Universal expression in a New Guinea village. New York: Garland.

Ekman, P. (1992). Facial expression and emotion. *American Psychologist,* Vol. 48, No. 4, (April 1992), pp. 376-379, ISSN: 0003-066X.

Ekman, P., Davidson, R. J., Friesen, W. V. (1990). The Duchenne smile: Emotional expression and brain physiology II. *Journal of Personality & Social Psychology,* Vol. 58, No. 2, (February 1990), pp. 342–353, ISSN: 0022-3514.

Fairhall, S.L., & Ishai, A.(2007). Effective connectivity within the distributed cortical network for face perception. Cerebral Cortex, Vol. 17, No. 10, (December 2006), pp. 2400–2406, ISSN: 1047-3211.

Fisher, H., Aron, A., & Brown, L.L. (2005). Romantic love: An fMRI study of a neural mechanism for mate choice. *The Journal of Comparative Neurology,* Vol. 493, No. 1, (December 2005), pp. 58-62, ISSN: 1096-9861.

Gobbini, M.I., & Haxby, J.V. (2007). Neural systems for recognition of familiar faces. *Neuropsychologia,* Vol. 45, No. 1, 32-41, ISSN: 0028-3932.

Grasso, D.J., & Simons, R.F. (2011). Perceived parental support predicts enhanced late positive event-related brain potentials to parent faces. *Biological Psychology,* Vol. 86, No. 1, (January 2011), pp. 26-30, ISSN: 0301-0511.

Grasso, D.J., Moser, J.S., Dozier, M., & Simons, R. (2009). ERP correlates of attention allocation in mothers processing faces of their children. *Biological Psychology,* Vol. 81, No. 2, (May 2009), pp. 95-102, ISSN: 0301-0511.

Haxby, J.V., & Gobbini, M.I. (2011). Distributed Neural Systems for Face Perception. In: *The Oxford Handbook of Face Perception,* Andrew J. Calder, Gillian Rhodes, Mark H. Johnson, & James Haxby, pp. 93-110, Oxford University Press, New York.

Herrmann, E., Call, J., Hernández_Lloreda, M.V., Hare, B., & Tomasello, M. (2007). Humans have evolved specialized skills of social cognition: The cultural intelligence hypothesis. *Science,* Vol. 317, No. 5843, (September 2007), pp. 1360-1366, ISSN: 0036-8075.

Herrmann, M.J., Ehlis, A.C., Ellgrin, H., & Fallgatter, A.J. (2005). Early stages (P100) of face perception as measured with event-related potentials (ERPs). *Journal of Neural Transmission,* Vol. 112, No. 8, (December 2004), pp. 1073-1081, ISSN: 0300-9564.

Herzmann, G.H., Schweinberger, S.R., Sommer, W., & Jentzsch, I. (2004). What's special about personally familiar faces? A multimodal approach. *Psychophysiology,* Vol. 41, No. 5, (September 2004), pp. 688-701, ISSN: 0048-5772.

Izard, C. (1971). *The face or emotion.* New York: Appleton-Century-Crofts.

Izard, C. (1977). *Human emotions.* New York: Plenum Press.

Izard, C. (1994). Innate and universal facial expressions: Evidence from developmental and cross-cultural research. *Psychological Bulletin,* Vol. 115, No. 2, (March 1994), pp. 288-299, ISSN: 0033-2909.

Jacobson, E. (1929). *Progressive Relaxation.* Oxford, England: University of Chicago Press.

Jansen, D.M., Fridja, N.H. (1994). Modulation of the acoustic startle response by film-induced fear and sexual arousal. *Psychophysiology,* Vol. 31, No. 6, (November 1994), pp. 565- 571, ISSN: 0048-5772.

Lang, P. J., Greenwald, M. K., Bradley, M. M., & Hamm, A. O. (1993). Looking at pictures: Affective, facial, visceral, and behavioral reactions. *Psychophysiology,* Vol. 30, No. 3, (May 1993), pp. 261–273, ISSN: 0048-5772.

Lang, P.J. (1995): The emotion probe: Studies of motivation and attention. *American Psychologist,* Vol. 50, No. 5, (May 1995), pp. 372-385, ISSN: 0003-066X.

Lang, P.J., & Bradley, M.M. (2010). Emotion and the motivational brain. *Biological Psychology,* Vol. 84, No. 3, (July 2010), pp. 437-450, ISSN: 0301-0511.

Lang, P.J., Bradley, M.M., & Cuthbert, B.N. (2008). *International affective picture system (IAPS): Affective ratings of pictures and instruction manual. Technical Report A-8.* University of Florida, Gainesville, FL.

Lang, P.J., Davis, M., 2006. Emotion, motivation, and the brain: reflex foundations in animal and human research. *Progress in Brain Research,* Vol. 156, pp. 3–29.

Lang, P.J., Davis, M., Öhman, A., 2000. Fear and anxiety. Animal models and human cognitive psychophysiology. *Journal of Affective Disorders,* Vol. 61, No. 3, (December 2000), pp. 137–159, ISSN: 0165-0327.

Lang, P.J.,Bradley,M.M.,&Cuthbert,B.N.(1997).Motivated attention: Affect, activation and action. In P.J.Lang, R.F.Simons, & M.T.Balaban (Eds.), Attention and orienting: Sensory and motivational processes. Hillsdale, NJ: Lawrence Erlbaum Associates, Inc.

Langeslag, S.J.E., Hansma, B.M., Franken, I.H.A. & Strien, J.W.V. (2007). Event-related potential responses to love-related facial stimuli. *Biological Psychology,* Vol. 76, No. 1-2, (September 2007), pp. 109-115, ISSN: 0301-0511.

Larsen, J.T., Norris, C.J., & Cacioppo, J.T. (2003). Effects of positive and negative affect on electromyographic activity over zygomaticus major and corrugator supercilii. *Psychophsysiology,* Vol. 40, No. 5, (September 2003), pp. 776-785, ISSN: 0048-5772.

Lenggenhager, B., Smith, S.T., & Blanke, O. (2006). Functional and Neural Mechanisms of Embodiment: Importance of the Vestibular System and the Temporal Parietal Junction. *Reviews in Neurosciences,* Vol. 17, No. 6, pp. 643-657, ISSN: 0306-4522.

Li, H., Chan, R.C.K., McAlonan, G.M., & Gong, Q. (2010). Facial emotion processing in schizophrenia: A meta-analysis of functional neuroimaging data. *Schizophrenia Bulletin,* Vol. 36, No. 5, pp. 1029-1039, ISSN: 745-1701.

Mehrabian, A., & Russell, J.A. (1974). *An approach to environmental psychology.* Cambridge, MA: M.I.T. Press.

Losin, E.A., Dapretto, M., & Iacobini, M. (2010). Culture and neuroscience: additive or synergistic? *Social Cognitive & Affective Neuroscience,* Vol. 5, No. 2-3, (January 2010), pp. 148-158, ISSN: 1749-5016.

McGuigan, F.J. (1978).*Cognitive psychophysiology: Principles of covert behavior.* Englewood Cliffs. NJ: Prentice-Hall.

Miltner, W. (1994). Emotional qualities of odors and their influence on the startle reflex in humans. *Psychophysiology,* Vol. 31, No. 1, (January 1994), 107– 110, ISSN: 0048-5772.

Niedenthal, P. M., Winkielman, P., Mondillon, L., Vermeulen, N. (2009). Embodiment of emotion concepts. *Journal of Personality and Social Psychology,* Vol 96, No. 6, (Jun 2009), pp. 1120-1136, ISSN: 0022-3514.

Öhman, A., Lundqvist, D., & Esteves, F. (2001). The face in the crowd: A threat advantage with schematic stimuli. *Journal of Personality and Social Psychology,* Vol. 80, No. 3, (March 2001), pp. 381-396, ISSN: 0022-3514.

Oloffson, J.K., Nordin, S., Sequeira, H., & Polich, J. (2008). Affective picture processing: An integrative review of ERP findings. *Biological Psychology,* Vol. 77, No. 3, (March 2008), pp. 247-265, ISSN: 0301-0511.

Osgood, C.E., Suci, G., & Tannenbaum, P. (1957) *The measurement of meaning.* Urbana, IL: University of Illinois Press.

Palomba, D., Angrilli, A., & Mini, A. (1997). Visual evoked potentials, heart rate responses and memory for emotional pictorial stimuli. *International Journal of Psychophysiology,* Vol. 27, No. 1, (July 1997), pp. 55-67, ISSN: 0167-8760.

Russell, J.A. (1994). Is there universal recognition of emotion from facial expression? A review of the cross-cultural studies. *Psychological Bulletin,* Vol. 115, No. 1, (January 1994), pp. 102-141, ISSN: 0033-2909.

Sabatinelli, D., Lang, P.J., Keil, A., & Bradley, M.M. (2007). Emotional perception: correlation of functional MRI and event related potentials. *Cerebral Cortex,* Vol. 17, No. 5, pp. 1085-1091, ISSN: 1047-3211.

Schupp, H.T., Cuthbert, B.N., Bradley, M.M., Cacioppo, J.T., Ito, T., & Lang, P.J. (2000). Affective picture processing: The late positive potential is modulated by motivational relevance. *Psychophysiology,* Vol. 37, No. 2, (March 2000), pp. 257-261, ISSN: 0048-5772.

Schupp, H.T., Junghöfer, M., Weike, A.I., & Hamm, A.O. (2004). The selective processing of briefly presented affective pictures: An ERP analysis. *Psychophysiology,* Vol. 41, No. 3, (May 2004), pp. 441-449, ISSN: 0048-5772.

Schwartz, G. E., Fair, P. L., Salt, P., Mandel, M. R., & Klerman, G. L. (1976a). Facial muscle patterning to affective imagery in depressed and nondepressed subjects. *Science,* Vol. 192, No. 4238, (April 1976), pp. 489–491, ISSN: 0036-8075.

Schwartz, G. E., Fair, P. L., Salt, P., Mandel, M. R., & Klerman, G. L. (1976b). Facial expression and imagery in depression: An electromyographic study. *Psychosomatic Medicine,* Vol. 38, No. 5, (September 1976), pp. 337–347, ISSN: 0033-3174.

Schweinberger, S.R. (2011). Neurophysiological correlates of Face Recognition. In: *The Oxford Handbook of Face Perception,* Andrew J. Calder, Gillian Rhodes, Mark H. Johnson, & James Haxby, pp. 345-366, Oxford University Press, New York.

Sperry, R.W. (1952). Neurology and the mind-brain problem. *American Scientist,* 40, No. 2, (April 1952), pp. 291-312, ISSN: 0003-0996.

Tomasello, M., Carpenter, M., Call, J., Behne, T., & Moll, H. (2005). Understanding and sharing intentions: The origins of cultural cognition. *Behavioral and Brain Sciences,* Vol. 28, No. 5, pp. 675-735, ISSN: 0140-525X.

Tomkins, S.S. (1962). *Affect, imagery and consciousness: Vol. I. The positive affects.* New York: Springer.

Voss, J.L., & Paller, K.A. (2006). Fluent conceptual processisng and explicit memory for faces are electrophysiologically distinct. *The Journal of Neuroscience,* Vol. 26, No. 3, (January 2008), pp. 926-933, ISSN: 1529-2401.

Voss, J.L., & Paller, K.A. (2007). Neural correlates of conceptual implicit memory and their contamination of putative neural correlates of explicit memory. *Learning and Motivation,* Vol. 14, pp. 259-267, ISSN: 1072-0502.

Vuilleumier, P. & Pourtois, G. (2007). Distributed and interactive brain mechanisms during emotion face perception: Evidence from functional neuroimaging. *Neuropsychologia,* Vol. 45, No. 1, pp. 174-194, ISSN: 0028-3932.

Washburn, M.F. (1928). Emotion and Thought: A Motor Theory of Their Relations. In: Martin L. Reymert (Ed.), *Feelings and Emotions: The Wittenberg Symposium.* Worcester, MA: Clark University: 104-115.

Watson, J.B. (1913). Psychology as the Behaviorist views it. *Psychological Review*, Vol. 20, No. 2, (March 1913), pp. 158-177, ISSN: 0033-295X.

Whalen, P.J., Rauch, S.L., Etcoff, N.L., McInerney, S.C., Lee, M.B., & Jenike, M.A. (1998). Masked presentations of emotional facial expressions modulate amygdala activity without explicit knowledge. *The Journal of Neuroscience*, Vol. 18, No. 1, (January 1998), pp. 411-418, ISSN: 0270-6474.

Xu, X., Aron, A., Brown, L., Cao, G., Feng, T., & Weng, X. (2011). Reward and motivation systems: A brain mapping study of early-stage romantic love in Chinese participants. *Human Brain Mapping*, Vol. 32, No. 2, (February 2011), pp. 249-257, ISSN: 1097-0193.

Yovel, G., & Paller, K.A. (2004). The neural basis of the butcher-on-the-bus phenomenon. When a face seems familiar but is not remembered. *NeuroImage*, Vol. 21, No. 2, (February 2004), pp. 789-800, ISSN: 10538119.

Zeki, S. (2007). The neurobiology of love. *FEBS Letters*, Vol. 581 No. 14, (June 2007), pp. 2575-2579, ISSN: 0014-5793.

21

Noninvasive Monitoring of Breathing and Swallowing Interaction

N. Terzi[1,2], D. Orlikowski[2,3], H. Prigent[2,4],
Pierre Denise[6], H. Normand[6] and F. Lofaso[2,4,5]
[1]INSERM, ERI27, Caen; Univ Caen, Caen; CHRU Caen
Service de Réanimation Médicale, Caen
[2]Centre d'Investigation Clinique - Innovations Technologiques, Hôpital Raymond Poincaré, AP-HP; Université de Versailles-Saint Quentin en Yvelines, Garches
[3]Centre d'Investigation Clinique - Innovations Technologiques 805, Service de Réanimation et Unité de Ventilation à Domicile, Hôpital Raymond Poincaré, AP-HP
[4]Services de Physiologie - Explorations Fonctionnelles
Hôpital Raymond Poincaré, AP-HP
[5]INSERM, U 955, Créteil
[6]INSERM, ERI27, Caen, Univ Caen; CHRU Caen
Service d'Explorations Fonctionnelles, Caen
France

1. Introduction

The evaluation of swallowing parameters and of interactions between breathing and swallowing is crucial to optimise the management of patients with chronic respiratory failure, as swallowing must occur in precise coordination with breathing. Various techniques have been used to study the physiology and biomechanics of the oral and pharyngeal stages of swallowing. Among them, the two most commonly used, videofluoroscopy and videoendoscopy, provide information on the motion of anatomic structures during swallowing. The determination of muscle activation patterns is best achieved with electromyography (EMG). Most of the initial EMG studies of swallowing used needle electrodes to record intramuscular EMG activity (Doty and Bosma 1956; Perlman, Palmer et al. 1999). Ertekin *et al.* (Ertekin, Pehlivan et al. 1995) were the first to describe an electrophysiological method for investigating swallowing in humans.
Recent advances in the management of respiratory failure have considerably improved the survival of patients with neuromuscular disease (Finder, Birnkrant et al. 2004). For example, the introduction in the 1990s of mechanical ventilation (MV) improved the survival of patients with Duchenne muscular dystrophy (DMD) from about 15 years in the 1960s to more than 30 years now. Quality of life, however, declines over time as the disease progresses. Malnutrition is common: in one study, for instance, 44% of patients had malnutrition (Willig, Bach et al. 1995). The main causes of malnutrition are prolonged swallowing, respiratory failure, and dysphagia, which jeopardize the patient's ability to meet intake needs. Feeding difficulties often develop insidiously, being frequently underestimated by family members and healthcare professionals (Hill, Hughes et al. 2004).

Aspiration is another important consequence of impaired swallowing that becomes increasingly common as the disease progresses (Finder, Birnkrant et al. 2004).
Studies have demonstrated that swallowing dysfunction is closely associated with impaired inspiratory muscle strength (Terzi, Orlikowski et al. 2007; Orlikowski, Terzi et al. 2009) and improve with tracheostomy and mechanical ventilation (Terzi, Prigent et al.; Terzi, Orlikowski et al. 2007). Swallowing and inspiratory muscle strength are being evaluated in patients with acute exacerbations of chronic obstructive pulmonary disease (COPD) requiring noninvasive ventilation.
Noninvasive methods for evaluating swallowing are useful to investigate various disorders and the interactions between breathing and swallowing. Here, after a review of swallowing physiology to explain the EMG evaluation and a discussion of interactions between breathing and swallowing, we describe the most commonly used electrophysiological method, which is noninvasive and easy to perform at the bedside. We do not address methods requiring the connection of measurement devices directly to the airway.

2. Physiology of swallowing

Swallowing is a complex physiological function that was generally investigated using videofluoroscopy, videoendoscopy, manometric methods, or invasive methods providing information on a single pair of muscles involved in swallowing. Swallowing was usually divided into three phases: an initial oral phase; a pharyngeal phase; and an esophageal phase (Dodds 1989). These phases of swallowing involve different in innervation patterns. Thus, the oral phase is usually described as voluntary, the pharyngeal phase as a reflex response, and the esophageal phase as controlled by both the somatic and the autonomic nervous system (Doty and Bosma 1956; Miller 1982).

2.1 Oral phase

The oral phase is mainly voluntary and highly variable in duration depending in humans on taste, environment, hunger, motivation, and consciousness. First, the tongue presses the bolus against the hard palate and initiates displacement of the bolus to the posterior part of the tongue and toward the oropharynx. This stage ends with the triggering of the pharyngeal phase of swallowing.
When the volume swallowed is small (1-2 ml, e.g., saliva), there is no preparatory phase and the oral and pharyngeal phases occur in sequence. In contrast, with large liquid boluses, the oral and pharyngeal phases overlap (Logemann, Kahrilas et al. 1992; Ertekin, Celik et al. 2000). The size of the bolus does not alter the sequence of events during oropharyngeal swallowing but modulates the timing of each phase of the swallow. As volume size increases, pharyngeal transit time increases, as do laryngeal closure and elevation (Ertekin, Aydogdu et al. 1997).
When 20 ml of water is placed in the mouth, normal individuals tend to divide the water into two or more parts, which are swallowed in sequence (Ertekin, Aydogdu et al. 1996). This phenomenon is called piecemeal deglutition.
From this stage to the end of the swallow, breathing is inhibited.

2.2 Pharyngeal phase

The pharyngeal phase is closely related to the oral phase, and the distinction between the two is often unclear. This intimate relationship is expressed by the widespread use of the terms oropharynx and oropharyngeal swallowing.

When the movement of the bolus from the oral cavity to the pharyngeal space triggers the swallowing reflex or response, several closely coordinated events occur in rapid overlapping sequence, transporting the bolus from the oropharynx to the esophagus without allowing aspiration. Coordination of these events may be chiefly under the control of the central pattern generator (CPG) in the brainstem (Miller 1982; Jean 2001). These events are as follows: (i) several reflexes governed by the CPG protect the nasal, laryngeal, and tracheal airways and support laryngeal closure; (ii) the tongue moves backward to push the bolus through the pharynx; (iii) and the upper esophageal sphincter relaxes and opens, allowing the bolus to descend into the esophagus.

Once the pharyngeal phase is initiated, the chain of events is irreversible. The entire oropharyngeal sequence takes only 0.6 to 1.0 second, and this duration is remarkably constant in humans (Ertekin, Pehlivan et al. 1995).

2.3 Esophageal phase

In comparison with the extraordinary complexity and rapidity of the oropharyngeal phase, the esophageal phase of swallowing is simpler and slower. It consists of a peristaltic wave of contraction of the striated and smooth muscles, which propagates to the stomach.

2.4 Neurological control of swallowing

The process of swallowing is an ordered sequence of sensory and motor events. Swallowing is a fundamental motor activity, since it serves two vital functions: by propelling food into the stomach, swallowing subserves the alimentary function; and the swallowing reflex protects the upper respiratory tract, thus preventing aspiration of food particles into the lungs (Miller 1982). Swallowing can occur voluntarily via cerebral cortex activation and/or as a reflex under brainstem control.

The central neural control of swallowing is also divided between the cortex and brainstem. Cortical centers in conjunction with afferent feedback from the musculature initiate and modulate the volitional swallow (Sumi 1969; Car and Roman 1970; Martin and Sessle 1993), whereas the brainstem swallowing CPG generates the sequence of reflex swallowing via the nuclei of the Vth, IXth, and XIIth cranial nerves. Normal swallowing requires coordinated interactions among these outputs. Any disruption in the process of coordination leads to swallowing dysfunction.

The importance of suprabulbar influences in regulating swallowing has been established in animal models in which cortical swallowing regions are disrupted by lesion induction, anesthesia, or cooling (Sumi 1969; Martin and Sessle 1993). In humans, the development of functional magnetic resonance imaging (fMRI) has allowed the identification of the cortical regions involved in voluntary swallowing. The primary motor and sensory areas are consistently active in healthy adults during swallowing. The anterior cingular cortex is also activated during swallowing (Hamdy, Mikulis et al. 1999; Humbert and Robbins 2007).

There is convincing evidence that the sequential and rhythmic patterns of swallowing are formed and organized by a central pattern generator (CPG) located within the medulla oblongata (Jean 2001). The CPG was first described as a swallowing center that can be subdivided into three systems: an afferent system composed of the central and peripheral inputs to the center; an efferent system composed of outputs from the center to various motor neuron pools involved in swallowing; and an organizing system composed of interneuronal networks that program the motor pattern.

Although the central regulation of swallowing is chiefly dependent on the brainstem, which receives sensory input from the oropharynx and esophagus, the initiation of swallowing is a voluntary action that requires the integrity of sensorimotor areas of the cerebral cortex. Therefore, both the brainstem and cortex must be intact to ensure normal swallowing.

3. Interaction between respiration and swallowing

The temporal coordination of pharyngeal and laryngeal swallowing events with breathing is essential to prevent aspiration of oropharyngeal contents into the lungs. Indeed, both breathing and swallowing occur continually, although at different frequencies. As the upper airway is used for both breathing and swallowing, the motor pattern generators for these two activities must work in tight coordination to prevent aspiration and to ensure clearance of lower airway secretions (Feroah, Forster et al. 2002).

The swallowing CPG may play a crucial role in coordinating swallowing and breathing. Within this CPG, some of the premotor and motor neurons can be involved in at least two different tasks, such as swallowing and breathing, swallowing and mastication, and swallowing and phonation (Jean 2001).

During swallowing, mechanisms that protect the airways include adduction of the vocal cords, inversion of the epiglottis, and the upward and forward movement of the larynx away from the flow of the bolus. Respiratory control during swallowing contributes to airway protection.

In 1985, Nishino et al. clarified the effects of swallowing on the pattern of continuous breathing in humans. In adults, approximately 80% of spontaneous or water-induced swallows occurred during the expiratory phase. Furthermore, breathing resumed at the point of the expiratory phase where the interruption had taken place (Nishino, Yonezawa et al. 1985). A striking finding was that most of the water-induced swallows occurred during expiration although the timing of water administration was determined at random. The mechanisms underlying these findings are unclear but may involve reflex-mediated responses, as all the study participants reported being unaware of the breathing phase during which their swallows occurred. One of the main hypotheses is that the timing of swallows is not entirely independent from volitional control. The effects of swallowing on the pattern of continuous breathing were analyzed in detail in this study. Spontaneous (automatic) and volitional (water-induced) swallows occurring during expiration were followed by a small increase in the duration of the interrupted expiration. As the time from expiration onset to swallowing increased, the duration of the expiration increased. Swallows that interrupted the inspiratory phase were followed by short expirations. Thus, swallowing was followed by resetting of the respiratory cycling with a return to the functional residual capacity before the initiation of a new inspiration. This alteration in the breathing pattern may help to clear the airway of secretions and foreign material before the next inspiration, thus contributing to prevent aspiration (Nishino, Yonezawa et al. 1985).

Breathing-swallowing interactions and the underlying mechanisms have been studied in healthy volunteers by measuring a variety of parameters including the duration of deglutition apnea (Nishino, Yonezawa et al. 1985; Selley, Flack et al. 1989; Martin, Logemann et al. 1994; Klahn and Perlman 1999) and the timing of breathing events relative to swallows (Perlman, Schultz et al. 1993; Martin, Logemann et al. 1994; Paydarfar, Gilbert et al. 1995; Klahn and Perlman 1999). Several factors that influence breathing-swallowing interactions were identified. Interestingly, many studies showed that breathing-swallowing coordination was influenced by neurological disorders affecting the brain, spinal cord, or peripheral nerves.

Studies in unconscious patients demonstrated that several mechanisms integrating breathing and swallowing remained operative, leading to changes in the breathing pattern during repeated swallows. These findings are consistent with a role for brainstem control (Nishino and Hiraga 1991), especially as both the respiratory center and the swallowing CPG are located in the same area of the brainstem. In contrast, other studies demonstrated that the cortex influences breathing-swallowing interactions in unconscious patients (Hadjikoutis, Pickersgill et al. 2000).

In the other direction, alterations in breathing patterns and ventilation may influence the coordination of swallowing and breathing. This effect is of particular importance in patients with chronic respiratory failure, in whom close breathing-swallowing coordination is essential to maintain adequate ventilation despite the limited ventilatory capacity. Alterations in breathing-swallowing coordination have been reported in patients with chronic obstructive pulmonary disease (COPD) (Shaker, Li et al. 1992) and in awake healthy volunteers subjected to added respiratory loads (Kijima, Isono et al. 1999). Tachypnea and lung volume have also been demonstrated to influence breathing-swallowing coordination.

Alterations in breathing-swallowing coordination chiefly affect temporal coordination. When temporal coordination is disrupted, most swallows are followed by an inspiration, which significantly increases the risk of aspiration.

4. Breathing-swallowing interaction in neuromuscular patients

Elucidation of breathing-swallowing interactions in patients with specific neuromuscular diseases is of considerable interest. Patients with neuromuscular disease have achieved substantial survival gains in recent years as a result of advances in the management of respiratory failure (Finder, Birnkrant et al. 2004). The introduction of mechanical ventilation (MV) in the 1990s improved survival in patients with Duchenne muscular dystrophy (DMD) from about 15 years in the 1960s to more than 30 years now. Quality of life, however, declines over time as the disease progresses. Malnutrition is common: in one study, for instance, 44% of patients had malnutrition (Willig, Bach et al. 1995; Finder, Birnkrant et al. 2004). The main causes of malnutrition are prolonged swallowing, respiratory failure, and dysphagia, which jeopardize the patient's ability to meet intake needs. Feeding difficulties often develop insidiously, being frequently underestimated by family members and healthcare professionals (Hill, Hughes et al. 2004). Aspiration is another important consequence of impaired swallowing that becomes increasingly common as the disease progresses (Finder, Birnkrant et al. 2004).

To the best of our knowledge, breathing-swallowing interactions initially received little research attention (Hadjikoutis, Pickersgill et al. 2000). Moreover, improvements in the management of chronic respiratory failure translate into differences in breathing conditions across patients and over time, and this variability is likely to complicate the evaluation of breathing-swallowing interactions. These breathing conditions are now well defined and include spontaneous breathing (SB), (Raphael, Chevret et al. 1994), noninvasive mechanical ventilation (NIV) (Bach, Alba et al. 1993; 1999; Mehta and Hill 2001; Annane, Orlikowski et al. 2007), tracheostomy with SB (Bach and Alba 1990; Chadda, Louis et al. 2002), and tracheostomy with MV (Bach and Alba 1990; Bach 1993; Simonds 2003).

In contrast to spontaneously breathing patients, tracheostomized patients receiving assist-control MV cannot prolong their expiratory phase. Consequently, the ventilator determines whether expiration or inspiration occurs after swallowing. Under normal breathing conditions, swallows are nearly always followed by expiration (Nishino, Yonezawa et al. 1985; Smith, Wolkove et al. 1989; Paydarfar, Gilbert et al. 1995), which may contribute to prevent aspiration.

In studies of breathing-swallowing interactions in neuromuscular patients with chronic respiratory failure, we found that SB was associated with piecemeal deglutition leading to an increase in the time needed to swallow a water bolus, as well as with inspiration after nearly half the swallows. These abnormalities may contribute to feeding difficulties. They correlated with the reduction in respiratory muscle performance, suggesting a relationship between breathing-muscle performance and swallowing-muscle performance. Accordingly, tongue strength and indices of global and respiratory strength varied in parallel throughout the course of Guillain-Barré syndrome (Orlikowski, Terzi et al. 2009). Tongue strength can be considered representative of the strength of the various muscles involved in swallowing. Another hypothesis is that respiratory failure alone may alter breathing-swallowing coordination. In keeping with this possibility, breathing-swallowing abnormalities were documented in COPD patients with respiratory failure but no upper-airway muscle-strength abnormalities. These findings indicated a need for evaluating the positive impact of MV on breathing-swallowing interactions in patients with respiratory failure.

First, in tracheostomized NM patients who were able to breathe spontaneously, we demonstrated that MV decreased both piecemeal deglutition and swallowing time per bolus (Terzi, Orlikowski et al. 2007).

Second, we evaluated the impact of tracheostomy with MV on swallowing performance in patients with DMD. To this end, we assessed swallowing performance and breathing-swallowing coordination before and after tracheostomy in the same patients. Piecemeal deglutition over several breathing cycles occurred in all patients. Before tracheostomy, half the swallows were followed by inspirations. Tracheostomy was associated with significant decreases in total bolus swallowing time and number of swallows per bolus, compared to the values before tracheostomy. These findings indicated that invasive ventilation via a tracheostomy improved swallowing. Several hypotheses can be put forward to explain this effect. Breathing and swallowing use the same initial pathway and, therefore, competition occurs between these two functions. Under physiological conditions, this competition is well controlled via close coordination of breathing and swallowing. Respiratory failure exacerbates the competition, giving preference to breathing over swallowing and altering the coordination between these two activities. Our results suggest that, by reversing the respiratory failure and separating the breathing and swallowing pathways, invasive MV may have a positive impact on swallowing in patients with respiratory failure.

The question is now whether treating the respiratory failure without separating the breathing and swallowing pathways, e.g., by using NIV, improves swallowing performance in patients with respiratory failure. We are currently studying the impact of NIV on swallowing in patients with chronic obstructive pulmonary disease (COPD) admitted to the intensive care unit for acute respiratory failure. The first results strongly support a beneficial effect of NIV on swallowing performance.

All these studies underline the clinical usefulness of noninvasive dynamic evaluations of breathing-swallowing interactions in order to detect patients at risk for swallowing dysfunction due to respiratory failure. All our studies were done using a previously described noninvasive method (see below).

5. From bench to the bedside

EMG can be used to demonstrate the sequential and orderly activity of the muscles involved in swallowing and breathing. The anatomical components of the swallowing apparatus include the bony and cartilaginous support structures, striated and smooth muscles, and neural elements.

The muscles involved in swallowing have been studied in experimental animals and, to some extent, in humans. In dogs, the pattern of EMG activity was studied in the oral and pharyngeal muscles during swallowing elicited reflexively by electrical and mechanical stimuli (Doty and Bosma 1956). Needle electrodes were used to record intramuscular EMG activity during swallowing from a large complex of oral, pharyngeal, and laryngeal muscles in anesthetized animals. Descriptive studies based on this technique consistently found that the nonvolitional component of swallowing was controlled by a CPG (Miller 1972; Suzuki, Tokuriki et al. 1977; Kobara-Mates, Logemann et al. 1995). In humans, most of the intramuscular EMG studies of the pharyngeal phase of swallowing focused on a single muscle or muscle pair (Basmajian and Dutta 1961; Perlman, Luschei et al. 1989). Such studies can shed valuable light on the properties of the muscle of interest. However, they provide no information on the dynamics of swallowing.

To evaluate the dynamics of swallowing, researchers used quantitative surface EMG of the submental complex (SM) composed of submandibular/suprahyoid muscles including the mylohyoid, genohyoid, and anterior digastric muscles. All the muscles in this complex contract simultaneously to initiate a swallow and function as laryngeal elevators (Miller 1982). Consequently, submental surface EMG activity provides considerable information about the onset and duration of the oropharyngeal swallowing phase, as contraction of the SM complex pulls the hyoid bone into an anterosuperior position, thereby elevating the larynx and initiating the other reflexive changes that constitute the pharyngeal phase of swallowing (Donner, Bosma et al. 1985; Dodds, Logemann et al. 1990; Ertekin, Pehlivan et al. 1995). However, pharyngeal and laryngeal EMG recording during swallowing was difficult to perform noninvasively and usually required the insertion of a needle electrode. However, laryngeal motion can be detected fairly easily using a mechanical sensor.

To evaluate swallowing, we used a method previously described by Ertekin et al. (Ertekin, Aydogdu et al. 1998). Skin-surface electrodes are placed on the chin to record submental muscle activity and a piezo-electric sensor is placed between the cricoid and thyroid cartilages on the midline to detect laryngeal motion (Figure 1) (Terzi, Orlikowski et al. 2007). Breathing-swallowing coordination is assessed by using respiratory inductive plethysmography to record thoracic and abdominal movements. All signals are digitized and recorded on a personal computer equipped with an MP 150 data acquisition system (Biopac Systems, Goleta, CA, USA). The system software (AcqKnowledge) is configured to display the EMG signals, laryngeal movements, thoracic and abdominal movements simultaneously on separate channels.

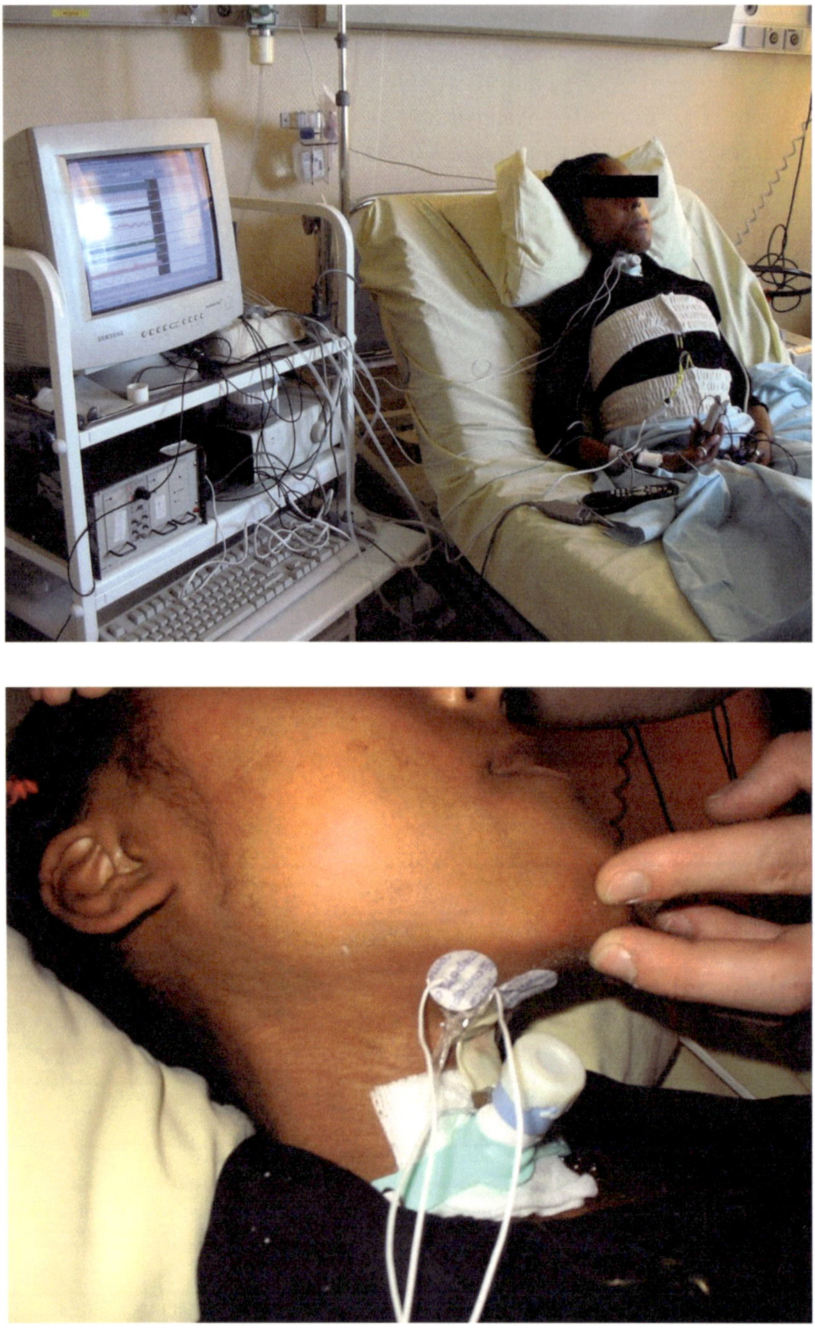

Fig. 1. Noninvasive monitoring. Extracted from Terzi et al. (Terzi, Orlikowski et al. 2007)

First, using this method we have demonstrated that the breathing-swallowing interaction was associated with piecemeal deglutition in neuromuscular patients, contrary to healthy subjects (Figure 2).

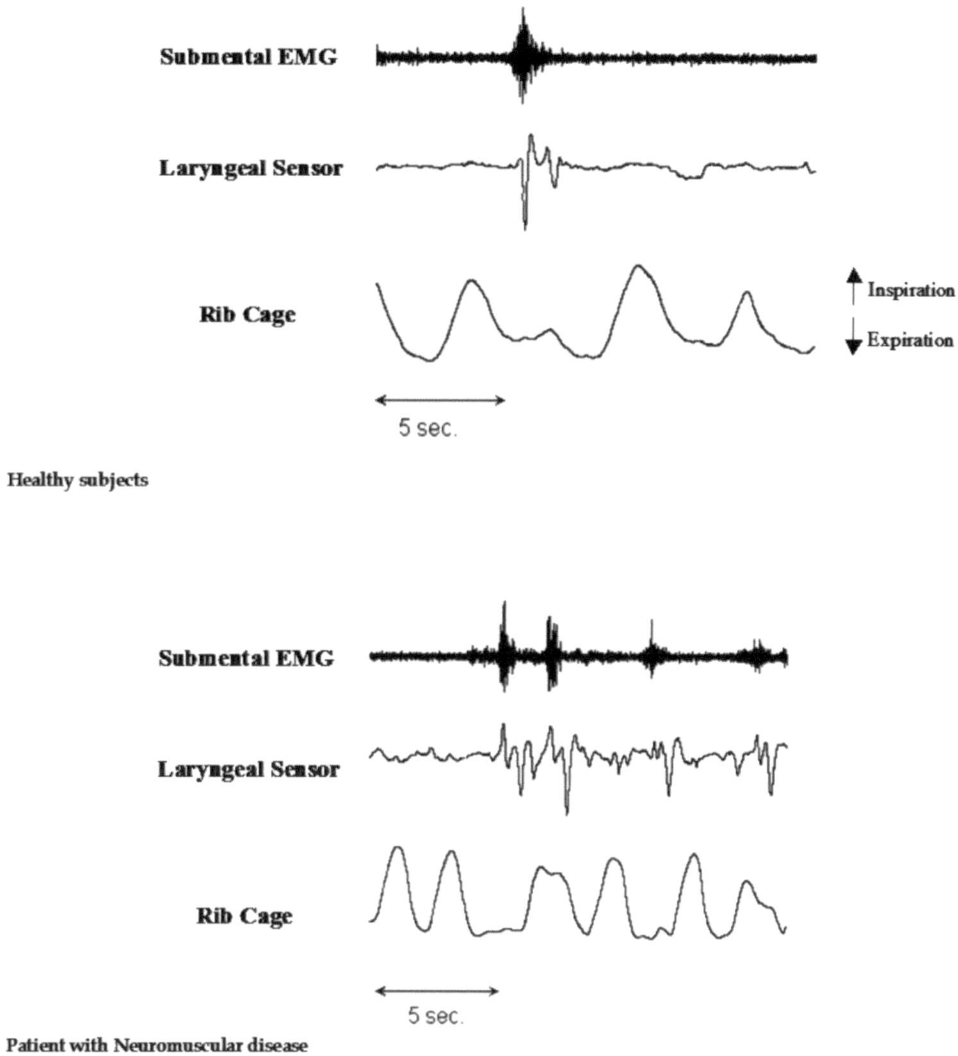

Fig. 2. Example of recordings in healthy subjects, and in patient with neuromuscular disorder. Extracted from Terzi et al. (Terzi, Orlikowski et al. 2007).

Piecemeal deglutition and breathing-swallowing anormalities was also demonstrated when neuromuscular patients were tracheostomized, however swallowing performance improved with mechanical ventilation (Figure 3).

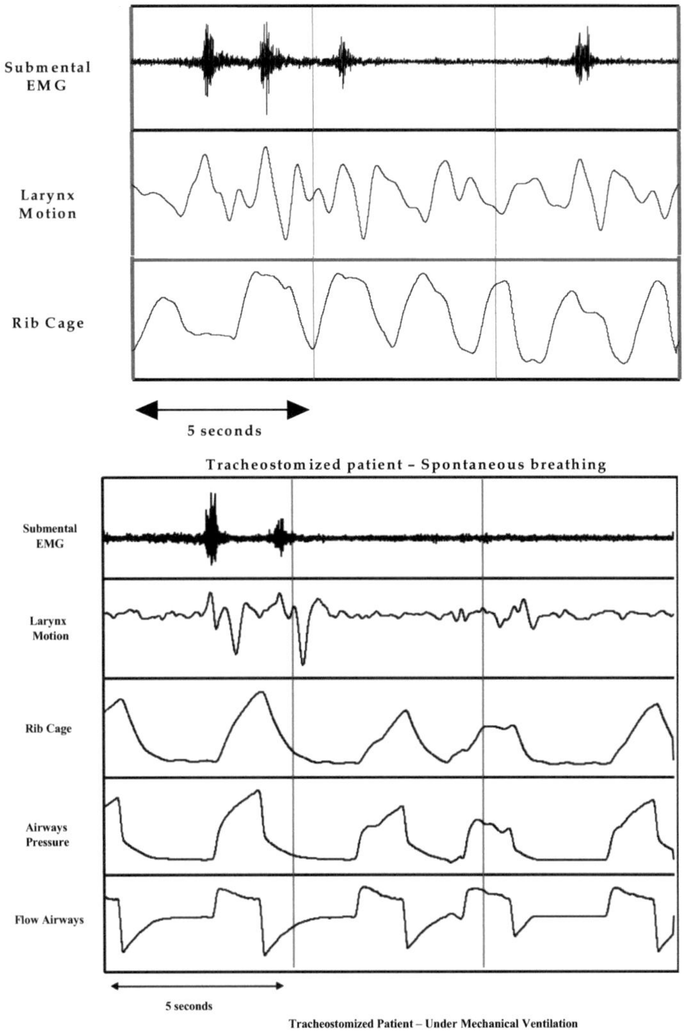

Fig. 3. Example of recordings with or without mechanical ventilation. Swallowing performance was improved by mechanical ventilation.

6. References

(1999). "Clinical indications for noninvasive positive pressure ventilation in chronic respiratory failure due to restrictive lung disease, COPD, and nocturnal hypoventilation--a consensus conference report." Chest 116(2): 521-534.

Annane, D., D. Orlikowski, et al. (2007). "Nocturnal mechanical ventilation for chronic hypoventilation in patients with neuromuscular and chest wall disorders." Cochrane Database Syst Rev(4): CD001941.

Bach, J. R. (1993). "A comparison of long-term ventilatory support alternatives from the perspective of the patient and care giver." Chest 104(6): 1702-1706.

Bach, J. R. and A. S. Alba (1990). "Tracheostomy ventilation. A study of efficacy with deflated cuffs and cuffless tubes." Chest 97(3): 679-683.

Bach, J. R., A. S. Alba, et al. (1993). "Intermittent positive pressure ventilation via the mouth as an alternative to tracheostomy for 257 ventilator users." Chest 103(1): 174-182.

Basmajian, J. V. and C. R. Dutta (1961). "Electromyography of the pharyngeal constrictors and levator palati in man." Anat Rec 139: 561-563.

Car, A. and C. Roman (1970). "[Deglutitions and oesophageal reflex contractions induced by electrical stimulation of the medulla oblongata]." Exp Brain Res 11(1): 75-92.

Chadda, K., B. Louis, et al. (2002). "Physiological effects of decannulation in tracheostomized patients." Intensive Care Med 28(12): 1761-1767.

Dodds, W. J. (1989). "Physiology of swallowing." Dysphagia 3(4): 171-178.

Dodds, W. J., J. A. Logemann, et al. (1990). "Radiologic assessment of abnormal oral and pharyngeal phases of swallowing." AJR Am J Roentgenol 154(5): 965-974.

Donner, M. W., J. F. Bosma, et al. (1985). "Anatomy and physiology of the pharynx." Gastrointest Radiol 10(3): 196-212.

Doty, R. W. and J. F. Bosma (1956). "An electromyographic analysis of reflex deglutition." J Neurophysiol 19(1): 44-60.

Ertekin, C., I. Aydogdu, et al. (1996). "Piecemeal deglutition and dysphagia limit in normal subjects and in patients with swallowing disorders." J Neurol Neurosurg Psychiatry 61(5): 491-496.

Ertekin, C., I. Aydogdu, et al. (1997). "Effects of bolus volume on oropharyngeal swallowing: an electrophysiologic study in man." Am J Gastroenterol 92(11): 2049-2053.

Ertekin, C., I. Aydogdu, et al. (1998). "Electrodiagnostic methods for neurogenic dysphagia." Electroencephalogr Clin Neurophysiol 109(4): 331-340.

Ertekin, C., M. Celik, et al. (2000). "The electromyographic behavior of the thyroarytenoid muscle during swallowing." J Clin Gastroenterol 30(3): 274-280.

Ertekin, C., M. Pehlivan, et al. (1995). "An electrophysiological investigation of deglutition in man." Muscle Nerve 18(10): 1177-1186.

Feroah, T. R., H. V. Forster, et al. (2002). "Effects of spontaneous swallows on breathing in awake goats." J Appl Physiol 92(5): 1923-1935.

Finder, J. D., D. Birnkrant, et al. (2004). "Respiratory care of the patient with Duchenne muscular dystrophy: ATS consensus statement." Am J Respir Crit Care Med 170(4): 456-465.

Hadjikoutis, S., T. P. Pickersgill, et al. (2000). "Abnormal patterns of breathing during swallowing in neurological disorders." Brain 123 (Pt 9): 1863-1873.

Hamdy, S., D. J. Mikulis, et al. (1999). "Cortical activation during human volitional swallowing: an event-related fMRI study." Am J Physiol 277(1 Pt 1): G219-225.

Hill, M., T. Hughes, et al. (2004). "Treatment for swallowing difficulties (dysphagia) in chronic muscle disease." Cochrane Database Syst Rev(2): CD004303.

Humbert, I. A. and J. Robbins (2007). "Normal swallowing and functional magnetic resonance imaging: a systematic review." Dysphagia 22(3): 266-275.

Jean, A. (2001). "Brain stem control of swallowing: neuronal network and cellular mechanisms." Physiol Rev 81(2): 929-969.

Kijima, M., S. Isono, et al. (1999). "Coordination of swallowing and phases of respiration during added respiratory loads in awake subjects." Am J Respir Crit Care Med 159(6): 1898-1902.

Klahn, M. S. and A. L. Perlman (1999). "Temporal and durational patterns associating respiration and swallowing." Dysphagia 14(3): 131-138.

Kobara-Mates, M., J. A. Logemann, et al. (1995). "Physiology of oropharyngeal swallow in the cat: a videofluoroscopic and electromyographic study." Am J Physiol 268(2 Pt 1): G232-241.

Logemann, J. A., P. J. Kahrilas, et al. (1992). "Closure mechanisms of laryngeal vestibule during swallow." Am J Physiol 262(2 Pt 1): G338-344.

Martin, B. J., J. A. Logemann, et al. (1994). "Coordination between respiration and swallowing: respiratory phase relationships and temporal integration." J Appl Physiol 76(2): 714-723.

Martin, R. E. and B. J. Sessle (1993). "The role of the cerebral cortex in swallowing." Dysphagia 8(3): 195-202.

Mehta, S. and N. S. Hill (2001). "Noninvasive ventilation." Am J Respir Crit Care Med 163(2): 540-577.

Miller, A. J. (1972). "Significance of sensory inflow to the swallowing reflex." Brain Res 43(1): 147-159.

Miller, A. J. (1982). "Deglutition." Physiol Rev 62(1): 129-184.

Nishino, T. and K. Hiraga (1991). "Coordination of swallowing and respiration in unconscious subjects." J Appl Physiol 70(3): 988-993.

Nishino, T., T. Yonezawa, et al. (1985). "Effects of swallowing on the pattern of continuous respiration in human adults." Am Rev Respir Dis 132(6): 1219-1222.

Orlikowski, D., N. Terzi, et al. (2009). "Tongue weakness is associated with respiratory failure in patients with severe Guillain-Barre syndrome." Acta Neurol Scand 119(6): 364-370.

Paydarfar, D., R. J. Gilbert, et al. (1995). "Respiratory phase resetting and airflow changes induced by swallowing in humans." J Physiol 483 (Pt 1): 273-288.

Perlman, A. L., E. S. Luschei, et al. (1989). "Electrical activity from the superior pharyngeal constrictor during reflexive and nonreflexive tasks." J Speech Hear Res 32(4): 749-754.

Perlman, A. L., P. M. Palmer, et al. (1999). "Electromyographic activity from human laryngeal, pharyngeal, and submental muscles during swallowing." J Appl Physiol 86(5): 1663-1669.

Perlman, A. L., J. G. Schultz, et al. (1993). "Effects of age, gender, bolus volume, and bolus viscosity on oropharyngeal pressure during swallowing." J Appl Physiol 75(1): 33-37.

Raphael, J. C., S. Chevret, et al. (1994). "Randomised trial of preventive nasal ventilation in Duchenne muscular dystrophy. French Multicentre Cooperative Group on Home Mechanical Ventilation Assistance in Duchenne de Boulogne Muscular Dystrophy." Lancet 343(8913): 1600-1604.

Selley, W. G., F. C. Flack, et al. (1989). "Respiratory patterns associated with swallowing: Part 1. The normal adult pattern and changes with age." Age Ageing 18(3): 168-172.

Shaker, R., Q. Li, et al. (1992). "Coordination of deglutition and phases of respiration: effect of aging, tachypnea, bolus volume, and chronic obstructive pulmonary disease." Am J Physiol 263(5 Pt 1): G750-755.

Simonds, A. K. (2003). "Home ventilation." Eur Respir J Suppl 47: 38s-46s.

Smith, J., N. Wolkove, et al. (1989). "Coordination of eating, drinking and breathing in adults." Chest 96(3): 578-582.

Sumi, T. (1969). "Some properties of cortically-evoked swallowing and chewing in rabbits." Brain Res 15(1): 107-120.

Suzuki, M., M. Tokuriki, et al. (1977). "Electromyographic studies on the deglutition movement in the goat." Nippon Juigaku Zasshi 39(3): 243-253.

Terzi, N., D. Orlikowski, et al. (2007). "Breathing-swallowing interaction in neuromuscular patients: a physiological evaluation." Am J Respir Crit Care Med 175(3): 269-276.

Terzi, N., H. Prigent, et al. "Impact of tracheostomy on swallowing performance in Duchenne muscular dystrophy." Neuromuscul Disord 20(8): 493-498.

Willig, T. N., J. R. Bach, et al. (1995). "Nutritional rehabilitation in neuromuscular disorders." Semin Neurol 15(1): 18-23.

Part 6

EMG New Frontiers in Research and Technology

22

Man to Machine, Applications in Electromyography

Michael Wehner
Wehner Engineering, Berkeley, USA

1. Introduction

The study of electrical signals due to muscle activation has been evolving since Francesco Redi found electrical generation in the muscles of the electric ray fish in 1666 (Fishman, Wilkins, 2011), Dubois discovered electrical activation in voluntary muscles in 1849 (Blanc, Dimanico, 2010), and Mari coined the term Electromyography in 1922 (Raz, et al., 2006). Evolving over the following decades, electromyography has found widespread use in clinical settings as well as extensive use in ergonomic assessment and biomechanics research laboratories.
As with many technologies, the discovery of electromyography occurred long before inexpensive and robust hardware was developed to utilize the vast amount of information available from myoelectric signals. Until recently, existing technology could not support efficient generation of repeatable robust signals for even highly sophisticated research laboratories, let alone the widespread availability of affordable, robust hardware required to propagate electromyography through the research communities. New high-speed computation tools make real-time analysis feasible. With the emergence of low cost hardware, high speed wireless communication technology, and low cost, high speed computing/signal processing equipment, Electromyography is becoming available to a whole new set of experimenter. With these advances making electromyography a feasible option in many situations, we see the emergence of a key period in the evolution of the technology. Surface electromyography (sEMG) provides a convenient and relatively non-invasive avenue for determining muscle activation, particularly as highly portable devices become available. Of course with the benefits of wider availability, we must consider the risks inherent in this spread, as the practitioners involved move from electromyography specialists, to technologists in other fields, using electromyography either part time, or only occasionally. Electromyography is a detailed art, and can easily lead to erroneous conclusions if not practiced carefully. With new applications, particularly where electromyography is employed as a means for humans to control electromechanical systems, care must be taken to insure that these systems are developed with robust safety systems, and improper assumptions about electromyography do not cause harm, injury, or even death.

2. Background

Recognized as a potentially powerful tool EMG was first used in measuring human movement at the turn of the 20th century (Medved, 2001). As use spread, techniques for recording, processing, and interpreting EMG signals varied widely. With a lack of standardization, various styles developed and the discipline became an art as much as it was a science (De Luca, 1997).Efforts have been underway to standardize the EMG process, with considerable efforts in the past decade to implement standards which 1) formalize scientific understanding of the concepts behind EMG (De Luca, 1997), 2) allow interpretation and repetition of previously published results (Hermens, et al., 2000) , and 3) provide standards going forward for generating as well as publishing EMG data (Hermens, et al., 2000). In the following sections, three major efforts to standardize the EMG recording, processing, interpreting, and publishing procedures are discussed

2.1 What is electromyography?

Muscle cells are surrounded by a selectively permeable membrane with a resting electrical potential of 70 to 90 millivolts. The outside of the cell is positive relative to the inside. Motoneurons carry impulses from the central nervous system to the muscle cells called the nerve action potential (NAP). All muscle cells (or fibers) innervated by one motoneuron are called a motor unit, and are stimulated simultaneously when the motoneuron fires. The muscle fibers of one motor unit are not bundled within a muscle. Rather they are spread throughout the muscle with a relatively uniform distribution. When a series of NAP's reach the cells of a muscle unit they cause a release of chemical transmitters which depolarize the cell to a threshold value, initiating an action potential as the cell wall permeability changes. This depolarization causes a brief contraction, or twitch, of the muscle cell (and all other cells in that motor unit) and comprises the basis of muscle movement. The depolarization that travels along the muscle fiber and can be detected on the surface of the muscle as a small electrical potential called the muscle action potential (MAP). Each muscle is comprised of many muscle motor units, which are comprised of many cells, and are connected to many motoneurons, thus a seemingly simple muscle contraction will correspond to a complex overall MAP waveform. An electrode properly positioned with respect to the muscle can record these MAP waveforms. The sensing and recording of these electrical waveforms is called electromyography (EMG). Though a motor unit is either on or off, based on whether or not it is being stimulated by a NAP, an increase in muscle tension beyond that caused by a single NAP can occur either from multiple NAPs stimulating the same motor unit, or from recruitment of additional motor units. Fortunately, both phenomena cause an increase in overall MAP waveform amplitude, corresponding to an increased EMG signal (Chaffin, Andersson, 1999). Properly recorded and processed EMG signal is known to correlate to muscle activation level, and in some cases can be used to determine muscle tension (De Luca, 1997). EMG recordings can be done through two basic methods; 1) Intramuscular, where needle based electrodes are inserted through the skin into the muscle of interest, or 2) Surface, where flat electrodes are adhered to the skin surface above the muscle of interest. Intramuscular EMG is the preferred method when measuring small muscles, particularly those surrounded by large muscles which may prevent accurate recording of the signal of interest or when attempting to measure only a few motor units. Surface EMG is preferred when studying large muscles, especially those near the surface and with few large muscles nearby. An added advantage of surface EMG is that the electrodes are adhered to the skin surface, thus piercing of the skin is not required.

2.2 EMG, proper signal detection and processing

In the Journal of Applied Biomechanics, De Luca details the factors affecting EMG signal and proper procedure for detecting and processing the signal (De Luca, 1997). These discussions are followed by a summary of recommendations in the use of EMG. In most biomechanics applications, EMG is used in three areas, 1) to identify the initiation of muscle activity, 2) as a surrogate for estimating muscle tension (force), and 3) as a method for estimating muscle fatigue. In this discussion we cover applications involving filtered and processed EMG signals, thus initiation and fatigue will serve only as tertiary topics of discussion, with the focus of this chapter on muscle activation level. In detecting and recording an EMG signal with maximum fidelity and minimum noise, one must consider a number of factors.

- Electrode configuration. This includes shape and area, material, and inter-electrode distance (IED) which determines the number of motor units being detected. Also to be considered are location of the electrodes on the muscle, laterally and longitudinally. This effects the amplitude and frequency of the signal detected as well as the level of cross-talk from other nearby muscle groups. An appropriate IED should be chosen which is small enough to minimize crosstalk, yet large enough to minimize risk of shunting (electrical contact between electrodes, in effect making them one larger electrode and reducing signal amplitude and signal to noise ratio).
- Intrinsic (muscle) factors. This includes the number of active motor units at any time, fiber type of the muscle, blood flow to the muscle, fiber diameter, and the depth of active muscle fibers. These considerations can affect amplitude and frequency characteristics of muscle response. Also of consideration are the amount and type of tissue between the muscle surface and the electrode. Signal may experience considerable spatial filtering due to interstitial tissue.
- Intermediate factors. These effects include electromechanical properties of the electrodes, and their ability to act as band-pass filters or integrators, and the tendency to record cross-talk from other muscles. Also of concern is the conduction velocity of action potentials and spatial filtering effects of relative electrode-muscle fiber position, as these tend to affect amplitude and frequency characteristics of an EMG signal. This is particularly important when considering anisometric EMG, as EMG signal varies as muscle fibers change in length.
- Deterministic factors. This includes the number of active and detected motor units, motor unit force twitch, fiber interaction, firing rate, characteristics of the action potentials, and recruitment characteristics.
- Other interstitial tissue properties. It can be understood that the movement of subcutaneous tissues including muscle and fat can cause signals erroneously. These signals should be considered in EMG data as a source of artifact error.

The recorded EMG signal can be used to determine muscle activation level in many situations and even to determine muscle force in some cases. These relationships are not automatic however, and care must be taken to design the experiment correctly and to draw only appropriate conclusions from the data. For the isometric case, the amplitude of the EMG signal is understood to increase with muscle force. This qualitative relationship however can not be extrapolated to a force magnitude for one subject or especially as a force comparison or magnitude measurement from subject to subject. In order to make force predictions or make comparison between subjects, EMG signals must be normalized to some applied force. This is usually done normalizing to maximum contraction of the muscle (MVC 100%) or to a reference voluntary exertion (RVE). Additionally, every time an electrode is moved (between sessions or simply due to electrode dislodging) normalization must be repeated. When electrodes are placed, no matter how carefully, they cover a slightly different set of motor units. As the muscle units under study and the spatial filtering characteristics will change with the new electrode placement, they will yield a slightly or even substantially different signal. Also, if the joint angle changes, the location of the electrodes relative to the muscle belly change. In comparing signals between subjects, the amount of subcutaneous fatty tissue can vary substantially and becomes a major concern. De Luca warns that all of these issues become magnified, and new issues arise when dynamic EMG is considered.

Several recommendations are given and are listed in an abridged form below.

- The preferred electrode configuration (general, not muscle specific) consists of two parallel bars, 1cm by 1-2 mm wide placed 1 cm apart, which record at a bandwidth 20-500 Hz.
- Locate the electrodes on the midline of the muscle belly.
- Use the RMS value of the signal for measuring amplitude of the EMG signal.
- Measure activation time of all contractions.
- Check for crosstalk
- Quantitative comparisons between EMG signals are to be performed in static cases only, and require additional precautions and procedures.
- Instantaneous EMG signals should be treated as stochastic. To obtain a force-EMG relationship, signal should be filtered over a 1 second window, among other precautions.
- In constant force isometric contractions, motor units should not be near their threshold.
- Avoid measurement of anisometric contractions. Additional considerations are required.
- Normalize EMG at values less than 80% of maximum voluntary contraction (MVC), but calibrate between electrode placements and between subjects at MVC.

2.3 EMG, and SENIAM (surface EMG for a non-invasive assessment of muscles)

European group SENIAM has a specific objective of creating collaboration, developing recommendations on sensors, sensor placement, signal processing and modeling. From 1996 – 1999, a major effort was conducted to scan the literature for existing surface-electromyography (SEMG) work, contact these researchers for details and clarifications on their SEMG work, and develop recommendations for SEMG in the future (Hermens, et al., 2000). This effort yielded results showing the breadth of hardware and procedures used, as well as those that were most common.

Based on this research as well as parallel investigation into optimum properties (as opposed to the most commonly reported ones discussed above), SENIAM generated the following recommendations for SEMG.

- There is no recommendation regarding electrode shape, but the size of the electrode should not exceed 10 mm in the direction of the muscle fiber.
- IED should be 20 mm, but this should be reduced for small muscles.
- Pre-gelled Ag/AgCl electrodes are recommended.
- Skin at the sensor location is to be shaved if covered with hair and is to be cleaned with alcohol prior to adhering the sensors.
- SENIAM refers to their CD data for proper subject posture during sensor attachment for specific muscles. This is also the case with determining proper sensor location on specific muscles.

2.4 Standards for reporting EMG data, ISEK

The International Society of Electrophysiology and Kinesiology (ISEK) has endorsed standards for reporting EMG data, and have published them in the Journal of Electromyography and Kineseology (Merletti, 1999). Standards applicable to the experiments conducted here are summarized below.

- Electrode material, shape, and size should be reported.
- Skin and electrode preparation should be given, including abrasion, shaving, cleaning, and use of gel or paste.
- Electrode orientation and location over the muscle should be given.
- Detection details, including gain range used should be given.
- Filtering details, hardware and software, should be given, and amplifier filters should be in the range of high pass 5 Hz, and low pass 500 Hz.
- If rectification and smoothing occur in hardware prior to sampling and storing data, sampling rates can be reduced to 50 - 100 Hz.
- Description of the A/D card used should be given.
- If the Mean Average Value (MAV) of the rectified signal over time T is used, then T should be given.
- EMG values should be normalized about MVC, and conditions should be described.
- When normalizing, the following information should be provided: Training, rate of rise of force, velocity of shortening or lengthening and range of angles if not isometric, load in non-isometric contractions.
- Efforts should be taken to determine that crosstalk did not contaminate the signal. And care should be taken in areas with subcutaneous adipose tissue (body fat).

In reviewing the recommendations from these sources, and especially when comparing them to published experiments, one sees some ambiguity and even some conflicting recommendations. For the most part, however, the guidelines allow the design of well organized experiments, and data can be taken with considerable confidence as to standards and repeatability. In using these agreed upon methods, EMG based devices and applications can anticipate good, robust, and recognizable result. These relatively consistent results can be used to control an array of devices.

As discussed above, EMG data is not a reliable method of predicting forces during individual events within a short task, because EMG signals do not correlate with muscle forces on a real time basis, and individual event measurement is understood as stochastic data only. De Luca expressed concern over the repeatability of tests based on calibration around maximum voluntary contraction and the consistency of subjects applying a truly maximum contraction. Depending on the application, calibration based on maximum or reference contractions are of varying importance. In many applications, truly real-time event recognition may not be necessary, so filtering over a relatively long timeframe (hundreds of milliseconds) may be perfectly acceptable. In other applications, higher speed may be necessary, but accuracy of signal magnitude may be of low concern. In such applications, different approaches to interpreting myoelectric signals should be undertaken. For yet other applications, very little lag is permissible, and high signal fidelity is also required. For such applications, EMG may not currently be the optimum sensing tool. As with most design projects, clearly understanding the parameters and scope of the endeavor is key to developing a successful device or tool. So while standards are in place for interpreting myoelectric signals, proper care and design structure is required to insure the best possible results.

3. Chapter organization

Electromyography is being used in a myriad of evolutionary and revolutionary ways, both alone and in conjunction with other technologies. Along with the widespread availability of high speed, robust computing and sensing equipment at a relatively low cost, EMG is pushing the forefront of human machine interface. We discuss several of the interesting applications of EMG, including current and emerging areas of EMG use, as well as mixed-use applications in which EMG is used in conjunction with other technologies to yield a suite of sensors providing robust signals for the application at hand. Next, we cover possible future applications of EMG, and we discuss the relative merits and cautions of using EMG in various applications.

4. Methods of utilizing EMG in engineering devices

Electromyography can be used in many ways for various applications, with various techniques and concerns corresponding to each new application. This chapter covers five of the most common methods of employing EMG. Each technique has advantages and disadvantages to be explored or avoided based on the specific application.
Methods of using EMG in engineering applications:
Method 1. Sense and emulate/amplify. Here, Electromyography is used to sense the activity of a muscle and the myoelectric signal is processed in order to determine an activation magnitude as a function of time. This magnitude is then used to determine a target force, position, or motion of a worn mechanical device emulating, or actually worn over the same limb. In this method, the myoelectric signal is interpreted in order to determine a discrete magnitude, not a target threshold value. This method is used in controlling the HAL exoskeleton discussed later (Kasaoka, Sankai, 2001)

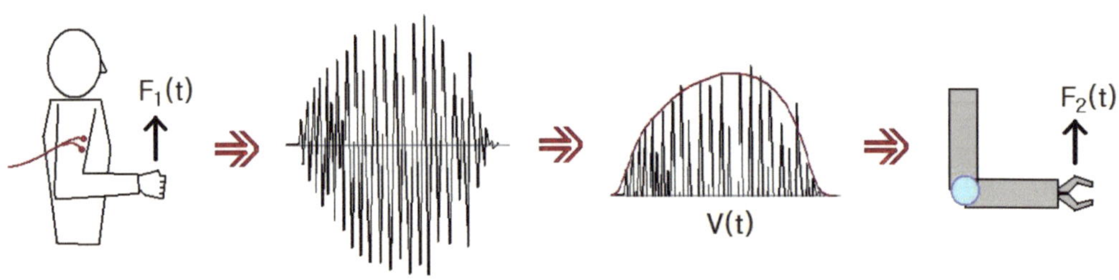

Fig. 1. Method 1 Schematic.

Method 2. Sense and interpret, proportional. Similar to method one, EMG is used to determine activation level of a muscle as a function of time. Rather than interpreting the signal in order to control a local device and directly emulate the limb being sensed, this method interprets the signal in order to provide input to another device, either locally or remotely. Signal strength is used to interpret a desired magnitude (such as speed, lift force, grip strength) For example, a prosthetic arm can not use EMG signals from the missing limb (an exception to this, using the emerging TMR techniques, will be discussed later in the chapter) but can be controlled by sensing the activity of other muscles. Likewise, myoelectric signals can be used as an input source for other devices, either locally or remotely. In this method, as in method one, signal strength is interpreted to determine a magnitude which changes over time rather than a threshold value.

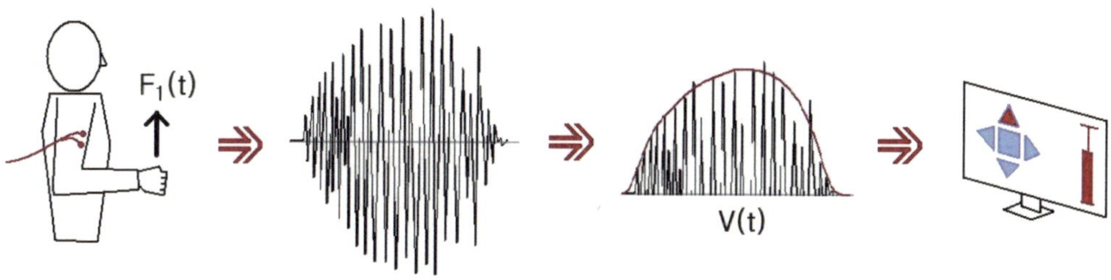

Fig. 2. Method 2 Schematic.

Method 3. Sense and interpret, threshold. A myoelectric signal is read, processed, and compared to a predetermined threshold value. When that value is reached, a condition is considered satisfied. Rather than interpreting a signal to determine a curvilinear magnitude with respect to time, this application is more similar to an on-off switch. EMG signal can be used to signal stop-go, open-close, or other two state situations. Other configurations such as three state situations or any number of two state situations are also possible. The matrix of possible states available is limited only by the number of EMG channels available, and user skill/endurance in operating the device. A simple two or three state device offers the advantage of being easier to operate and has a faster learning curve. This method is used in some prosthetic devices and is believed to cause less fatigue for users than the proportional control in method 2 when the system is designed properly with this goal in mind. This advantage is possible because with the threshold value technique, the controlling muscle is not required to maintain a consistent activation level to maintain the device state.

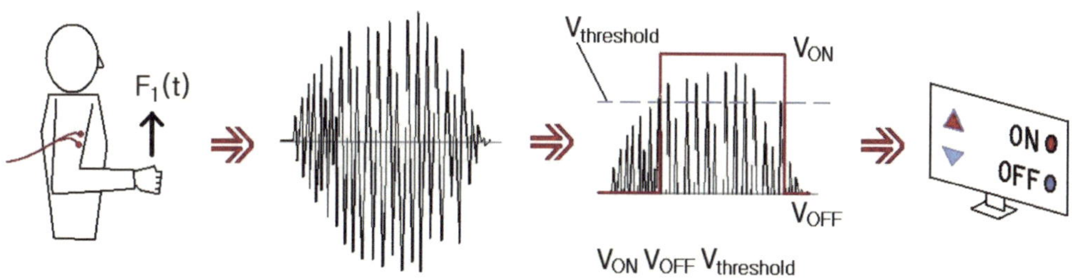

Fig. 3. Method 3 Schematic.

Method 4. Monitor to design. EMG signals are recorded and evaluated during the design and development phases of a device in order to optimize device effectiveness. After development is completed, the EMG tools are no longer used on the device. This use of EMG may be completely transparent to the end user or purchaser of the retail device. This method was used in the development of the Berkeley Lifting Exoskeleton device to evaluate the effectiveness of the device in reducing activation levels in the muscles of the lower back during lifting (Wehner, et al., 2009).

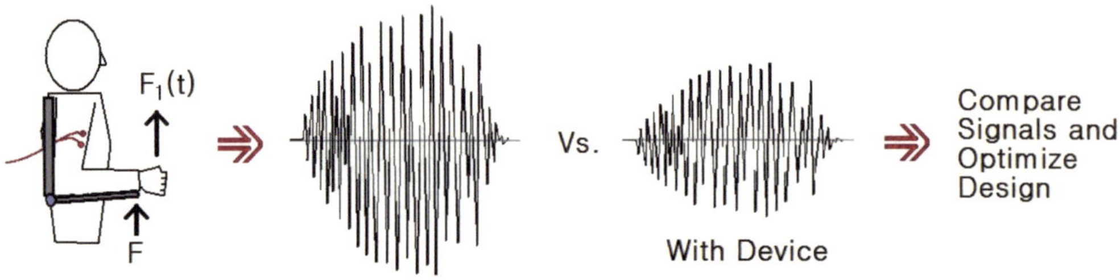

Fig. 4. Method 4 Schematic.

Method 5. Monitor to evaluate. EMG technology is used to study muscle activation levels and report on the effectiveness of a device after it has been designed, and possibly after it is already commercially available. In devices, procedures, or workplace layouts developed to reduce operator exertion or injury, this method can be used alone or with other tools such as surveys to gather data. In some of these cases, EMG was not used during the development of the device, and the developer may not even be aware of EMG technology or its use in evaluating the design. Ergonomic evaluations often fall under this method (Ulrey, Fathallah, 2011).

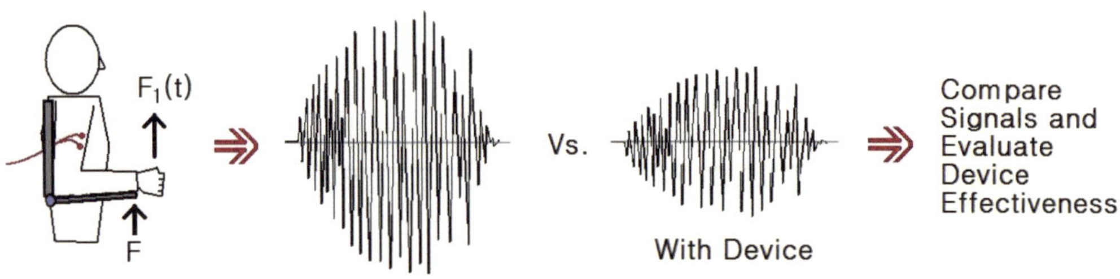

Fig. 5. Method 5 Schematic.

5. On-body devices (worn devices, human exoskeletons, and prosthetics)

Electromyography lends itself especially well to use in on-body devices, as the devices are by definition local to the user. In some applications, EMG provides a particularly intuitive and convenient interface, as the device is intended to perform an action very similar to the motion of the wearer. Because surface EMG is less invasive than some other options, it has natural advantages in non-clinical settings. EMG also has the advantage that the hardware required to record and process myoelectric signals can be relatively small and light, making it more convenient than other sensors which would be awkward or impossible to incorporate into mobile devices (MRI, fMRI). Because EMG electrodes are placed locally, it can anticipate a greater user acceptance than a full EEG sensor array, designed to cover the user's head. Social acceptance can be a considerable block to device use, so eliminating the requirement of wearing a sensor network on one's head can greatly affect a devices widespread success.

5.1 Human exoskeletons

Human exoskeletons have undergone rapid development recently, and are enjoying a surge in popularity. With the wide variety of applications for which human exoskeletons are utilized, use of EMG can fall under any of the five methods discussed earlier. For re-ambulation of patients with reduced ability due to illness or advanced age, method one can be the most suitable technology. To amplify the efforts of able bodied workers, providing additional strength, reach, or range of motion, method one may also be a valuable method and additional features can even be employed in which the wearer controls an additional device utilizing methods two or three. For paraplegic patients with no muscle signal to measure, or patients with other disorders causing spastic muscle behavior, method one would be an inappropriate and possibly dangerous choice. Many exoskeleton designs can utilize method four during the design optimization process or method five after development is complete. As with any application, the appropriate parameters must be set prior to deciding on a method.

The selection of muscle to measure and electrode placement is critical to effective use of EMG for exoskeleton and machine control, particularly if a worn device is intended to perform such complex tasks as interpreting a wearer's intent. A selection of muscles and sensor locations must maximize signal strength, and minimize noise/crosstalk. Additionally, the design must maximize sensitivity to desired signals, yet insure maximum specificity, and not read undesired signals as intended commands. In addition, the decision regarding sensor placement must consider variability in wearer physiology as well as gait variations. Body shapes and sizes vary and have a vastly varying amount of adipose tissue interfering with proper EMG sensing. Additionally, any electrode placement should not be overly invasive, cause discomfort, and can not obstruct proper use of the device. These often competing concerns make EMG sensor placement a difficult task. For example, perhaps the most readily measurable muscle contains high signal variability (false positives), and the most predictive muscle (both sensitivity and specificity) is either small, difficult to reach, or surrounded by larger muscles. Zhen, Songli, Yanan, and Jinwu discuss the relative merits of using sEMG signals of four ankle muscles for gait analysis and control (Zhen, Songli, 2007). The following is a discussion of some human exoskeleton projects, and their use of EMG.

5.1.1 Berkeley exoskeleton (BLEEX, Austin, HULC, etc)

The exoskeleton systems developed at the University of California at Berkeley are used for a variety of applications and come in both active and passive versions (application based). The Lifting Exoskeleton project employs a passive device, as it is used to reduce back forces in able bodied workers during lifting (Wehner, 2009). The Austin, medical exoskeleton, however, is active as it re-ambulates patients with no use of their lower extremities. Intended for paraplegic users, the Austin project would not be a suitable candidate for the direct use of EMG for control. Other exoskeletons, BLEEX, ExoClimber and HULC, are active exoskeleton systems, intended to amplify the movements and abilities of able-bodied users. While not using EMG for sensing or control, and not using EMG during development, method five is still a viable candidate for further experimentation, and can be incorporated with other techniques such as VO2 monitor and treadmill tests. Passive ExoHiker, shown below, uses active damping control based on stride, and swing/stance gait phase to support heavy weight, but actuation is performed by the able bodied wearer. This exoskeleton system does not use EMG for sensing or control, but could utilize method five during future experiments. The Lifting Exoskeleton project used EMG by method four to monitor and evaluate the device during design, development, and testing (Wehner, 2009). The device was developed as a research platform, intended to generate data which will serve as a knowledge base for the development of an eventual low-cost passive device to reduce back forces. It was never anticipated that the final device would include EMG capability.

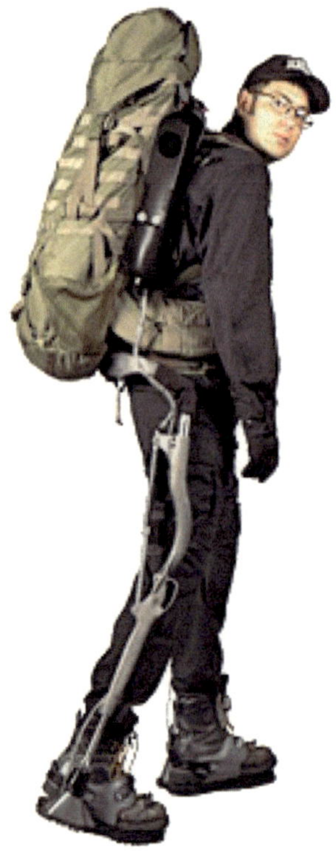

Fig. 6. Berkeley ExoHiker exoskeleton.

On the Lifting Exoskeleton project, a passive exoskeleton based device was developed to reduce back forces during lifting. During device development, a variety of techniques were used to optimize the design balancing effectiveness at reducing forces and user comfort. The device featured a spectrum of adjustable features including adjustable size of various features for wearers of varying height and body type. Additionally, the device featured adjustable overall restoring force, adjustable onset angle, and adjustable restoring moment profile, allowing wearers to vary the amount of restoring moment provided in various portions of the squat-lift cycle. Key techniques employed in optimizing the design were human subject comfort surveys, video motion tracking, force plate based lift analysis, and surface EMG, used during static squat postures and dynamic squat lifting. sEMG was used to track the activity of the lumbar erector spinae muscles during repeated lifting of objects with and without the assistance of the device. Use of these techniques facilitated tuning of the device using a variable stiffness spring profile, yielding a reduction of erector spinae muscle activity (as measured by EMG) of 27 to 52%. Tests were conducted in dynamic squat-lift scenarios as well as static squat-sustain postures. This allowed the utilization of the benefits of static EMG (well understood muscle contraction correlation, averaging over long periods, minimal electrode-to-muscle relative motion), but also generated valuable data over more realistic dynamic tasks. Issues such as crosstalk, relative muscle movement, and inability to determine momentary muscle activation were considered individually during experiment design, as should be done by any EMG practitioner.

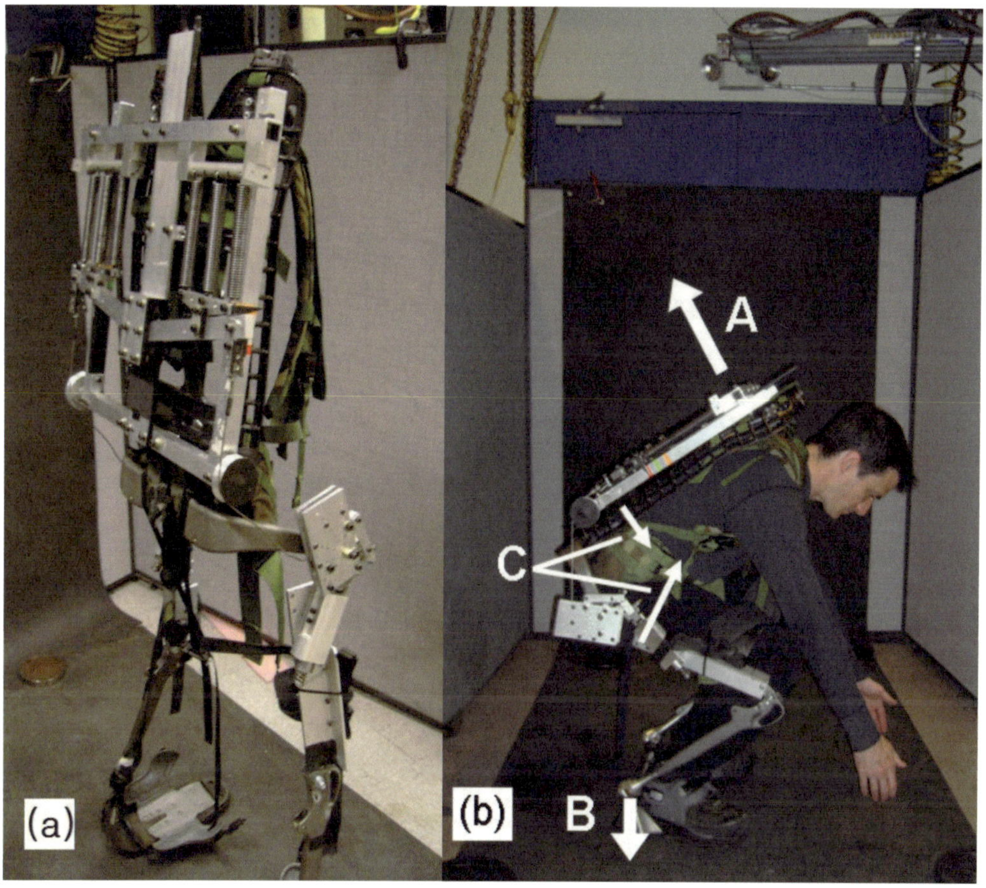

Fig. 7. Berkeley lifting exoskeleton. (a) device. (b) the device with a wearer in squat position. Forces illustrated.

5.1.2 HAL (hybrid assistive limb) exoskeleton by cyberdine

The HAL system by cyberdine (Kasaoka, Sankai, 2001) uses a number of innovative techniques in order to allow the device to function using EMG method one described above. Due to the inherent sensitivities, requirements, and considerations with EMG, specifically high noise rate, muscle movement relative to skin, and difficulty in determining momentary events (detailed in the background section), direct sensing-actuating can not be conducted with the confidence required of such a fault-intolerant application as bipedal walking. For this reason, HAL uses an assortment of techniques to anticipate user actions, adapt to each user's gait, and vary impedance in the knees of the HAL device. (Lee, Sankai, 2002). It is believed that the human limb moves most efficiently at its natural frequency, thus HAL uses the natural frequency/pendulum model to determine initial settings for the device, modifying the dynamics based on user behavior and EMG signal based feedback (Lee, Sankai, 2003). These techniques utilize known characteristics of EMG signals, standard human gait and gait variation, using a recursive least square (RLS) technique to optimize HAL's gait and impedance realtime. These techniques allow a more natural gait, reduced energy consumption by the exoskeleton device, a robust sensing/actuation loop, and reduced energy expenditure by the user (Kawamoto, Suwoong, 2003). Further refinement, including correlation between a large amount of data from many gait studies by biomedical research groups has allowed the HAL project to develop a calibration algorithm, further developing the natural gait capabilities based solely on sensors onboard the exoskeleton system (Fleischer, Hommel, 2008), and based mainly on surface EMG signals.

5.1.3 Other exoskeletons

Though the above exoskeletons use EMG for design optimization and force amplification, several exoskeleton devices are not currently using these methods. The Sarcos/Raytheon exoskeleton (Sarcos, 2011) MIT exoskeleton (MIT, 2011) and the Berkeley BLEEX exoskeleton (BLEEX, 2011) use direct force control to sense/anticipate user intention. Use of EMG for gait control is an exceedingly difficult task, as seen by the HAL system. Despite not using EMG to directly control the motion the exoskeleton actuators, these exoskeleton systems can incorporate EMG into the development and refinement of their devices (methods 4 and 5). There is no indication if such efforts are currently underway.

5.2 Lift assist devices

Numerous knee-to-shoulder lift assist devices have been designed and are at various levels of development (We hner et al., 2009). Professor Fathallah at UC Davis has conducted extensive tests on these devices, and an additional two person device (Ulrey & Fathallah, 2011; Paskiewicz & Fathallah, 2007). Research tools include extensive use of sEMG, inclinometers, electrogoniometers, and a lumbar motion monitor were used. The worn devices evaluated are shown in figures 8, 9, and 10 below. Figure 11 shows a two-person device, GRIPSystem™. Device effectiveness varies between devices, but sEMG proves to be an effective method of evaluating relative muscle activation and is relatively easy to switch test setups between subjects. While numerous variables must be considered, sEMG provides a highly quantifiable measure of back muscle activation (magnitude and variability from lift to lift and from subject to subject) with and without the device. Other factors such as user comfort and satisfaction as well as device adaptability to various body shapes are critically important to a lift assist device. These factors are not, however, as readily quantifiable as EMG based muscle activation information. Comfort surveys can yield valuable data, but uncertainty is much greater than with EMG muscle activation data. Even if a device is ineffective or yields highly varied results, which can be shown in a quantifiable manner with EMG based experiments, making sEMG particularly useful in this suite of data options. In testing the BNDR system, investigators were able to witness and quantify the flexion relaxation (FR) phenomenon, where some subjects are able to relax the erector spinae muscles of the lower back during sustained static stoop postures, where other subjects maintain high back stresses. The device under study (BNDR) reduced erector spinae forces by 26% ($p<.001$) among non-FR subjects, while those experiencing FR had such low erector spinae activation that the device did not cause a significant change in activation. Without a

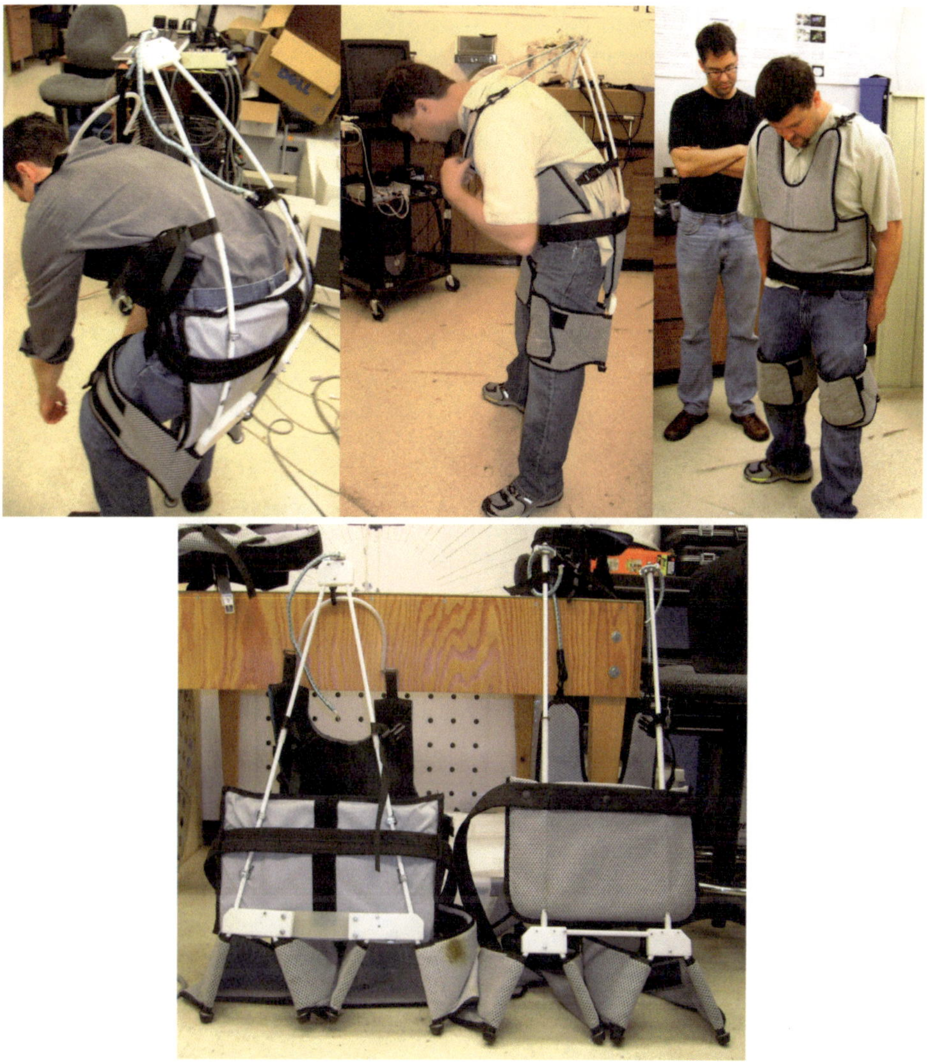

Fig. 8. Happy back, two versions. Top, in use. Bottom, both versions alone.

quantitative analysis tool such as EMG, this phenomenon would have been difficult to detect, let alone separate out the subjects experiencing FR. Device comfort and adjustability were major concerns (Ulrey, Fathallah, 2011). In a study of the GRIPSystem™, twelve subjects performed a variety of real-world lift scenarios, lifting 3 devices at various weights (weight adjusted with the addition of sandbags). EMG was used to monitor the activation levels of ten muscle groups (right and left erector spinae, latissimus dorsi, rectus abdominus, internal abdominal obliques, external abdominal obliques) with and without the use of the device. Erector spinae muscles of the low back saw reductions in low back muscle activation (erector spinae) of varying percentages, all yielding p values below 0.05. EMG allowed researchers to quantify the benefits of the device, but other concerns were evaluated through careful manual analysis. It was noted that the device couples the two workers and makes It more difficult to release an object. Thus, other safety concerns may arise from such a device.In both the GRIPSystem™ and the BNDR study, EMG was the conduit to valuable information, but the researcher was still required to make the observations and decisions which lead to the true discoveries.

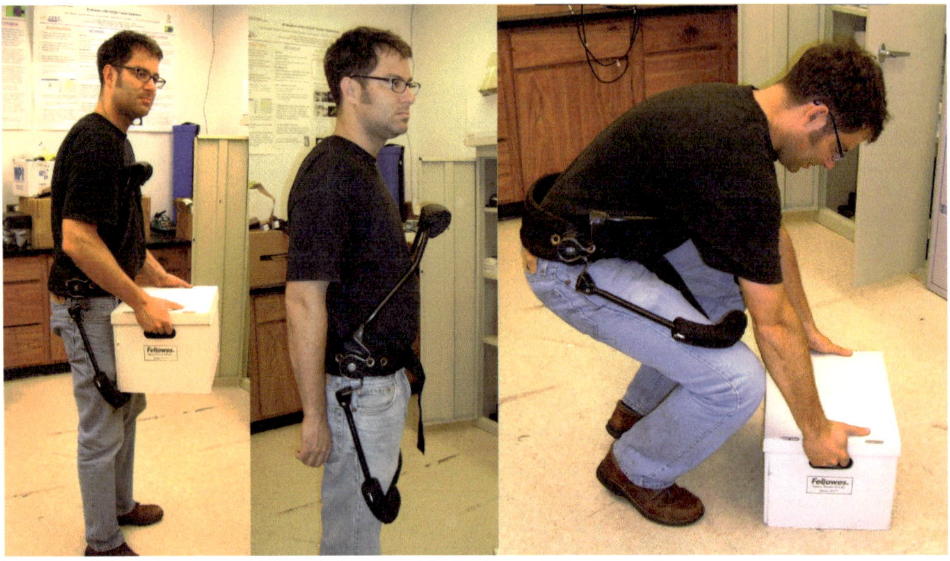

Fig. 9. BNDR lift assist system.

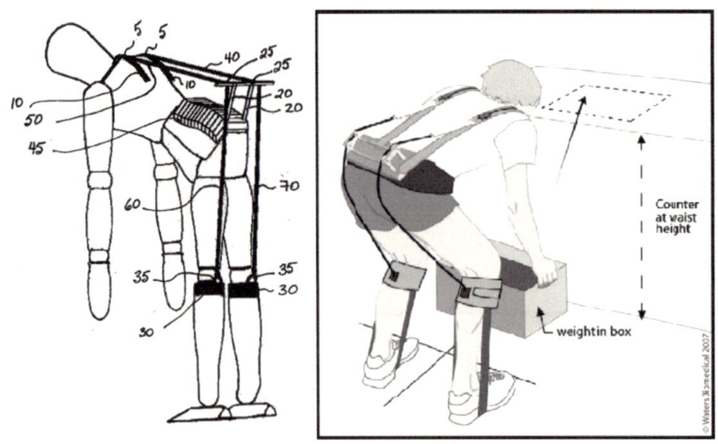

Fig. 10. PLAD lift assist system.

6. Prosthetics, upper limb

Upper limb prosthetics (hand, elbow) have been available in some form for millennia. In recent decades, these prosthetics have developed from fairly rudimentary rigid devices to single degree of freedom (DOF) devices, controlled by movment of the shoulder inside of a mechanical harness. More recently, modern upper limb prosthetics have used EMG to control much more advanced devices, incorporating more complex motion into reduced

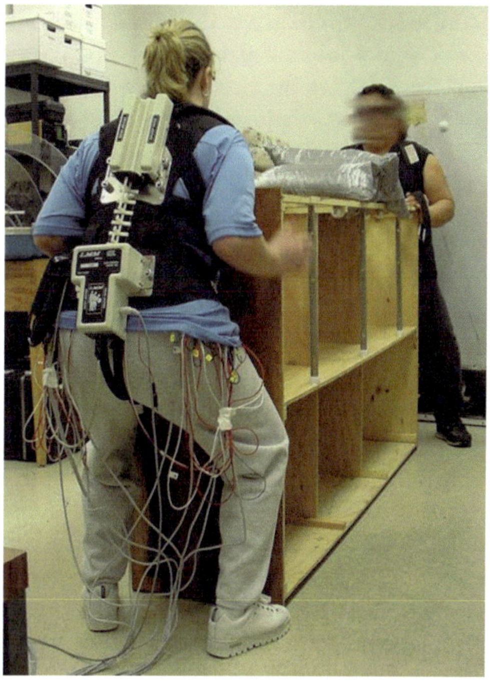

Fig. 11. GRIPSystem™.

order devices and multiple DOF devices more closely resembling actual hands and arms. EMG based prosthetic hands were first used in 1960 by Kobrinkski et al., and have been growing in popularity and capability ever since. In 1980, forty-three subjects were tested using Otto Bock EMG based as well as hook based hands. Results varied based on many factors, but overall observations included a desire for more durable fingers and finer control of the prosthetic's fingers (Northmore-Ball, et al., 1980). Since this time, of course, advances in materials science, controls, robotics, and other areas have permitted modern designs to greatly improve on the earlier models. In reviewing the five methods of using EMG in on-body devices, we can make several observations. Because prosthetics specifically deal with replacement of missing body parts, method one (amplifying existing motion) does not apply. An exception to this using emerging TMR technology is discussed below. Methods two and three (sense and interpret, proportional or threshold) are the most common use of EMG in prosthetics. Methods four and five (monitor to design or evaluate) can be used to evaluate/optimize designs, or determine metabolic cost of a design or configuration.

6.1 Proportional sensing versus threshold sensing

Upper extremity prosthetics present a considerably different set of challenges from lift assist devices and lower extremity/walking exoskeletons. Emulating a natural gait is not the goal, and precise measurement of muscle activation/muscle force is not necessarily a requirement or even a goal. One popular choice in EMG based upper limb prosthetic control is to use threshold sensing to achieve robust control of a reduced order (one or two DOF) prosthetic hand or hand/elbow system. Otto Bock has developed a full line of threshold based prosthetic hands (Ottobock, 2011a) using a myoelectric signal to activate a degree of freedom based on a threshold. Signal above a threshold initiates or ceases a command. Force is exerted based on yes/no value (breaking a threshold) rather than proportional to the signal strength. A variety of signal-logic structures are possible, the most basic of which causes a gripper to open/close based on presence of one EMG signal. More complex possible logic structures include a combination of signals all acting as 'switches' to indicate various states such as Signal 1: open, signal 2: close, signal 3: make the DOF go limp, no signal: lock DOF at present location. Of course, the matrix of possible logic states is limited only by the number of EMG sensors available, the available DOF's, and of course the ability/endurance of the patient. Another option in prosthetic control is proportional sensing. In this method, the speed or force of a DOF is controlled by the magnitude of a signal. This presents all of the traditional difficulties of EMG (crosstalk, filtering, realtime issues), and presents new challenges of safety, accuracy/repeatability, and user fatigue. While potentially much more elegant, and possibly capable of providing more realistic emulation of natural hand movement, proportional sensing includes the fundamental issue of requiring a much higher level of continuous engagement from the user. Proportional sensing, by its nature requires continuous stimulation of the controlling muscle by the user. User fatigue quickly becomes a major concern. Recent advancements in computer science and machine learning are addressing this. Current work uses EMG with downsampling techniques to reduce the exertion/fatigue issues (Castellini & Smagt, 2009) and use of a linear-nonlinear projection method to more effectively control myoelectric prosthetic hands real-time (Chu, et al., 2006).

6.2 Current research and commercial prosthetic hands

Currently, Otto Bock provides a variety of EMG based prosthetic hands to the commercial market (Ottobock, 2011b) including high speed (300mm/s) and high force (160N compression) options. i-Limb provides a hand with five independently powered digits, but is controlled by only two EMG electrodes (Touch Bionics, 2011). Antfolk et al. discuss controlling the SmartHand prosthetic using sixteen myoelectric sensors on able bodied and amputee participants (Antfolk, et al., 2010). 86% accuracy was reported on this extremely complex sixteen DOF system (three per finger plus one for thumb-opposition). Despite these considerable advances, EMG control of prosthetic hands is still far from natural hand motion, and some feel that a great deal of improvement is possible (Massa, et al., 2002).

Currently, feedback is a major concern in upper limb prosthetics. Clearly, existing prosthetics can not 'feel' in the traditional sense. While much research is underway to provide haptic touch/force feedback, for position, feedback is still obtained by visual examination of the prosthetic. Touch/force research is currently underway using vibration as a feedback mechanism to indicate contact, or even force feedback (Cipriani, et al., 2008).

6.3 Targeted Muscle Reinnervation (TMR)

Research is also underway to use targeted muscle reinnervation (TMR), in which residual nerves of an amputated limb are connected to spare muscle fibers of a target nerve. EMG signals from these newly innervated muscle fibers are then used to drive a prosthetic device (Zhou et al., 2005a) (Zhou et al., 2005b). Using this technique, a patient performs the mental action of moving the phantom extremity. The rerouted nerves stimulate the newly innervated fibers, generating a myoelectric signal. This signal can be measured similar to traditional EMG measurement of the original muscle fibers, allowing patients to generate a signal in a much more natural manner. With additional development, TMR could allow researchers to fundamentally rethink the control of prosthetics, and allow for innovative new designs. If successful, this promising technique would allow the use of EMG in prosthetics to move from Methods 2 and 3 to the highly preferable Method 1. Because TMR allows users to actuate prosthetics by "moving" their corresponding phantom muscles, prosthetics controlled by TMR based EMG signals have been shown to be much more intuitive. This new technique has been shown to yield a much shorter learning curve, and has allowed users to control far more sophisticated devices with a greatly increased number of DOF's. As this technology evolves, it will allow the development of considerably more realistic, higher order devices (Kuiken, et al., 2009). Emerging technology, targeted Sensory Reinervation (TSR) promises a complementary technique, providing a sense of touch to the missing limb. A segment of the skin over the TMR site is denervated and regenerating nerves from the TMR procedure reinnervate in this area. When this area is touched, the patient feels a touch sensation in the phantom limb Kuiken et al., 2007). These two emerging technique could allow the realistic closed loop control of multi DOF prosthetics.

7. Lower extremity prosthetics

Electromyography has been used extensively in upper limb prosthetics, and has enjoyed numerous advancements in myoelectric signal processing, as well as pattern recognition (PR) software algorithms. Rates as high as 97.4% EMG based recognition accuracy have been achieved (Chu, et al., 2007). While this is a major achievement in upper extremity control, in highly fault-intolerant tasks such as walking, a 2.6% error rate could prove disastrous. A great deal of effort has gone into EMG for lower extremity exoskeletons, and tremendous strides have been made in this extremely difficult task (see exoskeleton section for details). In EMG controlled prosthetic ankle/knee applications, where the limb is completely absent, patients would be required to control active prosthetics by enervating other muscles. This is considerably difficult in upper limb prosthetics, where real-time movement control (walking gait) is not required. For many applications, grasping can be completed at a modified pace, with position feedback being generated by observing the position of the prosthetic. This would provide overly cumbersome for EMG as a neural control system for lower limb prosthetics, and failures could be dangerous for the user. Due to the critical importance of real-time control and very fault-intolerant nature of walking, lower limb prosthetics are generally not EMG based, though recent research brings new hope about it's future viability. Even in research scenarios, there is a large variation between cycles, making PR difficult. Without the ability to sense or predict the user's intent, active control becomes difficult, because impedance and power must be varied in a feed-forward manner (Huang, et al., 2008). While several active prosthetic ankles and knees have been developed at a research level (Au, et al, 2009; Johansson, et al., 2005; Wilkenfeld, Herr, 2000). There has even been very preliminary work on the possibility of controlling an active ankle prosthetic using EMG, and it has shown promise over a neural network approach (Au, et al., 2006). For the most part, however, other techniques are largely used to control lower limb prosthetics. Despite not currently being suitable for methods one through three, methods four and five can be utilized in lower limb prosthetics development and evaluation. The Otto Bock C-Leg is a popular active lower extremity prosthetic, making it a prime candidate for EMG based gait research (Orendurff, et al., 2006).

8. Tele-operation and gesture based remote control

Just as EMG can be used to control on-body devices, it can be used to tele-operate remote devices from great distance or nearby. While tele-operation via EMG possesses the same restrictions and drawbacks of EMG control of worn devices, it can nevertheless be a powerful tool, and in certain situations the so-called drawbacks of EMG can be used as advantages. Current research in EMG teleoperation includes controlling a wheelchair through a combination of EMG and electroencephalography (EEG) (Han, et al., 2003). In this research, a novel application of EMG has been proposed. In addition to a neural control system for the wheelchair, EMG can be used as a monitoring and alarm system. Other research has used EMG and EEG to control a robot system, with the intent of future use by the handicapped (Ferreira, et al., 2008). In this application, eight subjects were able to control a computer algorithm designed to command devices, with a rightness rate of 95%. Experiments were undertaken to control a robotic arm by EMG signals in the forearm (Flexor Carpi Radialis), control a robotic wheelchair by EMG signals acquired from a neck muscle (elevator scapulae) to allow use by patients with upper and lower limb motor disabilities due to paralysis or amputation (Moon et al, 2003). Yet other research has investigated using EMG to control humanoid robots such as Honda's Asimo (Honda, 2011). Clearly, other possibilities exist, from remotely operating machinery in dangerous locations such as nuclear reactors or deep undersea, to a more intuitive control mechanism for any number of applications. Gesture based control of machinery and computer systems are well within the realm of EMG research, using methods 2 and 3 (Xu, et al., 2009). In these applications, monitoring, warning, and feedback control can be incorporated much more simply and effectively than in previously discussed applications. Each of these remotely operated applications would incorporate a method of feedback. An audio or video warning could be included indicating various states or warnings. An indicator could illuminate to indicate that the device has contacted an object. Complex haptics configurations can be eliminated or greatly reduced in these applications. In order to retain force magnitude "sensing", an array of strain gauges can record forces, and transmit this information to the controller. One is not limited to emulating human capability. Proximity sensors can also be installed to indicate when a remotely-operated device is approaching the desired object. Bar-graph style indicators could be included on a monitor to indicate magnitude based values such as force based control. In any of these applications, just as with worn devices, user comfort must be considered. To this end, a design/evaluate/optimize cycle can be included during the development process, and method four can be used to reduce user fatigue from operation.

9. Emerging applications in modern culture and technology based art

Electromyography is being used to illustrate muscle phenomena in the technology-based-art community. Experimental artists are using EMG to generate a signal from muscles to control audio or video signals, and to actuate electromechanical apparatus in performance settings. As has been the case with previous emerging technologies, artists are using EMG in creative new ways. With the availability of high-speed real-time wireless devices at ever increasingly high bandwidth and low cost, the same technology that allows convenient gathering of walking and running gate-data allows avant-garde dance troupes to collect EMG data during performances to control audio signals or video displays. Artistic applications are often more fault tolerant than traditional applications (In art, a bad myoelectric signal can hurt an artistic performance. In a prosthetic knee, a bad signal can cause injury or even death). The art community can therefore utilize technologies before the technologies are commercially viable for the mass market.

Australian performance artist Stelarc has been using technology in his art, and using the human body as an art medium since 1976 (Elsenaar & Scha, 2002). His work has explored the boundary between man and machine, using signals from his body to control machinery, and using external machinery to control parts of his body, through mechanical animation, and by electrically stimulating muscles, often using his own body as the art medium. Stelarc has used electromyography in conjunction with numerous other sensor technologies (EEG, ultrasound, electromechanical encoders, goniometers), along with other more broadly used sensors (accelerometers, thermistors, and contact microphones) to control devices in performances around the world. In one work, Stelarc developed a "Third Hand", a robotic appendage, attached to his own arm, but controlled via EMG sensors measuring activation of muscles in his abdomen and thigh. In another piece, Stelarc used a similar suite of sensors to create a variety of sounds, all generated, directly or indirectly, real-time by the human body. In this piece, he contrasted rhythmic sounds (heartbeat, breath) with more "chaotic" sounds such as those found in myoelectric signals (Elsenaar & Scha, 2002). Stelarc uses these techniques and sensors to blur the line between himself, electromechanical devices, and the audience. Many of his performances even blur the line between local and remote self, transmitting the body signals over the internet to control remote devices or manipulate audio-video displays at a performance site far from his physical body in order to question the localized self (Fleming, 2002). In another performance, Stelarc used an electromechanical device to allow audience members to manipulate his body via actuators. EMG was used to detect his muscle actuation, blurring the distinction between his voluntary movements and those caused by the audience. These myoelectric signals were then transmitted to a remote device, where a robotic actuator system was "controlled" by the signals. The audience input was done locally and remotely over the internet. In this piece, Stelarc used himself as a portion of the nonlinear control loop in which the audience indirectly controlled the robotic actuator. Additionally blurring the line between self, machine, and even location (Elsenaar & Scha, 2002).

Electronic/visual artist, Sean Clute often incorporates electronics and technology more traditionally found in other fields in his work. An upcoming piece for his performance group Double Vision (Jennings, 2011) uses EMG extensively. Professor Clute describes the piece as follows:

"Intermedia performance company Double Vision's work entitled Wishing for the Perfect Dorsiflexion depicts a solo performer controlling live-video via a wireless electromyogram interface. Conceptually, the work highlights two symptomatic conditions of Multiple Sclerosis; foot drop (dorsiflexion) and Uhthoff's phenomenon. The performer, who has MS, can be seen walking on stage with increased difficulty over time. Simultaneously, a rear video projection of a recreation trail in Stowe, Vermont can be seen. As the performer shows increased signs of weakened gait the video projection appears to both stumble and become unnaturally high in contrast. Thus, the real-time physical condition of the performer is projected visually for the audience to express the surreality of having a demyelinating disease such as MS.

Double Vision uses a wireless EMG attached to muscles in the anterior portion of the lower legs. The data is sent via the Open Sound Control (OSC) communication protocol developed at the Center for New Music and Audio Technologies at the University of California at Berkeley. The data is received by a computer using custom software created in the language Max/MSP Jitter. The software takes the incoming data, runs it through a band pass filter, and then maps to the x and y axis of prerecorded video footage. If the EMG activity is below a certain threshold then the video begins to "wiggle." This visually represents the foot drop. Additionally, the same data is used to control the contrast of the video. Artistically, this relationship is to demonstrate the unusual characteristics of Uhthoff's phenomenon including increased optic neuritis and vision abnormalities with nerve weakness.

This work is proof of the growing application of electromyography in the performing arts community. As the cost of producing works using electromechanical encoders decreases with an increase in the shared knowledge base of how to use such technologies, emerging groups such as Double Vision are experimenting with ways to map the human condition artistically" (Clute, 2011).

Such use of EMG in the art world helps expose the technology to ever growing numbers of people from more varied fields. Clute and Stelarc show that as previously arcane technologies become more robust, reliable, and affordable, the arts communities can provide a conduit to expose them to these populations. Figure 12 shows images from the work of Clute's group Double Vision (with co-director Pauline Jennings). Included are a preliminary image for the upcoming performance entitled Wishing for the Perfect Dorsiflexion, and a still image from a previous live performance.

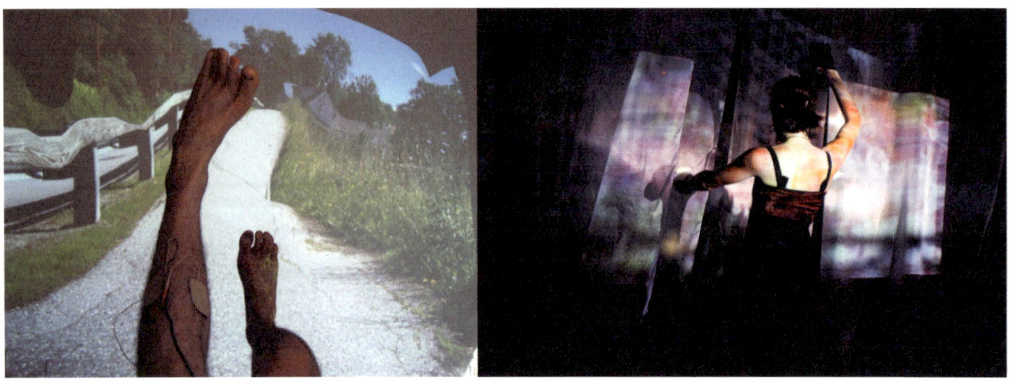

Fig. 12. Double Vision. Left, preliminary image from "Wishing for the Perfect Dorsiflexion". Right, image from a previous performance. (Jennings, 2011a, Jennings, 2011b).

10. Mixed applications - EMG in combination with other technologies

While a powerful tool on its own, some of the greatest benefits of EMG come when combined with other sensing technologies. If well planned, an application can be designed so that the weaknesses in EMG can be supplanted by strengths in other sensors, and the inherent strengths in EMG can be fully leveraged, often overcoming difficulties in other methods. Designers must also keep in mind that myoelectric signals can have a detrimental effect on other signals. Electroencephalography (EEG) practitioners have long found problems with EMG signals contaminating their data. As EEG detects brain signals of even smaller amplitudes (10 to 100 microvolts) noise from the relatively much larger EMG waves signals (10 to 100 milivolts) can completely drown out an EEG signal. As careful as EMG practitioners must be in minimizing crosstalk when studying EMG signals, EEG practitioners must deal with a much greater relative problem. Fortunately, muscles of the human body are either relatively small (cranio-ocular musculature) or relatively distant from the brain and EEG setup (shoulders, arms, back, legs) (Shackman, et al., 2009). With proper consideration, valuable data can be taken from different technologies simultaneously, valuable information can be learned, and innovative new devices can be developed, all of which would be impossible using only one type of sensor.

10.1 EMG with fMRI

Magnetic resonance imaging (MRI) and functional magnetic resonance imaging (fMRI) allow practitioners to generate detailed internal structures of the human body, often the brain. Of course, such valuable technology comes with features which can be drawbacks or even make the tool unusable in some applications. The devices are very large, not portable, and in the case of MRI, involve a very high dose of electromagnetic radiation. Additionally, the hardware and operation of the devices is very expensive. While tremendously valuable in many applications, these factors make MRI and fMRI prime candidates for mixed use applications, particularly those in which initial procedures can be completed with MRI fMRI, but can later be simplified to eliminate the large expensive machinery. It has been shown (Dai, et al., 2001) that fMRI, EMG, and joint muscle force can be correlated in some cases. Ten volunteer participants were asked to exert a hand grip force as measurements were taken. Brain images were acquired using FMRI, as participants gripped at 20, 35, 50, 65, and 80% of their maximal force. Concurrently, EMG signal data was taken on the activation levels of the flexor and extensor muscles. EMG based signals were directly proportional to brain signal amplitude. Both of these signal intensities also correlated with hand grip force. A novel technique, computed myography (CMG), uses a dense array of individual sEMG electrodes rather than traditional bipolar electrodes to determine muscle activation across several muscle groups. Multiple electrodes were attached to a human forearm to record a broad spectrum of EMG data during flexion/extension (number and locations of sensors were varied based on the experiment performed) Then, using the finite element method (on commercial analysis packages Comsol and Matlab), this array of electrode data is inverted to determine qualitatively and quantitatively the activation levels of the internal muscles. Concurrently, the arm is monitored with fMRI, yielding a well understood map of the desired muscle activation. It is believed that with further correlation, the fMRI can be eschewed completely, and an essentially fMRI level map can be generated using only EMG and this novel CMG method (Vand Den Doel et al., 2008). An EMG based prosthetic arm was used to study the mutual adaptation between the system and the human body. A 13 DOF prosthetic was used, including electrical stimulus for tactile feedback. fMRI data is recorded to clarify the plasticity of portions of the brain due to changes in the device. The experiments show adaptation in the studied areas (from fMRI data) of a phantom limb image to the prosthetic (Kato, et al., 2009).

10.2 EMG with EEG

Recently, great strides have been made in brain-machine interface using EEG. Unfortunately, because EEG signals are several orders of magnitude smaller than EMG, and because interstitial layers, particularly the skull, tends to damp out much of the frequency range of EEG signals, EEG signals are notoriously difficult to record, process, and interpret accurately (Saneei & Chambers, 2007). Just as advances have been made in interpreting EMG signals, the field of EEG has been rapidly evolving and hardware is becoming available at ever reduced cost to ever larger groups. Concurrently, much research has occurred developing a hybrid approach to human-machine interface utilizing EEG, EMG, fMRI, and recently even motion tracking systems such as the Kinect by Microsoft. EMG has been used in conjunction with EEG in a clinical setting to detect changes in sleep and shift between sleep stages in healthy patients and patients suffering from narcolepsy or other ailments, leading to increased ability to diagnose certain disorders and has lead to a greater understanding of sleep and the many musculo-physical issues associated with it (Ferri, et al., 2008; Rechtschaffen & Kales, 1968). This EMG EEG hybrid approach has also been used to control machinery and virtual conditions. Often, EEG is used as a source of multi-dimensional data, and EMG is used as a more reliable safety/backup system, utilizing the advantages of both systems. Research has been done on wheelchair control, allowing users to control the device with EEG. EMG was used to correlate desired commands with recorded EEG states. While research shows encouraging preliminary results, additional research and possible further hybridization with EMG is required (Blankertz, et al., 2006). This research was particularly encouraging, because it found that very little training was required before subjects could begin controlling the apparatus using only EMG and EEG. Robotic control using EMG and EEG has been proposed and is the subject of several experiments. A technique labeled Biopotential, using EMG and EEG to control machines was studied. Data acquisition rates in EMG and EEG realms are quite high and more work is required to process this magnitude of data real-time (McMillan, 1998). Flight control via EMG and EEG is far from a reality, as any fault could be catastrophic. However, virtual flight control research can readily be performed. EEG was used for control, with EMG as validation and backup signal (Friedman, et al., 2004). Yet another study into flight simulation via human-machine interface actually used both EMG and EEG to control the simulation. In this experiment, subjects showed the ability to control the single DOF simulation with relative accuracy (though some suffered cybersickness from immersion in the simulator). The study presented the questions of users' limits of control, suggesting future experiments including multi-DOF tasks. A program is now underway in the Netherlands to control a lower limb exoskeleton using EEG and EMG signals. Entitled MINDWALKER, the project attempts to develop a device primarily for use among those suffering from spinal cord and other injuries. An ambitious project, the use of both EEG and EEG EMG based controls will be implemented, because it is understood that those with spinal cord injuries may not be able to control such a device using EMG. The addition of EEG with EMG expands the realm of applications, and techniques used for voluntary and semi-voluntary control. Event-related potential (ERP), or the direct brain response to a perception/thought as well as P300, by which the patient can learn to control slow brain waveforms in order to control devices. These techniques along with measures of autonomic system balance (Heart Rate Variability, Skin Conductance) expand the use of EMG into entirely new realms of system control from gaming to dentistry.

11. Future directions

As technologies mature, additional applications become feasible. Just as many applications discussed above were the subject of wild fancy a short time ago, we will continue to see advancements including EMG as the primary driver, or one tool in a suite of technologies bringing us ever greater opportunities. Energy Harvesting/Scavenging is an ever growing field, in which low power and intermittently powered devices use available energy from the surroundings. Energy sources include heat and vibration, and are absorbed using pieso-electrics and thermopiles (Vullers, et al., 2009), often for applications in difficult to reach areas, where changing a battery or hard-wiring electricity is difficult or costly. In vivo devices are prime examples of such difficult to access applications. One highly plausible method for research is the study of EMG or EKG as a power source for energy harvesting. In such an application, signal clarity, timing, and interpretation are unimportant. Cross talk from other nearby muscles can actually be a benefit. The focus in this application is the magnitude of the signal. It has also been proposed that EMG and EEG can be used as a form of human/robot interaction where a robot/device would sense EMG/EEG signals to learn about nearby humans, not explicitly for control (Bien, et al., 2008). EMG techniques can also be used to monitor users for fatigue, alertness, or other variables in various situations. Work has already begun in user monitoring in wheelchair applications, in which the device will stop if EMG signals fall below a threshold or become abnormal, allowing a failsafe in wheelchair operation (Han, et al., 2003). Research has been conducted on using EMG signals to trigger a hands-free electrolarynx device (Goldstein et al., 2004), in which myoelectric signals are monitored to control initiation and termination of the device. Additional research includes EMG for voice/speech recognition even at the sub-auditory level (Jorgensen et al., 2003)

12. Discussion

The field of Electromyography is developing into new areas. As the necessary technology is developed and the devices become more reliable and less expensive, EMG can be used more reliably and at a reduced cost, making it feasible in an ever increasing range of applications. As the applications of EMG change, we must consider the benefits as well as the potential drawbacks inherent in this proliferation. The applications exploring the possible use of EMG have different priorities, and if used appropriately, many of them may use EMG as a powerful tool. If used improperly, however, erroneous data taken from a myoelectric signal can be useless, if not harmful or even fatal. In traditional applications, crosstalk is a major concern. In energy scavenging, or in spread array techniques such as CMG, crosstalk becomes less of a concern, or even an additional source of electrical energy. Some EMG applications rely on robust signal fidelity, divisible into fine resolution to obtain maximum data. Other applications, such as two state and three state conditions discussed as method three in this chapter, do not require such high signal fidelity. Table 1 below covers major applications of EMG, and addresses the relative importance of major factors for each.

When developing new devices or applications drawing EMG out of the traditional setting, one must consider the challenges, risks, drawbacks, and advantages involved in using EMG. Some challenges are being addressed through modern sensing, signal processing, and computational techniques, but other issues are inherent to the nature of the phenomenon. Advanced hardware now allows us to acquire and filter signals real-time in a ever more portable packages. Computer modeling and other software techniques are now allowing us to learn about myoelectric signal and even predict motions and muscle activity. EMG is being used in various suites of sensors to extract the best components of EMG as well as the other sensors such as fMRI, EEG, and motion tracking. As EMG becomes available to more

Application		Consideration				
		Signal Fidelity & Resolution	Realtime	Convenience	Crosstalk & Accuracy	cost
Worn Devices	Exo (lower extremities)	2	1	3	1	3
	Prosthetic hand, proportional (method 2)	2	1	3	1	3
	Prosthetic hand, gradient (method 3)	3	1	3	3	2
	Lower Limb Prosthetics	1	1	3	1	3
Device control	virtual environment control	2	2	1	3	1
	hybrid, fail-safe, signal check	3	3	3	3	2
Art/dance/culture		3	3	2	3	1
Design validation/ Optimization (methods4, 5)		2	4	2	2	2
Matrix devices/FEA/CMG		2	3	3	4	4
Energy Scavenging		4	4	4	4	3

Table 1. Relative importance, applications vs major areas of concern in EMG. 1. Critical. 2. Important. 3. Somewhat Important. 4. Not Important.

practitioners and applications, it becomes tempting to use the technology as a "black box" (simply extracting data without understanding the details), and not understand the background and limitations. As EMG becomes easier to use, it becomes easier to abuse. Untrained practitioners can draw erroneous conclusions, which can cause harm, injury, or even death. We must be mindful to maintain the integrity of EMG applications, along with the other sensing techniques used, in worn devices, devices to assist the elderly and handicapped, control machinery, and other new and emerging technologies.

13. Acknowledgment

The authors would like to thank: Professor Fadi Fathallah, Department of Biological and Agricultural Engineering, University of California at Davis for discussion of devices, models, and methodology; David Gessel of Black Rose Technology and the Massachusetts Institute of Technology for EMG concept discussion, procedures, and support; Professor Sean Clute and Pauline Jennings, department of fine and performing arts, Hohnson State College, for discussions of EMG in art and contribution of pre-release material from their upcoming performances.

14. References

Antfolk, C.; Cipriani, C.; Controzzi, M.; Carrozza, M.; Lundborg, G.; Rosen, B. & Sebelius, F. (2010) Using EMG for Real-time Prediction of Joint Angles to Control a Prosthetic

Hand Equipped with a Sensory Feedback System. *Journal of Medical and Biological Engineering*, vol 30 no 6, pp 399-406

Au,s.; Webber, J.; & Herr, H.; (2006) Initial experimental study on dynamic interaction between an amputee and a powered ankle-foot prosthesis. *Proceedings of Dyn. Walking: Mech. Control Hum. Robot Locomotion*, Ann Arbor, MI, Jul. 2006.

Au, S.; Weber, J, & and H. Herr, H (2009) Powered ankle-foot prosthesis improves walking metabolic economy. *IEEE Trans. Robotics*, vol. 25, no. 1, pp. 51–66.

Bien, Z.; Lee, H.; Do, J.; Kim, Y.; Park, K. & Yank, S. (2007) Intellignet Interaction for Human-friendly Service Robot in Smart House Environment. *International Journal of Computational Intellignece Systems*, vol. 1, no. 1, (Jan 2008), pp 77-93

Biswarup, N.; Soumyajit, M.; Soumya, G.; Sinchan, G. & Das, A. (2005) Simulation Techniques for Biologically Active Prosthetic feeet-an Overview. *International Journal of Information Technology and Knowledge Management* January-June 2011, Volume 4, No. 1, pp. 239-242

Blanc, Y.; & Dimanico, U. (2010) History of the Study of Skeletal Muscle Function with Emphasis on Kinesiological Electromyography. *The Open Rehabilitation Journal*, vol 3 pp 84-93.

Blankertz, B.; Dornhege, G.; Krauledat, M.; Müller, K.; Kunzmann, V.; Losch, F. and Curio, G. (2006) The Berlin Brain-Computer Interface: EEG-based communication without subject training. *IEEE Trans. Neural Sys. Rehab. Eng.* vol. 14 no.2. pp147-152.

BLEEX, (no date), accessed 2011, available from: <http://bleex.me.berkeley.edu/research/exoskeleton/bleex/ >

Carmena, J. M. et al. (2003) Learning to control a brain-machine interface for reaching and grasping by primates. *PLoS Biology*, Vol 1,(2003).

Castellini, C. & van der Smagt, P. (2009) Surface EMG in advanced hand prosthetics. *Biological Cybernetics*, (2009) 100, pp. 35–47.

Chaffin DB, Andersson G. Occupational Biomechanics. 3rd ed. New York: John Wiley & Sons; 1999

Chu, J-U.; Moon, I. & Mun, S. (2006) A real-time EMG pattern recognition system based on linear-nonlinear feature projection for a multifunction myoelectric hand. *IEEE Trans. Biomed. Eng.*, vol. 53, no. 11, pp. 2232-2239.

Chu, J-U.; Moon, I.; Lee, YJ.; Kim, K. & Mun, S. (2007) A supervised feature-projection-based real-time EMG pattern recognition for multifunction myoelectric hand control. *IEEE/ASME Trans. Mechatronics*, vol. 12, no. 3, pp. 282–290.

Cipriani, C.; Zaccone, F.; Micera, S. & Carrozza, MC. (2008) On the Shared Control of an EMG-Controlled Prosthetic Hand: Analysis of User Prosthesis Interaction. *IEEE Transactions on Robotics 2008*, vol 24, pp 170-184.

Clute, S. (2011) Personal conversation with Sean Clute, Assitant Professor of Fine and Performing Arts, Johnson State College. , accessed 2011, available from: < http://www.seanclute.com/bio/ >

Dai TH, Liu JZ, Sahgal V, Brown RW, Yue GH (2001) Relationship between muscle output and functional MRI-measured brain activation. *Exp Brain Res* 140:290–300

De Luca. C.J. (1997) The Use of Surface Eletromyography in Biomechanics. *Journal of Applied Biomechanics*, Volume 13, Pages 135-163, 1997

Ferreira, A.; Celeste, W.; Cheein, F.; Bastos-Filho, T.; Sarcinelli-Filho, M. and Carelli, R. (2008) Human-machine interfaces based on EMG and EEG applied to robotic systems. *Journal of NeuroEngineering and Rehabilitation*, pp. 5–10.

Elsenaar, A. and Scha, R. Electric Body Manipulation as Performance Art: A Historical Perspective. *Leonardo Music Journal, 12, 2002, 17-28.*

Ferri, R.; Franceschini, C. & Zucconi. M. (2008) *Searching for a marker of REM sleep behavior disorder: submentalis muscle EMG amplitude analysis during sleep in patients with narcolepsy/cataplexy*. Sleep. vol 31, pp 1409–17.

Fishman, L. & Wilkins, A. (2010) Functional Electromyography. (1st edition), Springer, 1607610191.

Fleischer, C. & G. Hommel, G. (2008) A Human--Exoskeleton Interface Utilizing Electromyography. *IEEE Transactions on Robotics*, vol. 24, pp. 872-882.

Friedman, D.; Leeb, R.; Antley, A.; Garau, M.; Guger, C.; Keinrath, C.;(2004). Navigating virtual reality by thought: First steps. *Proceedings of the 7th Annual International Workshop on Presence*, pp. 160–167.

Goldstein, EA.; Heaton, JT.; Kobler, JB.; Stanley, GB. & Hillman, RE. (2004) Design and implementation of a hands-free electrolarynx device controlled by neck strap muscle electromyographic activity. *IEEE Transactions on Biomedical Eng* 2004, vol 51, pp 325–332.

Han, J.; Bien, Z.; Kim, D.; Lee, H.; Kim, J.; (2003) Human–machine interface for wheelchair control with EMG and its evaluation. *Proceedings of the 25th IEEE International Conference on Engineering in Medicine and Biology Society, Cancun, Mexico, (September 2003)*, pp. 1602–1605.

Honda, (no date), accessed 2011, available from: <http://dreams.honda.com/robotics-mobility/ >

Huang, H.; Kuiken, A. & Lipschutz, R. (2008) A strategy for identifying locomotion modes using surface electromyography. *IEEE Trans. Biomed. Eng.*, vol. 56, no. 1, pp. 65–73, Jan. 2009.

Jennings, P. (2011a), accessed 2011, available from: <http://www.double-vision.biz/new/about/artistic-directors/>

Jennings, P. (2011b), Photo by Anne Peattie, Dancer: Mira Cook, accessed 2011, available from: <http://www.double-vision.biz/new/about/artistic-directors/>

Johansson, JL.; Sherrill, DM.; Riley, PO.; Bonato, P.; and Herr, H.; (2005). A clinical comparison of variable-damping and mechanically passive prosthetic knee devices. *Am. J. Phys. Med. Rehabil.* vol 84, pp 563-575.

Jorgensen, C.; Lee, D. & Agabon, S.;(2003) Sub Auditory Speech Recognition Based on EMG/EPG Signals. *Proc. of the International Joint Conference on Neural Networks*, 2003.

Kasaoka, K. & Sankai, Y. (2001)Predictive control estimating operator's intention for stepping-up motion by exo-skeleton type power assist system HAL. *Proceedings of International Conference on Intelligent Robots and Systems*, pp. 1578-1583, 2001.

Kato, R.; Yokoi, H.; Hernandez, A.; Yu, W.; and Arai, T. (2009) Mutual adaptation among man and machine by using f-MRI analysis, Robot. *Auton. Syst.* vol 57 no. 2, pp. 161–166.

Kawamoto, H.; Lee, S.; Kanbe, S. & Sankai, Y. (2003) Power assist method for HAL-3 using EMG-based feedback controller. *Proceedings of IEEE Int. Conf. Syst., Man, Cybern.*, 2003, pp. 1648–1653.

Kuiken, T. A.; Li, G.; Lock, B. A.; Lipschutz, R. D.; Miller, L. A.; Stubblefeld, K. A.; et al. (2009). Targeted muscle reinnervation for real-time myoelectric control of multifunction artifcial arms. *JAMA*, vol 301 no 6, pp 619-28.

Kuiken, T.; Miller, L.; Lipschutz, R.; Lock, B.; Stubblefield, K.; Marasco, P.; Zhou, P. & Dumanian, G. (2007) Targeted reinnervation for enhanced prosthetic arm function in a woman with a proximal amputation: a case study *The Lancet*, vol 369 pp 371-380.

Lee, S. & Sankai, Y. (2002) Power assist control for walking aid with hal-3 based on emg and impedance adjustment around knee joint. *Proceedings of IEEE/RSJ Int. Conf. Intelligent Robots and Systems*, pp. 1499–1504,2002.

Lee S. & Y. Sankai, Y. (2003) The Natural Frequency-Based Power Assist Control for Lower Body with HAL-3, *Proceedings of International Conference on Intelligent Robots and Systems*, pp. 1642-1647, 2003.

MIT, (no date), accessed 2011, available from: < http://biomech.media.mit.edu/research/research.htm>

Mcmillan, Grant. (1998) The technology and applications of biopotential-based control. *Proceedings of Alernative Control Technologies: Human Factors Issues*, Bretigny, France, Oct. 1998.

Massa, B.; Roccella, S.; Carrozza, M. C. & Dario, P. (2002) Design and Development of an Underactuated Prosthetic Hand. *Proceedings of the 2002 IEEE International Conference on Robotics and Automation*, pp. 3374-3379

Medved, V. (2001) *Measurement of Human Locomotion*, CRC Press, Boca Raton, Fl.

Merletti, R. (1999) Standards for Reporting EMG Data, *Journal of Electromyography and Kineseology*, vol 9, 1999.

Moon I, Lee M, Ryu J, Mun M: Intelligent Robotic Wheelchair with EMG-, Gesture-, and Voice-based Interfaces. *Proceedings of 2003 IEEE/RSJ International Conference on Intelligent Robots and Systems (IROS 2003)*, Las Vegas, Nevada 2003, 4:3453-3458

Northmore-Ball, D.; Heger, H. & Hunter, G. (1980) The below-elbow myoelectric prosthesis: a comparison of the Otto Bock myoelectric prosthesis with the hook and functional hand. *Bone Joint Surg.* vol 62B, pp 363-367.

Orendurff, M.; Segal, A.; Klute, G.; McDowell, M.; Pecoraro, J. & Czerniecki, J. (2006) Gait efficiency using the C-Leg. *J Rehabil Res Dev.* vol 43 no 2. pp239–46.

Ottobock, (2011a) accessed 2011, available from: <http://www.ottobock.com/cps/rde/xchg/ob_com_en/hs.xsl/384.html>

Ottobock (2011b) accessed 2011, available from: < http://www.ottobock.com/cps/rde/xchg/ob_com_en/hs.xsl/384.html>

Paskiewicz, J. & Fathallah, F. (2007) Effectiveness of a manual furniture handling device in reducing low back disorders risk factors. *Industrial Ergonomics.* vol 37, pp 93-102.

Raez, M.B.I.; Hussain, M.S.; & Mohd-Yasin, F. (2006). Techniques of EMG signal analysis: detection, processing, classification, and applications. *Biological Procedures Online*, vol 8, pp 11-35.

Rechtschaffen A, Kales A, eds. (1968) A manual of standardized terminology, techniques and scoring system for sleep stages of human subjects. Washington, D.C.: Government Printing Office, NIH publication no. 204. 1968.

Sanei, S. & Chambers, J. (2007) *EEG Signal Processing*. Hoboken, NJ: John Wiley & Sons, 2007.

Sarcos, (no date), accessed 2011, available from: < http://www.sarcos.com/>

Shackman, A.; McMenimin,B.; Slagter, H; Maxwell, J.; Greischar, L. & Davidson, R. (2009) Electromyogenic artifacts and Electroenecpalographic interferences. *Brian Topography*, 22(1), (June 2009), pp7-12.

Touch Bionics (2007) i-Limb system, accessed 2011, available from: <http://www.touchbionics.com>

Ulrey, B.L.; & Fathallah, F.A. (2011). Biomechanical Effects of a Personal Weight Transfer Device in the Stooped Posture. *Proceedings of the 55th Annual Meeting of the Human Factors and Ergonomics Society*. Santa Monica, CA: Human Factors and Ergonomics Society.

Van den Doel, K.; Ascher, U. & Pai, D. (2008) Computed myography: three dimensional reconstruction of motor functions from surface EMG data. *Inverse Problems*, vol 24 065010, 2008.

Vullers, R.; van Schaijk, R.; Doms, I.;van Hoof C. & Mertens, R. (2009) Micropower Energy Harvesting. *Solid-State Electronics*, vol. 53, no. 7, pp. 684 - 693.

Wehner (2009) Lower extremity exoskeleton as lift assist device. Wehner, M.; Kazerooni, H.; Ph.D. Thesis, University of California at Berkeley.

Wehner, M.; Rempel, D. & Kazerooni, H. (2009) Lower Extremity Exoskeleton Reduces Back Forces in Lifting. *Proceedings of ASME 2009 Dynamic Systems and Control Conference* October, 2009, Hollywood, California, USA,

Wilkenfeld, A.; Herr, H. (2000) "An auto-adaptive external knee prosthesis", PhD. Thesis, MIT

Zhang, X.; Chen, X.; Wang, W.; Yang, J.; Lantz, V.; & Wang, K. (2009) Hand Gesture Recognition and Virtual Game Control Based on 3D Accelerometer and EMG Sensors. *Proc ACM IUI* 2009, pp 401-406.

Zhen, Z.; Songli, Y.; Yanan, Z. & Jinwu, Q. (2007) On the surface electromyography sensor network of human ankle movement. Proceedings *of IEEE International Conference on Robotics and Biomimetics*, pp. 1688-1692, 2007.

Zhou, P.; Lowery, M.A.; Dewald, J. & Kuiken, T. (2005a) Towards Improved Myoelectric Prosthesis Control: High Density Surface EMG Recording After Targeted Muscle Reinnervation. *Conf Proc IEEE Eng Med Biol Soc.* 2005, 4:4064-7

Zhou, P.; Lowery, M.A. & Kuiken, T. (2005b) Elimination of ECG Artifacts from Myoelectric Prosthesis Control Signals Developed by Targeted Muscle Reinnervation. *Conf Proc IEEE Eng Med Biol Soc.* 2005;5:5276-9

23

Water Surface Electromyography

David Pánek, Dagmar Pavlů and Jitka Čemusová
Department of Physiotherapy, Faculty of Physical Education and Sport,
Charles University
Czech Republic

1. Introduction

Registration of electrical muscle activity with the use of surface electromyography (SEMG) is today already a routine neuro-physiological method. Over the course of a few decades it has moved from the field of the purely experimental to the area of rehabilitation medicine, kinesiology, and sports issues. Together with this trend, interest has begun to deepen in the study of all types of movement patterns stereotypes conducted in a water environment and in a dry environment. This has also opened a new area of electromyographic diagnostics that represents a modification of the basic methodology of surface EMG in a water environment, so-called Water Surface Electromyography -WaS-EMG (Pánek et al., 2010).
Although current modern technology allows a huge number of computer post-processing of an acquired native recording, a key phase of the actual recording of electrical activity remains in the hands of the experimenter. For these reasons significant attention is paid to the methodology and issue of correct placement and fixing of electrodes in all neuro-physiological methods. In general approach, recording an EMG signal in a water environment is no different from the common methodology of surface EMG, but there are certain specifics in that case. Currently, great attention is paid in the literature to the issue of the different effect of water and dry environments on the nature of the EMG recording itself (Kelly et al., 2000; Masumoto et al., 2004, 2008; Rainoldi et al., 2004; Veneziano et al., 2006), and thus on the course of a defined movement stereotype (Kelly et al., 2000; Masumoto et al., 2004, 2005, 2008; Pavlů & Panek, 2008; Holländerova, 2011; Sladká, 2011).
In this work we take up the issue of Water Surface Electromyography (WaS-EMG), both in terms of research and the practical, including a summary of the results of several of our experiments.

2. WaS-EMG methodology

In our workplace we use a telemetric EMG instrument, the TelemyoMini 16, which is made by the Neurodata company. We evaluate and process the acquired data with the help of MyoResearch XP Master Edition software for concurrent video monitoring. However, the following items are also needed to complement the equipment for recording an EMG signal in a water environment (Fig. 1):

1. Water-resistant sac for the EMG amplifier and transmitter.
2. Special bipolar electrodes with a set of two-sided adhesive patches that are necessary for solidly affixing the electrodes to the skin.

3. Covering, waterproof patches for the electrodes, which prevent moistening and the subsequent release of electrodes into the water.
4. An abrasive and conductive paste.
5. Alcohol benzine.
6. Electrode conductive cream (from GE Medical System).
7. Universal Silicone.

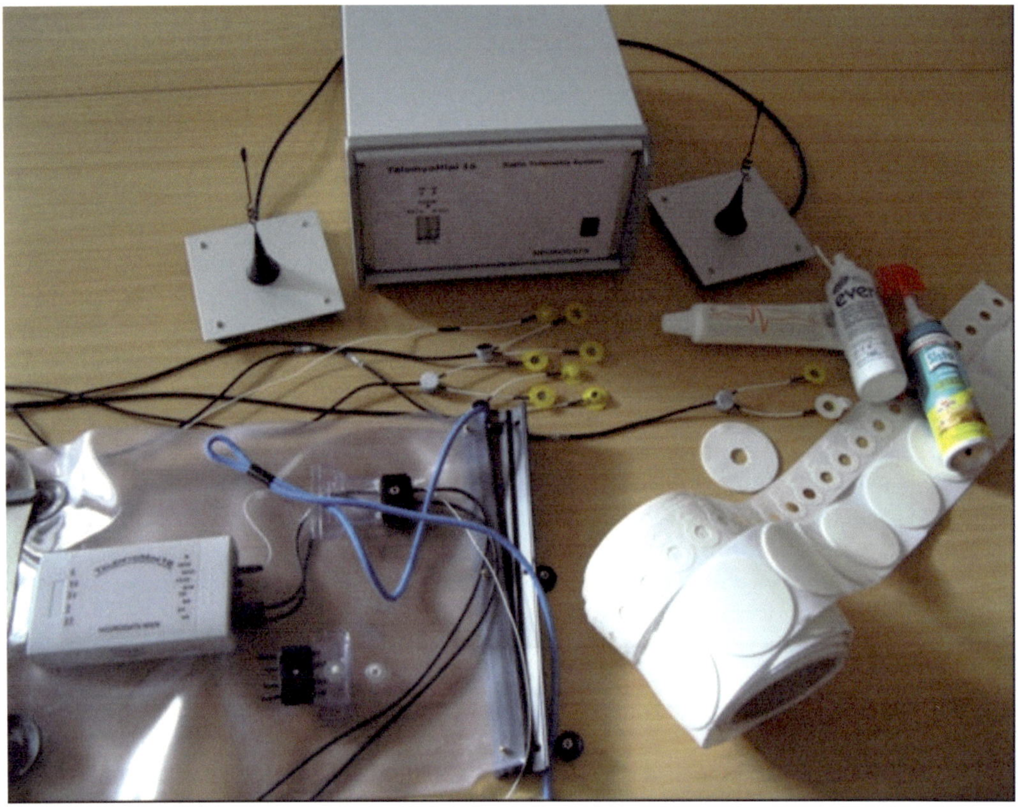

Fig. 1. The equipment for recording EMG singnal in a water environment (Pánek et al., 2010).

2.1 Preparatory phase of measurement

Significant attention must be paid to placing the EMG transmitter in the water-resistant sac. Unless we ensure proper sealing of the sac, the damage will reach large financial sums. Closing the main opening of the sac poses no problems, but sealing the openings for the bipolar electrode cables is more complicated. Because this involves relatively complex and precise work, we recommend immediately preparing all the cables that we have at our disposal. If we do not use all the cables in the measurement, we can secure the remaining cables with water-resistant adhesive tape right to the sac. We place the cables in grooves already prepared in the sealing rubber, which is divided into two halves and secured with a screw. Nevertheless, it is still necessary to assure that it is water-resistant by sealing the cables in the grooves with common Universal Silicone. This method makes it possible to later free up the cables and clean the grooves in the sealing rubber without problems. Before closing the main opening of the sac it is good to place the transmitter on a polystyrene board, which will allow the transmitter to float. In this way we can avoid loss of the EMG signal at the moment when the proband is moving actively in the water, which can lead to the EMG transmitter being submerged below water level (Pánek et al., 2010).

2.2 Application of electrodes on the skin

For recording an EMG signal in a water environment we use special bipolar electrodes (Fig.2). This involves Ag/AgCl disk electrodes that are 5 mm in diameter, which are embedded in plastic periphery so that only the central part, which is placed against the skin, remains free.

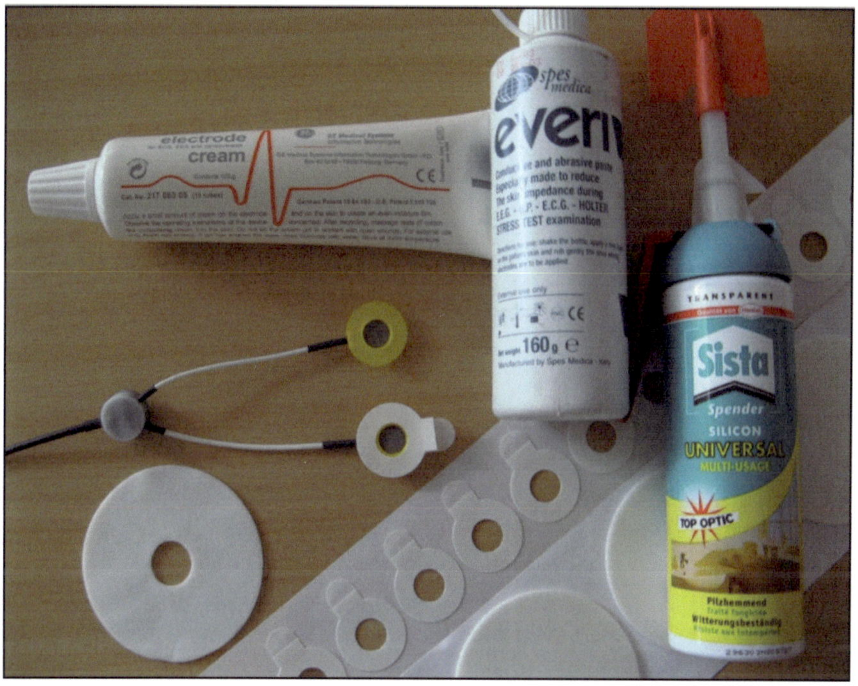

Fig. 2. WaS- EMG electrodes intended for water environments with accessories (Pánek et al., 2010).

Here, too, the basic rule applies that the electrodes are affixed to thoroughly cleaned and degreased skin. In our case, we used an abrasive tape and alcohol benzine. We stick two-sided adhesive tape, which copies the round shape of the electrode and is supplied together with the electrodes, to the plastic disk of the electrode, which is placed against the skin. Only then do we apply the conductive gel to the electrode. In our experience this phase is very important, because too much gel markedly increases the risk of the electrode coming loose during the course of the experiment. Of course a small amount does not ensure proper adherence of the electrode to the skin, it increases the impedance between the electrodes and the skin, and there is a weakening and disruption of the electrical signal. Each subsequent correction of the attachment to the skin is, due to the wet environment, significantly complicated. After sticking the electrode to the skin, we cover it with a special round sealing patch with a central opening, which we place precisely over the electrode. We also paste over the electrode cable; passing the cable through the central opening has not worked, as in water the electrode itself always came unstuck. Maintaining the recommended distance between electrodes at 1cm (DeLuca, 2002) is impossible for use of this methodology, as any decrease in the diameter of the covering patch leads to the electrode becoming unstuck. However, it follows from our experience that covering the individual patches by about 1/3 of their diameter is stable, and the electrodes do not fall off in water.

2.3 Affixing the water-resistent sac to the body, and entering the pool

After applying all the electrodes on the skin we can proceed to affixing the water-resistant sac to the body. It seemed to us that the best option is to pull the sac's blue hanger (Fig. 3) over the head and loosen it sufficiently so that during movement in water it will slip into the C-Th area and not cause an unpleasant feeling of pulling in the area of the neck. We adjust the sac's strap in the area of the torso in such a way that during movements the sac can be above water surface level.

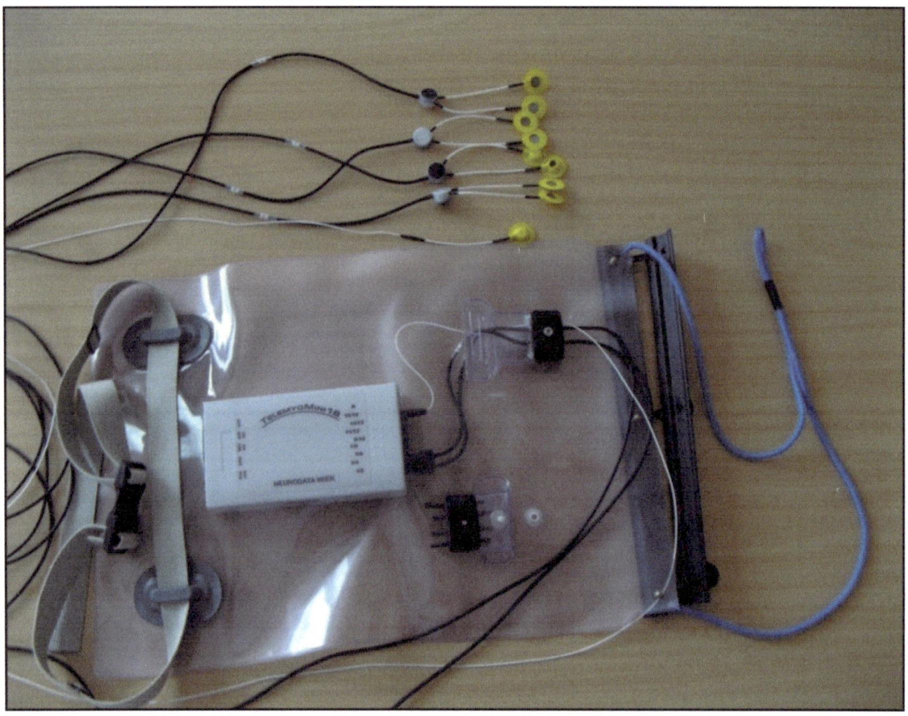

Fig. 3. Water-resistant sac with EMG transmitter and electrodes (Pánek et al., 2010).

It is necessary to affix the loose cables from the bipolar electrodes placed on the skin to the proband's body, because they can both obstruct movement and lead to detachment of the electrode from the preamplifier placed for the electrode itself, and their free movement can also affect the EMG signal (Rainoldi et al., 2004). It is possible to use water-resistant straps that are used in various water sports for affixing loose cables, but there is the possible risk of allergic contact reactions. One variant appears to be to cut patches for the electrodes that do not come unstuck in water or cause allergic reactions.

Because we are working in a wet environment, we must protect the EMG instrument itself and the notebook against damage. We select a place that is relatively well protected against

direct contact with water. For this reason, most of the affixing of electrodes and the overall preparation of the proband proceed further from optimal entry into the water.
In Figure 4 we see how the proband climbs over the side area of the pool only with the help of an assistant who holds the sac and the loose cables. We consider this method of entering the pool to be simply unsuitable, because its result can be only yanking or unsticking an electrode.

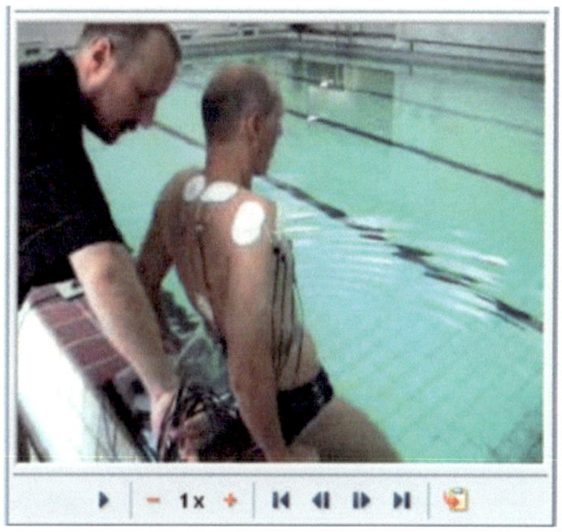

Fig. 4. Unsuitable entry into swimming pool

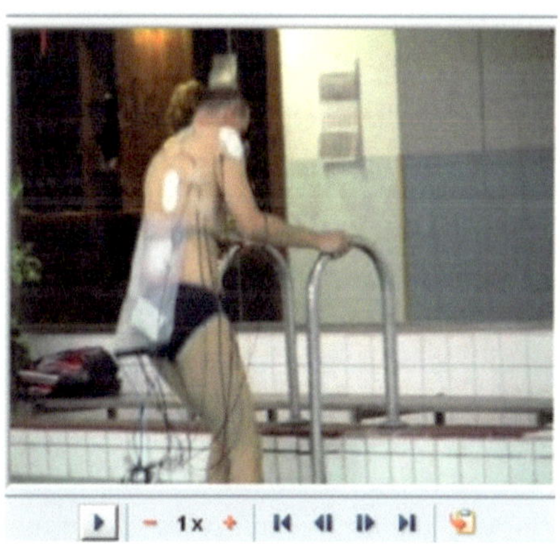

Fig. 5. Recommended entry into pool.

For this reason we recommend that the proband enter the pool in a freely accessible place, in our case by the steps, and on the side of the pool, where it is possible to comfortably stand on the bottom (Fig. 5). In this way the proband can´t demage the loose cables and the water-resistant sac, which remains on the water surface behind the proband. When using the telemetric EMG instrument it is necessary to ensure that the water-resistant sac remains above the water level during the course of the experiment. We achieved this by placing lightening floats right in the sac (Fig. 6), or we used an assistant who always kept the sac above water level, thereby limiting increased movement of loose cables during the course of the probands' motor activity (Sladká, 2011).

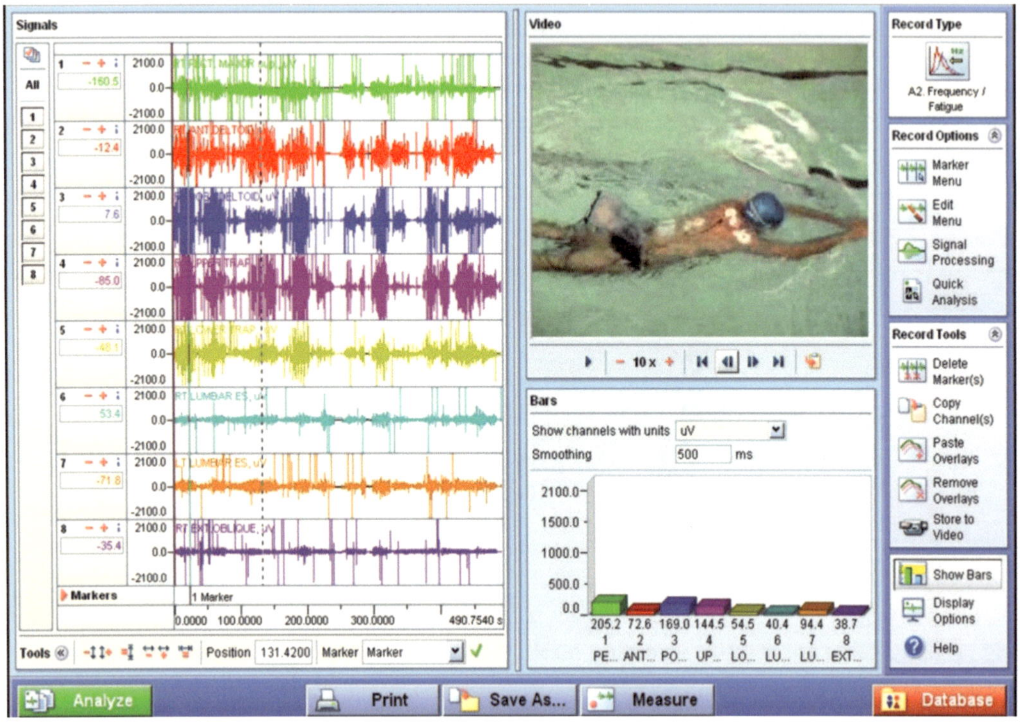

Fig. 6. WaS-EMG: Recording of swimming (Pánek et al, 2010).

The issue of the difference between telemetric measurement and direct connection of the EMG instrument and the electrodes by cables has already been dealt with in the study by Clarys et al. (Clarys et al., 1985). When using both methods for registering an EMG signal no difference was found. And for this reason, due to the more advantageous manipulation with the telemetric system, this method is primarily recommended for recording electrical activity of muscles.

Other technical parameters of registration are also taken up by Masumoto and Mercer (Masumoto & Mercer, 2008), who evaluated whether it is better to use a water-resistant suit or to affix each electrode covered by water-resistant tape with a foam cushion. Although a water-resistant suit appears to be better, there are also many disadvantages. The suit must both fit every individual, thereby increasing the price of the measurement, and the cables must leave through holes in the suit, resulting in potential places for leaks. And, last but not least, it is not entirely clear whether the suit limits the proband's dynamic movement. For these reasons, according to Masumoto and Mercer it is better to apply each electrode separately, with covers of waterproof tape.

3. Effect of water environment on the amplitude and spectral characteristics of an EMG signal

During electromyographic studies in a water environment, and especially when comparing the motor behaviour of an individual in water and on a dry land, the relevant question arises as to how the water environment affects the native EMG signal, and what the specific changes are in muscle activity caused by the change in gravitation and by the resistance of the water environment.

The original studies by Clarys et al. (Clarys et al., 1985) and Pöyhönem et al. (Pöyhömen et al. 1999) pointed to decreased amplitude of the EMG signal in the course of maximal voluntary contraction (MVC) in water compared to EMG activity on a dry land. But it was not clear whether this result was affected by methodological limitations or physiological changes caused by the water environment. That is to say, in both cases the authors did not use waterproof attachment of electrodes or attachment of electrode by means of adhesive tape (Sulkova, 2011).

A significant contribution to the solution of this problem is the study by Rainoldi et al. (Rainoldi et al., 2004). The authors monitored the EMG activity of the brachial biceps muscle during maximal voluntary contraction on a dry land, in standing water, and in a flowing water at 25° C. In all cases they compared the individual parameters of the EMG signal (average rectified value, root mean square, mean frequency, median frequency) during isometric contraction with and without attachment of electrodes by means of water-resistant adhesive tape and with attachment of free electrode cables. The results of the study indicated that without the covering tape over the electrodes, the amplitude of the signal is recorded in standing and flowing water as lower (by 6.7%) than during contractions on a dry land. A dramatic change appeared during isometric contractions in flowing water without the covering tape, when there was a significant increase of the frequency component in the low frequency band of 0-20Hz, which affected all of the monitored parameters. The incidence of this artefact was caused by the movement of free cables, and after they were affixed and the electrodes were glued on it disappeared. The conclusion of this study was to recommend the use, when registering EMG activity in water, water-resistant adhesive tape, whereby we can rule out the occurrence of marked artefacts and ensure constant conditions during the course of the entire experiment.

Da Silva Carvalhoa et al. (Da Silva Carvalhoa et al., 2010) present many studies that stress the importance of water-resistant tape when measuring EMG in a water environment, but also several practices that cast this fact in doubt. They conducted an experiment that should have clarified the inconsistency. We can see the following from the results: during isometric contractions in water without taping, there was a EMG amplitude decreased in to 50%. When comparing isometric contractions in a water environment with the use of covering tape, the results were in accord with those that were measured on a dry land with and without tape. So according to them, the covering tape used on a dry surface does not affect the EMG amplitude, yet it had a marked effect on the EMG recording in a water environment.

Similarly, Veneziana et al. (Veneziano et al., 2006) also recommend the use of covering tape in a water environment and on dry land, because among other things, the covering tape also develops a certain mechanical pressure on the skin and the muscle tissue under the electrode.

Many authors thus agree on the necessity of attaching the electrodes with water-resistant tape, which eliminates the artificially lowered amplitude of the EMG recording and the spectral changes in water. We thus ensure that the EMG signals acquired on a dry land and in water can be correctly reproduced and compared. When adhering to the correct methodology for attaching the electrodes the water environment does not affect the registered electrical activity of the muscle or the maximum muscle contraction.

Another discussed question is whether we should normalise the EMG data to the maximal voluntary contraction (MVC) in water or on a dry land. Masumoto and Mercer (Masumoto

& Mercer, 2008) recommend that it all be normalised to MVC on a dry land, because most prior studies were conducted in precisely by this way. Silvers and Dolny (Silvers & Dolny, 2001) tested maximal voluntary contraction on a dry land and in water on 12 probands. From the results they conclude that no marked difference was found between individual MVC values on a dry land and under water. So they also recommend normalisation to MVC values registered on a dry surface.

4. Effect of water temperature on the native EMG signal

The heat conductivity of water is 23 times higher than the conductivity of air. Dewhurst et al. (Dewhurst et al., 2005) documents that the temperature of a muscle is, under ordinary conditions, always higher than the temperature on the surface of the body. In a water environment there is a faster exchange of heat between the water and tissues, and therefore the organism cools earlier than on the air.

Proximal muscles are warmer at rest, by an average of 4.1° C, than distal muscles. Muscle temperature changes the most in the first 5 minutes after being submerged in water, and in 15 minutes their temperature equals the temperature of ambient water (Petrofsky J, 2005).

Petrofsky and Laymon (Petrofsky & Laymon, 2005) tracked the effect on an EMG signal in connection with water temperature on 7 probands. They registered EMG activity from the upper and lower extremities (m. biceps brachii, m. brachioradialis, m. quadriceps femoris, m. gastrocnemius) after 20 minutes of submersion in water at temperatures of 24°, 27°, 34° a 37° C. For all four examined muscles there was no statistically significant difference between the MVC values and the median frequency among the three highest water temperature. Nevertheless, after submersion in the coolest water (24° C), all of the monitored muscles showed a significant MVC decrease (by up to 44.8%), a shift of the median frequency by 32 Hz in the direction of lower values, and a slower speed of action potential conduction in the muscle fibre by 2m/s in comparison with the value achieved in the warmest water.

A similar issue was taken up in the diploma thesis by Stejskalová (Stejskalová, 2011), where she evaluated the amplitude changes in isometric contraction after 5 minutes in water at temperatures of 15° C, 24° C, 35° C for 30%, 50%, and 70% of the maximum output muscle strength measured by pressing a hand dynamometer. She registered EMG activity from finger flexors and the wrist of the right upper extremity, which was submerged in a water bath at the level of half the forearm. The results of the study, as opposed to the work of Petrofsky and Laymon (Petrofsky & Laymon, 2005), did not show any effect of water temperature on the EMG recording. This finding explains the shorter period of the extremity's submersion in water, when for the first time after 15 minutes the temperature between the ambient water and the muscle stabilize which subsequently appears in cool water as changes of electromyographic activity.

The water temperature and duration of submersion are significant factors that affect the EMG record. For these reasons, the stimulation of the water temperature must be stated and considered. According to Jandová (Jandová, 2009), after an isothermic bath the water bath temperature was designated as 34-35° C. But this involved baths in their entirety for which no physical activity was assumed. At a temperature of 25-32° C, the bath was cooling, hypothermal. At a temperature of 25° C there was already a decline in body temperature of 1° C after 7 minutes (Jandová, 2009). Most electromyographic studies in a water environment work at temperatures between 27 and 34° C (Miyoshi et al., 2004; Masumoto et al., 2004, 2009; Veneziano et al., 2006; Shono et al., 2007; Kaneda et al., 2008; Pavlů & Pánek, 2008).

5. Comparison of movement in a water environment and on a dry land

The growing popularity of all sorts of rehabilitation and fitness procedures in water has led to many studies that deal with dynamic regimens of muscle activity and their comparison when done on dry land or in water. The specificity of the water environment leads, in comparison with dry surfaces, to different muscle timing through a change in the proportional representation of activity agonistic-antagonistic muscles, and through a different compensation mechanism that follows from a certain postural "instability" in movements in water. Most published works deal with the issue of normal or modified gait or the monitoring of activity of muscles of the lower extremities in variously defined movements. Less attention is paid to the activity of muscles of the upper extremities, mostly with a focus on the shoulder girdle.

5.1 WaS-EMG analysis of walking in water

Movements in a water environment are affected by the viscosity of the water, which is eight hundred times as great as that of air. Bodies submerged in water are lighter than in air thanks to the buoying force. This buoying force of water decreases the vertical burden in a water environment against to walking on a dry land. This result was objectivised on the basis of treading on a Kistler pressure-sensitive surface in a water environment (Miyoshi et al., 2004).
Masumoto et al. (Masumoto et al., 2004) monitored muscle activity during walking on a treadmill in a water environment with the use of an water counterflow and without, and they compared it with walking on a dry land. They monitored muscles in the lower extremities (m.gluteus medius, m.rectus femoris, m.vastus medialis, m.biceps femoris, m.gastrocnemius lateralis, m.tibialis anterior) and bilaterally on the trunk (mm.paravertebrales in the area of the fourth lumbar vertebra and the m.rectus abdominis). The gait speed in a water environment (30 m/min, 40 m/min, 50 m/min) was half that of the gait speed on a dry surface. The depth of the water in the pool reached the level of the processus xiphoideus. Significantly lower electrical activity values were found in the monitored muscles when walking in a water environment with a counterflow and without a counterflow in comparison with identical movement on a dry land, the difference amounting to 10-20%. These results corresponded to previous studies, which also describe decreased EMG activity in a water environment compared with identical movement on a dry land (Clarys et.al., 1985; Fujisawa et al., 1998; Pöyhömen et al., 1999; Kelly et al., 2000). The following year Masumoto et al. (Masumoto et al., 2005) published a further study. In which, while keeping the previous conditions, they again monitored the activity of muscles of the lower extremity and trunk musculature while walking on a treadmill backwards on a dry land and in a water environment (with and without a water counterflow). They arrived at similar reasults. The sole exception was heightened activity of paravertebral muscles in the area of the fourth lumbar vertebra. They explained the increase in their activity in water by citing the greater resistance of the water environment, greater demands on balance, and backwards walking.
In the work of Shono et al. (Shono et al., 2007), electrodes were placed on muscles of the right lower extremity: m.tibialis anterior, m.gastrocnemius medialis, m.vastus medialis, m.rectus femoris, m.biceps femoris. Gait was measured among sixty years old women at speeds of 20 m/min., 30 m/min, and 40 m/min in a water environment, and then at twice these speeds on a dry land. The gait cadence was lower (by nearly one-half) and the stride length was longer in a water environment, if the same gait speeds in both environments were compared. However, when comparing the same intensity of movement, i.e.,

approximately 30 m/min in a water environment against 60 m/min on a dry land, the stride length was not significantly different. At a corresponding intensity of movement, nearly identical activity for the m. tibialis anterior, m. vastus medialis, and m. biceps femoris was recorded, but the m. gastrocnemius medialis and m. rectus femoris showed lower activity in a water environment. When comparing the results of the same speeds, activity of the tibialis anterior, vastus medialis, and biceps femoris was higher in a water environment, while activity of the gastrocnemius medialis and the rectus femoris was the same.
Pöyhönen (Pöyhönen T, 2001) evaluated the muscle activity of the m. quadriceps femoris and the m. biceps femoris during flexing and extension of the knee on a dry land and in a water environment. In the water environment the test was run with and without the use of a "Hydro Boot." Eighteen persons without any physical problems took part in the study. The underwater EMG results showed a decline in time in the concentric activity of the agonist muscles with concurrent activity of the antagonist muscles without the "Hydro Boot." When measuring activity in a water environment with and without the resistance boot the probands were seated on a chair so that they are submerged up to the mid-sternum level. In the results, the EMG amplitudes were similar in both cases. The authors are of the opinion that with and without the use of the boot the size of the EMG amplitude was similar, especially thanks to the "power-speed" relationship of the muscle contraction. But it was pointed out that if a muscle acts as an agonist it is active in roughly the first 50-60% of the extent of the movement. If it is acting as an antagonist it is active in roughly the last 50-60% of the extent of the movement, while on a dry surface an agonist is active throughout the entire period of movement and an antagonist shows only a little activity.

5.2 WaS-EMG analysis of muscle timing during cycling on dry land and in a water environment

In the work of Sladká (Sladká, 2011), with the help of surface EMG, was compared the timing of muscles of four probands aged 23-24, while riding a bicycle on a dry land and in a water environment. In the experiment she used two identical Sapilo water bicycles (Fig. 7). She placed WaS-EMG electrodes on the right and left paravertebrales muscles and the m. biceps femoris, m. gastrocnemius lateralis, m. vastus medialis, and m. tibialis anterior of the left, non-dominant extremity.

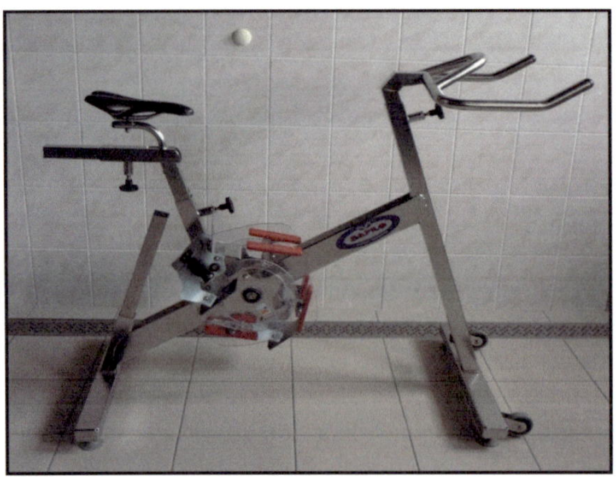

Fig. 7. Sapilo water bicycle.

The temperature of the water in the pool was 32° C (±0.5° C), and the temperature of the air was 28° C (±0.5° C). The depth of the water was up to 125 cm. The measurement itself of the EMG recording was made while riding on the water bicycle, first on a dry surface and then in the water. The pedalling speed was 60 revolutions per minute. The pedalling time on the dry land and in the water was one minute.

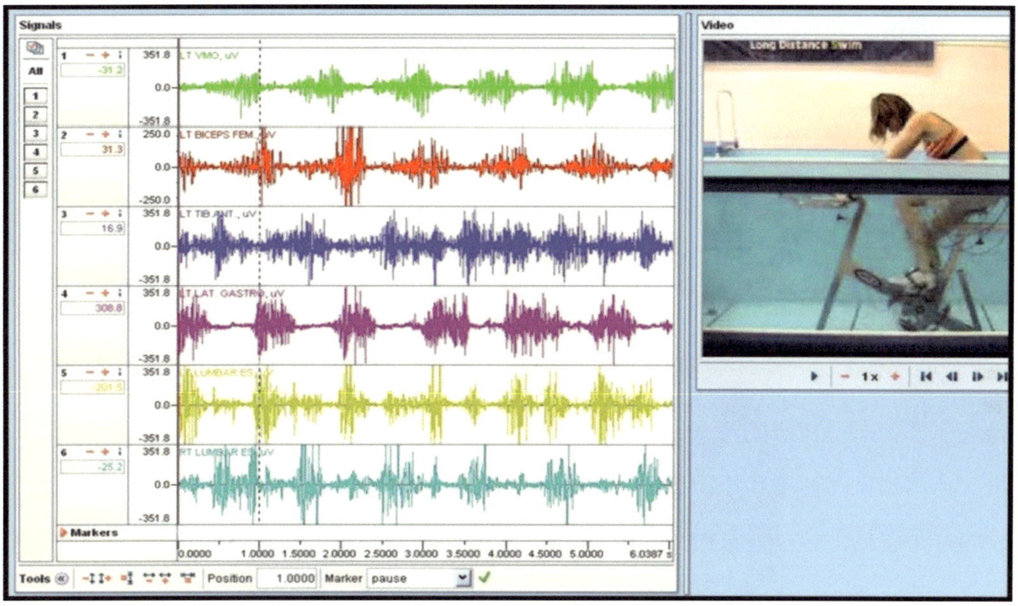

Fig. 8. EMG recording with a synchronized video recording. The interrupted vertical line captures the left lower extremity at the beginning of the pedal revolution (Sladká, 2011).

The results of the study did not show changes in the timing of the monitored muscles of the lower extremity when riding a bicycle on dry land and in a water environment. Due to greater demands related to stabilizing the pelvis in the water environment, there was co-contraction of both paravertebral muscles. On dry land this tendency was not recorded. At the same time, it was found that in the water environment pedalling was more regular than pedalling on dry land.

5.3 Analysis of muscles of the pectoral girdle with the help of WaS-EMG

The already outlined general trend towards decreasing electromyographical activity for identical movements in water versus dry land has also been described by many authors studying muscle activity in the area of the pectoral girdle (Rouard & Clarys, 1995; Fujisawa et al., 1998; Pavlů & Pánek, 2008).

Kelly et al. (Kelly et al., 2000) broadened their question to include the issue of the speed of abduction in the shoulder joint with a concurrent comparison of the activity of muscles of the rotator cuff and the synergies of the shoulder during exercise on dry land and in water. Six probands took part in the research. In the water environment, the probands were submerged up to neck level. In both environments they caused abduction in their shoulder joints at speeds of 30°/s, 45°/s, and 90°/s. The results showed that when the selected speed corresponded to 30°/s and 45°/s, the activity of the muscles (supraspinatus, infraspinatus, subscapularis, and the front, middle and back parts of the deltoideus) was smaller than on dry land. At 90°/s, the muscle activity especially of the m. subscapularis, increased markedly.

Holländerová (Holländerová, 2011), during the course of her study, which was conducted in our workplace, evaluated the timing and size of activation of muscles during abduction in the shoulder joint as opposed to the resistance of a flexible pull on dry land and in water. The flexible resistance was provided with the help of Thera-Band yellow dye. Four probands took part in the study. EMG activity was registered from the m. trapezius pars superior et inferior and the m. deltoideus pars medialis muscles (Fig. 9).

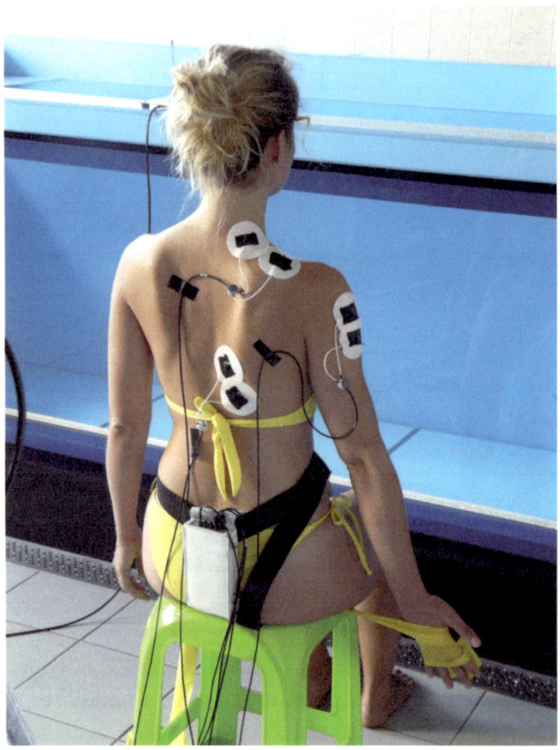

Fig. 9. Localization of WaS-EMG electrodes during study of muscle activity against flexible resistance with the help of Thera-Band yellow dye (Holländerová, 2011).

The water temperature was 32° C. The probands caused abduction in the shoulder joint at a speed of 30°/s to the horizontal position of the brachium, first on a dry surface and then in water, which reached the level of the procesus spinosus vertebra C5. They continually repeated abduction of the brachium 10 times, and 7 stable cycles were evaluated (Fig. 10). The results of the study indicated a decrease in monitored muscle activity in the water environment; the most marked change was captured in the m. trapezius pars superior muscle - 47-57% - in the other two muscles the change ranged between 19 and 29%. She also found different muscle timing, coinciding with an earlier study (Pavlů & Pánek, 2008), between movement in water and on dry land, but this was individual and there was no common trend.

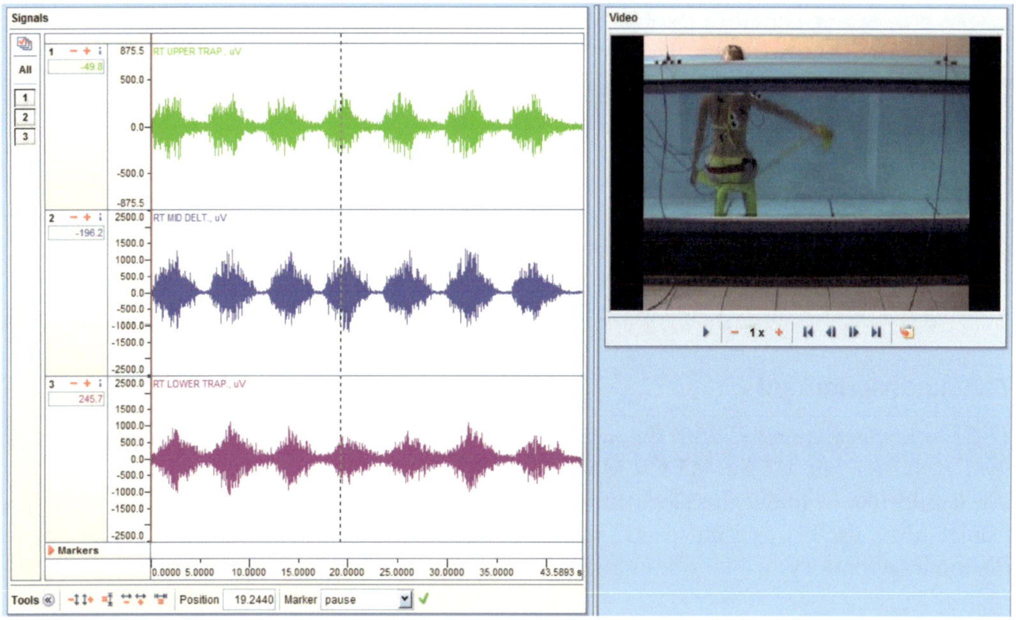

Fig. 10. EMG activity in the course of 7 cycles of brachial abduction in a water environment (Holländerová, 2011).

6. Conclusion

WaS-EMG is a relatively modern method for studying electrical muscle activity in an environment that was formerly rather inaccessible for neuro-physiological methods. Nevertheless, there are many studies that make it possible to follow up on acquired knowledge relating primarily to methodological measurement and the effect of a captured biological signal. In summary, here are the most basic of them:

1. For registering electrical activity it is best to use separate electrodes. Water resistant suits and garments are mainly more expensive, they place greater limitation on the probands' activity, and they are more likely to leak water onto the electrodes.
2. Electrodes should be attached with water-resistant tape, which should also affix loose cables. This limits the occurrence of artefacts from cable movements that appear in the 0-20 Hz frequency band.
3. Pasted on electrodes should be used for measurements on dry land as well, because this does not change the character of the EMG signal between the water environment and on a dry land.
4. For measurement of the maximal voluntary contraction (MVC) should be used movements on a dry land. This is a simple method, and furthermore, is also in standard use in prior publications.
5. In dynamic modes it is good to engage in a defined movement activity in water at half the speed of that on dry land. The greater viscosity of water as against air can lead, especially during faster movements, to the change in the native EMG recording.
6. The optimal water temperature is between 27 and 34° C. Cooler water leads to lower electrical muscle activity. Higher temperatures are uncomfortable for the performance

of movement activities. Stable temperatures of muscles and the ambient water are reached in approximately 15 minutes.

7. When making an identical movement in water and in a dry environment, in the water environment there is decreased muscle activity versus the identical movement on a dry land.
8. The change on the size of muscle activity in a water environment depends on the speed of the movement on a dry land, and primarily for fast movements, when greater effect of water's viscosity is emphasized.
9. If we study movements that are more demanding on posture, the activity of trunk muscles, which must adjust to this burden, is increased.

7. Acknowledgment

This work was elaborated with the help of the research plan of the Ministry of Education of the Czech Republic **VZ MŠMT ČR MSM 0021620864.**

We would like to thank the Department of Swimming of the FTVS UK, and namely Mgr. Daniel Jurák for his assistance and making possible measurement in the Aquatic Sports Research Laboratory.

8. References

Clarys, J.; Robeaux, R.& Delbeke, G. (1985). Telemetrical versus conventional EMG in air and water. *Biomachnics IX: Human Kinetics,* pp.286-294, ISBN:0-931250-52-8, Champaign, France, 1985

Da Silva Carvalhoa, R.; Amorimb, C.&Perácioa L.&Coelhoa H.&Vieiraa, A.& Menzelc, H.& Szmuchrowski, A. (2010). Analysis of various conditions in order to measure electromyography of isometric contractions in water and on air. *Journal of Electromyography and Kinesiology.* Vol. 20, No. 5, (2010), pp.988-993, ISSN 1050-6411

DeLuca, C. (2002). Surface Electromyography: Detection and Recording. In: Delsys, 2.3.2006, Available from http://delsys.com/KnowledgeCenter/Tutorials.html.

Dewhurst, S.; Riches, P. & Nimmo, M. & De Vito, G. (2005). Temperature dependence of soleus H-reflex and M-wave in young and older women. *European Journal of Applied Physiology.* Vol. 94, No. 5-6, (2005), pp. 491-499, ISSN 8750-7587

Fujisawa, H,; Seunaga, N.& Minami, A. (1998). Electromyographic study during isometric exercise of the shoulder in head-out water immersion. *Journal of Shoulder and Elbow Surgery.* Vol. 7, No.5, (1998), pp. 491-494, ISSN 1058-2746

Holländerova, D. (2011). *Evaluation of EMG Activity of the Shoulder Girdle Muscles during Exercises with Thera-Band in the Aquatic Environment and on the Land.* Diploma thesis, Departmen of Physiotherapy. Faculty of Physical Education and Sport, Charles University, Prague, Czech Republic, 2011 (in Czech)

Jandová, D. (2009). *Balneologie.* Grada Publishing a.s., ISBN 978-80-247-2820-9, Prague, Czech Republic (in Czech)

Kaneda, K.; Wakabayashi, H.& Sato, D.& Uekusa, T.& Nomura, T. (2008). Lower extremity muscle activity during deep-water running on self-determined pace. *Journal of Electromyography and Kinesiology.* Vol.18, No. 6, (2008), pp. 965-972, ISSN 1050-6411

Kelly, B.; Roskin, D.& Kirkendall, D.& Speer, K. (2000). Shoulder muscle activation during aquatic and dry land exercises in nonimpaired subjects. *Journal of Orthopaedic & Sports Physical Therapy*. Vol.30. No.4, (2000), pp. 204-210, ISSN 0190-6011

Masumoto, K.; Takasugi, S. & Hotta, N. & Fujishima, K. & Iwamoto, Y. (2004). Electromyographic Analysis of Walking in Water in Healthy Humans. *Journal of Psychiological Anthropology and Applied Human Science*. Vol. 23, No. 4, (2004), pp. 119-127, ISSN 1345-3475

Masumoto, K.; Takasugi, S. & Hotta, N. & Fujishima, K. & Iwamoto, Y. (2005). Muscle activity and heart rate response during backward walking in water. *European Journal of Applied Physiology and Occupation Physiology*. Vol. 94, No. 1-2, (2005), pp. 54-61, ISSN 0301-5548

Masumoto, K. & Mercer, J. (2008). Biomechanics of Human Locomotion in Water: An Electromyographic Analysis: Methodological Considerations for Quantifying Muscle Activity During Water Locomotion. *Exercise and Sport Sciences Reviews.*, Vol. 36, No.3, (2008), pp.160-169, ISSN 0091-6331

Masumoto, K.; Delion, D. & Mercer, J. (2009). Insight into Muscle Activity during Deep Water Running. *Medicine & Science in Sports & Exercice*. Vol. 41, (2009), pp. 1958-1964, ISSN 0195-9131

Miyoshi, T.; Shirota, T. & Yamamoto, S. & Nakazawa, K. & Akai, M. (2004). Effect of the walking speed to the lower limb joint angular displasments, joint movements and ground reaction force during walking in water. *Disability & Rehabilitation*. Vol. 26, No. 12, (2004), pp. 724-732, ISSN 0963-8288

Pánek, D.; Jurák, D. & Pavlů, D. & Krajča, V. & Čemusová, J. (2010). Water Surface Electromyography -WaS-EMG. *Rehabilitation and Physical Medicine*.Vol. 17, No. 1, (2010), pp.21-25, ISSN 1211-2658 (in Czech)

Pavlů, D. & Pánek, D. (2008). EMG - Analysis of Selected Muscles of Upper Extremity Moving in Water Environment and Motion against Elastic Rezistance. *Rehabilitation and Physical Medicine*. Vol. 15, No. 4, (2008), pp. 167-173, ISSN 1211-2658 (in Czech]

Petrofsky, J. & Laymon, M. (2005). Muscle Temperature and EMG Amplitude and Frequency During Isometric Exercise. *Aviation, Space and Environment Medicine*. Vol. 76, No.11., (2005), pp. 1024- 1030, ISSN 0095-6562

Pöyhömen, T.; Kyrolainen, H. & Keskinen, K. & Hautala, A. & Savolainen, J. & Mälkiä, E. (1999). Isometric force production and electromyogram activity of knee extensor muscles in water and on dry land. *European Journal of Applied Physiology and Occupation Physiology*. Vol. 80, No. 1, (1999), pp. 52-56, 1999, ISSN 1432-1025

Pöyhönen, T.; Keskinen, K. & Kyröläinen, H. & Hautala, A. & Savolainen, J. & Mälkiä, E. (2001). Neuromuscular function during therapeutic knee exercise under water and on dry land. *Archives of Physical Medicine and Rehabilitation*. Vol. 82, No. 10, (2001), pp. 1446-1442, ISSN 0003-9993

Rainoldi, A.; Cescon, C. &, Bottin, A. & Casale, R. & Caruso, I. (2004). Surface EMG alteration induced by undewater recording. *Journal of Electromyography and Kinesiology*. Vol. 14, No.3, (2004), pp. 325-331, ISSN 1050-6411

Rouard, A. & Clarys, J. (1995). Cocontraction in the Elbow and Shoulder Muscles During Rapid Cyclic Movements in an Aquatic Environment. *Journal of Electromyography and Kinesiology. Vol.* 5, No. 3, (1995), pp. 177-183, ISSN 1050-6411

Shono, T.; Masumoto, K. & Fujishima, K. & Hotta, N. & Ogaki, T. & Adachi, T. (2007). Gait Patterns and Muscle Activity of the Lower Extremities of Elderly Women during Underwater Treadmill Walking againts Water Flow. *Journal of Physiological Anthropology*. Vol. 26, No. 6, (2007), pp. 579-586, ISSN 1880-6791

Silvers, W. & Dolny, D. (2001). Comparison and reproducibility of sEMG during manual muscle testing on land and in water. *Journal of Electromyography and Kinesiology*. Vol. 21, No.1, (2001), pp. 95-101, ISSN 1050-6411.

Sladká, H. 2011. *Compare of muscle timing during cycling on land and in water*. Diploma thesis. Departmen of Physiotherapy. Faculty of Physical Education and Sport, Charles University, Prague, Czech Republic, 2011 (in Czech)

Stejskalova, P. (2011). *Effect of water temperature on muscle contraction*. Diploma thesis. Departmen of Physiotherapy. Faculty of Physical Education and Sport, Charles University, Prague, Czech Republic, 2011 (in Czech)

Sulková, I. (2011). *Possibility of using Aquatherapy for shoulder stabilization*. Diploma thesis. Department of Physiotherapy, Faculty of Physical Education and Sport, Charles University, Prague, Czech Republic, 2011 (in Czech)

Veneziano, W.; da Rocha, A. & Goncalves, C. & Pena, A. & Carmo J. & Nascimento, F. & Rainoldi, A. (2006). Confounding factors in water EMG recordings: an approach to a definitive standard. *Medical & Biological Engineering & Computing*. Vol. 44, No. 4, (2006), pp. 348-351, ISSN 0140-0118

24

Scanning Electromyography

Javier Navallas[1], Javier Rodríguez[1] and Erik Stålberg[2]
[1]*Department of Electrical and Electronic Engineering, Public University of Navarra, Pamplona*
[2]*Institute of Neuroscience, Department of Clinical Neurophysiology, Uppsala University Hospital, Uppsala*
[1]*Spain*
[2]*Sweden*

1. Introduction

The study of the anatomy and physiology of the motor unit has important implications in the diagnosis and follow-up of neuromuscular pathologies. Muscle action potentials allow the use of electrophysiological techniques based on electromyography (EMG) to make inferences about muscle structure, state and behaviour. Scanning EMG is one such technique that can record the temporal and spatial distribution of electrical activity of a single motor unit, allowing for deep insight into the structure and function of motor units.

In this chapter, we describe the scanning EMG technique in detail, both from a technical and clinical point of view. A brief review of the motor unit anatomy and physiology is provided in Section 2. The technique, the apparatus setup, the recording procedure and the signal processing required are described in Section 3. Key results of studies using scanning EMG are reviewed in Section 4, including findings related to motor unit organisation in normal muscle and how changes due to pathology are reflected using this electrophysiological technique. Finally, Section 5 provides some hints regarding the use of scanning EMG in research.

2. Investigation of the motor unit structure

The motor unit is the functional building block of skeletal muscle and the target of scanning EMG. In this section, the main concepts regarding the anatomy and physiology of the motor unit are described. Several electrophysiological techniques that allow the investigation of the structure of motor units are also introduced.

2.1 Motor unit anatomy

The motor unit is the smallest functional structure in skeletal muscle, comprising a motoneuron and the set of muscle fibres innervated by its axon. An action potential propagating through the axon eventually arrives at motor end-plates at the presynaptic side of the neuromuscular junctions. The electrical stimulus is then converted into a chemical signal that subsequently induces an action potential in the muscle fibre. This single fibre action potential (SFAP) propagates in both directions toward the ends of the muscle fibre, inducing a contraction of the fibre itself. The motor unit fibres, i.e., all the muscle fibres belonging to the same motor unit, contract synchronously given upon receiving the motor control command from the same motoneuron through the arborisations of its axon.

Viewing the muscle longitudinally (Fig. 1), motor unit fibres generally run in parallel between two musculotendinous junctions, although some muscle fibres have tapered fibre-to-fibre ends (Lieber, 1992). Motor end-plates of corresponding neuromuscular junctions tend to concentrate in the central portion of the fibres, halfway between their two ends. In a muscle like the biceps brachii, motor end-plate zone occupies a thin strip about 6-10 mm in width (Aquilonius et al., 1982; Amirali et al., 2007). Action potentials generated under motor end-plates propagate through the muscle fibre at a certain conduction velocity (Stålberg, 1966); the conduction velocity of a muscle fibre is directly related to its diameter (Nandedkar & Stålberg, 1983a).

Views of muscle cross-sections (Fig. 2) reveal that fibres belonging to the same motor unit occupy only a fraction of the cross-section area (Kugelberg et al., 1970); this area is referred to as the motor unit territory, and is generally irregular, mainly rounded, although it has also been described to be oval-shaped (Bodine et al., 1988) or crescent-shaped closer to the fascia. Within this territory, fibres of the same motor unit are scattered and intermingled with fibres belonging to other motor units (Burke et al., 1974). Hence, territories of different motor units overlap. The size and shape of a single motor unit territory is considerably preserved throughout the entire length of the motor unit, as shown in three-dimensional reconstructions of complete motor units (Roy et al., 1995).

The technique employed to study motor unit cross-sections is based on glycogen depletion (Edström & Kugelberg, 1968). Briefly, a single axon is repeatedly stimulated to ensure that all the glycogen is depleted from the muscle fibres innervated by the axon. Next, the muscle is excised and stained with a glycogen reagent. In the microtome cross-section, the glycogen-depleted fibres that belong to the same motor unit can be traced. The glycogen depletion technique provides a picture of the motor unit cross-section that enables a

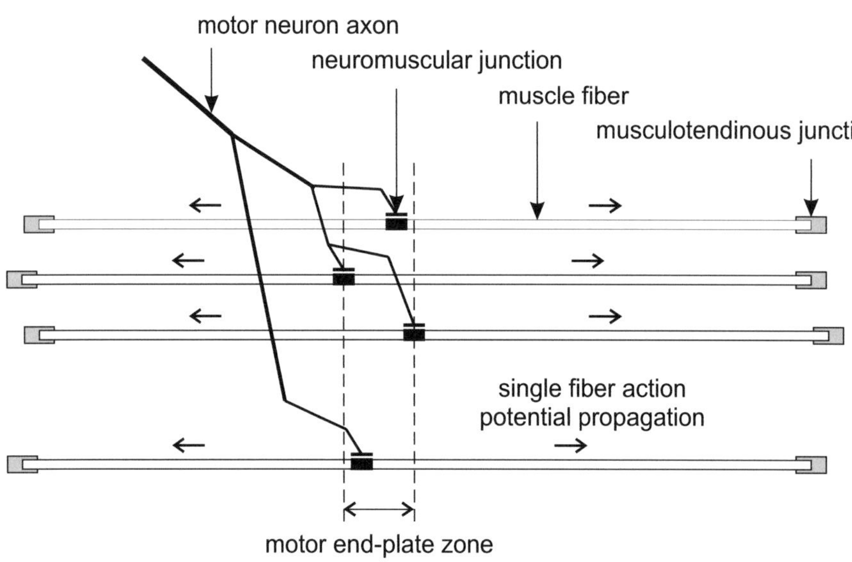

Fig. 1. A schematic representation of a motor unit with the motoneuron axon branching to innervate a set of muscle fibres.

visualisation of individual motor unit fibres. The technique also makes it possible to count individual motor unit fibres and to study their spatial distribution (Venema, 1994).

Several glycogen depletion studies have demonstrated that the number of motor unit fibres greatly varies not only among muscles (Enoka, 1995; Feinstein et al., 1955) but also within the same muscle, where the number of motor unit fibres can vary up to 10-fold (Bodine et al., 1988; Burke & Tsairis, 1973; Burke et al., 1974; Edström & Kugelberg, 1968). For example, in the medial gastrocnemius of the rat, the observed number of motor unit fibres ranges from 40 to 350 (Kanda & Hashizume, 1992). The area of the motor unit territory has also been measured in several glycogen depletion studies (Ansved et al., 1991; Bodine et al., 1988; Kanda & Hashizume, 1992; Rafuse & Gordon, 1996), which also show a broad range of variation. For example, motor unit territories of the tibialis anterior of the rat account for 10% to 24% of the muscle cross-sectional area, whereas territories of the soleus account for 25% to 75% of the cross-sectional area (Kugelberg et al., 1970).

Given the number of motor unit fibres and the area of the motor unit territory, the motor unit fibre density can be calculated (Kanda & Hashizume, 1992). Fibre density seems to be rather independent of the size of the motor unit (Weijs et al., 1993) and constant throughout the length of the motor units (Roy et al., 1995). However, fibre density can vary for different motor unit types, with smaller motor units having lower fibre densities (Kanda & Hashizume, 1992).

The spatial distribution of motor unit fibres within a motor unit territory has become a controversial issue. This spatial distribution has been described as uniform without localised collections (Burke et al., 1974), quasi-Gaussian (Miller-Larsson, 1980), evenly distributed (Willison, 1980), uniform (Gath & Stålberg, 1982), and random (Gates & Betz, 1993). A thorough statistical analysis of spatial point patterns obtained by glycogen depletion has provided more insight into this discrepancy. Short-range analysis based on adjacency tests and nearest-neighbour distributions suggest a random distribution (Bodine et al., 1988).

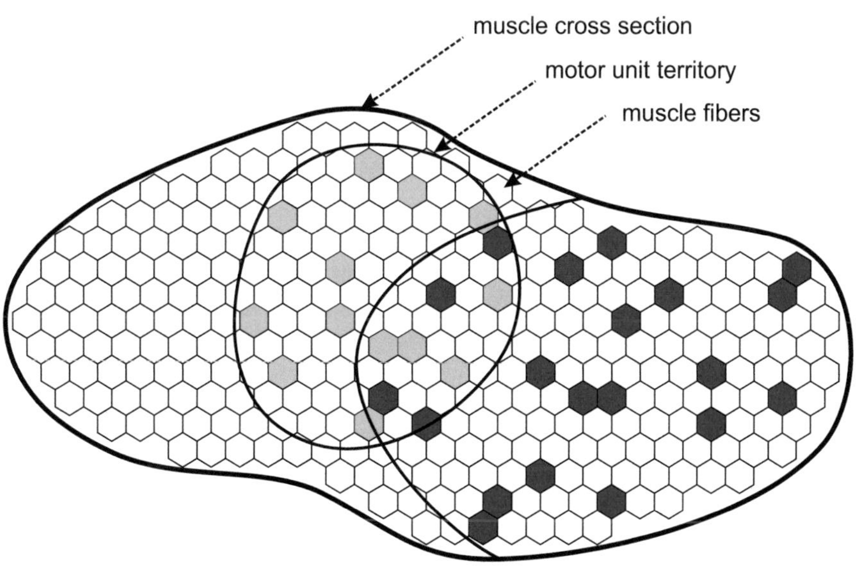

Fig. 2. A schematic representation of two motor units with overlapping territories within a muscle cross-section, and their corresponding muscle fibers.

However, long-range analysis based on quadrat analysis, point-to-nearest-neighbour distributions and inter-fibre distance distributions suggest the existence of holes within the territory and some degree of clustering in motor unit fibre distribution (Bodine-Fowler et al., 1990). The spatial clustering can be related to the axonal branching pattern established during the development of the neuromuscular system (Monti et al., 2001; Pffeifer & Friede, 1985). Other results show that, in the long-range, the randomness of the distribution may depend on the age and type of the motor unit (Ansved et al., 1991).

2.2 Electromyographic investigation of the motor unit structure

The electrical activity of the muscle can be recorded using intramuscular or surface electrodes. Intramuscular recordings are usually performed using needle electrodes. Depending on the type of needle and the recording procedure, EMG can measure the activity of muscle fibres by recording SFAPs, the activity of motor units by recording motor unit potentials (MUPs) or the activity of the entire muscle by recording the interference pattern.

2.2.1 Motor unit potentials obtained in concentric needle EMG

MUPs reveal many properties of motor unit structure because MUPs are made up of superimposed SFAPs of motor unit fibres. MUP characteristics depend on the number and relative positions of the muscle fibres generating the SFAPs and the temporal alignment of individual SFAPs (Nandedkar et al., 1988b).

The number of muscle fibres, especially within the closest uptake area of the electrode, determines the size of the resulting MUP (Nandedkar et al., 1988a). Several parameters reflect the size of MUPs, like the amplitude, the area, or the size-index (Sonoo & Stålberg, 1993). The duration of MUPs also reflects the number of fibres, but within a larger uptake area (Nandedkar et al., 1988b). A misalignment of the SFAPs contributing to an MUP increases the waveform complexity of the resulting MUP. This temporal misalignment can be caused by spatial dispersion of motor end-plates, temporal dispersion the initial depolarisation of motor end-plates, and differences in muscle fibre conduction velocities in different motor unit fibres (Navallas & Stålberg, 2009). The complexity of MUPs can be assessed with parameters like the number of phases, the number of turns (Pfeiffer & Kunze, 1992; Stålberg, 1986; Willison, 1964), or the irregularity coefficient (Zalewska & Husmanova-Petrusevich, 1995).

2.2.2 Specific techniques to estimate motor unit parameters

Quantitative analysis of MUPs is a valuable tool in diagnosis. In addition, there are other specific EMG techniques that allow us to estimate some of the physiological and anatomical parameters of the muscle and motor units. Because the glycogen depletion technique requires excising the muscle, it is unsuitable for human research, although some restricted experiments have been performed using muscle biopsies (Gollnick et al., 1973; Garnett et al., 1979). Hence, all available data pertaining to complete muscle cross-sections correspond to small mammalians. Alternative techniques based on electrophysiological recordings have been developed allowing the investigation of motor unit structures in human muscles.

The number of motor units in a certain muscle can be estimated by incrementally stimulating the nerve while simultaneously recording the compound muscle action potential (CMAP) with a surface electrode, a technique called motor unit number estimation

(MUNE) (McComas et al., 1971). This basic concept was later developed into a number of MUNE methods.

The number of motor unit fibres cannot be estimated quantitatively using electrophysiological techniques, but a relative measure can be assessed using macro EMG (Stålberg, 1980; Stålberg & Fawcett, 1982). It has been demonstrated that the amplitude of motor unit potentials recorded using the macro EMG technique is highly correlated with the number of muscle fibres involved in the generation of the signal and hence the number of motor unit fibres (Nandedkar & Stålberg, 1983b; Roeleveld et al., 1997a, 1997b).

The density of motor unit fibres can also be estimated using single fibre EMG (Gath & Stålberg, 1982). This technique relies on the assumption of a homogeneous Poisson distribution of muscle fibres (Gath & Stålberg, 1981, 1982) and provides an average measure of fibre density of different motor units (Stålberg, 1986). Although this technique may average the differences in fibre densities for different motor units, recent studies in humans show no change in fibre density with a recruitment threshold up to 50% of the maximum voluntary contraction (Lukács et al., 2009).

2.2.3 Multipoint EMG techniques

The previously presented electrophysiological techniques share one thing in common: the recordings are made using electrodes with a single channel, and hence all the information is recorded from a single spatial location. Using special multilead electrodes, or multielectrodes, simultaneous recordings from different locations can be obtained, enhancing the scope of the electrophysiological technique for studying the muscle. A straightforward example is the use of a special multielectrode to assess muscle fibre conduction velocity *in situ* (Stålberg, 1966).

Using multielectrodes with recording sites lined up along the length of the needle, the main axis of the needle defines a recording corridor. It is common to position the corridor perpendicular to the muscle fibres, so that different recording sites gather information from different regions of the muscle cross-section or the motor unit territory under study.

One of the most straightforward applications of multipoint techniques is the investigation of motor unit territories. Motor unit territories have been have been studied using various EMG multielectrode configurations, one containing twelve 1.5 mm long leads distributed over 25 mm (Buchthal et al., 1957, 1959) and another containing 14 different recording sites of 25 µm diameter allowing 40 recording sites spaced 150 µm apart over 14 mm (Stålberg et al., 1976; Schwartz et al., 1976). Scanning EMG was developed as an extension of multielectrode techniques (Stålberg & Antoni, 1980), allowing higher flexibility both in the spatial interval of detection and in the type of of electrode used. In this case, any type of conventional needle electrode can be used; therefore, the technique is not restricted to a single fibre-like recording.

In addition to the investigation of motor unit topography using scanning EMG (Diószeghy, 2002; Gootzen, 1990; Gootzen et al., 1992; Stålberg & Antoni, 1980; Stålberg & Diószeghy, 1991; Stålberg & Eriksson, 1987; Tonndorf, 1994), motor end-plate topography has also been studied using this technique (Navallas & Stålberg, 2009).

3. Scanning EMG technique

In this section, the methods, procedure, and set-up required to perform scanning EMG will be reviewed. Special attention will be paid to the recording procedure and the signal processing required to condition the signal after it is recorded.

3.1 Recording setup

The main objective of scanning EMG is to record the electrical activity of a motor unit from different locations along a scanning corridor as the needle electrode passes through the motor unit territory (Fig. 3). A very important aspect is that, although a single recording is made at each location, all recordings must be synchronised in relation to the firing of the motor unit, equivalent to simultaneously recording from all the sites. To extract the firing pattern of the motor unit, a second needle electrode, called the triggering needle, is inserted into the muscle. This electrode records localised activity, ideally from a single fibre, to minimise interference from other motor units. Hence, single fibre EMG needles or facial concentric needles are used for this purpose. A given motor unit is separated from others using an amplitude trigger.

If a concentric needle is used as the scanning electrode, the signal recorded in each location corresponds to an MUP. As the scanning needle moves through the scanning corridor, the relative geometry of motor unit fibres in relation to the active region of the electrode changes; hence, the recorded MUPs will be different, reflecting these changes. However, because the triggering needle is maintained at a fixed location, all the MUPs recorded by the scanning needle will be synchronised with the firing pattern of the motor unit.

The signals from both the triggering needle and the scanning needle are amplified and digitised, and transmitted to a personal computer running specific scanning EMG software (Fig. 4). This software must provide a way to establish a voltage threshold for the signal acquired from the triggering electrode. Whenever the signal exceeds this threshold voltage, the scanning software performs three operations:

1. Records a trace of the scanning signal within the predefined bounds of a temporal window, i.e., a buffer gathering the samples some milliseconds before and after the trigger event.

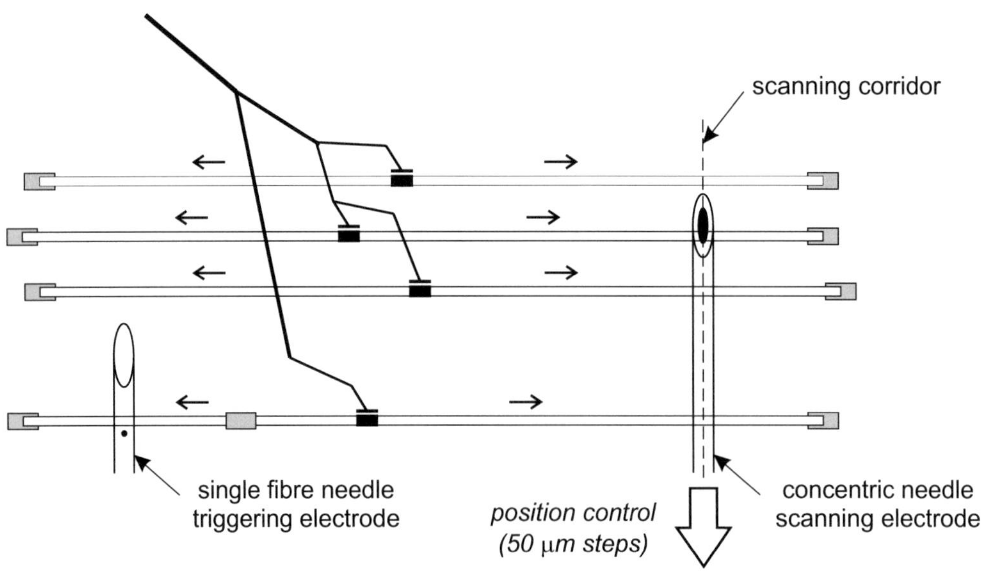

Fig. 3. A schematic representation of the recording procedure with the triggering needle in a fixed position and the scanning needle moving along the scanning corridor throughout the motor unit territory.

2. Sends a command to a micromotor controller to advance one step.
3. Waits until a new threshold event occurs. The micromotor controller is responsible for translating software commands into electrical signals that instruct the step-motor to advance a predefined distance, e.g., 50 μm.

The recorded signal is 2-dimensional in nature (Fig. 5(a)); the first dimension represents the spatial location of the recording in the scanning corridor and the second dimension represents the temporal duration of the recorded MUP. Both dimensions are discretised, the spatial dimension according to the step length controlled by the micromotor, and the temporal dimension according to the sampling time, i.e., the inverse of the sampling frequency of the acquisition system. Therefore, the signal can be thought of as a collection of MUPs from the same motor unit, where each trace is an individual MUP recorded from a different position along the scanning corridor, but also as a picture of the spatiotemporal distribution of the electric potential generated by the motor unit.

3.2 Recording procedure

In the first step, the triggering needle, a single fibre EMG electrode or facial concentric needle, is inserted to record the activity from one motor unit during slight voluntary contraction. The electromyographer should look for a stable waveform with good amplitude that is free of interference from other motor units. Next, the needle should be maintained in a fixed position to ensure a stable recording during the remainder of the process. The voltage level of the trigger must be adjusted so that a single trigger event is recorded each time the selected motor unit discharges.

The scanning needle is inserted a few centimetres away (20 mm is recommended) from the triggering electrode along the direction of the muscle fibres. The tip of the electrode must be sharp to ensure a smooth movement through the scanning corridor. The electrode must be inserted as close to perpendicular to the muscle fibres as possible (Stålberg & Antoni, 1980) to record from the actual cross-section of the muscle. Once the needle is inserted, the electromyographer should move it while looking for electrical activity synchronised with

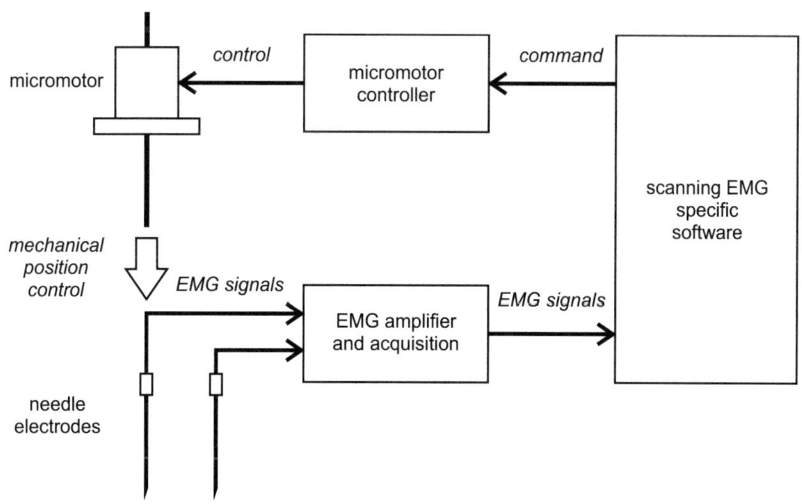

Fig. 4. A schematic representation of a scanning EMG system consisting in acquisition (needles and amplifier), processing, and control devices (micromotor and controller).

that of the triggering electrode (time-locked activity). To obtain good recordings and to ensure that the scanning needle is completely inside the motor unit territory, this time-locked activity should satisfy the same recording criteria applied to standard recordings; if a concentric needle is used for the scanning, the recorded signals should have high amplitude and a short rise-time.

Once the scanning needle is inside the motor unit territory, the electromyographer should push the needle until it reaches a position where spike activity is no longer detected. This ensures that we have completely passed through the motor unit territory. This procedure of selecting the triggering signal and finding synchronous activity with the scanning needle should take little more than one minute.

The next step is to physically connect the scanning needle to the step-motor, which should be mounted in a holder with an electrode grip and a wide-foot plate. The foot plate is held tightly against the skin over the muscle during the recording to ensure no relative movement between the step-motor and the muscle. Once the recording procedure begins, the step-motor pulls the scanning needle in small spatial increments until the recorded signal decays in amplitude or the needle exits the skin. The complete procedure should take less than five minutes.

3.3 Signal processing

The scanning EMG signal as initially recorded is a raw signal (Fig. 5(a)) that must be post-processed to obtain a cleaner version that is free of noise and interferences. There are two steps in the enhancement of the raw signal. First, a temporal filter is applied individually to each of the scanning traces (Stålberg & Antoni, 1980). A low-pass or band-pass filter can be applied to remove baseline noise produced by the needle or muscle movement and a band-pass filter will also subtract high frequency noise from the signal. The resulting signal (Fig. 5(b)) presents a smoother profile in the spatial dimension with fewer and smaller baseline jumps. Actual filter settings, like filter order and cut-off frequencies, will depend on the recording needle and should follow the recommendations for conventional recording using the needles.

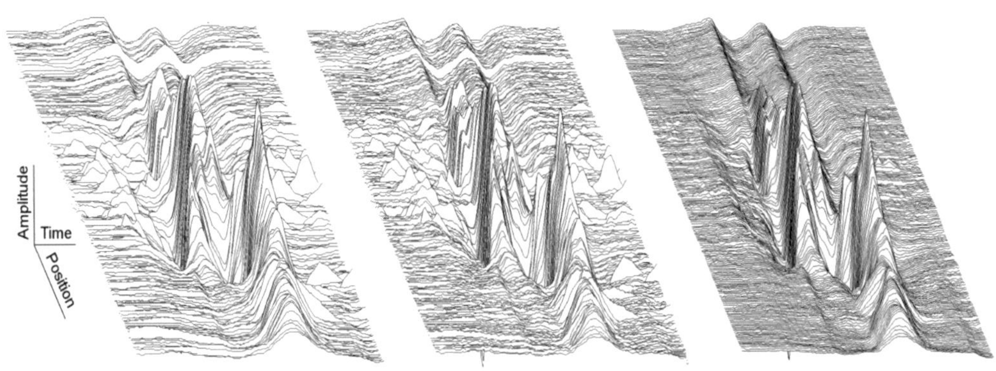

(a) (b) (c)

Fig. 5. A three-dimensional representation of a scanning EMG signal: (a) a raw signal, (b) the pervious signal filtered in the temporal domain, and (c) the previous signal filtered in the spatial domain.

Significant interference due to the coactivation of other motor units may still exist in the signal, represented by superimposed MUPs scattered alongside the MUP being tracked. However, superimposed discharges are not synchronised with the firing of the tracked motor unit. Therefore, these interfering discharges are not consistently repeated and, in a trace corrupted with such an artefact, superimposed MUPs are usually found between two clean traces in the spatial domain. For this reason, a median filter is applied in the spatial dimension during the second processing step (Stålberg & Antoni, 1980). Median filters preserve smoothly changing values of synchronised activity in motor units being tracked, removing all artefacts generated by other motor units (Fig. 5(c)).
Although median filtering is a very useful technique to eliminate interfering MUPs, its influence on the signal it is not negligible. The larger the size of the median filter, the greater the reduction in the amplitude of the peaks compared to the raw data. When a 3-point median filter is used, peaks are reduced by about 10%, and when a 5- or 7-point median filter is used, peaks are reduced up to 30% (Gootzen, 1990). This should be taken into account when extracting quantitative data from the signals.

4. Scanning EMG results

Scanning EMG provides valuable information not only about the territory and arrangement of muscle fibres within a motor unit, but also about the spatiotemporal distribution of the electrical activity of a motor unit, information no other EMG technique can provide (Diószeghy, 2002). We will introduce some key aspects for qualitative interpretation of scanning EMG signals and several parameters for quantitative analysis.

4.1 Interpretation of the scanning EMG signal

In the most straightforward interpretation, a scanning EMG signal is a collection of MUPs recorded from slightly different locations through a scanning corridor. Hence, it shows the evolution of MUPs as the location of the needle electrode changes relative to the motor unit fibres of the motor unit being tracked. However, a scanning EMG signal can also be interpreted as a picture of the spatiotemporal distribution of the electric potential generated by a motor unit. Fig. 6 shows a 2-dimensional signal as a contour map that allows us to distinguish between peaks and valleys corresponding to the negative and positive phases of MUPs. In this figure, four spatial locations within the corridor are selected, and the corresponding traces representing the MUPs recorded at these sites are depicted.
Due to the recording procedure, the first part of the scanned recording corresponds to a section of the corridor outside the motor unit territory. In this case, the recording tip of the needle electrode is too far away from the generators to record their signals. However, the cannula, which is used as reference electrode in concentric needle recordings, is almost completely inside the motor unit territory. The result is that an inverted potential is recorded, similar to that of a macro EMG recording (first selected MUP in Fig. 6). This causes a trough at the beginning of the scan referred to as the cannula effect. In this way, it is possible to obtain the equivalent of an inverted macro EMG recording from the motor unit under study by averaging 50 to 100 traces that are recorded before the tip of the needle is inside the motor unit territory (Stålberg & Diószeghy, 1991). It is important to note that this method is not identical to conventional macro EMG, as the cannula used in the scanning procedure may not be partially insulated (Stålberg & Diószeghy, 1991).

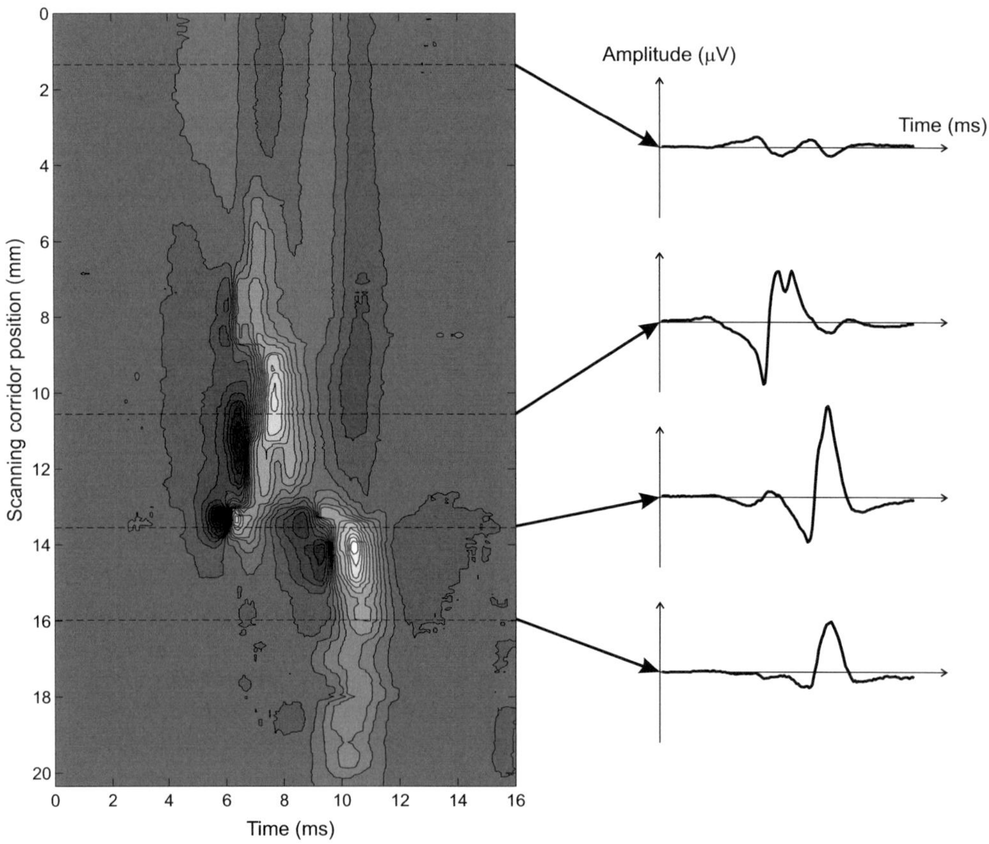

Fig. 6. A topographic representation of a scanning EMG signal in a contour plot (left) and selected MUPs at four different positions along the scanning corridor (right), with the uppermost MUP being a clear example of the cannula effect.

Once the active area of the electrode enters the motor unit territory, the recorded electric field increases and takes the shape of a conventional MUP (second to fourth MUPs in Fig. 6). Remarkably, the high variability of MUPs becomes apparent in scanning EMG recordings; as we move through the scanning corridor, the MUP waveform changes dramatically, reflecting the changes in the geometrical disposition of the set of generators, i.e., the set of motor unit fibres.

The length of the recording is characterised by regions of high activity separated by regions where the potential amplitude decays considerably. Regions of high activity are called motor unit fractions, or simply fractions, and the regions of low activity are called silent areas.

Clearly, the fractions correspond to regions close to motor unit fibres, whereas silent areas correspond to holes in the motor unit territory, or regions depleted of motor unit fibres. This arrangement of motor unit fibres, where motor unit fibres are not evenly distributed throughout the motor unit territory, is in agreement with glycogen depletion findings suggesting a certain degree of clustering of the muscle fibres within its motor unit territory (Bodine et al., 1998). Furthermore, fractions observed in scanning EMG recordings from normal muscle more commonly present distinct latencies rather than spatial separation. This observation points to the existence of different average temporal latencies of fibres belonging to different fractions (Stålberg, 1986; Navallas & Stålberg, 2009) and supports the hypothesis that each fraction represents a set of fibres innervated by a common axonal branch; therefore, the end-plates of these fibres will be in close proximity to one another compared to the overall motor end-plate zone dispersion (Stålberg, 1986; Nandedkar & Stålberg, 1986; Stålberg & Diószeghy, 1991; Navallas & Stålberg, 2009).

Sudden amplitude changes may also occur in scanning EMG profiles. These can be produced either by small uncontrolled jumps of the scanning needle or by changes in the properties of the volume conductor as the needle passes through a tendon layer or through a fascia (Stålberg & Eriksson, 1987; Diószeghy, 2002).

4.2 Analysis and parameterisation of the signal

Quantification of the EMG waveforms establishes objective criteria for comparing signals and for subsequent diagnosis. Several parameters have been proposed to quantify scanning EMG waveforms, most based on characteristics that cannot be observed in conventional EMG recordings. It is important to note that because the individual traces of scanning signals are MUPs themselves, all the conventional MUP parameters, like amplitude, area, duration, size index, etc., can be calculated in these traces. However, we will focus on specific scanning EMG parameters that exploit the two-dimensional nature of the signal and the recording through the spatial corridor.

4.2.1 Length of the motor unit cross-section

The length of the motor unit cross-section (Hilton-Brown & Stålberg, 1983a, 1983b ; Stålberg, 1986) is defined as the maximal distance between traces with amplitudes of at least 50 µV (Fig. 7). This distance represents an estimation of the length of the scanning corridor that runs inside the motor unit territory, given that as soon as the active area of the electrode enters the territory, the amplitude of the recorded MUP will exceed the 50 µV threshold. The length of the motor unit cross-section can alternatively be defined as the length between the two most distant traces with amplitudes above 15% of the maximum positive amplitude of the scan (Gootzen, 1990). However, this definition may under- or overestimate the measured length because it is relative to the amplitude of the largest MUP recorded during the scanning procedure (Stålberg & Diószeghy, 1991).

Measured length can be used as a lower bound to estimate the diameter of motor unit territories (Stålberg, 1986). It has to be noted that an actual estimation of the motor unit diameter is not feasible with this parameter, as it is not evident whether or not the recording has being done through a maximal arc of the motor unit territory bounds (Fig. 8). Statistically, the average measured length of the motor unit cross-section would be 87% of the true transverse motor unit diameter for territories with round cross-sections (Stålberg & Eriksson, 1987).

4.2.2 Number and length of silent areas

The number of silent areas (Stålberg, 1986) is defined as the number of areas within the length of a motor unit cross-section with amplitudes below 50 µV (Fig. 7). The length of the silent areas corresponds to the length measured over the cross-section of the corresponding silent areas (Stålberg and Diószeghy, 1991).

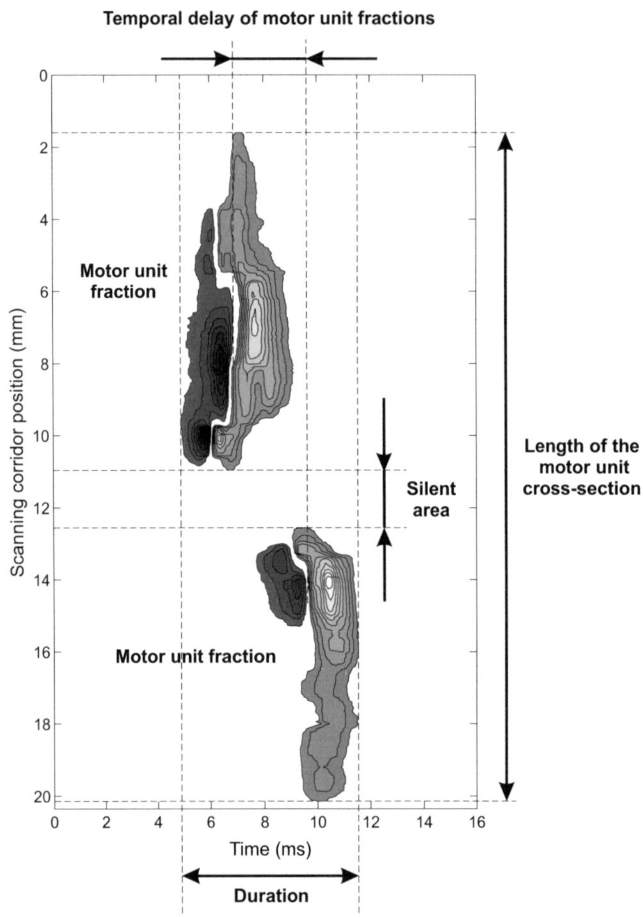

Fig. 7. Parameterisation of a scanning EMG signal after removing the signal content below the 50 μV threshold for the sake of clarity.

4.2.3 Number and length of fractions

The number of fractions (Stålberg, 1986) is defined as the number of areas within the length of a motor unit cross-section with amplitudes above 50 μV and either separated by silent areas or having clearly separated maxima along the time axis (Fig. 7). The length of the fractions corresponds to the length measured over the cross-section of the corresponding motor unit fractions (Navallas & Stålberg, 2009).

4.2.4 Number and length of polyphasic fractions

An MUP is defined a polyphasic or complex if it has more than 4 phases or more than 5 turns. Hence, the number of fractions containing polyphasic MUPs can be counted (Stålberg, 1986), and the overall length of these fractions can be measured (Stålberg & Diószeghy, 1991).

4.2.5 Temporal dispersion of fractions

The temporal dispersion of the motor unit fractions (or motor unit time dispersion) is defined as the latency difference between the earliest and latest MUP traces recorded within

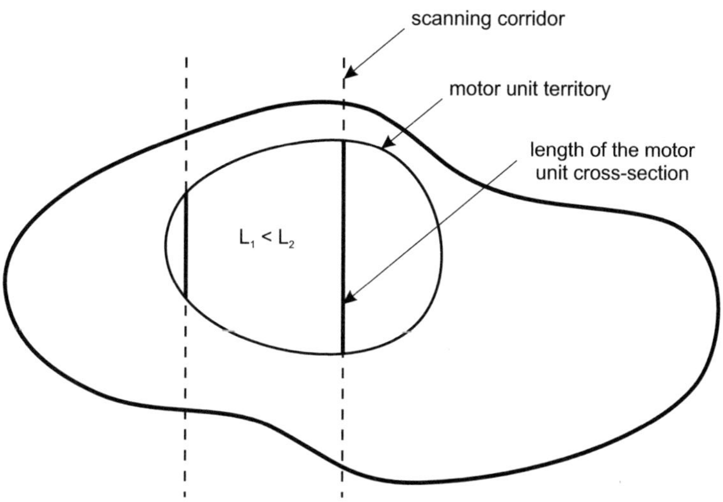

Fig. 8. An illustration of the problem regarding motor unit territory diameter estimation: how can we ensure that we are crossing a maximal arc?

a motor unit cross-section, where the latency of an MUP is measured at the steepest downward slope (Gootzen, 1990) or at the time point corresponding to 50% of the energy of the envelope signal (Navallas & Stålberg, 2009). Temporal dispersion measurements are slightly affected when the needle is not inserted orthogonally into the muscle fibres, which can produce up to 0.5 ms of error for a 20° angle deviation (Gootzen et al., 1992).
It is important not to confuse this parameter with the temporal dispersion of individual SFAPs contributing to MUPs when observed from a single point (Gootzen, 1990). Rather, this parameter gives information about the average temporal dispersion of groups of SFAPs contributing to different fractions, which reside in different parts of motor unit territories and are observed essentially from different locations throughout the scanning corridor (Navallas & Stålberg, 2009).

4.2.6 Depth of the motor unit territory

Although not a parameter of a scanning EMG signal, it is important to note that the depth of the motor unit territory under study can also be estimated using the scanning procedure. A stereotactic location system can be used to assess the location of the moving EMG needle relative to the internal tendinous boundaries within the muscle under study (Tonndorf, 1994) by combining magnetic resonance imaging, scanning needle electrode optical tracking, and stereotactic reconstruction.
Furthermore, by taking into account the beginning and ending positions of the scanning electrode and the number of steps taken for each trigger, the electrode location can be estimated. Using this information, the position of the motor unit can be defined as the position in the scans corresponding to a contribution of 50% of the signal within the length of the cross-section (Roeleveld et al., 1997a, 1997b). The position of the motor unit provides an estimation of the depth of the centre of the motor unit territory.

4.3 Findings in normal conditions

A limited number of muscle types has been investigated using scanning EMG, including the biceps brachii (Hilton-Brown & Stålberg, 1983a, 1983b; Stålberg & Diószeghy, 1991; Navallas

& Stålberg, 2009), the tibialis anterior (Hilton-Brown & Stålberg, 1983a, 1983b; Stålberg & Diószeghy, 1991), the masseter (Stålberg & Eriksson, 1987), and the quadriceps (Gootzen, 1990; Gootzen et al., 1992).

The length of the motor unit cross-section has been measured in normal conditions in various muscles. In the biceps brachii, the length of the motor unit cross-section has been reported as 6.0 ± 3.9 mm (mean ± SD) (Hilton-Brown & Stålberg, 1983a, 1983b), 4.64 ± 2.14 mm with a range of 1.69 to 10.17 mm (n=59) (Stålberg & Diószeghy, 1991), and 4.39 ± 2.29 mm with a range of 1.55 to 10.70 mm (Navallas & Stålberg, 2009). In the tibial anterior, the length has been reported as 7.9 ± 1.3 mm (Hilton-Brown & Stålberg, 1983a) and 5.26 ± 2.18 mm with a range of 1.53 to 10.33 mm (n=70) (Stålberg & Diószeghy, 1991). In the masseter, the length has been reported as 3.7 ± 0.6 mm with a range of 0.6 to 12.5 mm (Stålberg & Eriksson, 1987) and 3.7 ± 2.3 mm with a range of 0.4 to 13.1 mm (Tonndorf et al, 1994b). Finally, in the quadriceps, the length has been reported with a range of 2.0 to 8.0 mm (Gootzen, 1990; Gootzen et al., 1992).

As previously stated, motor unit fractions and silent areas, which are structural properties that can only be observed using scanning EMG, suggest that adjacent motor unit fibres have adjacent motor end-plates with a lower spatial dispersion than the overall muscle motor end-plate zone width (Navallas & Stålberg, 2009). Each fibre group would correspond to a distinct axonal branch reflecting a distinct motor unit fraction in a scanning EMG recording (Stålberg, 1986; Navallas & Stålberg, 2009).

The number of fractions and silent areas gives an indication of the degree of grouping or clustering of motor unit fibres in a normal muscle. The number of fractions generally ranges from 1 to 4 fractions per scan (Stålberg, 1986), although exact counts may vary among muscles. In the biceps brachii, 3.25 ± 1.49 (mean ± SD) fractions with the range of 1 to 6 fractions (Stålberg & Diószeghy, 1991) and 1.65 ± 1.02 fractions with a range of 1 to 5 fractions (Navallas & Stålberg, 2009) have been reported. In the tibialis anterior, 3.73 ± 1.74 fractions with a range of 1 to 8 fractions have been reported (Stålberg & Diószeghy, 1991). The number of silent areas has also been measured in the biceps brachii. A mean of 0.5 silent areas (Hilton-Brown & Stålberg, 1983b) and 0.15 ± 0.36 silent areas with a range of 0 to 1 (Stålberg & Diószeghy, 1991) have been reported. In the tibialis anterior, a mean of 0.2 silent areas (Hilton-Brown & Stålberg, 1983b) and 0.19 ± 0.47 silent areas with a range of 0 to 2 (Stålberg & Diószeghy, 1991) have been reported. The length of the individual motor unit fractions in the biceps brachii has been reported as 1.56 ± 1.07 mm with a range of 0.35 to 5.10 mm (Navallas & Stålberg, 2009).

Furthermore, temporal dispersion between fractions (see section 4.2.5) has provided valuable information about innervation patterns of motor units. The temporal dispersion measured in the biceps brachii has been reported as ranging from 0.5 to 5.0 ms (Gootzen, 1990) and 0.55 ± 0.98 ms with a range of 0.01 to 4.70 ms (Navallas & Stålberg, 2009). These temporal differences can be justified by assuming 1) a variation in the depolarisation delay in different fractions due to length differences among the innervating axonal branches and/or 2) different mean motor end-plate positions along the muscle fibres (Fig. 9) (Navallas & Stålberg, 2009).

The complexity of MUPs, measured in terms of the number of phases, number of turns, or irregularity coefficient, is a key feature used to distinguish normal conditions from pathology (Zalewska et al., 2004). In scanning EMG recordings from normal muscles, the complexity parameters of individual MUP traces extracted from a scan are within the range of values of conventional multi-MUP studies. The following complexity parameters of the

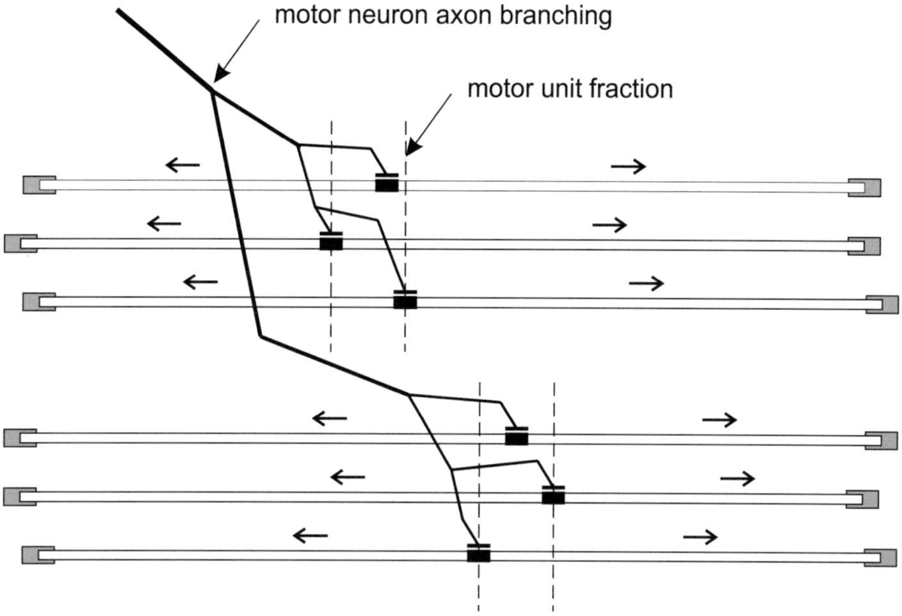

Fig. 9. The motor unit fractions hypothesis states that motor unit fractions are representing groups of motor unit fibres innervated by different axonal braches that may have a shifted motor end-plate location.

biceps brachii have been reported: a mean (± SD) of 3.26 ± 1.18 phases, a mean of 4.17 ± 1.87 turns, and an irregularity coefficient of 3.61 ± 0.82 (Navallas & Stålberg, 2009). The number of polyphasic fractions reported in the biceps brachii was 0.21 ± 0.41 with a range of 0 to 1 polyphasic sections (Stålberg & Diószeghy, 1991), and the number of polyphasic fractions reported in the tibialis anterior was 0.41 ± 0.58 with a range of 0 to 2 polyphasic sections (Stålberg & Diószeghy, 1991). Therefore, the proportion of polyphasic fractions, as the proportion of polyphasic MUPs in conventional quantitative EMG studies, is relatively low in normal conditions.

4.4 Findings in pathological conditions

In a study conducted with subjects suffering from a variety of neuropathies (including ALS, SMA, postpolio, polyneuropathy, and syringomyelia), the most relevant changes in scanning EMG recordings taken from the biceps brachii and the tibialis anterior were related to an increased complexity of motor units (Stålberg & Diószeghy, 1991). Specifically, the length of motor unit cross-sections and the number of fractions were slightly increased in both muscles, although only significant in the tibialis anterior. The number and length of silent areas were not significantly different from controls. Finally, the number and the length of polyphasic sections were significantly increased in both muscles.

These changes in scanning parameters are related to a reorganisation of motor units that occurs in neuropathies. Reorganisation is essentially due to reinnervation by collateral sprouting of surviving axons (Kugelberg et al., 1970). During reinnervation, collateral sprouts tend to be confined to the originally innervated fascicles, what derives in the observation of non increased motor unit cross-sections (Stålberg & Sanders, 1984). The increase in the number of motor unit fibres creates more compact and dense motor units;

therefore, the increase in motor unit fibres does not lead to a significant increase in silent areas or motor unit fractions (Diószeghy, 2002). However, reinnervation does cause an increase in fibre diameter variation and the dispersion of motor end-plates, which results in an increased waveform complexity throughout the region and an increased length and number of polyphasic fractions (Stålberg & Diószeghy, 1991).

Another study conducted with subjects suffering from various myopathies (including muscular dystrophies and polymyositis) found that the most relevant changes in scanning EMG recordings of the biceps brachii and the tibialis anterior were related to increased fractioning and an increased complexity of motor units (Stålberg & Diószeghy, 1991). The length of motor unit cross-sections was not significantly different from normal muscles. The number of fractions was significantly increased in both muscles. The length and number of silent areas was also significantly increased in both muscles, although more prominently in the tibialis anterior. Note that this significant change among myopathies is not identifiable using conventional EMG because, using this technique, an area with no activity cannot be ascribed to loss of muscle fibres within a given motor unit. Finally, the length and number of polyphasic sections was also significantly increased in both muscles. These results agree with previous findings in patients suffering from muscular dystrophy. The muscles of these patients showed no difference in the length of motor unit cross-sections but showed an increased number of silent areas and an increased variability in the amplitude profile and shape of scanning EMG recordings (Hilton-Brown & Stålberg, 1983a, 1983b).

Myopathic processes cause several structural changes, including fibre loss, fibre atrophy and hypertrophy, and fibre splitting (Hilton-Brown & Stålberg 1983a). Hence, an increased fibre grouping due to fibre splitting and an appearance of motor unit territories depleted of motor unit fibres explains the increased number of fractions and length and number of silent areas (Stålberg & Diószeghy, 1991; Diószeghy, 2002). The increased variability in fibre diameter due to hypertrophy and atrophy causes increased MUP complexity, which is observed as an increased length and number of the polyphasic fractions within scans (Diószeghy, 2002).

One study of juvenile myoclonic epilepsy (Gooker et al., 2009b, 2010) revealed that patients suffering from the disorder have enlarged motor unit territories compared to healthy subjects. The enlargement of motor units is not due to a reinnervation process but to a preponderance of genetically determined large lower motor units (Ertas et al., 1997).

Another study of both neuropathic and myopathic muscles (Gootzen, 1990; Gootzen et al., 1992) measured the length of motor unit cross-sections and the temporal dispersion of motor unit fractions in the biceps brachii. The results showed that scans from both patients and healthy subjects largely overlap with respect to the length of cross-sections. Both neuropathic and myopathic recordings showed an increased temporal dispersion of fractions. The temporal dispersion ranged from 0.5 ms to 6 ms in scans of healthy patients, 0.5 ms to 9 ms in scans of neuropathic patients, and 1 ms to 12.5 ms in scans of myopathic patients. Additionally, a strong positive correlation between the length of cross-sections and the temporal dispersion of the fractions was detected for the neuropathic group. Using these two parameters as a diagnostic tool, normal and pathological scans can be reliably separated, although parameters fail to distinguish between myopathy and neuropathy (Gootzen, 1990; Gootzen et al, 1992).

5. Future trends

The scanning EMG technique has evolved as a versatile and informative tool for the investigation of motor unit architecture. In combination with other EMG techniques, such as

fibre density measurements, a detailed description of motor units can be obtained using scanning EMG (Stålberg, 1986).
Further research should focus on extracting more information from the scanning signals. For example, the analysis of pathological signals suggests that parameters describing motor unit integrity, the complexity of motor end-plate zones or the variability in propagation velocities may soon be identified (Gootzen et al., 1992).
Several possible applications have been suggested in previous studies. Scanning EMG may be used to quantify the background activity of a muscle for a given degree of contraction to determine whether some regions account for many recruited motor units while others remain inactive (Stålberg, 1986). This could lead to studies relating functional compartmentalisation and recruitment strategies of muscles.
It has been also suggested that scanning EMG may be applied to verify volume conductor models by observing SFAPs (Gootzen, 1990), as scan recording profiles provide a reliable description of amplitude decay with distance. However, care must be taken to eliminate possible fibre movements to ensure there is no potential blocking.
In conclusion, scanning EMG is a valuable technique used in studies of motor unit anatomy and physiology and to study the structural and functional parameters in normal muscle and the changes that occur in pathology.

6. Acknowledgment

This work was supported by the Regional Health Ministry of the Government of Navarre under the project 1312/2010.

7. References

Amirali, A., Mu, L., Gracies, JM., & Simpson, DM. (2007) Anatomical localization of motor endplate bands in the human biceps brachii. *J Clin Neuromuscul Dis*, Vol. 9, No. 2, pp. 306-312.

Ansved, T., Wallner, P., & Larsson, L. (1991). Spatial distribution of motor unit fibres in fast- and slow-twitch rat muscles with special reference to age. *Acta Physiol Scand*, Vol. 143, No. 3, pp. 345-354.

Aquilonius, SM., Arvidsson, B., Askmark, H., & Gillberg, PG. (1982). Topographical localization of end-plates in cryosections of whole human biceps muscle. *Muscle Nerve*, Vol. 5, No. 5, pp. 418.

Bodine, SC., Garfinkel, A., Roy, RR., & Edgerton, VR. (1988). Spatial distribution of motor unit fibres in the cat soleus and tibialis anterior muscles: local interactions. *J Neurosci*, Vol. 8, No. 6, pp. 2142-2152.

Bodine-Fowler, S., Garfinkel, A., Roy, RR., & Edgerton, VR. (1990). Spatial distribution of muscle fibres within the territory of a motor unit. *Muscle Nerve*, Vol. 13, No. 12, pp. 1133-1145.

Buchthal, F., Erminio, F., & Rosenfalck, P. (1959). Motor unit territory in different human muscles. *Acta Physiol Scand*, Vol. 45, No. 1, pp. 72-87.

Buchthal, F., Guld, C., & Rosenfalck, P. (1957). Multielectrode study of the territory of a motor unit. *Acta Physiol Scand*, Vol. 39, No. 1, pp 83-104.

Burke, RE., Levine, DN., Salcman, M., Tsairis, P. (1974). Motor units in cat soleus muscle: physiological, histochemical and morphological characteristics. *J Physiol*, Vol. 238, No. 3, pp. 503-514.

Burke, RE., & Tsairis, P. (1973). Anatomy and innervation ratios in motor units of cat gastrocnemius. *J Physiol*, Vol. 234, No. 3, pp. 749-765.

Diószeghy, P. (2002). Scanning electromyography. *Muscle Nerve*, No. S11, pp. 66-71.

Edström, L., & Kugelberg, E. (1968). Histochemical composition, distribution of fibres and fatiguability of single motor units. Anterior tibial muscle of the rat. *J Neurol Neurosurg Psychiatry*, Vol. 31, No. 5, pp. 424-433.

Enoka, RM. (1995), Morphological features and activation patterns of motor units. *J Clin Neurophysiol*, Vol. 12, No. 6, pp. 538-559.

Ertas, M., Uludag, B., & Araç, N., Ertekin, C., & Stålberg E. (1997). A special kind of anterior horn cell involvement in juvenile myoclonic epilepsy demonstrated by macro electromyography. *Muscle Nerve*, Vol. 20, No. 2, pp. 148-152.

Feinstein, B., Lindegard, B., Nyman, E., & Wohlfart, G. (1955). Morphologic studies of motor units in normal human muscles. *Acta Anat (Basel)*, Vol. 23, No. 2, pp. 127-142.

Garnett, RAF., O'Donovan, MJ., Stephens, JA., & Taylor, A. (1979). Motor unit organization of human medial gastrocnemius. *J Physiol*, Vol. 287, pp. 33-43.

Gates, HJ., & Betz, WJ. (1993). Spatial distribution of muscle fibers in a lumbrical muscle of the rat. *Anat Rec*, Vol. 236, No. 2, pp. 381-389.

Gath, I., & Stålberg, E. (1979). Measurements of the uptake area of small-size electromyographic electrodes. *IEEE Trans Biomed Eng*, Vol. 26, No. 6, pp. 374-376.

Gath, I., & Stålberg, E. (1981). In situ measurement of the innervation ratio of motor units in human muscles. *Exp Brain Res*, Vol. 43, No. 3-4, pp. 377-382.

Gath, I., & Stålberg, E. (1982). On the measurement of fibre density in human muscles. *Electroencephalogr Clin Neurophysiol*, Vol. 54, No. 6, pp. 699-706.

Goker, I., Baslo, MB., Ertas, M., & Ulgen, Y. (2009a). Design of an experimental system for scanning electromyography method to investigate alterations of motor units in neurological disorders. *Digest Journal of Nanomaterials and Biostructures*, Vol. 4, No.1, pp. 133-139

Goker, I., Baslo, MB., Ertas, M., & Ulgen, Y. (2009b). Motor unit territories in juvenile myoclonic epilepsy patients. *Conf Proc IEEE Eng Med Biol Soc*, 2009, pp. 819-822.

Goker, I., Baslo, MB., Ertas, M., & Ulgen, Y. (2010). Large motor unit territories by scanning electromyography in patients with juvenile myoclonic epilepsy. *J Clin Neurophysiol*, Vol. 27, No. 3, pp. 212-215.

Gollnick, PD., Armstrong, RB., Saubert, CW., Sembrowich, WL., Shepherd, RE., & Saltin, B. (1973). Glycogen depletion patterns in human skeletal muscle fibers during prolonged work. *Pflugers Arch*, Vol. 344, No. 1, pp. 1-12.

Gootzen, TH. (1990). *Electrophysiological investigation of motor unit structure by means of scanning EMG*, University of Nijmegen, ISBN 90-9003335-1, Nijmegen.

Gootzen, TH., Vingerhoets, DJ., & Stegeman, DF. (1992). A study of motor unit structure by means of scanning EMG. *Muscle Nerve*, Vol. 15, No.3, pp. 349-357.

Hilton-Brown, P., & Stålberg, E. (1983a). The motor unit in muscular dystrophy, a single fibre EMG and scanning EMG study. *J Neurol Neurosurg Psychiatry*, Vol. 46, No. 11, pp. 981-995.

Hilton-Brown, P., & Stålberg, E. (1983b). Motor unit size in muscular dystrophy, a macro EMG and scanning EMG study. *J Neurol Neurosurg Psychiatry*, Vol. 46, No. 11, pp. 996-1005.

Kanda, K., & Hashizume, K. (1992). Factors causing difference in force output among motor units in the rat medial gastrocnemius muscle. *J Physiol,* Vol. 448, pp. 677-695.

Kugelberg, E., Edström, L., & Abbruzzese, M. (1970). Mapping of motor unit in experimentally reinnervated rat muscle. *J Neurol Neurosurg Psychiatry,* Vol. 197, No. 33, pp. 319-329.

Lieber, RL. (1992). *Skeletal Muscle Structure and Function: Implications for Rehabilitation and Sports Medicine* (1st ed.), Williams and Wilkins, ISBN 978-0683050264, London.

Lukács, M., Vécsei, L., & Beniczky, S. (2009). Fibre density of the motor units recruited at high and low force output. *Muscle Nerve,* Vol. 40, No. 1, pp. 112-114.

McComas, AJ., Fawcett, PR., Campbell, MJ., & Sica, RE. (1971). Electrophysiological estimation of the number of motor units within a human muscle. *J Neurol Neurosurg Psychiatry,* Vol. 34, No. 2, pp. 121-131.

Miller-Larsson, A. (1980). A model of spatial distribution of muscle fibres of a motor unit in normal human limb muscles. *Electromyogr Clin Neurophysiol,* Vol. 20, No. 4-5, pp. 281-298.

Monti, RJ., Roy, RR., & Edgerton, VR. (2001). Role of motor unit structure in defining function. *Muscle Nerve,* Vol. 24, No. 7, pp. 848-866.

Nandedkar, SD., Barkhaus, PE., Sanders, DB., & Stålberg, EV. (1988a). Analysis of amplitude and area of concentric needle EMG motor unit action potentials. *Electroencephalogr Clin Neurophysiol,* Vol. 69, No. 6, pp. 561-567.

Nandedkar, SD., Sanders, DB., Stålberg, EV., & Andreassen, S. (1988b). Simulation of concentric needle EMG motor unit action potentials. *Muscle Nerve,* Vol. 11, No. 2, pp. 151-159.

Nandedkar, SD., & Stålberg, E. (1983a). Simulation of single muscle fibre action potentials. *Med Biol Eng Comput,* Vol. 21, No. 2, pp. 158-165.

Nandedkar, SD., & Stålberg, E. (1983b). Simulation of macro EMG motor unit potentials. *Electroencephalogr Clin Neurophysiol,* Vol. 56, No. 1, pp. 52-62.

Navallas, J., & Stålberg, E. (2009). Studying motor end-plate topography by means of scanning electromyography. *Clin Neurophysiol,* Vol. 120, No. 7, pp. 1335-1341.

Pfeiffer, G., & Friede, RL. (1985). The localization of axon branchings in two muscle nerves of the rat. A contribution to motor unit topography. *Anat Embryol (Berl),* Vol. 172, No. 2, pp. 177-182.

Pfeiffer, G., & Kunze, K. (1992). Turn and phase counts of individual motor unit potentials: correlation and reliability. *Electroencephalogr Clin Neurophysiol.* Vol. 85, No. 3, pp. 161-165.

Rafuse, VF., & Gordon, T. (1996). Self-reinnervated cat medial gastrocnemius muscles. II. analysis of the mechanisms and significance of fiber type grouping in reinnervated muscles. *J Neurophysiol,* Vol. 75, No. 1, pp. 282-297.

Roeleveld, K., Stegeman, DF., Vingerhoets, HM., & Van Oosterom, A. (1997a). Motor unit potential contribution to surface electromyography. *Acta Physiol Scand,* Vol. 160, No. 2, pp. 175-183.

Roeleveld, K., Stegeman, DF., Vingerhoets, HM., & Van Oosterom, A. (1997b). The motor unit potential distribution over the skin surface and its use in estimating the motor unit location. *Acta Physiol Scand,* Vol. 161, No. 4, pp. 465-472.

Roy, RR., Garfinkel, A., Ounjian, M., Payne, J., Hirahara, A., Hsu, E., & Edgerton, VR. (1995). Three-dimensional structure of cat tibialis anterior motor units. *Muscle Nerve*, Vol. 18, No. 10, pp. 1187-1195.

Schwartz, MS., Stålberg, E., Schiller, HH., & Thiele, B. (1976). The reinnervated motor unit in man. A single fibre EMG multielectrode investigation. *J Neurol Sci*, Vol. 27, No. 3, pp. 303-312.

Stålberg, E. (1966). Propagation velocity in human muscle fibers in situ. *Acta Physiol Scand*, Suppl. 287, pp. 1-112.

Stålberg, E. (1980). Macro EMG, a new recording technique. *J Neurol Neurosurg Psychiatry*, Vol. 43, No. 6, pp. 475-482.

Stålberg, E. (1986). Single fibre EMG, macro EMG, and scanning EMG. New ways of looking at the motor unit. *CRC Crit Rev Clin Neurobiol*, Vol. 2, No. 2, pp. 125-167.

Stålberg, E., & Antoni, L. (1980). Electrophysiological cross section of the motor unit. *J Neurol Neurosurg Psychiatry*, Vol. 43, No. 6, pp. 469-474.

Stålberg, E., & Dioszeghy, P. (1991). Scanning EMG in normal muscle and in neuromuscular disorders. *Electroencephalogr Clin Neurophysiol*, Vol. 81, No. 6, pp. 403-416.

Stålberg, E., & Eriksson, PO. (1987). A scanning electromyographic study of the topography of human masseter single motor units. *Arch Oral Biol*, Vol. 32, No. 11, pp. 793-797.

Stålberg, E., & Fawcett, PR. (1982). Macro EMG in healthy subjects of different ages. *J Neurol Neurosurg Psychiatry*, Vol. 45, No. 10, pp. 870-878.

Stålberg, E., & Karlsson, L. (2001). Simulation of the normal concentric needle electromyogram by using a muscle model. *Clin Neurophysiol*, Vol. 112, No. 3, pp. 464-471.

Stålberg, E., & Sanders, DB. (1984). The motor unit in ALS studied with different neurophysiological techniques, In: *Research Progress in Motor Neurone Disease*, pp. 105-122, FC Rose (Ed), Pitman Books, London.

Stålberg, E., Schwartz, MS., Thiele, B., & Schiller, HH. (1976). The normal motor unit in man. A single fibre EMG multielectrode investigation. *J Neurol Sci*, Vol. 27, No. 3, pp. 291-301.

Sonoo, M., & Stålberg, E. (1993). The ability of MUP parameters to discriminate between normal and neurogenic MUPs in concentric EMG: analysis of the MUP "thickness" and the proposal of "size index". *Electroencephalogr Clin Neurophysiol*, Vol. 89, No. 5, pp. 291-303.

Tonndorf, ML., & Hannam, AG. (1994). Motor unit territory in relation to tendons in the human masseter muscle. *Muscle Nerve*, Vol. 17, No. 4, pp. 436-443.

Venema, HW. (1994). Motor unit innervation patterns and fiber type grouping. *Muscle Nerve*, Vol. 17, No. 3, pp. 360-362.

Weijs, WA., Jüch, PJ., Kwa, SH., & Korfage, JA. (1993). Motor unit territories and fiber types in rabbit masseter muscle. *J Dent Res*, Vol. 72, No. 11, pp. 1491-1498.

Willison, RG. (1964). Analysis of electrical activity in healthy and dystrophyic muscle in man. *J Neurol Neurosurg Psychiatry*, Vol. 27, No. 5, pp. 386-394.

Willison, RG. (1980). Arrangement of muscle fibers of a single motor unit in mammalian muscles. *Muscle Nerve*, Vol. 3, No. 4, pp. 360-361.

Zalewska, E., & Hausmanowa-Petrusewicz, I. (1995). Evaluation of MUAP shape irregularity--a new concept of quantification. *IEEE Trans Biomed Eng*, Vol. 42, No. 6, pp. 616-620.

Zalewska, E., Husmanova-Petrusewicz, I., & Stålberg, E. (2004). Modeling studies on irregular motor unit potentials. *Clin Neurophysiol*, Vol. 115, No. 1, pp. 543-556.

25

EMG PSD Measures in Orthodontic Appliances

Şükrü Okkesim[1], Tancan Uysal[2], Aslı Baysal[3] and Sadık Kara[1]
[1]*Fatih University, Institute of Biomedical Engineering, İstanbul*
[2]*İzmir Katip Çelebi University, Faculty of Dentistry, İzmir*
[3]*Kocaeli University, Faculty of Dentistry, Kocaeli*
Turkey

1. Introduction

The human body consists of different systems which include the nervous system, the cardiovascular system, the musculoskeletal system, etc. Each system performs some kind of vital task and carries on many physiological processes. For example, the primary functions of the musculoskeletal system can be summarized as generating forces, producing motion, moving substance within the body, providing stabilization, and generating heat. Physiological processes are multifaceted fact and most of them manifest themselves as signals that reflect their nature and activities. These types of signals may be hormonal, physical or electrical. The general name of the electrical signals taken from the related organ or physiologic process with invasive or non-invasive methods is called Biomedical Signals. This signal is normally a function of time and is definable in terms of its amplitude, frequency and phase (Rangayyan, 2002).
The electromyography (EMG) signal is a biomedical signal that detects the electrical potential generated by muscle cells when these cells contract, and also when the cells are at rest. Three types of muscle tissue can be identified. One of them is the skeletal muscle, and the others are the smooth muscle and the cardiac muscle. The EMG is applied to the study of skeletal muscle (Reaz et al., 2006).
Skeletal muscles are comprised by nearly parallel cells and the muscle fibers which constitute the contractile structural units. Muscle fibers are activated by the central nervous system through electrical signals transmitted by motoneurons. A single motoneuron together with the muscle fibers that it contacts is called a motor unit which is the smallest functional subdivision of the neuromuscular system (Moritani, et al. 2004) The central nervous system controls the activation of motor units to optimize the interaction between our body and the surrounding environment. When the motor units are activated by the central nervous system, they produce an action potential trains of the active motor units add together to generate the interference EMG signal.
Surface and needle electrodes have been used to detect EMG of muscles. Surface electrodes have been widely used to investigate neuromuscular functions because of their several advantages, for example, it is noninvasive, easy to adhere to the skin and to detect the total activities of the muscle and it was called Surface EMG (SEMG). Bu the real advantage of this technique is that it is more beneficial in studies, in which simultaneous movement of many muscles is examined in vast muscle groups. On the other hand, surface electrodes have disadvantages as well. Due to the broad area for receiving signals on respective muscle

bundle, signals received by surface electrodes may stem from proximal muscle groups. This situation leaves questions about the accuracy of records. Although a great deal of effort is spent to determine and characterize the effect of such artefacts, a technique of analysis that completely allays questions has not been developed yet (Cobbold, 1974).

SEMG has advantages and disadvantages; they are used widely for several issues. SEMG signals are used widely for diagnosis and to assess the treatment of some neuropathic, myopathic and neuromuscular junction diseases in the hospital and in research about biomechanics, sport medicine and rehabilitation ...etc.

Orthodontics is the branch of science dealing with teeth, jaw and face structure in terms of treatment of abnormalities/irregularities.

In orthodontics treatment performed with two different 'point of views'. One of them is the jaw orthopaedics in which the malposition of the jaws related to face or related to each other is corrected with special appliances. The other is called orthodontics and related with the correction of teeth. Generally patients are treated simultaneously with orthodontic and orthopaedic approaches.

Malocclusion is the general name of the orthodontic abnormalities arising from misalignment of teeth and incorrect relation between the upper and lower jaw and divided into Class I, II and III. Class II malocclusion is one of the most common orthodontic problems, and it is reported to constitute nearly one-third of all orthodontic disorders (Kraus, 1956 ; and Kleissen et al., 1998).

Class II malocclusions can be skeletal or dental. In skeletal Class II malocclusions the maxilla and the maxillary arch may be positioned anteriorly related to cranial base, the mandibula and the mandibular arch may be positioned posteriorly related to cranial base or the combination of these two factors. Treatment of Class II malocclusions achieved with orthopaedic and orthodontic approaches (Riedel, 1952; McNamara, 1981; Renfroe, 1948; Blair, 1954). Dental Class II malocclusions are arising from the increase in the inclination of upper incisor, crowding etc. As dental Class II malocclusion does not include skeletal problems, orthodontic corrections are sufficient for this type of malocclusions. The variability of Class II malocclusions cause to arise a lot of treatment options. Treatment options include non-oral or oral appliances, arch expansion mechanics and treatment with dental extractions (Proffit et al., 1998).

Non-oral appliances are one of the oldest treatment methods that are used widespread. The most common widespread non-oral appliance is headgear. As headgear can be used for steering or curbing the growth of upper jaw to the forward and downward (overbite), it can also be used for activating teeth in distal direction. Therefore, it can be said for this appliance that it has both orthopaedic and orthodontic effects. In addition to such advantages, the use of this appliance being difficult and the length of its service life diminish its chance for success. Additionally, the sight formed because of the appliance being placed upon the face and skull causes aesthetic considerations and for this reason, adaptation problems with patients come into existence. Non-oral appliances entail cooperation of patients given that they both pay attention to service life of apparatus and ignore the abovementioned disadvantages. Oral appliances were designed that do not entail cooperation with patients, increase his/her quality of life to be able to prevent this situation called patient cooperation (McNamara & Brudon, 2001; Hunter, 1967; Rogers, 1984).

The aim of treatment using oral appliances is to change the bone structure of the face and direction of development. Although oral appliances are designed to treat each type of malocclusion, they are most successful in the Class II malocclusion. Oral appliances can be divided three groups, called active, passive and functional (Basciftci et al., 2003).

Limiting maxillary growth, the possible development in mandibular position and its growth and the change in teeth position and muscle structure are the expected effects of functional appliances (Clark, 2002). In addition to that the use of functional appliance leads to alterations in tissues around teeth and mouth of patients, it was observed in conducted studies that it can restrict the growth of mid-face to forward, bring about a change in the location of the glenoid fossa and also changes that increase bone construction and destruction in the neuromuscular anatomy and function (Jena et al., 2006 ; Harvold, 1985 ; Pancherz, 1982 ; Birkeback et al., 1984)

Functional appliances are designed for the available pace of adaptive skeletal growth in people keeping the mandible forward (McNamara, 1981). Additionally, it produces a reciprocal effect between the maxillary and mandibular structures and the appliance itself by stimulating muscular and circulatory systems.

It is stated in the Orthodontic literature that Herbst and Twin-Block appliances are the most frequently used functional appliances. Both appliances are effective in correction of class II malocclusions (Lund & Sandler, 1998). In particular, the studies conducted in the last 10 years proved the effectiveness of Twin-Block appliance (Mills C & McCulloch, 1998).

Albeit the Twin-Block appliance is placed within the mouth, it is an appliance having unrestraint in fulfilling normal functions of mouth, at the same time providing higher level freedom in anterior and lateral movements in comparison with other appliances and that is used the whole day (Clark, 1982; Clark, 1988).

The Twin-Block appliance consisting of bite blocks and acrylic artificial palate pertaining to mandibular and maxillary bones was presented by Clark in 1970's. This appliance consists of sub and upper parts arriving to the contact point (junction) at a 70-degree angle. These parts provide stability in closing the jaw (Clark, 1982; Clark, 1988) (Figure 1.)

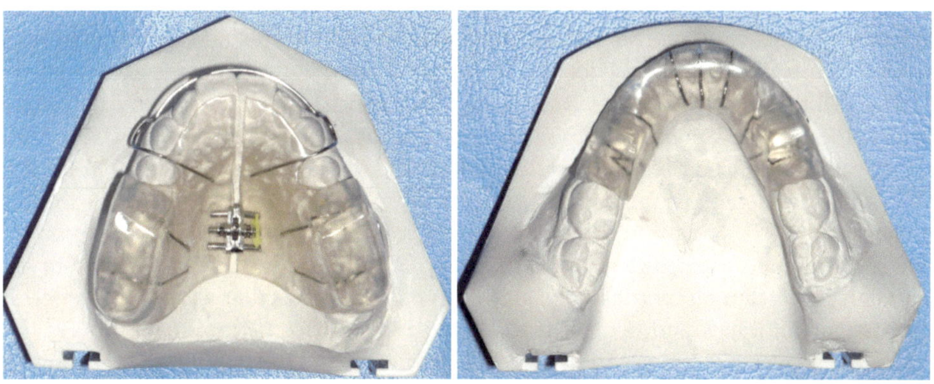

Fig. 1. Sub and Upper Parts of the Twin-block Appliance.

This appliance was preferred in our study owing to these advantages provided by the Twin-Block appliance and they being used incrementally by dentists in the last 10 years. Orthodontists are obliged to inform their patients about the different appliances, duration of treatment and about the possible changes in this period. For this aim, image of the skull is obtained; using X-ray or ultrasound techniques, thereafter jaw and teeth abnormalities are diagnosed. The name of this method is cephalometry (Figure 2). However, advantages of the appliances compared to one another and which one is more useful for one kind of abnormalities is determined by only experiences of Orthodontists.

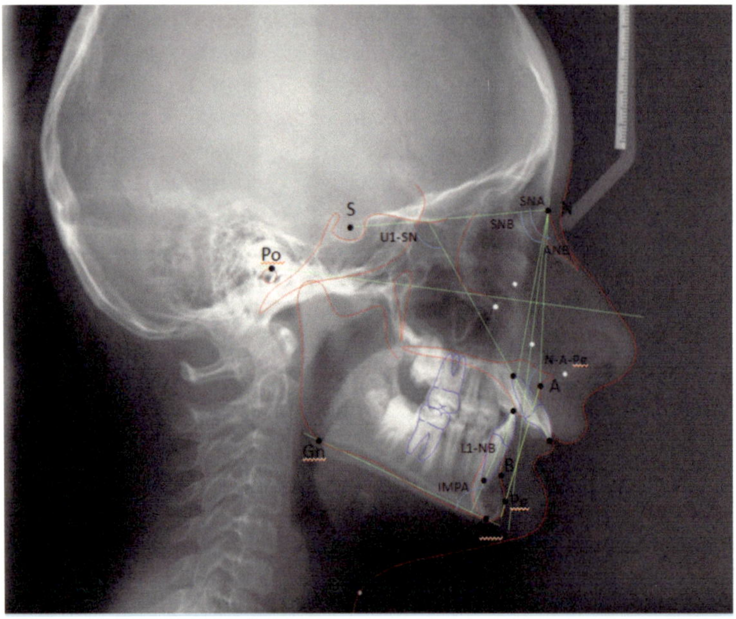

Fig. 2. Cephalometry image and some points of measurement.

Results taken from cephalometric records proved that functional appliances used in the treatment of malocclusion allay the abnormality in the mouth by affecting the alignment of teeth and bone tissue (Graber, 1985). Having said that, many different approaches/hypotheses are proposed regarding how neuromuscular periphery of teeth and bone tissue adapt to the change developed after treatment and the interaction between functional appliance and neuromuscular structure. Protraction in sizes of muscle fibers after the start of use of appliances (Woodside, 1983), the change in muscle dimensions caused by rotation of bone structure and hypertrophy of muscle structure can be given as examples to these hypotheses (McNamara, 1973).

One of the most important reasons for this difference between hypotheses is that there is no reliable and precise reference line in cephalometric image analysis used in evaluating treatment results. This situation complicates the assessment of significant changes occurring in skeletal and tooth structure (Pancherz, 1984). Additionally, it is impossible to obtain information about cephalometric image analysis and neuromuscular adaptation process and be informed about the changing muscle and bone structure during treatment process.

The principle objective of this study is to be able to put forth the interaction between functional appliances and neuromuscular structure with more scientific findings. If treatment can be assessed by quantitative data, as orthodontists can inform their patients about the issues such as treatment process, possible success ratio and etc. and also they can clearly decide which appliance is more suitable for patient as well. The electrophysiological signal that allows non-invasive assessment for changes in muscle structure is EMG. For these reasons, EMG studies continue with an increasing interest to find quantitative solutions such as problems and to measure of muscular activity changes because of the appliances.

In order to achieve this aim, we use EMG signals and their appropriate features to measure and evaluate Twin-Blok related muscular activity changes in Anterior Temporal and Masseter muscles in children with Class II malocclusion.

For this aim power spectral density (PSD) graphics were obtained using EMG and maximum power spectral density value (Max PSD) and area of the PSD graphics (Area PSD) were calculated and changes between before treatment and at the end of the six months were analyzed statistically. Furthermore, Cephalometric images were taken before treatment and at the end of six months and changes in the position with respect to base of the skull were measured to make a comparison.

1.1 Advancement of functional appliances

Albeit first trials were worthy of note, treatment with functional appliances progressed by Roux's studies pertaining to natural forces and functional stimulation. Subsequently, Rogers advocated functional treatment and associated facial muscles with the development and form of the masticatory system (Woodside, 1983).

In 1920's, Andreasen set out to use the appliance that he developed in Class II malocclusions. Emil Herbst introduced the Herbst appliance in 1905 and published findings in 1935. In 1970's, Pancerz's studies on the Herbst appliance and findings that he attained led to this appliance used by dentists more frequently. The advantages of the Herbst appliance are that it is fixed on teeth and treatment period is short. Many studies have been conducted on short and long term effects of the appliance (Pancherz, 1991;. Mcnamara & Fränkel, 2002; Pancherz & Fackel, 1990). Following the introduction of the Herbst appliance, different disadvantages caused the development of various appliances to be used in treatment of Class II malocclusion (Vogt, 2003; Awbrey, 1999). disadvantages experienced in treatment by the Herbst appliance can be summarized as that it is not hygienic, it is rigid and therefore, it restricts lateral movements of the mandible quite a lot (Pancherz, 1985). Another functional appliance similar to this appliance is the Jasper Jumper appliance. This appliance brings about food accumulation inside as well due to its structure. The Bite Fixer appliance was developed to be able to overcome such disadvantages. The Bite Fixer appliance is more flexible and does not allow food accumulation thanks to polyurethane tube situating inside but it was observed to cause open bite in the posterior area in some cases (open bite: occlusion not being able to materialize between the mandible and maxilla in the respective region) (Awbrey, 1999).

Inspired by a case in which the left gonial area disappeared, Bimler saw that mandible movements deliver force to the maxilla and the maxillary arch broadened. The Bimler appliance appeared in the literature in 1949 after many modifications since the day this study was conducted to the present day (Rogers, 1984).

Kesling presented the positioner appliance in 1944. In 1950, Balters began to modify the appliance that Andreasen developed and ensured via modifications he made that talking with this appliance is achieved in a more comfortable fashion (Pancherz et.al, 1989). In 1957, taking into account the structure of skeletal-muscular system that leads to structural and functional changes, Frankel designed his appliance (Proffit & Fields, 2000). Different than other functional appliances, the appliance he named as Kinetor and defined by Stockfish incorporates elastic tubes between two plaques and is considered to optimize oral muscle pressures.

2. Materials and methods

2.1 Measurement of surface EMG signals

EMG recordings were extracted from patients fitting Class II malocclusion criteria below, from the right anterior temporal and right masseter muscles of 15 patients whose ages varied 8 and 13. Treatments of patients, who fit the criteria, were launched via the Twin-Block appliance in the Department of Orthodontics of the Faculty of Dentistry in Erciyes University [Figure 3]. None of the participants underwent orthodontic treatment before. Before each recording session, the procedure was explained in detail to the patient and their parents to allay anxiety.

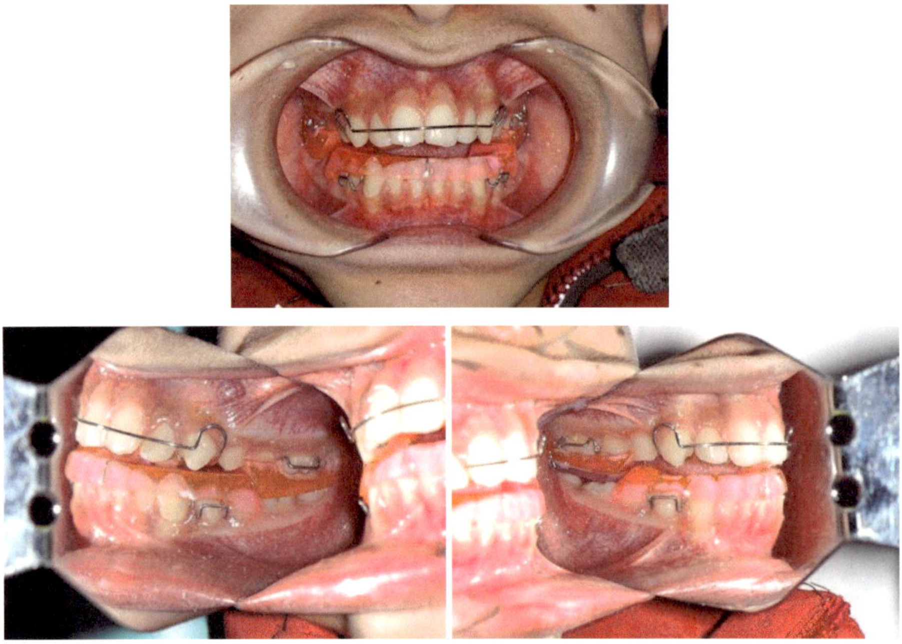

Fig. 3. Twin-block placement in situ.

Class II malocclusion criteria applied in our study:

Inclusion criteria

- Skeletal Class II relationship (ANB > 4°)
- Mandibular retrognathy (SNB < 78°)
- Overjet ≥ 5 mm
- Minimal crowding in dental arches (≤4 mm)
- Bilateral Class II molar and canine relation (at least 3.5 mm)

Exclusion criteria

- Previous history of orthodontic treatment
- Congenitally missing or extracted permanent tooth (except third molars)
- Posterior crossbites or severe maxillary transverse deficiency
- Severe facial asymmetry determined by clinical or radiographical examination
- Systemic diseases that may affect the orthodontic treatment results

Patients were asked to wash their faces with soap for face grease not to affect recordings and then recorded regions were wiped with alcohol and dried. Patients were suggested to sit up straight and look across while recordings were being kept. Electrodes were attached on the muscle bundles, which were found by palpating, by surgical plastic strips (adhesive washers) that do not irritate the skin. Filling silver-surfaced, bipolar electrodes with 4 mm. radius with electrode gel, they were sticked in a way that inter-electrode distance will be 2 cm. The common ground electrodes were adhered onto the forehead of the subject and the active electrodes were placed on the right anterior temporal and right masseter muscles as shown in Figure 4.

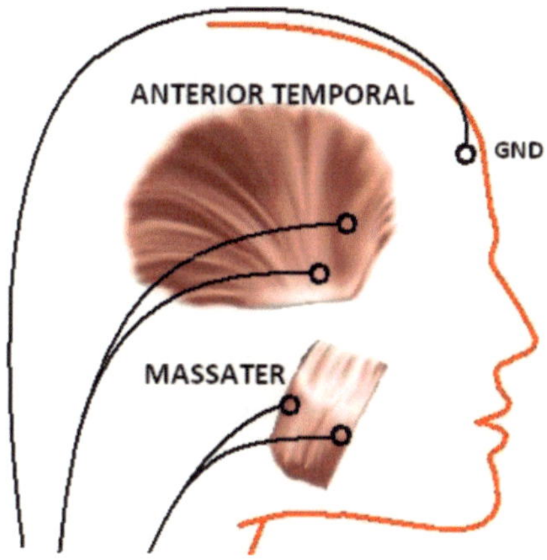

Fig. 4. Placement of surface electrodes on the anterior temporal and masseter muscles.

An important factor that affects recording quality is whether the spot where electrodes adhered and the region where muscle bundle is situated is the same. When the muscle, whose EMG recordings are sought to be taken, possesses a small area, electrodes also perceive signals coming from adjacent muscles and appear as noisy within EMG signals pertaining to the interested muscle bundle (Duchêne & Gouble 1993). Such noises can be avoided by selecting the electrode surface proportional with inter-electrode distance. The selection of appropriate electrode surface size and inter-electrode distance to be kept small diminishes the affect that will stem from the distance between electrode and source and shifts EMG bandwidth to high frequency region. Electrode diameter for bipolar recording should be as big as that can perceive muscle activity in acceptable amounts and at the same time as small as that does not pick activities of other muscles. Inter-electrode distance is described as the distance between the centres of conductive surfaces of electrodes. Inter-electrode distance recommended for bipolar recording is 20 mm (Pozzo, 2004).

Temporal and masseter muscles are muscles taking a part in the mandibular protrusion and EMG recording was extracted from these muscles considering that they may be effective in re-positioning of the mandible during treatment, ensure the mandibular growth and their adaptations may have an impact on treatment results. Mouth activity, in which these muscles play the most active role, is the jaw clenching. Therefore, recordings were taken during clenching activity. The movement was previously practiced by copying the observer.

The signals were recorded in two periods: before the treatment (0 month) and at the end of 6 months [Figure 5]. At each session, EMG recordings were made during the appliances is not in situ.

The MP150 biomedical data acquisition unit (Biopac Systems, Goleta, CA, USA) was used for recording signals. All of the signals were sampled at 5000 Hz and digitized (A/D converted) at a resolution of 12 bits per sample by the MP150 unit.

The EMG100C amplifier module of the MP150 unit was used to amplify and filter with the following settings: 500 Hz Low-Pass (LP) filter, 1.0 Hz High-Pass (HP) filter, and 2000 gain.

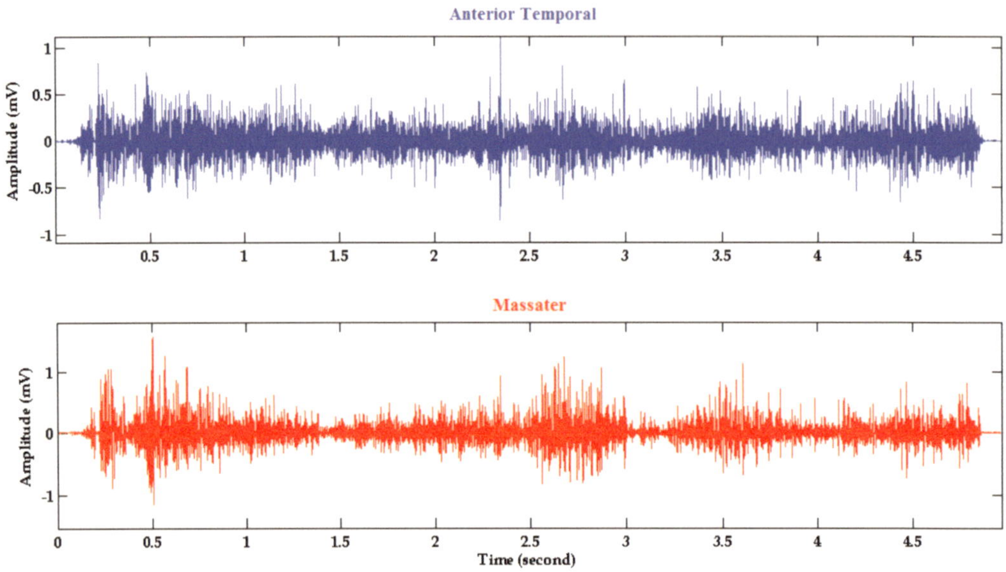

Fig. 5. Raw EMG Signals.

2.2 Analysis of surface EMG signals

There are two usual methods that have been used for the processing of EMG signals: frequency and time domain signal processing method. Some of the time domain signals processing methods are integration, linear envelope, and root mean square (RMS). However, these are are commonly not suitable, since obtained results depend on the selection of threshold [9].

The most powerful and generally used method for signal analysis in frequency domain had been the Fourier Transform (FT). FT is a method that assumes any signal is stationary. However, EMG signals are non-stationary (Panagiotacopulos, 1998)

Hence, the Fourier Transform cannot present satisfactory frequency resolution. In some respects, the Short Time Fourier Transform (STFT) is not perfectly suitable for processing of EMG signals. The main weakness inherent in the STFT is that trade off is inevitable between temporal and spectral resolution (Kim, 1989; Farina, 2004). If one uses a longer sliding time window to obtain higher spectral resolution, the underlying non-stationary will be smeared out, resulting in lower temporal resolution. Conversely, using a shorter window to achieve better temporal resolution will give lower spectral resolution. Because of these signal processing of the EMG signals were achieved using autoregressive (AR) model which is appropriate for non stationary signals and not having windowing problem (Kay, 1981). AR method is a parametric signal analysis method and first, model parameters of the available signal are estimated for such spectrum projection and then, the power spectral density value is calculated from these projection values (Kay, 1988). AR method is one of the most commonly used parametric methods owing to the fact that projection of AR parameters can be carried out easily with the resolution of linear equations. Signal that is modelled in AR method is causal.

The analysis conducted to demonstrate the distribution of power, which any physical signal that is carried to the frequency axis comprises, over frequency field is called as spectral analysis. In this way, graphs exhibiting the power density in frequency axis are denominated as the power spectral density (PSD) graph (Figure 6.).

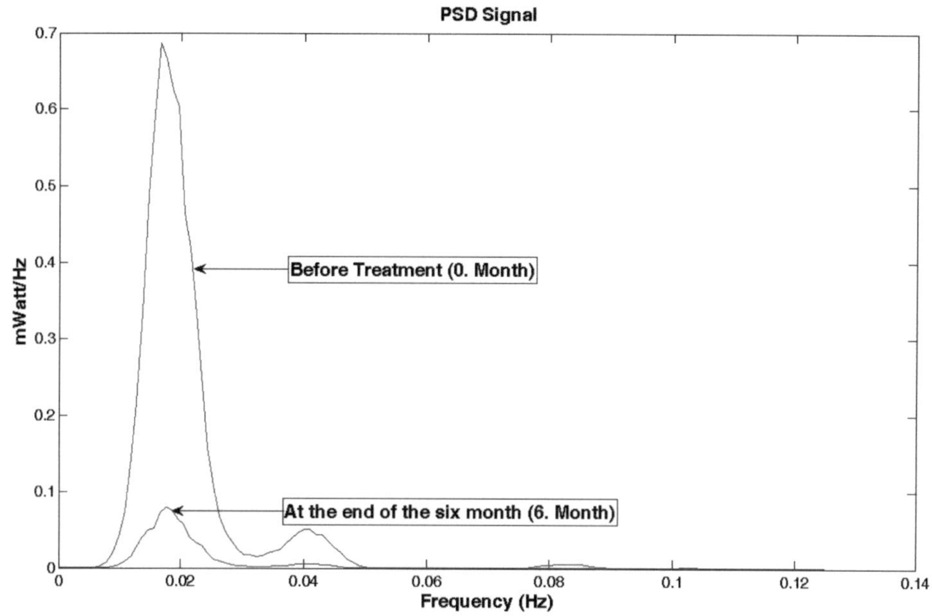

Fig. 6. The comparative display of PSD graphs calculated from EMG signals received at the end of the first and 6. Months.

EMG signal analysis that will be performed by addressing the power spectral density displaying the distribution of signal's energy capability in the frequency spectrum provides information about the neuromuscular conditions of motor units taking part during the activity (Okeson, 1998). The PSD values of EMG signals form as a result of the sum of spectral characteristics of action potentials of motor units. Consequently, it can be said that there is a characteristic power spectrum pertaining to every muscle (Blinowska, 1979). For these reasons, the PSD was used as a criterion in assessing the effect of appliance.

The maximum power spectral density value, which is a value of the PSD graph at its maximum point, varies by contraction density of motor units becoming active within that signal. The area below the PSD graph provides information about strain productivities of motor units carrying out contraction activity (Kwatny, 1970). Therefore maximum power spectral density value and area of the PSD graphics were calculated as a feature.

The AR model is a model revealing important informations in signal by using signal information in the past. It is employed widespread in biomedical signal processing because it responds well against noise. The dependence of past values to the future values is defined as autocorrelation function.

$$\Gamma_{xx}(k) = \frac{1}{N}\sum_{n=1}^{N-k} x[n]x[n+k] \quad (1)$$

where $\Gamma_{xx}[k]$ displays the signal's sample, which is shifted as much as k, and its autocorrelation. The AR model;

$$x[n] = \sum_{i=1}^{p} a_i x[n-i] + \varepsilon[n] \quad (2)$$

$x[n]$ shows the current value of time series, $a_1, \ldots, a_p$ displays the AR model parameters, which are weighting coefficients, and p is the model degree showing the number of past values that will be used to estimate the current value and $\varepsilon[n]$ displays the approximate error with 1 scale.
By using the AR method, the power spectrum is attained as;

$$P_{xx}^{AR}(f) = \frac{q_e^2}{\left|1 - \sum_{i=1}^{p} a_i e^{-j2\pi fi}\right|} \quad (3)$$

Where q_e^2, is the variance of $\varepsilon[n]$ error.
To calculate the AR parameters, whether numerical signal samples, whose spectral analysis will be directly conducted, are employed or autocorrelation function pertaining to these signal parameters is used. The Burg method was used for estimating the AR parameters (Marple, 1987).
One of the significant issues for employing the AR method is the selection of model degree. Many researchers studied on this problem and the Akaike Information Criteria (AIC) introduced by Akaike is used most commonly in the literature (Kaluzynski, 1989). The selection of AIC model degree is in the form of making the below statement minimum.

$$AIC(p) = \ln \sigma_{wp}^2 + 2p/N \quad (4)$$

Here, σ_{wp}^2 is the estimated variance of linear prediction error and N is the data length. σ_{wp}^2 decreases with the increase of the AR model degree and therefore, $\ln\sigma_{wp}^2$ decreases as well. That being said, 2p/N increases too with the increase of p. In this case, a minimum value should be designated for p (Kay, 1988; Kaluzynski, 1989). The p value calculated via the AIC criteria was obtained as 12.
In order to take the fact that measurements were obtained from the same subjects into account, we used paired sample t-test for statistical comparison between 0 month and 6 months. A p-value of less than 0.05 was considered as statistically significant.
All of the data processing was carried out using in-house programs developed under MATLAB R2009b Software (MathWorks Inc., Natick MA, USA).

3. Results and discussion

The aim of present study is to use EMG signals and their appropriate features to measure and evaluate Twin-Blok related muscular activity changes in Anterior Temporal and Masseter muscles in children with Class II malocclusion.
For this aim power spectral density (PSD) graphics were obtained using EMG and Max PSD and Area PSD were calculated and changes between before treatment and at the end of the six months were analyzed statistically. Furthermore, Cephalometric images were taken before treatment and at the end of six months and changes in the position with respect to base of the skull were measured to make a comparison.

Subject	Anterior Temporal			
	Before the Treatment		**At the end of 6 months**	
	Max PSD	Area PSD	Max PSD	Area PSD
1	0,00015	0,01137	0,00001	0,00109
2	0,00009	0,00638	0,00001	0,00101
3	0,00028	0,02380	0,00001	0,00076
4	0,00031	0,02548	0,00002	0,00128
5	0,00008	0,00492	0,00001	0,00072
6	0,00033	0,02871	0,00001	0,00049
7	0,00011	0,00956	0,00011	0,00811
8	0,00015	0,01323	0,00009	0,00549
9	0,00023	0,01278	0,00012	0,00668
10	0,00048	0,02936	0,00005	0,00217
11	0,00054	0,03590	0,00000	0,00006
12	0,00026	0,02064	0,00001	0,00106
13	0,00003	0,00250	0,00001	0,00047
14	0,00032	0,01215	0,00004	0,00259
15	0,00027	0,01883	0,00001	0,00062
Mean±SEM	0,00024±0,00004	0,01704±0,00258	0,00003±0,00001	0,00217±0,00065

Table 1. Max PSD and Area PSD values calculated from EMG signals received right before placing the Twin Block appliance in the mouth over anterior temporal muscle and after 6 months treatment.

The mean values of Max PSD and Area PSD values, calculated from EMG signals for each patient, appear in the last lines of tables. The abbreviation SEM in the tables refers to "standard error of the mean."

Subject	Massater			
	Before the Treatment		**At the end of 6 months**	
	Max PSD	Area PSD	Max PSD	Area PSD
1	0,00012	0,01055	0,00017	0,01362
2	0,00014	0,00997	0,00001	0,00018
3	0,00011	0,01032	0,00001	0,00018
4	0,00006	0,00593	0,00004	0,00327
5	0,00007	0,00565	0,00015	0,01131
6	0,00035	0,02834	0,00031	0,02579
7	0,00011	0,01028	0,00073	0,06498
8	0,00002	0,00148	0,00007	0,00557
9	0,00083	0,05027	0,00037	0,02382

Subject	Massater			
	Before the Treatment		**At the end of 6 months**	
	Max PSD	Area PSD	Max PSD	Area PSD
10	0,00012	0,00925	0,00001	0,00088
11	0,00015	0,01340	0,00001	0,00035
12	0,00016	0,01464	0,00012	0,00843
13	0,00012	0,00945	0,00018	0,01456
14	0,00032	0,02377	0,00003	0,00270
15	0,00006	0,00497	0,00002	0,00046
Mean±SEM	0,00018±0,00005	0,01388±0,00315	0,00015±0,00005	0,01174±0,00438

Table 2. Max PSD and Area PSD values calculated from EMG signals received right before placing the Twin Block appliance in the mouth over masseter muscle and after 6 months treatment.

Before the treatment values (0. month) are greater for both the anterior temporal and masseter muscles, as seen in Table 1 and 2. However, the difference between 0. month and 6 months values more pronounced for anterior temporal. This difference is statistically significant for both features for anterior temporal but there was no significant difference for the masseter muscle (Table 3).
In addition, changes in the position with respect to base of the skull are significant (p: 0.001).

	Max PSD	Area PSD
Anterior Temporal	**0.00014**	**0.00012**
Masseter	0.5689	0.65591

Table 3. p-values for "across treatment time" comparisons.

These observations are in-line with the results in the literature that "as a consequence of the use of functional appliances the length of the muscles around the jaw gets longer" (Du & Hägg, 2003).
The PSD values of the EMG signals are depending on the power of the motor unit action potentials which makes up these EMG signals (Blinowska, 1979). Six-month-long treatment leads to a decrease in the amplitude and narrowing in the frequency range of motor unit action potentials and so PSD.
Looking at results obtained for anterior temporal muscle, it is seen that there is a significant difference between the onset of treatment and its values after 6 months for both attributes. This result is not valid for the masseter muscle. Albeit both muscles lie among jaw-closing muscles, the Twin-Block Appliance had a different impact.
It is known that the lower jaws of the people who have Class II malocclusion is placed behind their upper jaws. Twin Block appliances tries to keep lower jaw and upper jaw in the same position due to the fact that lower palate and upper palate have a contiguous structure. This can only be accomplished by forcing the lower jaw through forward. In this case, length of the jaw closing muscles must be changed so that the new position of the jaw becomes permanent. For that reason, it is a natural result for jaw closing muscles to clench

with lower power density after 6 months. This result is matching the when the functional appliances is placed in the mouth, the jaw closing muscles become elongated ((Du & Hägg, 2003; Miles et al., 1986; Woodside et al., 1983). Hence, the brawn of the jaw closing muscles reduces and the PSD values tend to decrease to lower amplitude.

However, this outcome was not realized for the masseter muscle. Therefore, it can be inferred that the effect of the Twin-Block Appliance on the masseter muscle did not come into existence in the first 6 months.

The critical objective of treatment by the Twin -Block appliance is to trigger the formation of an additional extension on jawbone. This objective can be achieved by increasing the development of cartilage belonging to condyle and also restricting the maxillary growth. The change also seen in the sizes of proximal muscles as a result of elongation of jawbone particularly reflected to EMG signals extracted for anterior temporal muscle. The reason why a similar difference did not form on the masseter muscle can be explained by that a position shift materialized on jawbone rather than an actual growth. Likewise, in studies carried out on Twin-Block treatment, it is seen that the question whether the observed change is an actual growth or a position shift has been debated. (Baccetti et. al. 2000; Trenouth, 2000). Additionally, it is observed that posterior teeth do not still contact one another when the appliance is removed at the end of 6 months in patients treated by the Twin-Block. This case brings about more intensive occlusion of anterior teeth of patients and further contraction on front fibers of the masseter muscle. This impact hinders the occurrence of adaptation coming into being in masseter muscles in EMG recordings received during jaw closing/ constriction.

The patient must be observed in a longer period in order to follow the consequences which will be resulted from this condition.

4. Conclusion

The use of EMG signals in studies related to face muscles continues with an increasing interest. Muscle structure responsible for masticatory function and soft tissue belonging to face does not only affect bone development but also affects the period of orthodontic treatments and permanency of success achieved after treatment. EMG is a primary instrument to record this functional process and for the effect of skull traction. For these reasons, analysis of non-invasive EMG by appropriate methods can provide further information regarding the effect of treatment and service lives of appliances (Eckardt et al. 1997).

In the literature, there are some EMG studies that they are based one removable appliances. However, these kinds of appliances are worn only during night time (Tallgren et al. 1998; Ahlgren , 1960). Hence, the appliances act as a splint rather than an activator. On the other hand, the functional appliances that are worn full-time like the Twin-Block stimulate greater than those worn only part-time. For that reason, this study which is about the EMG and the Twin-Block, is important in order to investigate the muscle response.

The PSD is the feature regularly used for frequency domain analysis of EMG. An integration of the PSD over all frequencies yields the entire power. PSD value was chosen as a feature in order to evaluate the effects of the appliances. That's because PSD value is a parameter which is frequently used in the evaluation of the EMG signals and it gives information on power of total action potential formed by the muscles during tightening.

EMG and PSD are quite successful in showing the change occurred in the muscles. However, criteria must be determined for different age groups in using different trainers.

Moreover, if an expert system, which evaluates the functionality of the orthodontic appliances for the orthodontists; which estimates the treatment period; and which enables a follow-up for the effect of the applied orthodontic appliances on the person, is desired to be developed with artificial intelligence applications, PSD attribution will be insufficient for the input value. For that reason, orthodontists and engineers must enable different parameters to become evaluable by continuing their interdisciplinary studies.

5. Acknowledgment

The authors are grateful for the grant support provided by The Scientific & Technological Research Council of Turkey - TÜBİTAK, contract number 106E144.

6. References

Rangayyan R. M., (2002). Introduction to Biomedical Signals, In: *Biomedical Signal Analysis: A Case-Study Approach*, Akay, M., (Ed),. pp. 1-14, Wiley-IEEE Press, ISBN 0-471-20811-6, New York

Reaz, M. B. I., Hussain M. S., Mohd-Yasin F., (2006). Techniques of EMG signal analysis: detection, processing, classification and applications. *Biological Procedures Online* Vol.8, No. 1, pp. 11 - 35.

Moritani, T., Stegeman, D., Merletti R., (2004). Basic physiology and biophysics of EMG signal generation . In: *Electromyography: Physiology, Engineering, and Non-Invasive Applications*, Merletti, R., Parker, P. (Eds), pp. 1 - 26, Wiley-IEEE Pres,

Cobbold, R. S. C., Transducers for Biomedical Measurements: Principles and Applications, John Wiley & Sons, Inc., New York, (1974).

Kraus F., (1956) Vestibular and oral screens. Trans Eur Orthod Soc.; 32: 217–224

Kleissen R.F., Buurke J.H., Harlaar J., Zilvold G., Electromyography in the biomechanical analysis of human movement and it clinical application, Gait Posture, 8, 143–158, (1998).

Riedel R. A., The relation of maxillary structures to cranium in malocclusion and normal occlusion. Angle Orthod;22:142-145, (1952).

McNamara J. A. Components of Class II malocclusion in children 8-10 years of age. Angle Orthod.; 51:177-202 (1981).

Renfroe EW. A study of the facial patterns associated with Class I, Class II division 1 and Class II, division 2 malocclusions Angle Orthod;19:12-15, (1948).

Blair E.S. A cephalometric roentgenographic appraisal of the skeletal morphology of Class I, Class II, division 1 and Class II, division 2 malocclusion. Angle Orthod.;24:106-119, (1954).

Proffit W. R., Fields H. W., Moray L. J., Prevelance of malocclusion and orthodontic treatment need in the United States: estimates from the N-HANES III survey Int. J. Adult Orthod. Orthog. Surg.;13:97-106 (1998).

McNamara JA Jr. Brudon WL. Orthodontics and dentofacial orthopedics. Ann Arbor: Needham Pres;:67-80 (2001).

Hunter W. S., The vertical dimensions of the face and skeletodental retrognatizm. Am J Orthod; 53:586-595, (1967).

Rogers A. Concepts of functional jaw orthopedics. In: Graber TM, Neumann B, editors. Removable orthodontic appliances. 2nd ed. Philadelphia: Saunders;. p. 87. (1984).

Basciftci F. A., Uysal T, Büyükerkmen A, Sarı Z. (2003) "The effects of activator treatment on the craniofacial structure of Class II division 1 patients". Eur J Orthod.;25:87–93.
Clark WJ. Twin block functional theraphy applications in dentofacial orthopedics. 2nd ed. Mosby-Wolfe Press, St Louis (2002).
Jena AK, Duggal R, Parkashc H. Skeletal and dentoalveolar effects of Twinblock and bionator appliances in the treatment of Class II malocclusion: A comparative study. Am. J. Orthod. Dentofacial Orthop. 130:594-602, (2006).
Harvold EP. Bone remodelling and orthodontics. Eur J Orthod;7:217-230, (1985).
Pancherz H. The mechanism of Class II correction in Herbst appliance treatment. A cephalometric investigation. Am J Orthod;82:104-113, (1982).
Birkeback L, Melsen B, Terp S. A laminographic study of the alterations in the temporomandibular joint following activator treatment Eur J Orthod;6:267-276, (1984).
Lund D. L., Sandler P.J., The effects of Twin Blocks: a prospective controlled study. Am J Orthod Dentofacial Orthop;113: 104-10, (1998).
Mills C, McCulloch K. Treatment effects of the Twin-block appliance: a cephalometric study. Am J Orthod 1998;114:15-24.
Toth LR, McNamara JA, Jr. Skeletal and dentoalveolar adaptations produced by Twin-block appliance treatment. AmJ Orthod Dentofacial Orthop 1999;116:597-609.
Clark WJ. The Twin-block traction technique. Eur J Orthod 1982;4:129-38.
Clark WJ. The Twin-block technique. Am J Orthod Dentofacial Orthop 1988;93:1-18.
Graber TM, Rakosi T, Petrovic AG. "Dentofacial orthopedics with functional appliances". St Louis: CV Mosby; 1985.
Graber TM. Physiologic principles of functional appliances. St Louis: CV Mosby; 1985
Woodside DG, Altuna G, Harvold E, Herbert M, Metaxas A. Primate experiments in malocclusion and bone induction. Am J Orthod 1983;83:460-8.
McNamara Jr JA. Neuromuscular and skeletal adaptations to altered function in the orofacial region. Am J Orthod 1973;64:578-606.
Pancherz H. A Cephalometric analysis of skeletal and dental changes contributing to Class II correction in activator treatment. Am J Orthod 1984;85:125-34.
Pancherz H., The nature of Class II relapse after Herbst appliance treatment: a cephalometric long-term investigation. Am J Orthod Dentofacial Orthop;100:220-33, (1991).
Mcnamara JA Jr. Rolf Fränkel, 1908-2001 (in memoriam). Am. J. Orthod. Dentofacial Orthop.;121:238-9 (2002).
Pancherz H, Fackel U. The skeletofacial growth pattern pre- and post-dentofacial orthopaedics. A long-term study of Class II malocclusions treated with the Herbst appliance. Eur J Orthod;12:209-18, (1990).
Vogt W. A new fixed interarch device for Class II correction, J. Clin. Orthod. 2003;37:36-41
Awbrey J.J. The Bite-Fixer, Clinical Impressions, Ormco/A Company. 1999;8:10-16.
Pancherz H. The Herbst appliance. Its biologic effects and clinical use, Am. J. Orthod. 1985;87:1-20
Pancherz H., Malmgren O, Ha¨gg U, Omblus J, Hansen K. Class II correction in Herbst and Bass therapy. Eur J Orthod;11:17-30, (1989).
Proffit WR, Fields HW, editors. Contemporary orthodontics. 3rd ed. St Louis: Mosby; (2000).
Duchêne J. and Gouble F. Surface electromyogram during voluntary contraction: Processing tools and relation to physiological events. Critical Reviews in Biomedical Engineering 21(4): 313–397, (1993).

Pozzo M., Farina D., Merletti R., Electromyography:Detection, Processing and Applications Biomedical Technology and Devices Handbook, CRC press, 2004.
Panagiotacopulos N. D., J. S. Lee, M. H. Pope, K. Friesen, (1998) Evaluation of EMG signals from rehabilitated patients with low back pain using wavelets. J. of Electromyog. and Kinesiology, vol. 8, pp. 269 - 278,.
Kim, R. B. Hanson, T. L. Abell, and J. R. Malagelada. (1989) Effect of inhibition of prostaglandin synthesis on epinephrine-induced gastroduodenal electromechanical changes in humans. Mayo Clinic Proc. 64:149–157,.
Farina D., R. Merletti, D. F. Stegeman, (2004) Biophysics of the generation of EMG signals. In: Electromyography: Physiology, Engineering, and Non-Invasive Applications, New York, Wiley-IEEE Pres. , pp. 81 - 107.
Kay, S.M. , and Marple, S.L., (1981) Spectrum Analysis—A Modern Perspective, Proceedings of IEEE Transactions 69(11):1380–1419.
Kay S.M., Modern Spectral Estimation: Theory and Application. Prentice Hall-Englewood Cliffs, NJ, (1988).
Okeson J. P.,: "Management of Temporomandibular disorders and occlusion", Mosby, St. Louis Fourth edition (1998), pp:160-162.
Blinowska, A., Verroust, J., Cannet, G., "The Determination of motor unit characteristics from the low frequency electromyographic power spectra". Electromyography and Clinical Neurophysiology, 19, 281 - 290, (1979).
Kwatny, E., Thomas, D., Kwatng, H., (1970). An application of signal processing techniques to the study of myoelectric signals. IEEE Transactions on Biomedical Engineering 17, 303 - 312.
Marple S.L., Digital Spectral Analysis with Applications. Prentice Hall-Englewood Cliffs, NJ, 1987.
Kaluzynski K., Order Selection in Doppler Blood Flow Signal Spectral Analysis Using Autoregressive Modelling, Medical & Biological Engineering & Computing, 27, 89-92, (1989).
Du X., Hägg U. "Muscular adaptation to gradual advancement of the mandible". Angle Orthod., vol. 73, pp. 525 - 531, (2003).
Miles T. S., Nordstrom M. A., Turker K. S., "Length - related changes in activation threshold and waveform of motor units in human massater muscle", Journal of Physiology (London) vol. 370, pp. 457 - 465, (1986).
Baccetti T. et al. Treatment timing for Twin-block therapy. Am J Orthod dentofacial Orhop 2000;118:159-70.
Trenouth M. Cephalometric evaluation of the Twin block appliance in the treatment of Class II Division 1 malocclusion with matched normative growth data. Am J Orthod Dentofacial Orthop 2000;117:54-59.
Eckardt, L., Harzer, W., Schneevoigt, R., 1997. Comparative study of excitation patterns in the masseter muscle before and after orthognathic surgery. Journal of Cranio-Maxillojacial Surgery 25, 344-352
Tallgren, A., Christiansen, R., Ash, M. M., Miller, R. L., (1998) Effects of a myofunctional appliance on orofacial muscle activity and structures. Angle Orthodontists. 3, 249–258.
Ahlgren J., (1960) An Electromyographic analysis of the response to activator therapy. Odontol Revy 11, 125.

26

New Measurement Techniques of Surface Electromyographic Signals in Rest Position for Application in the Ophthalmological Field

Edoardo Fiorucci, Fabrizio Ciancetta and Annalisa Monaco
Università dell'Aquila,
Italy

1. Introduction

The Stomatognatic apparatus is a component of the craniomandibular system, and it represents an entryway to external stimuli: relationship among occlusion, masticatory muscle system (Murch, 1974; Oddsson, 1989) and head posture (Barber & Sharpe, 1988) have been recently confirmed.

Proprioception messages from the neck muscles are integrated in the central nervous system and contribute to control balance and body orientation. Centripetal impulses from neck proprioceptors cooperate with the labyrinth impulses to promote oculomotor muscular activity through the cervical–vestibular–ocular reflex (Ito, 1995). Some important encephalic nuclei (trigeminal nuclei, oculomotor nuclei, vestibular nuclei, accessorial nerve nuclei) are integrated in the medial longitudinal fasciculus.

Ocular proprioceptive receptors send afferent signals to trigeminal and cuneate nuclei. The anatomic and physiologic links of these anatomical structures imply a co-ordinated integration of proprioceptive ocular and stomatognathic afferences.

The ocular system and the stomatognathic one are anatomically and physiologically connected. Vision plays an important role in the multi-sensorial process of postural stabilisation: among visual inputs, the postural one allows to draw a moving object ocular nuclei control the eye position in the orbit; the ocular nuclei send fibers to nuclei which control neck and head movements and receive afferences from vestibular nuclei.

It has been observed that a modification of ocular proprioception modifies head and body posture (Donaldson & Knox, 1991; Buisseret-Delmas & Buisseret, 1990; Schmid et al., 1981).

Ocular proprioception is linked with stomatognathic muscular system: neuromuscular spindles and myotendinous receptors (Rose et al., 1991; Lukas et al., 1994; Rose & Abrahams, 1975) of extraocular muscles send afferences to trigeminal and cuneate nuclei (Porter, 1986). Moreover oculomotor, vestibular, trigeminal and accessorial nerve nuclei are connected through the medial longitudinal fasciculus. The role of trigeminal afferences on tonic-postural regulation has been underlined too (Meyer & Baron, 1976)

Several studies supported anatomical linkage between stomatognathic and ocular systems. Patients with Temporomandibular disorders (TMD) and this prevalence increase in those patients with head, neck, and shoulder pain. A similar association has been found in children with a mandibular functional lateral-deviation respect to healthy subjects in pediatric age. It is also stated that in TMD subjects, head rotation (as a compensatory adjustment for the eye dominance) is significantly associated to a mandibular shifting toward the contralateral side. These relationships, recorded by measuring transverse head postural change by means of temporary eye dominance change, have been confirmed (Lin SY & White, 1996). Passive soft-tissue viscoelasticity and stretch reflexes in the jaw-closing muscles are involved in mandibular postural stability during locomotion as a consequence of the influence of head support and body posture on the mandibular rest position. Relationship between oculomotors and neck cephalogyric muscles have been reported by Meyer & Baron, 1976. These authors showed that desmodontal receptors and temporo-mandibular joint, like sternocleidomatoid, trapezius and cervical muscles are connected with oculomotor muscles. A study confirmed that the alteration of dental occlusion can induce some fluctuations in visual focusing (Sharifi et al., 1998)

Electromyography has been widely applied to estimate oro-facial muscle function or dysfunction.

Association between EMG activity of jaw and neck muscles with TMD signs/symptoms as well as malocclusion, parafunctions and posture has been investigated

Some works shows the effects of body position on the EMG activity of sternocleidomastoid and masseter muscles in healthy subjects. Many sEMG studies are concerned with functional activity, such as clenching, and few of them have studied the rest position and the difference between the anterior temporalis sEMG in open and closed eye conditions.

Patients with myogenous facial pain show that the open eyes condition, compared with the closed eyes one, is associated with a change in the head and neck sEMG activity in the mandibular rest position (Monaco et al., 2010). This behaviour is not present in the healthy control subjects. A recent study (Spadaro et al., 2010) involving young healthy subjects with normal occlusion and without visual defects, compared the EMG values of the the anterior temporalis area at mandible rest position, in the closed eyes and open eyes conditions: the results showed no significant difference in the EMG values, suggesting that subjects with class I without myogenous facial pain signs or symptoms and with clinically verified correct vision, accept the exteroceptive visual input without an adaptive mechanism on the sEMG pattern of the stomatognathic system.

These observations suggest that the visual input effect could be a good provocation test for assessing a neuromuscular reply that will be more significant in neurogenic facilitation areas (Schmid & Mongini , 1985) .

The alteration of dental occlusion can induce some fluctuations in visual focusing, and the visual input effect on the EMG activity of Sternocleidomastoid and Masseter muscles at rest has been proved too. The different pattern of EMG activity of anterior temporalis with respect to masseter, sternocleidomastoid, and anterior digastric observed at rest, upon variation in the visual input, suggests a differential innervation of stomatognathic muscles. In fact the innervations of the sternocleidomastoid and anterior digastric muscles is provided by spinal and hypoglossal (XI and XII) nerves, while that of masseter and anterior temporalis muscles is provided by the trigeminal (V) nerve.

Interactions between neck and the extraocular muscles in the myopic eye have been reported (Valentino & Fabozzo, 1993). Monaco et al., 2006 confirmed that myopic defects can induce some alterations on EMG activity of masticatory muscles.

Nevertheless, there is a low interest about the influence of visual inputs on EMG values, as well about the relationship between visual defects and EMG values.

Among the neuromuscular factors that are able to affect the EMG values of the jaw elevators, the activity of the extraocular muscles, that is explicated by the activity of anterior temporalis, could be of interest.

2. Electrical characteristics of SEMG signals in rest position

In the intramuscular EMG, the contribution of each different motor units (UM) is distinguished according to the morphology of the electrical potentials. On the contrary, in the surface EMG (SEMG), the filtering effect of human tissues drastically reduces the morphological difference between the voltages that cannot be used as a classification element.

The human body is a good electrical conductor, but unfortunately the conductivity varies with tissue thickness. Because the of amplitude EMG signals is inversely proportional to the square of the distance from the source, the Ums, whose activity is possible to detect, are those located at a maximum distance of 15 mm from the electrodes. The interposed tissues can attenuate the high-frequency of component signals, and generally this mitigation is proportionally to the UM depth.

Moreover, in case of size-recuded muscles, neighbouring muscles may produce a significant amount of EMG noise (crosstalk); this issue is omnipresent when dealing with SEMG signals. However, all possible efforts must be made to eliminate or reduce the presence of the crosstalk. Despite this disadvantage, the use of surface electrodes simplifies the signal pick-up, making possible to record the signals in static and dynamic conditions, such as during the execution of functional movements or exercises.

The isometric activities generate electrical voltages whose root mean square (rms) values range from less than 50 μV to 20-30 mV, depending on the investigated muscle. The typical amplitude of noise amount at 5 μV rms, so the S/N is enough for the correct evaluation of the muscle activity with an acceptable accuracy (Fig. 1). The signal is generally amplified by a factor from 500 to 2000.

The frequency range of a SEMG amplifier is from 10 Hz to 500 Hz. The typical repetition rate of UM firing is about 7 to 20 Hz, depending on the size of the muscle. The high frequency cut-off corresponds to the maximum frequency of the SEMG signals. Moreover, because of the movement of electrodes and cables, the low frequency components of the collected signal should be removed. The SEMG signal is filtered, to eliminate the disturbances and highlight the relevant components (e.g. a low-pass filtering to analyze low-frequency components, or a high-pass filtering to analyze high frequency components, or a notch-filtering to eliminate components at a specific band). Therefore, the signal is processed to extract the desired quantity concerning the muscular fibres.

The Study of the activities of superficial muscles in rest position has been considered with scant regard, for two main reasons: i) the activity of signals is not measured with needle electrodes during rest time, with a consequently worsening in the transmission of the signal; ii) the amplitudes of the acquired electromyographic signals in rest conditions are in the same range of the noise (1 to 5 μV rms), and are difficult to evaluate.

Nevertheless, some interesting phenomena were observed during the application of surface electromyography in rest position (Ferrario et al., 1993; Rilo et al., 1997). For example, the records of electrical signal from the anterior temporal muscle showed different results in rest condition of the mandible, according to the open or closed eyes condition. Those signals varied by subject, but were constant for the same person, during the same recording session and without changing the recording apparatus or the electrodes themselves; furthermore, this variation was independent from the state of the eyes. In the electromyographic measurement practice, keeping open or closed the eyes is usually required for about 15 s at a time (Miralles et al., 1998; Kawamura, 1967).

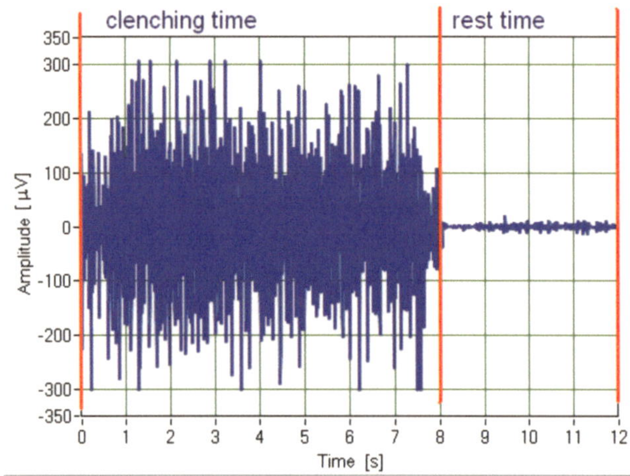

Fig. 1. The amplitude of electromyographic signal during the clenching and rest time.

From the preliminary measurements, the voltage amplitude of the investigated signals seems to be related to the sequence of the open-eyes and closed-eyes conditions. The signals appeared to be in the range of 1 to 6 µV rms, comparable with the noise level, and with a frequency lower than 20 Hz. This effect of movement could not be recorded because of the band pass (20 to 500 Hz filter), usually integrated in surface electromyographic equipment. Due to the limitation of these instruments, the clinical analysis of subjects could not unequivocally highlight the real cause of the obtained results (Bucci et al., 2009; Monaco et al., 2006; Shahani, 1977; Sharifi et al., 1998).
Considering that several clinical report questionated this issue, we decided to investigate the phenomenon with an ad hoc measurement station, that is capable to fully capture and analyze these signals. Briefly, the main goal of our research was the implementation and characterization of suitable measurement techniques for the identification of the biological signals, by reducing the effect of the superimposed noise without removing the signals related to non isometric muscle activities.

3. First preliminary study: evaluation of the influence of ocular defects on of the activity of stomatognatic muscles

The aim of this first preliminary study was to determine how the activity of the stomatognatic muscles is influenced by ocular defects. We expect a significant modification of SEMG values by changing visual input and visual defects.
A total of 20 children aged between 7 and 13 years (mean age 9±8 months), was evaluated.
In the study group 10 children with myopic defects were enlisted, selected among the patients afferent to the Pediatric Dentistry Department of the University of L'Aquila.

Ten subjects with normal vision, the control group, were chosen through the Pair Matching procedures, so that each myopic child had a matching age case control. All subjects were investigated by SEMG. Each subject underwent to two recordings of SEMG at rest: during the first SEMG each child was asked to keep his/her eyes closed, while during the second SEMG recordings each child was asked to keep his/her eyes open while looking straight ahead and to keep the lips in normal soft contact. The group of myopic children performed the recordings without lenses.Time for each recording was 15 seconds. Each individual was seated in a wooden chair with headrest in a comfortable stance. SEMG activity was recorded by K7 (Myotronic Inc.; Seattle,Washington, USA), using bipolar surface electrodes at single differential with interelectrode distance of 1 cm. The surface electrodes were placed with adhesive tape to the skin over the superficial masseter (LMM, RMM), anterior temporal (LTA, RTA), anterior digastric (RDA, LDA) and sternocleidomastoid (LSC, RSC) bilaterally and parallel to the muscle fibres. Eight channel surface electromyographic equipment was used (Myotronic Inc.; Seattle,Washington, USA). The obtained signals were amplified, recorded and computed using a clinical aimed software (K7- Myotronic Inc.; Seattle,Washington, USA); the Root Mean Square (RMS), expressed in µvolt, was used as amplitude indicator of the signal. SEMG of the subjects was examined by the same operator without knowledge of the recording purpose. A paired t-test for independent samples was performed to obtain a comparison between mean and variance values of electromyographic data. The p value $< .05$ was assumed as the level of significance. To facilitate the introduction of the data in the statistic software program, all the absolute values expressed in µvolt RMS were multiplied by 10.
Comparison according to the age of the individuals showed no significant differences between the groups ($p > .05$). Tables 1 and 2 illustrate the mean values, in µvolt, and standard deviations (parenthesis) of SEMG activity at rest with closed and open eyes for the anterior temporal, masseter, sternocleidomastoid and anterior digastric muscles of the children with normal vision (control group).

	LTA	LMM	RMM	RTA	LSC	LDA	RDA	RSC
Observations	10	10	10	10	10	10	10	10
Mean	17.2	13.6	14.5	17.7	23.6	24.5	32.0	24.7
SD	7.4	3.6	4.6	6.2	6.8	11.2	19.5	10.3

Table 1. Mean Value and Standard Deviation of Electromyographic Activity at Rest with closed eyes in the Stomatognatic Muscles of Control subjects.

	LTA	LMM	RMM	RTA	LSC	LDA	RDA	RSC
Observations	10	10	10	10	10	10	10	10
Mean	18.7	13.0	12.8	17.8	23.1	24.4	26.8	22.9
SD	8.6	3.8	2.5	10.2	10.2	10.7	8.5	8.5

Table 2. Mean Value and Standard Deviation of Electromyographic Activity with opened eyes in the Stomatognatic Muscles of Control Patients.

Tables 3 and 4 show the mean values and standard deviation of EMG activity at rest with closed eyes and open eyes for the anterior temporal, masseter, sternocleidomastoid and anterior digastric muscles of the children with myopic vision (study group). In myopic patients (study group) a significant difference was observed in LTA muscles.

	LTA	LMM	RMM	RTA	LSC	LDA	RDA	RSC
Observations	10	10	10	10	10	10	10	10
Mean	22.5	16.2	15.3	19.5	24.6	24.3	22.4	22.3
SD	11.5	8.1	10.4	7.2	8.3	11.2	8.05	10.9

Table 3. Mean Value and Standard Deviation of Electromyographic Activity with closed eyes in the Stomatognatic Muscles of Control Patients.

	LTA	LMM	RMM	RTA	LSC	LDA	RDA	RSC
Observations	10	10	10	10	10	10	10	10
Mean	32.6	17.3	14.6	24.2	20.8	27	25.9	18.4
SD	13.3	7.9	9.7	9.8	6.5	10.7	10.2	6.3

Table 4. Mean Value and Standard Deviation of Electromyographic Activity with opened eyes in the Stomatognatic Muscles of Control Patients.

In the closed eyes condition it is possible to observe an identical pattern of SEMG activity in both control and study group. SEMG values of left and right anterior temporal muscles were significantly different. These results underline that: i) a change in the visual input does not induce a modification in the basic tone of the stomatognatic system in children with normal vision; ii) the myopic children showed an increase of anterior temporal activity at rest. the activity of masticatory muscles, controlled by the trigeminal nerve, is regulated by several inputs coming from the proprioception of neuromuscular spindles. These inputs have an important role in the maintenance and in the modifications of muscular basal tone. Proprioception messages coming from the muscles of the neck are integrated in the central nervous system and contribute to control the balance and the body orientation in the space-time. Centripetal impulses from the muscles of the neck proprioceptors cooperate with the labyrinth impulses to promote the oculomotor muscular activity through the cervical-vestibular-ocular reflex.

Some important encephalic nuclei (trigeminal nuclei, oculomotor nuclei, vestibular nuclei, accessorial nerve nuclei) are integrated in the medial longitudinal fasciculus. Moreover, ocular proprioceptive receptors send afferences to the trigeminal and cuneate nuclei.

This study confirms the physiologic link of these anatomical structures: a modification of the proprioceptive ocular afferences can be reflected on the stomatognatic one. The EMG evaluations comported different RMS values as a consequence of the proprioceptive input change.

The results suggest that the relation between stomatognatic and oculomotor system is underestimated and the use of EMG could permit the integrate study of the two systems.

4. Second preliminary study: evaluation of the electromyographic activity of stomatognathic muscles at rest with eyes closed and with eyes open

The aim of the second preliminary study was to evaluate the electromyographic activity of stomatognathic muscles at rest with eyes closed and with eyes open and the effects of ocular correction on electromyographic activity and muscular balance. This knowledge could be clinically relevant in order to evaluate if, in subjects with functional lateral deviation, the ocular correction could contribute to variations of muscular tone and its symmetry.

The study was performed at the Dental Clinic of the University of L'Aquila. This study included 32 subjects with functional lateral-deviated mandible selected among children with tooth midline deviation, listed to paediatric dentistry clinic for dental care. All the patients presented natural dentition, an observable deviation of mandibular and anterior tooth midlines on functional base diagnosed by clinical examination, frontal and basal tele-radiographs. The subjects were chosen according to the following parameters: deviated chin from mid-sagittal plane (recognized by perpendicular line to horizontal bipupillary and bicommisural lines); the lack of alignment of the upper and lower labial frena; asymmetry of interincisive lines and molars/canine classes; deviation of incisor midline in maximal intercuspidation both in centric relation and at rest position; mandibular deviation during opening; noise and tenderness referred to temporomandibular joint (TMJ). The frontal teleradiograph, taken at open mouth, confirmed the symmetry of maxillary and mandibular structures. In order to be considered for the study, the following characteristics had to be present: i) negative history of orthodontic treatment; ii) observable deviation of anterior tooth midlines >1,5 mm with alignment at mouth open; iii) absence of skeletal asymmetry; iv) absence of any anterior or posterior/lateral crossbite; v) muscular ocular-extrinsic tone alteration. In the first visit all subjects underwent complete ophthalmological and orthoptical evaluation by the same ophthalmologist.

The oculo-extrinsic muscular tone disorders were classified as eso (convergence latent strabismus) and exophories (divergence latent strabismus) and measured by using cover test and Berens prisms. The values expressed as angle of deviation were measured in prismathic diottries (DP). Thirthy-two children with functional mandibular lateral deviation and muscular extrinsic ocular tone disorders, 19 girls and 13 boys, ranging from 8 to 12 years of age, with mean age of 10.1 (sd 1.1) in study group and 9.6 (sd 1.6) in control group (Table 1), were selected. No statistical differences were observed in the mean age for the two groups. Therefore, all subjects received a prescription for their ocular alterations. The subjects were randomly divided into two groups: study and control. The study group received ocular correction that needed to be balanced upon EMG control at the next visit, while the control group received a conventional ocular correction through lenses.

At second visit, all subjects were investigated by SEMG. Recordings were performed by placing bipolar surface electrodes (Instruments Co. Seattle) on the left and right anterior temporal, masseter, sternocleidomastoid and digastric muscles. During the recordings, EMG was monitored using a system K7 (Myotronic Inc., Seattle, Washington, USA). Each subject underwent three recordings of the integrated SEMG activity at rest, with eyes open and closed and after ocular correction. During the first SEMG recording each child was asked to keep his/her eyes closed. During the second SEMG recording, each child was asked to keep his/her eyes open while looking straight ahead and to keep the lips in normal soft contact. During the third SEMG recording children in the control group wore glasses for ocular correction through orthoptic examination only, while children in the the study group wore lenses centred and balanced through orthoptic evaluation integrated by means electromyography control. Recordings were performed with previous instruction to the children. SEMG recording time for each trial was 15 seconds. Two-samples paired comparison test (t-test) was performed on SEMG at rest, with and without visual input and with ocular correction, for each investigated muscle. The SEMG values are based on RMS measured in μvolt and using Symmetry Index (rightleft / right+left) (SI). SI values range from 0 to 1 (0 = perfect symmetry).

Each patient was seated in a wood chair with headrest in a comfortable stance, and patients were asked to closed the eyes, to avoid enviromental input. SEMG activity was recorded by

K7 software (K7 Myotronic Inc.-Seattle, Washington, USA) using bipolar surface electrodes at single differential with interelectrode distance of 1 cm. The surface electrodes were affixed with adhesive tape to the skin over the superficial masseter (LMM,RMM), anterior temporal (LTA,RTA), anterior digastric (RDA, LDA) and sternocleidomastoid (LSC, RSC), bilaterally and parallel to the muscle fibers. Eight channel surface electromyographic equipment was used (Myotronics). The signal obtained were amplified, recorded and computed using a clinical aimed software (K7-Myotronics); the Root Mean Square (RMS), expresses in μvolt, was used as amplitude indicator of the signal. SEMG of the subjects were examined by the same operator without knowledge of recording purpose.

The subjects of both groups were analysed with respect to the rate of lateral deviation from tooth midline and electromyographycally examined. Therefore the subjects of the study gruop wore lenses centred and balanced by means SEMG, the control group wore lenses fabricated according to conventional orthoptic evaluation.

The SEMG values were compared and statistically analysed. A paired t-test for independent samples was performed to obtain a comparison between mean and variance values of electromyographic data. The level of significance was set at the p value of $<.05$. A correlation analysis was performed between the rate of lateral deviation and the DP rate. A correlation coefficient (r) equal or greater than 0.600 was considered significant. A linear regression statistics coefficient was performed between the rate of lateral deviation and the DP rate.

To facilitate the introduction of the data in the statistic software, all absolute values expressed in μvolt rms were multiplied by 10. Tables 5 and 6 illustrate the mean values, in μvolt, of SEMG activity at rest with closed eyes for the anterior temporal, masseter, sternocleidomastoid and anterior digastric muscles respectively of the study and control group. Tables 7 and 8 show the mean values of SEMG activity at rest for the anterior temporal, masseter, sternocleidomastoid and anterior digastric muscles with eyes open in the study and the control groups, respectively.

Tables 9 and 10 report the mean values of SEMG activity at rest for the anterior temporal, masseter, sternocleidomastoid and anterior digastric muscles with ocular correction in the study and the control group, respectively. The comparison between the results in Tables 5 and 7 shows that EMG activity of the anterior temporal increases significantly in children with conventional ocular correction (control group) ($p<0.05$). In the study group children the ocular correction obtained by means SEMG did not show an increase of muscular values of TA.

	LTA	LMM	RMM	RTA	LSC	LDA	RDA	RSC
Observations	16	16	16	16	16	16	16	16
Mean	20.3	19.5	19.9	17.5	22.9	29.0	36.5	22.4
SD	10.5	13.0	13.7	6.7	6.4	18.1	22.7	10.5

Table 5. Mean Value and Standard Deviation of Electromyographic Activity at Rest with closed eyes in the Stomatognatic Muscles of study subjects.

	LTA	LMM	RMM	RTA	LSC	LDA	RDA	RSC
Observations	16	16	16	16	16	16	16	16
Mean	20.5	13.6	11.6	18.9	18.0	17.9	19.4	18.0
SD	9.4	7.0	5.1	8.0	10.9	8.6	8.2	8.7

Table 6. Mean Value and Standard Deviation of Electromyographic Activity at Rest with closed eyes in the Stomatognatic Muscles of control subjects.

	LTA	LMM	RMM	RTA	LSC	LDA	RDA	RSC
Observations	16	16	16	16	16	16	16	16
Mean	24.5	19.5	18.1	27.9	22.5	30.7	30.6	22.0
SD	12.4	12.3	13.2	15.1	8.5	21.5	18.5	9.7

Table 7. Mean Value and Standard Deviation of Electromyographic Activity at Rest with opened eyes in the Stomatognatic Muscles of study subjects.

	LTA	LMM	RMM	RTA	LSC	LDA	RDA	RSC
Observations	16	16	16	16	16	16	16	16
Mean	25.3	13.6	12.0	27.9	19.4	19.4	19.9	18.2
SD	12.7	6.3	5.2	15.1	10.0	8.9	8.1	9.2

Table 8. Mean Value and Standard Deviation of Electromyographic Activity at Rest with opened eyes in the Stomatognatic Muscles of control subjects.

	LTA	LMM	RMM	RTA	LSC	LDA	RDA	RSC
Observations	16	16	16	16	16	16	16	16
Mean	22.2	19.4	16.3	20.8	20.5	30.7	25.8	25.0
SD	10.4	8.0	5.7	9.0	6.7	21.5	10.8	17.3

Table 9. Mean Value and Standard Deviation of Electromyographic Activity at with ocular correction by means EMG in the Stomatognatic Muscles of study subjects.

	LTA	LMM	RMM	RTA	LSC	LDA	RDA	RSC
Observations	16	16	16	16	16	16	16	16
Mean	22.2	19.4	16.3	20.8	20.5	30.7	25.8	25.0
SD	10.4	8.0	5.7	9.0	6.7	21.5	10.8	17.3

Table 10. Mean Value and Standard Deviation of Electromyographic Activity at with conventional ocular correction in the Stomatognatic Muscles of control subjects.

5. The new measurement equipment

To extract useful information about the effect of incorrect lenses, the electromyographic signal in rest conditions should be suitably acquired and processed, in order to reduce the effect of the noise and to supply the oculist with a reliable quantitative indication.
To this aim, we developed an ad hoc measurement system, whose block diagram is reported in Fig. 2; the proposed system can operate in parallel with the conventional instrument to compare the supplied results.

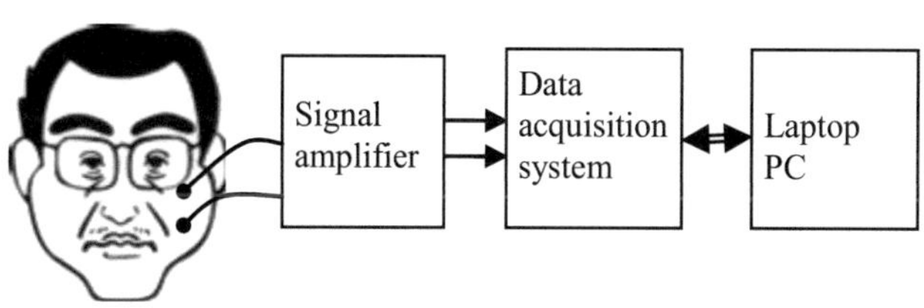

Fig. 2. The block diagram of the measurement setup.

The bio-electrical signal can be detected using two single electrodes (one active electrode located in correspondence of the muscle under analysis and another reference electrode located on a neutral point), or a bipolar electrode (two active electrodes located on the muscle). This last differential configuration has a better noise immunity, even if it presents some difficulties with muscles of reduced dimensions.

Because the SEMG signal is low in amplitude, with respect to other ambient signals on the surface of the skin, we decided to detect it with a differential configuration. The electrodes are placed in the midline of the belly of the muscle, where the signal has the maximum amplitude.

The electrode signal is amplified, acquired and processed. The amplifier is the EG&G PARC 113 Low-Noise Preamp, with a bandwidth from DC to 300 kHz. Its main features are: i) adjustable high and low frequency rolloffs; ii) two input channels, AC or DC coupled, with single-ended or differential input section; iii) maximum input voltage of 1 Vrms; iv) gain ranging from x10 to x10000, in the 1-2-5 sequence; v) input impedance of 1 GΩ, shunted by 15 pF; vi) common mode rejection of 100 dB in the range from DC to 1 kHz; input DC drift < 10 μV/°C, output DC drift < 1 mV/°C.

The amplified signal has been acquired by a USB data acquisition module, the Keithley KUSB-3108 High Gain Multifunction, whose main features are: i) resolution of 16 bits, effective number of bits of 14.1; ii) sampling rate of 50 kSamples/s; iii) accuracy of +/- 0.04 %; iv) nonlinearity of +/- 4 LSB; v) input impedance of 100 MΩ, 100 pF; vi) common mode rejection > 74 dB; vii) A/D converter noise of 0.4 LSB rms. A Laptop PC supplied by a battery has been used; data acquisition and processing have been programmed using the NI LabVIEW tool (Bucci et al, 2009; Fiorucci et al., 2011).

In order to analyze the behaviour of the proposed system, a plot of the signal acquired during the sequence closed-open-closed eyes, is shown in Fig. 3, while Fig. 4 reports the same signal acquired with a traditional instrument.

The effects produced by the internal blocks of a standard SEMG that, practically, processes this signal as a noise, are evident.

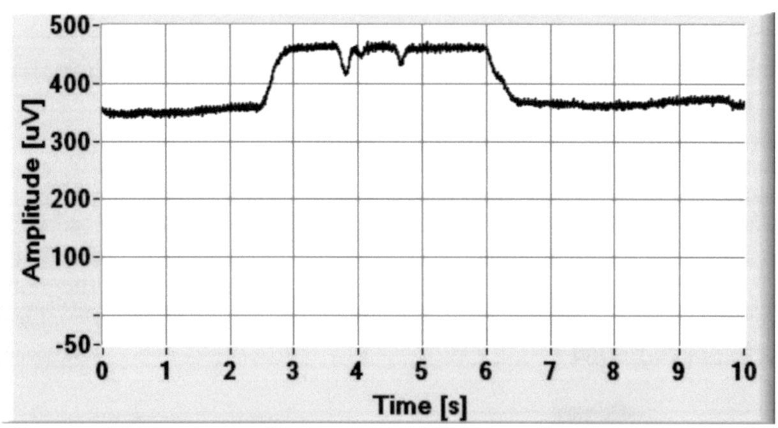

Fig. 3. Signal v(i) corresponding to the sequence closed-open-closed eyes, acquired with gain 10000.

Fig. 3 also shows that suitable signal processing techniques should be implemented in order to: i) detect the signal transitions that indicate the beginning (closed-open in the figure) and the ending (open-closed) of the time interval of interest; ii) process the signal during this time interval (up time) in order to extract the useful information.

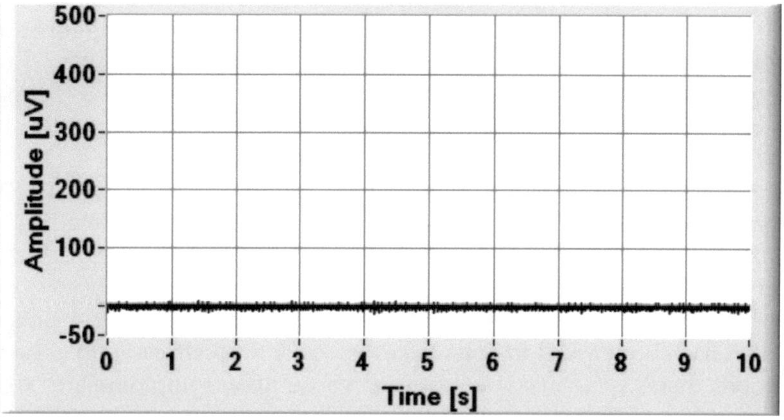

Fig. 4. Signal vemg(i) corresponding to the sequence closed-open-closed eyes (traditional SEMG) acquired with gain 10000.

6. The measurement technique and the signals analysis

The goal of the present research is the analysis of the surface electromyographic signals on patients wearing eyeglasses (Miralles et al., 1998; Kawamura, 1967; Shahani, 1977;). In detail, our experimental activity has been focused on the acquisition and analysis of the SEMG signals of anterior temporalis muscles at mandible rest conditions, in occurrence with some particular voluntary and involuntary movements of the patient, such as closed-open eyes condition; those signals can not be acquired with a traditional SEMG measurement apparatus, because of the presence of pass-band filters and of the electronic noise, which could mask the closed-open eyes effect (Airi Oksanen et al., 2007; Sharifi et al., 1998).
The acquisitions are performed in both dark and illuminated rooms, and each patient has been asked to open the eyes after 1 s and, after 3 s, to close them; the voluntary movement of opening and closing the eyes produces a rectangular shape in the digitized input voltage v(i).
With the aim to emphasize the low frequency voltage variations, we adopted the rms sliding window technique. In SEMG techniques, the rms of the signal can be considered as an index of the power of the signal itself, and it can be correlated to the muscular stress. We are interested in evaluating the variation of that stress during the time, to identify the conditions in which it is higher or lower; the adoption of the rms sliding window technique allows the observation of that variation. Moreover, the rms signal is filtered by the DEMG high frequency components, so it can be adopted to implement a threshold technique for the automatic identification of the time interval corresponding to the opened-eyes, in which the muscular stress must be measured.
Specifically, the input voltage v has been digitized and processed to calculate the rms voltage waveform v_{rms}. At any instant of time i, a new rms voltage value has been calculated from n samples of the acquired voltage v (j), using the formula:

$$v_{rms}(i) = \sqrt{\frac{1}{n}\sum_{j=i}^{i+n-1} v(j)^2} \quad (1)$$

where n is the number of samples contained in each summation interval (variable from 20 ms to 100 ms). The new value $v_{rms}(i+1)$ has been calculated by sliding forward a sample of the input voltage.

This technique improves the transitory response and guarantees a better temporal resolution: the $v_{rms}(i)$ is updated at each sampling point, so it is possible to directly compare v(i) and $v_{rms}(i)$.

During the experimental activity, by analyzing the features of the acquired SEMG signals and comparing them with the movements of the patients, we identified two stress symptoms, that can be directly related with the incorrect prescription of eyeglasses; they can be described comparing Figs. 5 and 6.

Fig 5 shows the SEMG signal acquired, in an illuminated room, on a patient without eyeglasses, that have been asked to open the eyes, to try to focalize and to close the eyes. In those conditions there is the maximum stress, whose main symptoms are: A) the partial closing and opening of the eyes due to the winking movement as a consequence of the difficulty in focusing the image; B) the amplitude increasing of the SEMG high frequency components, that is related to the increased activity of the masticatory muscles. The signal in Fig. 6 shows the minimum stress conditions, as it has been acquired in an illuminated room, on a patient wearing the correct eyeglasses: the A and B phenomena are absent.

To quantify the patient stress, we introduced a new signal, v*(i), calculated as the point-by-point difference between v(i) and $v_{rms}(i)$:

$$v^*(i) = v(i) - v_{rms}(i) \tag{2}$$

It represents the dynamic component of the muscle activity, that takes into account the winking movement (high frequency components). We observed that two quantitative parameters of the v*(i) signal can be adopted as indexes of the stress of a patient wearing incorrect eyeglasses: the average power and the voltage range in open-eyes condition. We verified that these parameters are smallest when the muscle stress is minimum, that is when the prescription of eyeglasses is correct. The measurement of the average power and voltage range was performed only in the time interval in which the rms signal $v_{rms}(i)$ is higher than a suitable threshold.

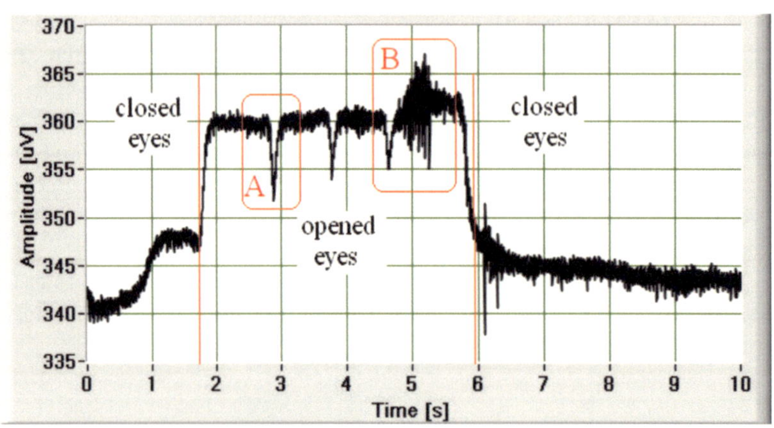

Fig. 5. Results in case of no lenses (maximum stress).

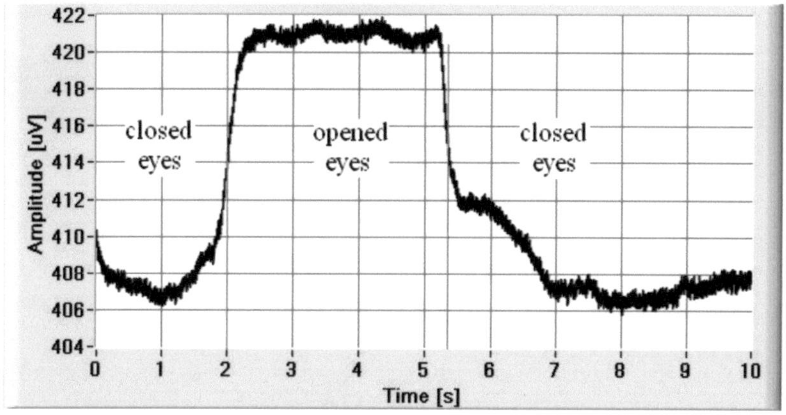

Fig. 6. Results in case of correct lenses (minimum stress).

We also performed the amplitude spectrum measurement, in order to investigate about the possible presence of frequency components whose amplitude could be related to the muscular stress.

In Fig.7 a flowchart of the signal processing algorithm implemented on the proposed measurement system is synthesized. Figs. 8 to 11 show $v_{rms}(i)$ and $v^*(i)$ signals obtained with the proposed technique starting, respectively, in dark and illuminated rooms. The acquisitions in an illuminated room have been performed asking the patient, without sight defects, to open the eyes, to try to focalize a sign and then to close the eyes. Fig. 10 shows the voltage level variations due to the voluntary movement of opening and closing the eyes, superimposed to the high-frequency signal due to the muscle stress; the voltage drop at 2.2 s is due to the focalizing movement involving a partial closing of the eyes.

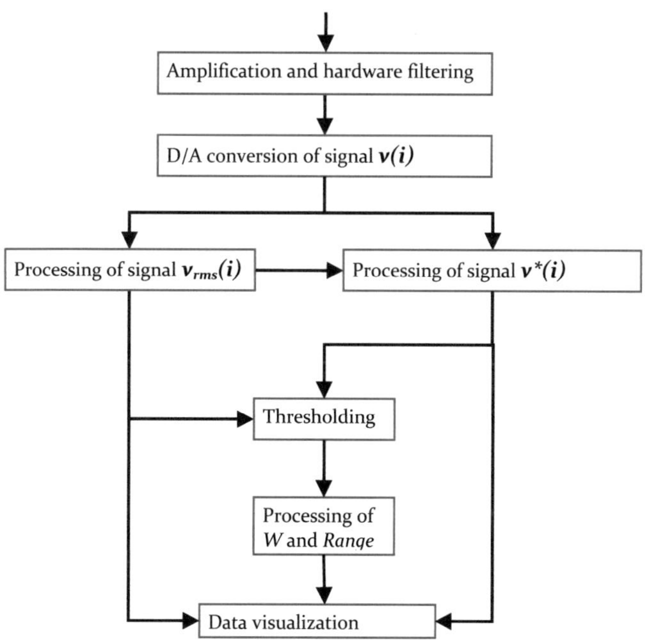

Fig. 7. Data analysis procedure.

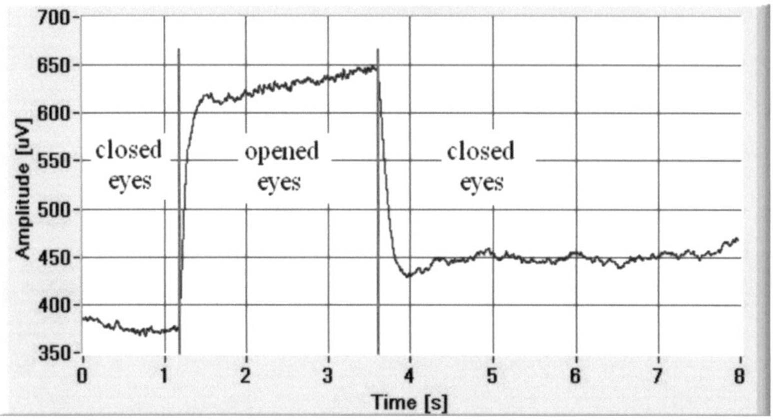

Fig. 8. Rms signal $v_{rms}(i)$ corresponding to the sequence closed-opened-closed eyes in a dark room.

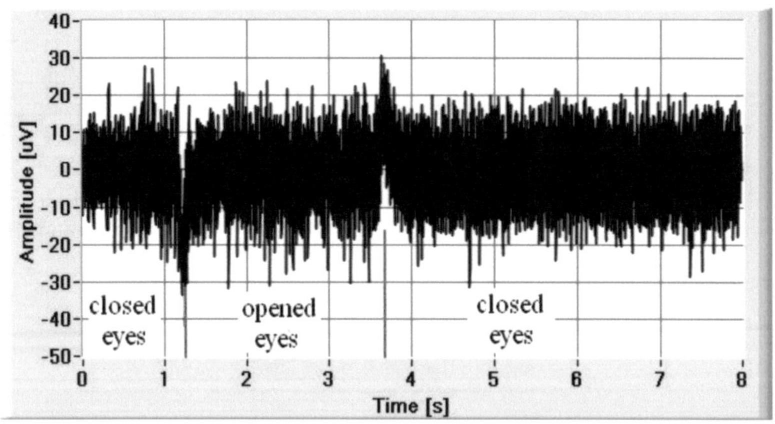

Fig. 9. Dynamic component $v^*(i)$ of the signal, corresponding to the sequence closed-opened-closed eyes in a dark room.

As part of the development phase, the measurement system has been tested to investigate its performance. The first test was the measurement of the frequency response, with different gain values: 500, 1000, 2000, 5000 and 10000. The reference signal has been generated using the Stanford Research DS360 Ultra Low Distortion Function Generator, whose main specifications are: i) output range from 20 μVpp to 40 Vpp; ii) THD 0.001%; iii) frequency accuracy of 25 ppm; iv) 20 bit D/A converter. The tests have been carried out by varying the amplitude and the frequency of a sinusoidal waveform in the ranges (50 to 500) μVrms, (5 to 5000) Hz. Successively we measured the total RMS noise voltage and the noise figure for the selected gains. The measurement of the total RMS noise, the noise figure and the system noise spectrum have been performed according to (Van Putten, 1988). In detail, the total RMS noise voltage eN , measured in the frequency range DC-1 kHz, adopted for all our experimental activity can be expressed as:

$$e_N = \sqrt{e_n^2 + i_n^2 R_{gen}^2 + e_R^2} \cdot \sqrt{1000} \tag{3}$$

where e_n is the equivalent short-circuit input RMS noise voltage, in is the equivalent open circuit RMS noise current, R_{gen} is the internal resistance of the voltage source, and e_R is the thermal noise voltage developed across R_{gen}.
As suggested in (Gerleman & Cook, 1992) a typical value of surface electrode impedance is R_{gen} = 20 kΩ, en has been measured by shunting a 20 kΩ resistor across the input terminals of the EG&G PARC 113, at 290 K, measuring the preamp output rms voltage and dividing it by the amplifier gains reported in Tab III. The Noise Figure has been calculated as:

$$NF = 10\log\left[\frac{e_N^2}{e_R^2}\right] \tag{4}$$

where:

$$e_R^2 = 4kT\,RB \tag{5}$$

K is the Boltzmann's constant, T the temperature, B the bandwidth and R the considered resistance. The obtained results, tabulated in Table 11, show a good response of the instrument, because the noise amplitude is quite irrelevant for the bio-electrical signal detection.
We also calculated the system dynamic range, considering that the CMRR of the EG&G PARC 113 in the range from DC to 1 kHz is greater than 100 dB; and that the 16 bits data acquisition board presents a theoretical dynamic range of 96 dB; from the tests we carried out that the overall system dynamic range can be assumed as 86 dB.

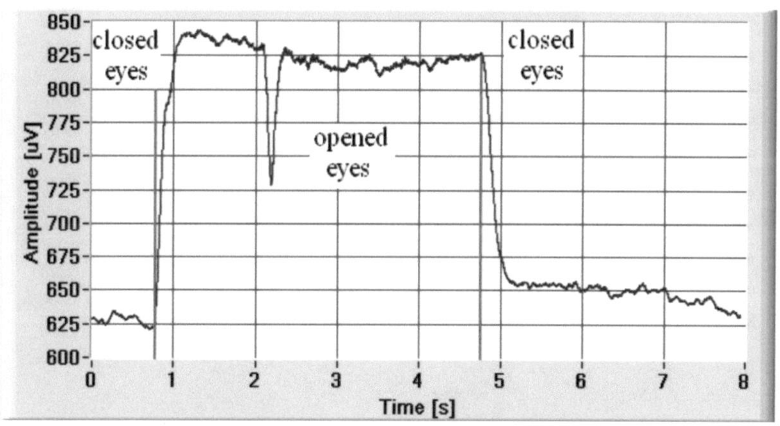

Fig. 10. Rms signal $v_{rms}(i)$ corresponding to the sequence closed-opened-closed eyes in an illuminated room with no eyeglasses.

Gain	Noise Figure [dB]	Total RMS noise voltage [nV rms]
500	2.56	952
1000	2.04	897
2000	7.60	1702
5000	3.10	1014
10000	2.15	908

Table 11. Noise figures and total RMS noise voltages for different gain settings.

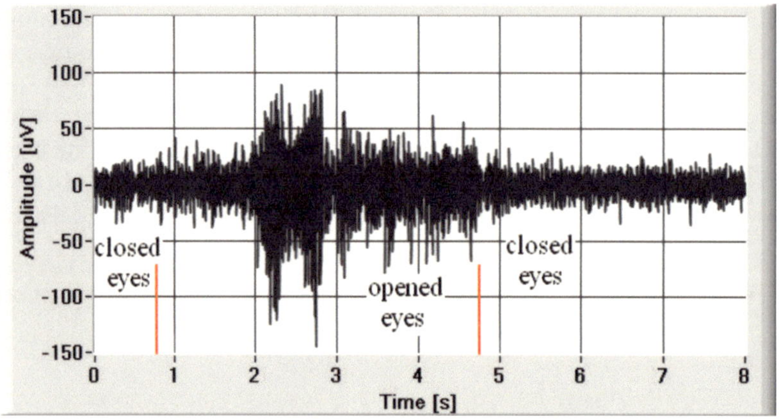

Fig. 11. Dynamic component v*(i) of the signal, corresponding to the sequence closed-opened-closed eyes in an illuminated room, without eyeglasses.

7. Experimental results

We conducted some test to investigate about the effectiveness of the processed parameters to provide useful information concerning the eyeglass prescription. To evaluate the stress of wearing eyeglasses, an experimental activity has been carried out in the Dental Clinic of the University of L'Aquila on a group of 30 patients with different visual defects.

As a first step, the correct eye glasses prescription is detected by the ophthalmologist of our team, by using a set of optical test lenses and a trial frame (Fig.12).

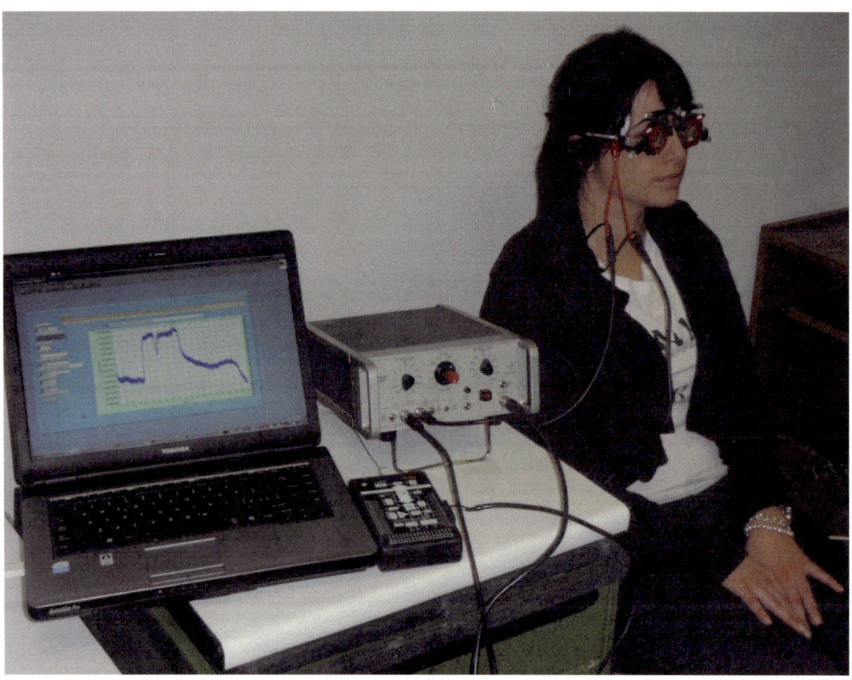

Fig. 12. A measurement session with optical test lenses and a trial frame.

After that, the closed-open-closed EMG signals are acquired while the patient is wearing correct and wrong (obtained by adding +/-0.25, +/-2 and +/5 cylindrical correction degrees) lenses. In all the tests, both the increasing and decreasing of the corrective lenses graduation have been characterized by an increase of the average power and by the presence of focalizing movements, involving an increase of the SEMG signal range. In other words, the minimum values of both the parameters are reached when the correct prescription is applied. To underline the relation between muscular stress and incorrect eyeglasses, the SEMG signals v(i) acquired on the same patient are presented in Figs. 13-17, with the previously described correction degrees; they have been obtained by adding respectively the following cylindrical correction degrees: +0.25, -0.25, + 2, -2, +5, -5. The measured values of voltage range and average power are reported in Table 12; it is possible, by using the proposed measurement and analysis approach, to determine the eyeglasses prescription minimizing the muscular stress. In Figs. 19-24 we propose the comparison between the amplitude spectrum of signal in Fig. 6, adopted as a reference for the minimum stress conditions, and the amplitude spectra of the signals in Figs. 13-18. It is possible to identify two frequency bands, in which the effect of the muscular stress seems to be more evident: 10-400 Hz, and 720-740 Hz.
In all the figures, the correct eyeglasses reduce the amplitude of the frequency components.

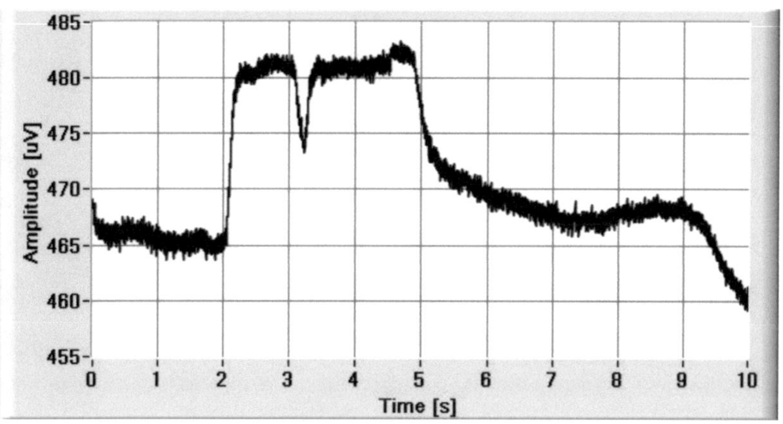

Fig. 13. Signal acquired in case of +0.25 degrees.

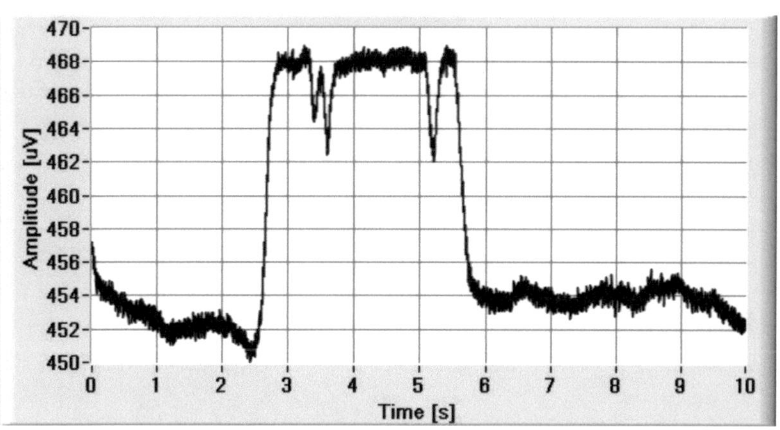

Fig. 14. Signal acquired in case of -0.25 degrees.

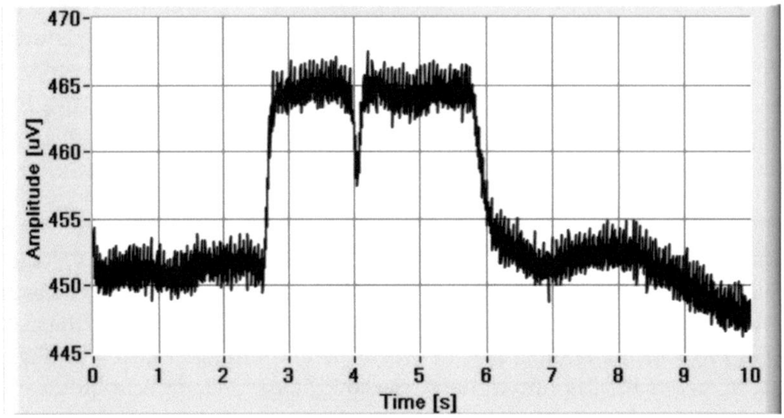

Fig. 15. Signal acquired in case of +2 degrees.

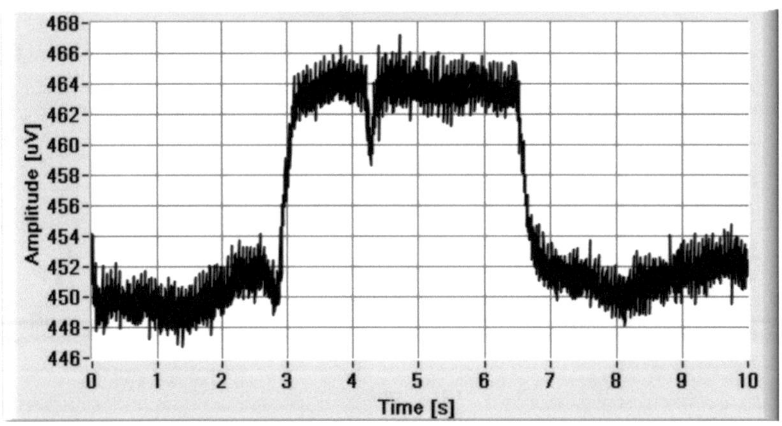

Fig. 16. Signal acquired in case of -2 degrees.

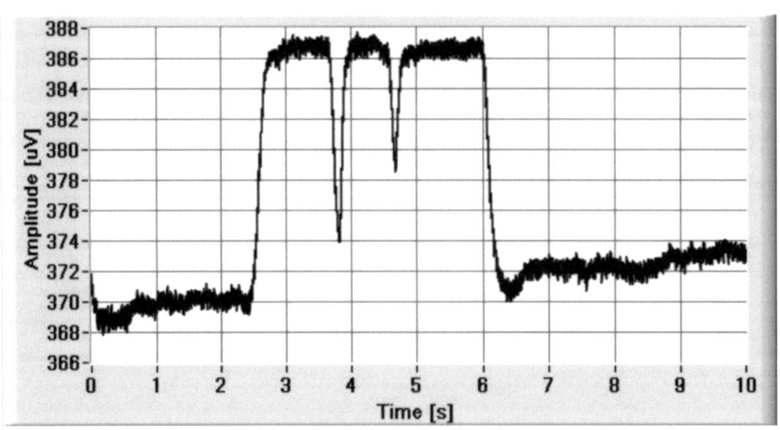

Fig. 17. Signal acquired in case of + 5 degrees.

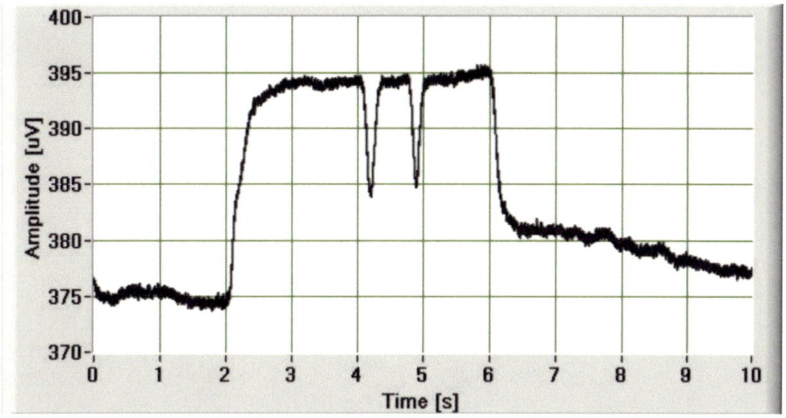

Fig. 18. Signal acquired in case of - 5 degrees.

Deviation from correct prescription [cylindrical correction degrees]	Range [uV]	Average power [pW]
-5	6.8	0.61
-2	6.7	0.35
-0,25	5.0	0.28
0	1.5	0.04
0,25	4.3	0.31
2	6.3	0.40
5	8.5	0.72

Table 12. Measured voltage range and average power values.

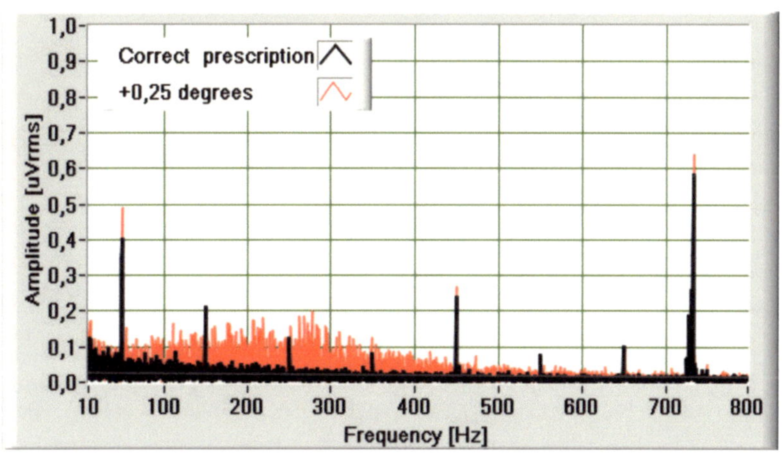

Fig. 19. Spectra comparison of signals for correct lenses and +0,25 degree lenses.

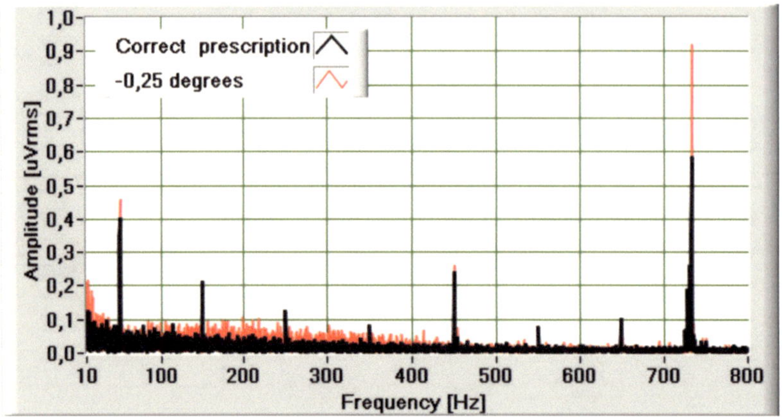

Fig. 20. Spectra comparison of signals for correct lenses and -0,25 degree lenses.

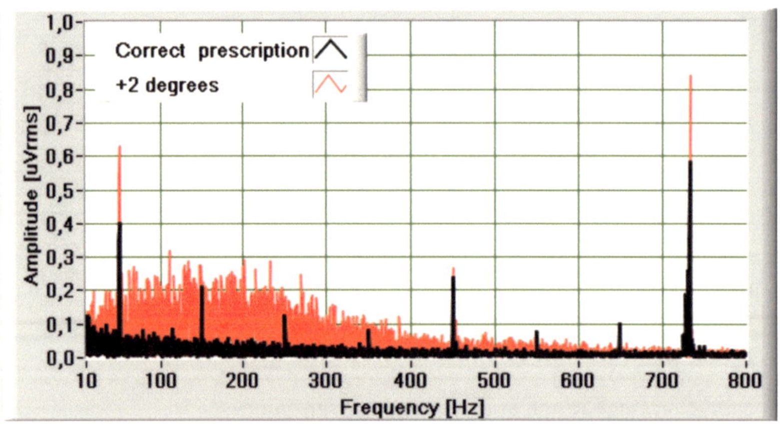

Fig. 21. Spectra comparison of signals for correct lenses and +2 degree lenses.

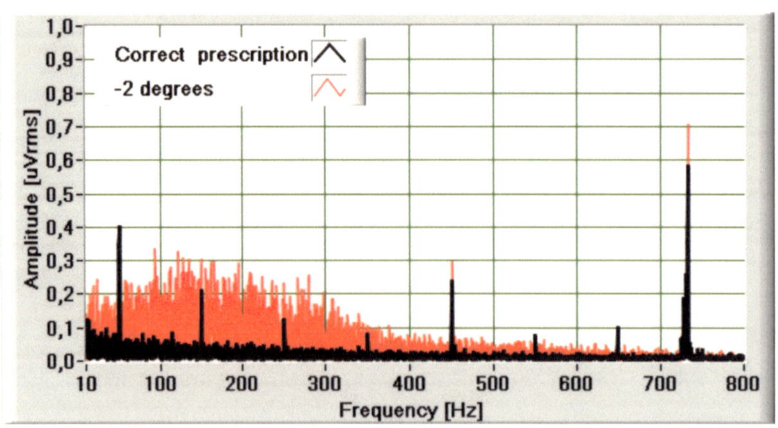

Fig. 22. Spectra comparison of signals for correct lenses and -2 degree lenses.

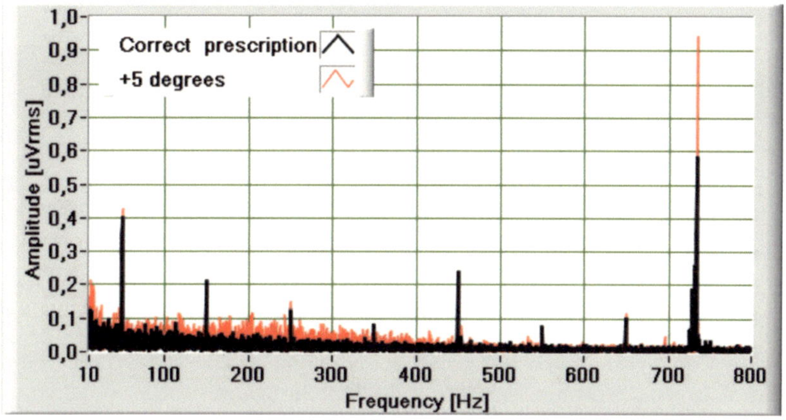

Fig. 23. Spectra comparison of signals for correct lenses and +5 degree lenses.

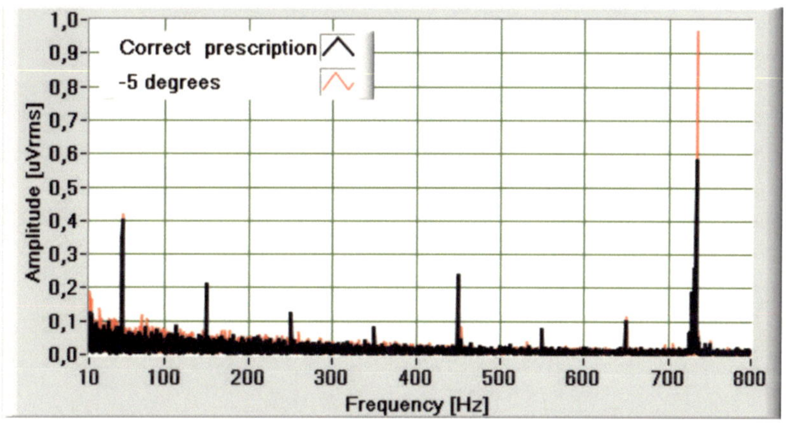

Fig. 24. Spectra comparison of signals for correct lenses and -5 degree lenses.

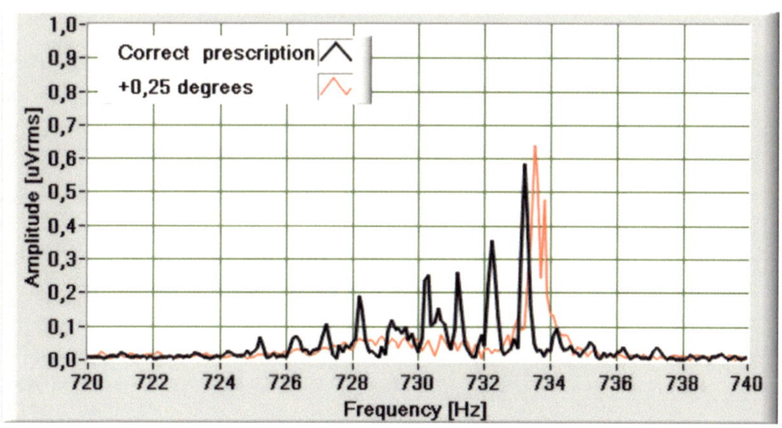

Fig. 25. Spectra comparison of signals for correct lenses and +0,25 degree lenses, in the range 720-740 Hz.

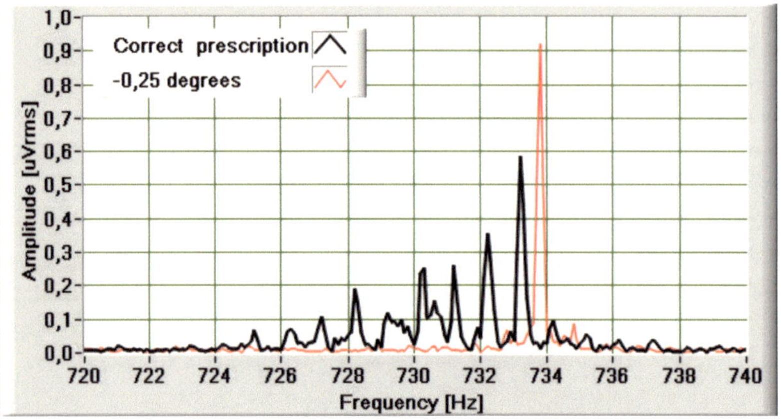

Fig. 26. Spectra comparison of signals for correct lenses and -0,25 degree lenses, in the range 720-740 Hz.

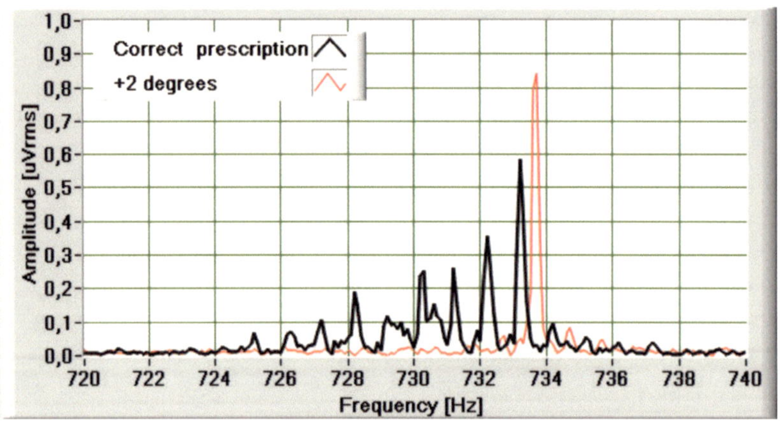

Fig. 27. Spectra comparison of signals for correct lenses and +2 degree lenses, in the range 720-740 Hz.

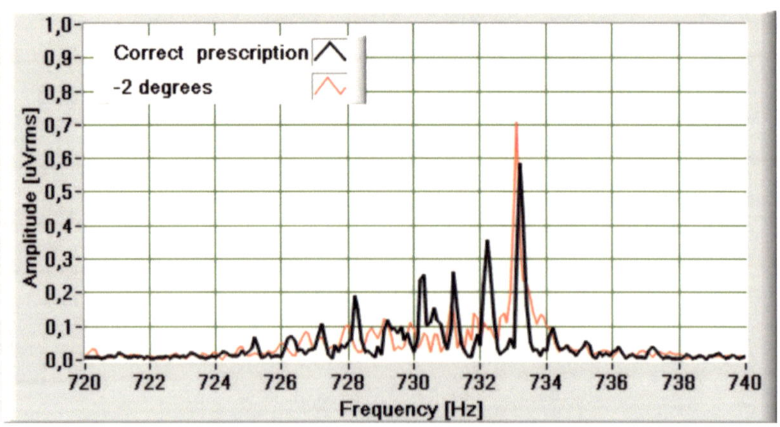

Fig. 28. Spectra comparison of signals for correct lenses and -2 degree lenses, in the range 720-740 Hz.

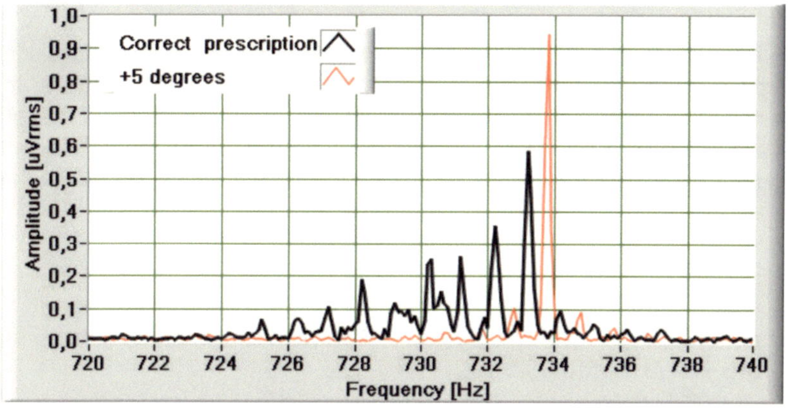

Fig. 29. Spectra comparison of signals for correct lenses and +5 degree lenses, in the range 720-740 Hz.

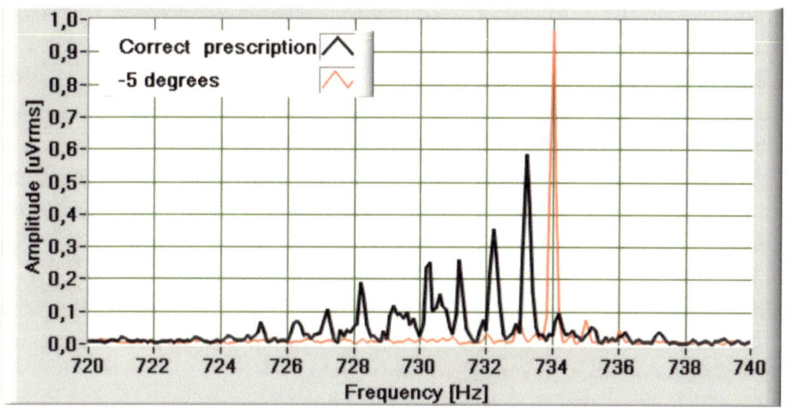

Fig. 30. Spectra comparison of signals for correct lenses and -5 degree lenses, in the range 720-740 Hz.

8. Conclusion

The main aim of this chapter was the implementation of new measurement techniques of surface electromyographic signals, that are of great importance for the analysis of neuromuscular functions. Traditional SEMG apparatuses can not be adopted for this application, mainly because of the presence of built-in filtering sections that eliminate the related signal components (Ferdjallah et al., 2000), but also because it is required a special signal processing. By adopting the proposed technique, it is possible to acquire the raw signals, to identify the presence of voluntary movements during the acquisition period with the proposed rms sliding window technique, and to calculate some indexes of the signal v*(i), such as average power and the voltage range in open-eyes conditions. The proposed approach has been applied to evaluate the effects of the graduation of eyeglasses and contact lens on the muscle stress in rest conditions. By processing the SEMG, it is possible to define the right choice for the grade of glasses or contact lenses, with a direct and objective evaluation of the generated muscular stress. Currently, we are working to elaborate a protocol by analysing a greater number of patients. Further improvement of the present paper will investigate the relation between the eyeglasses and contact lens and the amplitude spectrum of the SEMG signal in the frequency range 720 – 740 Hz, in which the amplitudes of the frequency components can supply information about the stress of the patients as suggested by Figs. 23-28. Finally, the adoption of an image acquisition device will be possible to directly compare the EMG signals to the filmed movement of the patient's face.

9. References

Barber HO. & Sharpe JA. (1988) *Vestibular disorder*. Year Book Medical Publisher Inc. Chicago, ISBN 0815104197.

Buisseret-Delmas C & Buisseret P. (1990) Central projections of extraocular muscle afferents in cat. C. *Neuroscience Letters*. Vol. 109, No. 1-2, pp.48-53, ISSN 0304-3940

Bucci G., Fiorucci E., Monaco A. & Cattaneo R. (2009), Development of an ad hoc measurement station for the human surface electromyography in rest position" *Proceedings of IEEE MEMEA 2009*, ISBN: 978-1-4244-3599-9, Cetraro Italy, May 2009

Donaldson IM & Knox PC. (1991) Afferent signals from pigeon extraocular muscles modify the vestibular responses of units in the abducens nucleus. *Proceedings Biological Sciences*. Vol. 244, No. 1311, pp.233-239, ISSN 09628452

Ferrario VF, Sforza c, Miani JR, D'Addona & Barbini E. (1993) Electromyographic activity of human masticatory muscles in normal young people. Statistical evaluation of reference values for clinical applications. *Journal of Oral Rehabilitation*. Vol. 20, No. 3, pp. 271-280, ISSN 1365-2842

Ferdjallah M.; Myers K., Starsky A. & Harris G.F. (2000) Dynamic electromyography. *Pediatric Gait, 2000. A new Millennium in Clinical Care and Motion Analysis Technology*, ISBN 0-7803-6469-4, Chicago USA , July 2000.

Fiorucci E., Bucci G., Ciancetta F. & Monaco A. (2011) Measurement and analysis of surface electromyographic signals on patients wearing eyeglasses *Proceedings of IEEE MEMEA 2011*, BARI Italy, May 2011

Gerleman D. G. & Cook T. M., (1992) *Selected Topics in Surface Electromyography for Use in the Occupational Setting: Expert Perspectives- Chapter 4: Instrumentation* U.S. Department of Health and Human Services.

Ito S., Taketomi M. &Hirano M. (1995) Effects on tonic neck reflex on optokinetic nystagmus in rabbits. *Acta Otolaryngologica* , Vol. 115, No. 2, pp 134–136.

Kawamura Y. (1967), Neurophysiologic background of occlusion. *Periodontics*. 1967; Vol.5:, pp. 175-183.

Lin SY. & White GE. (1996) Mandibular position and head posture as a function of eye dominance. *Journal of Clinical Pediatric Dentistry*, Vol. 20, No. 2, pp. 133-140, ISSN 1053-4628

Lukas JR. & Aigner M, Heinzl H, & Mayr R. (1994) Number and distribution of neuromuscular spindles in human extraocular muscles. *Investigative Ophtalmology & Visual Science*, Vol. 35, No. 13 , pp. 4317-4327, ISSN 1552-5783

Meyer J. & Baron JB. (1976) Participation of trigeminal afferences in tonic postural regulation. Static and dynamic aspects. *Aggressiologie* , Vol. 17, pp:33-40, ISSN 00021148

Miralles R., Gutierrez C., Zucchino G., Cavada G., Carvajal R., Valenzuela S. & Palazzi C. (1998) Visual input effect on EMG activity of sternocleidomastoid and masseter muscles in healthy subjects and in patients with myogenic cranio-cervical-mandibular dysfunction. *Cranio*, Vol. 16, No. 3, pp. 168-184, ISSN 0886-9634

Monaco A., Cattaneo R., Spadaro A., Giannoni M., Di Martino S. & Gatto R. (2006) Visual input effect on EMG activity of masticatory and postural muscles in healthy and myopic children. *European Journal of Paediatric Dentistry*, Vol. 7, No.1, pp. 18-22, ISSN 2035-648X .

Monaco A, Spadaro A, Cattaneo R. & Giannoni M. (2010) Effects of myogenous facial pain on muscle activity of head and neck. *International Journal of Oral & Maxillofacial Surgery* ; Vol. 39, No. 8, pp. 767-773, ISSN 0901-5027

Murch GM. (1973) *Visual and Auditory Perception*. New York: Bobbs-Merril Company Inc.;

Oddsson L. (1989) Motor patterns of a fast voluntary postural task in man: trunk extension in standing. *Acta physiologica Scandinavica*, Vol. 136, No. 1, pp. 47-58, ISSN 0302-2994

Oksanen A., Ylinen J., Pöyhönen T., Anttila P., Laimi K., Hiekkanen H. & Salminen J. (2007) Repeatability of electromyography and force measurements of the neck muscles in adolescents with and without headache. *Journal of Electromyography and Kinesiology*, Vol.17, No. 4, pp.493-503, ISSN 1050-6411

Porter JD. (1986) Branstem terminations of extraocular muscle primary afferent neuron in the monkey. *Journal of Comparative Neurology*, Vol. 247, No.2, pp. 133-143, ISSN 1096-9861

Rilo B., Santana U., Mora MJ. & Cadarso CM., (1997) Myoelectrical activity of clinical rest position and jaw muscle activity in young adults. *Journal of Oral Rehabilitation*. Vol. 24, No. 10, pp. 735-740, ISSN 1365-2842.

Rose PK. & Abrahams VC. (1975) The effect of passive eye movement on unit discharge in the superior colliculus of the cat. *Brain Research*, Vol 97, No. 1, pp 95-106, ISSN 00068993

Rose PK., Mac Donald J. & Abrahams VC, (1991) Projections of the tectospinal tract to the upper cervical spinal cord of the cat: a study with the anterograde tracer PHA-L. *Journal of Comparative Neurololgy* ; Vol. 314, No. 1, pp. 91-105, ISSN 0021-9967

Schmid W & Mongini F. (1985) Orthodontic treatment and mandibular modelling in growth. *Fortschr Kieferorthop* , Vol. 46, No. 5, pp. 352-357, ISSN 0015-816X

Schmid R., Zambarbieri D. & Magenes G. (1981) Modifications of vestibular nystagmus produced by fixation of visual and nonvisual targets. *Annals of the New York Academy of Sciences*, Vol. 374, pp. 689-705, ISSN 1749-6632

Shahani M, (1977) Influence of visual input on monosynaptic reflex. *Electromyography and Clinical. Neurophysiology*, Vol. 17, No. 1, pp. 3-11 ISSN

Sharifi Milani R, Deville de Periere D. & Micallef JP, (1988) Relationship between dental occlusion and visual focusing. *Cranio*. Vol. 16, No. 2, pp. 109-118, ISSN 0886-9634

Spadaro A, Monaco A, Cattaneo R., Masci C. & Gatto R. (2010) Effect on anterior temporalis surface EMG of eyes open-closed condition. *European Journal of Paediatric Dentistry* Vol. 11, No. 4, pp. 210-212, ISSN 2035-648X

Valentino B. & Fabozzo A. (1993) Interaction between the muscles of the neck and the extraocular muscles of the myopic eye. An electromyographic study. *Surgical and Radiologic Anatomy* , Vol. 15, No. 4, pp. 321-323, ISSN 0930-1038

Van Putten A. F. P. (1988) *Electronic Measurement Systems*, Prentice Hall, ISBN 9780132518857